P9-DFF-214

High-Resolution Electrocardiography

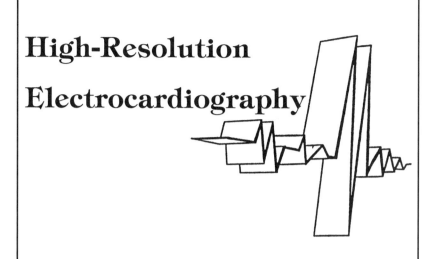

Edited by

Nabil El-Sherif, M.D.
Professor of Medicine and Physiology
Director of Electrophysiology
State University of New York
Health Science Center at Brooklyn
Chief, Cardiology Division
The Veterans Administration Medical Center
Brooklyn, New York

Gioia Turitto, M.D.
Associate Research Director
Wichita Institute for Clinical Research
Wichita, Kansas

FUTURA

**Futura Publishing
Company, Inc.**
Mount Kisco, NY

Library of Congress Cataloging-in-Publication Data

High resolution electrocardiography / edited by Nabil El-Sherif, Gioia Turitto.
   p. cm.
   Includes index.
   ISBN 0-87993-365-8
   1. Electrocardiography. I. El-Sherif, Nabil, 1938– II. Turitto, Gioia.
   [DNLM: 1. Electrocardiography—methods. WG 140 H638]
   RC683.5.E5H495 1992
   616.1'207547—dc20
   DNLM/DLC
   for Library of Congress   91-6530
                                                          CIP

Copyright 1992
Futura Publishing Company, Inc.

Published by
Futura Publishing Company, Inc
2 Bedford Ridge Road
Mount Kisco, New York 10549

L.C. No.: 91-6530
ISBN No.: 0-87993-3658

Every effort has been made to ensure that the information in this book is as up to date and accurate as possible at the time of publication. However, due to the constant developments in medicine, neither the author, nor the editor, nor the publisher can accept any legal or any other responsibility for any errors or omissions that may occur.

All rights reserved.
No part of this book may be translated or reproduced in any form without written permission of the publisher.

Printed in the United States of America

Contributors

Shimon Abboud, PhD   Senior Lecturer in Biomedical Engineering and Medical Physics, Biomedical Engineering Program, Faculty of Engineering, Tel Aviv University, Tel Aviv, Israel

Richard Adamec, MD   Medicin-Adjoint, Policlinic of Medicine, University Hospital, Geneva, Switzerland

David Albert, MD   Corazonix Corporation, Oklahoma City, Oklahoma

H. Dieter Ambos   Research Associate Professor of Medicine, Washington University School of Medicine, St. Louis, Missouri

Soad Bekheit, MD   Clinical Professor of Medicine, State University of New York Health Science Center at Brooklyn, Director, Coronary Care Unit, Veterans Administration Medical Center, Brooklyn, New York

Bernard Belhassen, MD   Professor in Cardiology, Sackler School of Medicine, Tel Aviv University; Director, Cardiac Electrophysiology Laboratory, Tel Aviv Medical Center, Ichilov Hospital, Tel Aviv, Israel

Edward J. Berbari, PhD   Associate Professor of Medicine, University of Oklahoma Health Science Center, Veterans Affairs Medical Center, Oklahoma City, Oklahoma

J. Thomas Bigger, Jr, MD   Professor of Medicine and Pharmacology, College of Physicians and Surgeons of Columbia University, Director, Arrhythmia Control Unit, Columbia-Presbyterian Medical Center, New York, New York

Dennis A. Bloomfield, MD   Clinical Professor of Medicine, New York Medical College, Chairman, Department of Medicine, St. Vincent Medical Center of Richmond, Staten Island, New York

Joseph Borbola, MD   Chief of Electrophysiology, Hungarian Institute of Cardiology, Budapest, Hungary

Martin Borggrefe, MD   Director of Electrophysiology, Medizinische Klinik and Poliklinik, Innere Medizin C (Cardiologie/Angiologie), Westfalische Wilhelms Universitat, Munster, Germany

Gunter Breithardt, MD   Professor of Medicine (Cardiology), Chief, Division of Cardiology, Medizinische Klinik and Poliklinik, Innere Medizin C (Cardiologie/Angiologie), Westfalische Wilhelms Universitat, Munster, Germany

Alfred E. Buxton, MD   Associate Professor of Medicine, University of Pennsylvania School of Medicine; Director, Clinical Electrophysiology Laboratory, Hospital of the University of Pennsylvania, Philadelphia, Pennsylvania

Michael E. Cain, MD   Associate Professor of Medicine, Washington University School of Medicine; Director, Clinical Electrophysiology Laboratory, Barnes Hospital, St. Louis, Missouri

René Cardinal, PhD   Assistant Professor of Pharmacology, University of Montreal; Centre de Recherche, Hopital du Sacre-Coeur, Montreal, Quebec, Canada

Edward B. Caref, MA   Biomedical Engineer, Veterans Administration Medical Center, Brooklyn, New York

William Craelius, PhD   Associate Professor, Department of Biomedical Engineering, Rutgers University, Piscataway, New Jersey

Pablo Denes, MD   Chief, Section of Cardiology, St. Paul-Ramsey Medical Center, St. Paul, Minnesota

Alan Robert Denniss, MD   Clinical Lecturer in Medicine, University of Sidney; Cardiologist, Westmead Hospital, Westmead, Australia

Nabil El-Sherif, MD   Professor of Medicine and Physiology and Director, Clinical Electrophysiology Program, State University of New York Health Science Center at Brooklyn; Chief, Cardiology Division, Veterans Administration Medical Center, Brooklyn, New York

Gerard Faugère, MD   Division of Cardiology, Hopital de la Timone, Marseille, France

Riccardo R. Fenici, MD   Associate Professor of Clinical Physiology and Cardiology, Cardiovascular Biomagnetism Unit, Catholic University, Roma, Italy

Nancy C. Flowers, MD   Professor of Medicine, Medical College of Georgia; Director, Electrophysiology Laboratory and Cardiology Training Program, Augusta, Georgia

John M. Fontaine, MD   Associate Professor of Medicine, Director of Cardiac Arrhythmia Services, Medical College of Pennsylvania, Philadelphia, Pennsylvania

Roger A. Freedman, MD.   Assistant Professor of Medicine, University of Utah School of Medicine, Division of Cardiology, University of Utah Medical Center, Salt Lake City, UT

J. Anthony Gomes, MD   Professor of Medicine, Mount Sinai Medical School; Director, Section of Electrocardiography and Electrophysiology, Mount Sinai Medical Center, New York, New York

William B. Gough, PhD   Assistant Professor of Medicine, State University of New York Health Science Center at Brooklyn; Cardiac Supervisory Physiologist, Veterans Administration Medical Center, Brooklyn, New York

Ralph Haberl, MD   Medizinische Klinik I, Ludwig-Maximilians-Universitat Munchen, Klinikum Grosshadern, Munchen, Germany

Raphael Henkin, PhD   Research Associate, Cardiology Research Program, Veterans Administration Medical Center, Brooklyn, New York

Vinzenz Hombach, MD   Professor of Medicine (Cardiology), Chief, Department of Cardiology-Angiology-Pneumology, University Hospital of Ulm, Ulm, Germany

Leo G. Horan, MD   Professor of Medicine, Medical College of Georgia; Chief, Cardiology Section, Veterans Affairs Medical Center, Augusta, Georgia

Bassiema Ibrahim, MD   Clinical Instructor in Medicine, State University of New York Health Science Center at Brooklyn; Director, Coronary Care Unit, Kings County Hospital, Brooklyn, New York

Gerhard Jilge, MD   Medizinische Klinik I, Ludwig-Maximilians-Universitat Munchen, Klinikum Grosshadern, Munchen, Germany

George J. Kelen, MD   Attending Physician, St. Vincent Medical Center of Richmond, Staten Island, New York

Denniss L. Kuchar, MD   Cardiologist, Coronary Care Unit, St. Vincent's Hospital, Darlinghurst, Australia

Dominique Lacroix, MD   Hopital Cardiologique, University of Lille, Lille, France

Paul Lander, PhD   Assistant Professor of Research Medicine, University of Oklahoma Health Science Center, Veterans Affairs Medical Center, Oklahoma City, Oklahoma

Ralph Lazzara, MD   Professor of Medicine, Chief, Section of Cardiovascular Diseases, University of Oklahoma Health Science Center, Oklahoma City, Oklahoma

Bruce D. Lindsay, MD   Assistant Professor of Medicine, Washington University School of Medicine; Associate Director, Clinical Electrophysiology Laboratory, Barnes Hospital, St. Louis, Missouri

Luisa Lopez, MD   Assistant in Clinical Physiology, Cardiovascular Biomagnetism Unit, Catholic University, Roma, Italy

Antoni Martinez-Rubio, MD   Medizinische Klinik and Poliklinik, Innere Medizin C (Cardiologie/Angiologie), Westfalische Wilhelms Universitat, Munster, Germany

Mariella Masselli, MD   Assistant in Clinical Physiology, Cardiovascular Biomagnetism Unit, Catholic University, Roma, Italy

Rahul Mehra, PhD   Senior Staff Scientist, Medtronic, Inc., Minneapolis, Minnesota

Guido Melillo, MD   Assistant in Clinical Physiology, Cardiovascular Biomagnetism Unit, Catholic University, Roma, Italy

Pierre Pagé, MD   Research Associate, Department of Surgery, University of Montreal; Staff Cardiovascular Surgeon, Hopital du Sacre-Coeur, Montreal, Quebec, Canada

Mark Restivo, PhD   Senior Research Associate, Veterans Administration Medical Center, Brooklyn, New York

Jean Richez, PhD   Electronic Engineer, Department of Electronics, Faculty of Medicine of the University of Geneva, Geneva, Switzerland

Pierre Savard, PhD   Institut Genie Biomedical, Ecole Politechnique, Montreal, Quebec, Canada

Benjamin J. Scherlag, PhD   Professor of Medicine, University of Oklahoma Health Science Center; Research Career Scientist, Veterans Affairs Medical Center, Oklahoma City, Oklahoma

Mohammad Shenasa, MD   Medizinische Klinik and Poliklinik, Innere Medizin C (Cardiologie/Angiologie), Westfalische Wilhelms Universitat, Munster, Germany

Michael B. Simson, MD   Associate Professor of Medicine, Hospital of the University of Pennsylvania, Philadelphia, Pennsylvania

Ann-Marie Starr, MD   Cardiology Fellow, St. Vincent Hospital of Richmond, Staten Island, New York

Gerhard Steinbeck, MD   Medizinische Klinik I, Ludwig-Maximilians-Universitat Munchen, Klinikum Grosshadern, Munchen, Germany

Jonathan S. Steinberg, MD   Assistant Professor of Clinical Medicine, College of Physicians and Surgeons of Columbia University; Director, Arrhythmia Service, St. Luke's/Roosevelt Hospital Center New York, New York

Peter Steinbigler, MD   Medizinische Klinik I, Ludwig-Maximilians-Universitat Munchen, Klinikum Grosshadern, Munchen, Germany

Gioia Turitto, MD   Associate Research Director, Wichita Institute for Clinical Research, Wichita, Kansas

Shantha N. Ursell, MD   Clinical Associate Professor of Medicine, Director, Coronary Care Unit, State University of New York Health Science Center at Brooklyn, Brooklyn, New York

Stephen L. Winters, MD   Assistant Professor of Medicine, Mount Sinai Medical School; Director, Arrhythmia Clinic, Mount Sinai Medical Center, New York, New York

Anita C. Wylds, BS   Medical College of Georgia, Medicine/Cardiology, Augusta, Georgia

Waiqun Yang, MS   Medical College of Georgia, Medicine/Cardiology, Augusta, Georgia

Marc Zimmermann, MD   Medicin-adjoint, Cardiology Center, University Hospital, Geneva, Switzerland

Preface

High-resolution electrocardiography (HRE) is a technique that allows detection and analysis of low-amplitude electrocardiographic signals that may not be detected on the body surface by routine measurements. The term "signal-averaged electrocardiogram," which is frequently used synonymously with HRE, refers to one signal processing technique that enhances the detection of low-amplitude electrocardiographic signals. Interest in HRE started in the early 1970s, and the goal was to record the His-Purkinje signal noninvasively. Interest in the technique would probably have waned if it was not for the observation made in the mid-70s by El-Sherif, Scherlag, and Lazzara that low-amplitude "fractionated" diastolic potentials are a potential marker for the anatomic-electrophysiologic substrate of reentrant arrhythmias. Although this was shown in an experimental model of ischemia, the clinical counterpart of this observation was later made by a number of clinical investigators and these potentials were called "late potentials." The 1980s witnessed an expanded interest in the theoretical, technical, and clinical aspects of HRE.

This book is intended to provide a state-of-the-art review of HRE. The book is organized into six separate sections. Theoretical and technical principles of HRE are discussed in detail in the first section. The second section reviews the data on beat-to-beat recordings of HRE, a potentially powerful technique but one that is still in need of further technical refinement before it is introduced to routine clinical use. The electrophysiologic principles of late potentials and their clinical application to risk stratification for arrhythmic events in the post-infarction period are extensively discussed in the

ix

third and fourth sections. This area currently represents the major application of HRE. The fifth section discusses the use of HRE in patients with nonsustained or sustained ventricular tachyarrhythmias, syncope, bundle branch block, and those patients on antiarrhythmic therapy. The final section evaluates the still evolving field of frequency-domain analysis of HRE, including the most recent spectro-temporal techniques.

This book was made possible because of the collaborative efforts of a large number of basic and clinical scientists who have contributed to the development of this field. Because HRE is a young and growing field, further technical improvements and expanded clinical applications are expected in the coming years. It is hoped, however, that what is included here provides a proper perspective of the subject that will prove valuable to medical students, primary care physicians, and cardiovascular specialists.

Nabil El-Sherif, M.D.
Gioia Turitto, M.D.

Contents

Section VI. Frequency-Domain Analysis of the Signal-Averaged Electrocardiogram

Section I.

Principles and Techniques

High-Resolution Electrocardiography: Historical Perspectives

Benjamin J. Scherlag, Ralph Lazzara

Introduction

Historians are beset with unavoidable bias because they must first select the chronology and personages of their history; and then because most of the events have occurred so long ago, they must provide, at best, a second-hand narrative since the original players have passed on. In writing a history of high-resolution electrocardiography, the bias on the second account fortunately can be mitigated since all of the major players are actively on the scene. Thus it was possible to contact them and get their unique impressions of this relatively new and exciting field of experimental and clinical research. Throughout this account direct passages or paraphrases from the movers in the field of high-resolution electrocardiography will be included for the purpose of adding historical perspective and to reduce bias.

In 1968, Cranefield and Hoffman,[1] in their kickoff editorial for the *Journal of Electrocardiology,* stated that the "electrocardiogram itself provides very little direct information about the electrical

From El-Sherif N, Turitto G (eds): *High-Resolution Electrocardiography.* Mount Kisco, NY, Futura Publishing Co., Inc., ©, 1992.

activity of the heart." Table I from that editorial details the basis for that statement. Just as the light microscope reveals important cell structures, i.e., the cell membrane, cytoplasm, and nucleus, it gives us little, if any, information on mitochondria, Golgi apparatus, ribosomes, etc., and conventional electrocardiograms only provide waveforms P, QRS, and T which correspond to electrical depolarization of the atria, ventricles, and repolarization of the ventricles in that order. However, only with higher resolution techniques, the electron microscope for anatomic studies, high-resolution electrocardiography in our case, can we obtain other "crucial events in the electrical activation of the heart" which are not represented by waveforms on the standard ECG.[1]

Cranefield and Hoffman called for a physiologic reevaluation of concepts and mechanisms made by inference from the electrocardiogram. This charge did not fall on deaf ears for in the next few years the introduction of His bundle electrocardiography[2,3] opened the way for new, basic and clinical studies to test previously deduced electrocardiographic theories. Areas of investigation included atrioventricular and intraventricular conduction defects, the pre-excitation syndromes, and multiple forms of ectopic impulse formation. It was in this setting that several laboratories entered the field of high-resolution electrocardiography in order to do noninvasively

Table I

Direct Electrocardiographic Evidence of Cardiac Activity

Site of Activity	Onset of Activity	Onset of Recovery
Sinoatrial node	No direct information	No direct information
Spread to atrium and atrioventricular node	No direct information	No direct information
Activation of atrium	P wave	Ta wave
Spread through atrioventricular node	No direct information	No direct information
Spread through His-Purkinje system	No direct information	U wave (?)
Activation of ventricle	QRS complex	T wave

(Reprinted with permission from the *Journal of Electrocardiology*.)

what was being done by invasive electrophysiologic studies using proximity electrodes to record from the specialized conduction system of the heart.

Signal averaging, the cornerstone of the initial studies on high-resolution electrocardiography, was first used in the neural sciences with some success in extracting encephalographic signals from noise.[4] The fiducial event for such recordings was a light flashed into the eyes which evoked an electrical response from recording sites on the scalp in the area of the visual cortex. Others have used signal averaging to differentiate the electrocardiogram of the fetus from the maternal electrocardiogram,[5] enhancement of P waves,[6] and clarification of electrocardiographic signals during exercise in which movement artifacts obscure repetitive cardiac activity.[7]

Signal averaging can be briefly described as a "signal processing technique, usually done digitally, whereby repeated or periodic waveforms which are contaminated by noise can be enhanced. That is, the signal-to-noise ratio can be improved. By summating successive noisy waveforms the random components, i.e., noise, will decrease while the deterministic components, i.e., the desired signal, will be unchanged."[8]

Edward J. Berbari arrived at the catheterization laboratory of Mt. Sinai Hospital in Miami Beach, FL, in 1971 as a graduate student in search of a suitable subject for a Master's thesis. His bundle electrocardiography for the study of atrio-ventricular block was reaching its zenith and in the forefront was Philip Samet's cardiology team headed by Onkar Narula. After observing several of the clinical His bundle studies, Berbari and William (Bill) Oliver, the senior technician in the laboratory, discussed the possibility of recording His bundle activity from the body surface. That discussion led to the animal laboratory where Berbari related his ideas to Ralph Lazzara, staff physician and Benjamin Scherlag, cardiovascular physiologist. Scherlag et al had initiated the growing field of clinical electrophysiology by establishing a consistent recording technique for the His bundle electrogram in dogs[2] then in man.[3] Berbari explained his approach using signal averaging to record His bundle activity from the body surface in the same way as evoked potentials were recorded in the neural sciences. To test the idea Berbari, showing the resourcefulness of the atypical graduate student, was able to obtain a hardwired signal averager from the Princeton Applied Research Company. Within a month, a series of dog studies were performed in which signal-averaged leads from the body surface showed reproducible waveforms coincident with His-Purkinje system activation.[9] The technique was not wholly noninvasive since an atrial pacing spike from a catheter positioned in the heart provided the trigger to start the data acquisition.

Berbari and his colleagues received invaluable support from the clinical sector when Philip Samet's successful appeal for $30,000 allowed the purchase of a Hewlett-Packard 21 computer. With the aid of a QRS detector constructed in-house, an A/D converter, and appropriate software, Berbari now could trigger the averaging sequence using a portion of the QRS as a fiducial point. These early investigations in dogs and in man culminated in several papers published in the early and mid 1970s.[9-11] All the studies concerned body surface recordings of His-Purkinje and atrio-ventricular nodal potentials.

At the same time other groups of investigators were bringing together their own approaches to the recording of His-Purkinje activity by means of high-resolution electrocardiography. Nancy Flowers became interested in the subject as a fellow in cardiology as early as 1963:

> I became intrigued with a device called the Nimetron (a cheaper version of the Computer of Averaged Transients [CAT]). Body surface mapping had begun in the laboratory (of Dan Brody) in Tennessee and was in its infancy before I arrived . . . Being the low-man on the totem pole I inherited the task of recording the maps row after row on Grass kymographic camera film and then having to spend literally hours, days, and weeks in the darkroom achieving a temporal reconciliation and the final output product of the body surface map. I thought there must be an easier way, and with the significantly greater knowledge of Leo Horan and Dan Brody, we embarked on signal averaging. It turned out that the Nimetron was not satisfactory . . . , but it did lead to the development of a signal-averaging system for electrocardiograms which has been modified through the years for signal enhancement and noise reduction.
>
> The second phase of my interest in high resolution electrocardiography was when . . . I became interested in "high frequency notching." The detailed notches and slurs that occurred as a result of cleaning signals with signal averaging, or even with just rapid speed recordings in a quiet environment were intriguing to me. I began to look at what others had done in this

area and discovered Paul Langner's work[12] and realized that we had a unique opportunity. We had already begun to accumulate (without applying a name to it) 'high resolution electrocardiograms' on a number of patients we were following longitudinally. . . .

"The third phase had to do with the surface recognition of His-Purkinje activity . . . [based on the] description of recording from an endocardial catheter His bundle activity from a dog,[2] and a short time later from man.[3] At that particular time, I was involved in looking at an experimental model for clues as to the origin of human deaths in the sudden sniffing death syndromes that had been described by Bass[13] a little while earlier, where kids sniffed aerosol propellants to get high, and died suddenly. We were exposing anesthetized dogs to various concentrations of halogenated hydrocarbons and had multiple electrocardiographic recordings on these animals in an extremely quiet environment. During one particularly electrically quiet day, I noticed on some electrocardiograms that had been amplified and filtered, little bumps in the PR segment that did not occur in the TP segment. These dogs were remarkably relaxed as a result of the Freon compound to which they were exposed and myotonic noise was virtually nonexistent. This dog conveniently developed 2:1 atrio-ventricular block and I noticed that after the first blocked P wave there were no such oscillations as occurred following the conducted P waves. Either at that experimental setting or at one shortly thereafter we tried our luck at recording His bundle activity transvenously . . . and were fortunate in being able to do so. We could then see some concordance between the mysterious surface blips in the PR segment and the internal His deflection. However, we had difficulty in doing this in every animal. At that point we realized we needed something further, and embarked on signal averaging in addition to amplification and filtering. The work done from 1972 to 1974 resulted.[14,15] We attempted to test the observations with pacing and with pharmacologic interventions and it appeared that what we were seeing were real phenomena. At about the same time we learned that Ed Berbari and some of his coworkers in the Miami area were employing not identical but similar enhancing techniques, and were further encouraged that these observations appeared to be real, not only to us, but to responsible investigators in totally different laboratories.

Independently, Marius Stopczyk at the Institute of Biocybernetics and Biomedical Engineering, in Warsaw, Poland, also received inspiration from his reading on studies of evoked potentials in neurophysiology using signal-averaging techniques. He was the first to use atrial pacing via a transesophageal approach to trigger the signal averager. In this way he was able to detect His-Purkinje system activity from the body surface. This work was published in 1973.[16] In 1974 Dr. Stopczyk was invited to Detroit, Michigan, to work with Dr. W.J. Wajszczuk and his colleagues. Several publications resulted from this collaboration relating to recordings from the sinoatrial node and His-Purkinje system.[17,18]

A key event in the early stages of development of noninvasive techniques for recording latent electrical events was the convening of the first international symposium on high amplification electrocardiography.[19] Andre Varenne had recorded his first body surface His-Purkinje potential in 1977 and quickly realized from the literature that there was no consensus among workers on leads, sampling algorithms, averaging techniques, or validation of signals. More than 200 participants gathered in Nice, France, in an attempt to define and standardize terminology and techniques.

> We were not recording artifacts, but cardiac signals belonging to the His-Purkinje system . . . I was convinced that . . . the right way [was to develop] a software-based system . . . it was premature to . . . propose a standardization of signal recording parameters. We were yet in a research field.

This first symposium introduced many of the participants to other waveforms that could be detected with noninvasive signal averaging. There was Stopczyk's body surface recording of pre-P wave activity[20] and Guy Fontaine's recording of late potentials in patients with right ventricular dysplasia[21] which supplemented a previous report from his group in a patient with resistant ventricular tachycardia.[22]

The recording of late potentials, i.e., low level electrical signals occurring after the end of the conventionally recorded QRS complex, also had its beginning in the animal research laboratory. In 1969, Han[23] recorded electrical activity from the heart surface of dogs with acute myocardial ischemia. Ventricular pacing induced delayed activation beyond the QRS complex. Similar delayed potentials were recorded by Durrer et al[24] in 1971. The close association of these delayed potentials and ventricular arrhythmias was shown by Boineau and Cox and Waldo and Kaiser in 1973[25,26] and by Scherlag et al in 1974.[27]

Perhaps the strongest evidence linking fractionation and delay of electrical activation on the surface of the heart to reentrant ectopic beats was the recording of continuous electrical activity bridging the diastolic interval between a normal beat and an ectopic beat and then between subsequent ectopic beats. This phenomenon of reentrant excitation theoretically proposed by Harris and Guevera-Rojas in 1943,[28] schematized by Boineau and Cox in 1973,[25] and actually recorded by Waldo and Kaiser[26] in the same year provided a new way to document reentrant excitation. The demonstration of reentry in the mammalian heart had eluded workers for more than half a century. Although these recordings of continuous electrical activity could be made during ventricular arrhythmias associated with acute infarction with the use of punctate and composite electrodes,[26,29-31] their patterns were evanescent and variable. In 1977, the use of composite electrodes and provocative pacing procedures in the subacute stages of myocardial infarction in the dog provided the stable substrate to consistently record late potentials which delay and fractionate and connect beats as bigeminy or ventricular tachycardia.[32-36]

The late potential, the low level signal, that occurred after the end of normal ventricular depolarization was the pathophysiologic marker of a reentrant substrate. This consistent delayed activation could be recorded from the body surface using signal averaging of sinus beats in the same way as the cryptic His-Purkinje waveform was detected with the same methodology. Berbari et al[37] in 1978 clearly brought the late potential from the heart to the body surface and established its importance as a marker of reentrant arrhythmias (Figure 1).

The clinicians were not far behind, indeed, they were in some respects well advanced in recording late potentials. As mentioned above, Fontaine and his colleagues recorded late potentials in patients with ventricular tachycardia,[21,22] Josephson and his associates used electrode catheters to record subendocardial late potentials and continuous electrical activity in patients with chronic myocardial infarction and ventricular aneurysm.[38-41]

Dr. Fontaine described his transition from direct myocardial recordings to high-resolution electrocardiography:

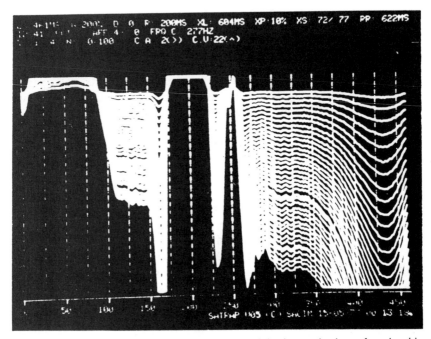

Figure 1. First recording of late ventricular activity from a body surface lead in a dog with 4-day-old myocardial infarction. The top trace is the highly filtered (60–300 Hz) and highly amplified surface averaged lead (SAL). The arrow points to the late activity which occurs after the end of the QRS in the conventional ECG lead (bottom trace). Note all of the early part of the QRS is shown. (Reproduced with permission from Berbari et al, In Hombach B, Hilger HH (eds): Signal Averaging Technique in Clinical Cardiology. Stuttgart-New York: FK Schattauer Verlag, 1981, pp. 163–176).

After recording delayed potentials on the endocardium as well as on the epicardium, it was interesting to consider the possibility of their detection from the surface electrocardiogram. The preliminary approach was to use a high-gain Tektronix differential amplifier with built-in filtering. The patient had a probable arrhythmogenic right ventricular dysplasia. Consistent beat-to-beat reproducible waveforms were hardly seen emerging from the skeletal muscle background noise (Figure 2). Analog filtering allowed better signal identification (Figure 3).

The technique of summation-averaging was considered to be the next logical step, this technique being already used for

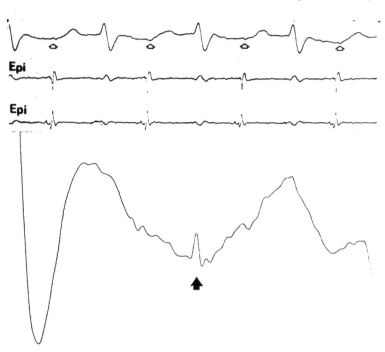

Figure 2. Four sweeps are recorded, displaying simultaneously a regular ECG lead (lower trace) and a bipolar chest lead after introduction of analogic filtering (upper trace). Note the exact superposition of the fragmented activity occurring after the end of the QRS complex.

His bundle recording.[42] The initial attempt was made in the recovery room in a patient with Uhl's anomaly after the operation. In this case delayed potentials were observed on the epicardium (Figure 4). The chest bipolar ECG signal was first recorded on a magnetic tape. This tape was later processed in the computer laboratory of the "Ecole Nationale Superieure des Telecommunications" in Paris. The result presented in Figure 4 was questionable. Nevertheless, it was considered encouraging and prompted us to engage a computer engineer to devote full-time on the project. After several months a software program written in assembly language was developed on a DEC PDP11/20 computer. This was presented in 1977.[22] The software was progressively improved and modified to include among other things, digital filters and Fourier transform analysis.

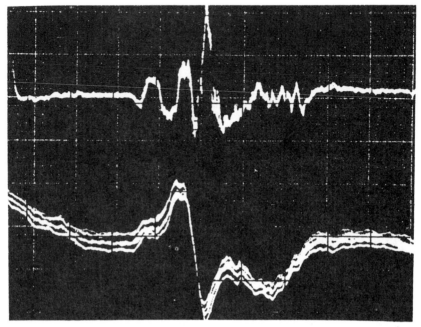

Figure 3. Recording of a delayed epicardial potential obtained at surgery in a case of Uhl's anomaly. The patient was operated on April, 1975. A few days later, a bipolar chest lead was recorded on tape and processed on a digital computer. The amplified QRS chest lead record was drawn on a graphic plotter and showed a potential recorded on the surface which was similar to the epicardial signal.

"Recording of delayed potentials in arrhythmogenic right ventricular dysplasia was relatively easy because of the proximity effect as well as the histologic structure of the myocardium, providing relatively organized strands of conducting layers within the adipose tissue.[43] As far as the delayed potentials after myocardial infarction are concerned, they were more difficult to record, occurring deeper in the thorax and the histologic pattern suggested a more diffuse phenomenon.[44]

"However, further attempts to improve the technique were not effective enough. Incorporation of a buffer amplifier, different kinds of grounding, were only partially successful. A research grant submitted to the French National Institute of Health (INSERM) prepared in collaboration with mathemati-

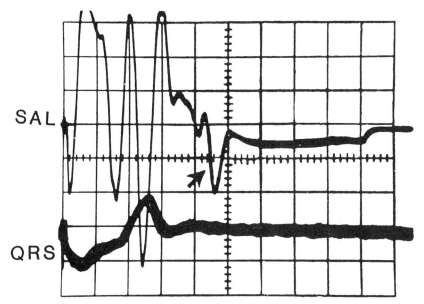

Figure 4. Tracing obtained with a computer system during the development phase. The summation of successive QRS complexes is displayed from top to bottom, from a bipolar chest lead in a patient with arrhythmogenic right ventricular dysplasia. It is possible to observe on the lower tracing delayed potentials and a probable His bundle potential.

cians and computer experts for developing a more sophisticated program was not accepted. Finally the move to Jean Rostand Hospital led us to use a new computer which needed too much work to redesign the program. An overview of the results obtained with this technique was nevertheless published in two book chapters.[21,45]

In 1981, two international symposia were held which were organized by Varenne in Nice and Hombach and Hilger in Cologne.[46,47] These meetings helped to establish the scope of high-resolution electrocardiography for recording low level signals generated by the heart under physiologic and pathologic conditions. From these sessions emerged a clear focus of clinical interest in late potentials that could be detected by signal averaging or beat-to-beat high-resolution electrocardiographic techniques.

One of the most important advances which contributed to the

preeminence of clinical interest in late potentials was the technical contribution of Michael Simson. Working with a population of patients with myocardial infarction, many of whom had ventricular aneurysms, he was able to establish quantitative measures of late potentials which allowed separation of those patients who had spontaneous and inducible sustained ventricular tachycardia from those that did not.[48] Key features of his signal processing system was the use of a bidirectional filter that mitigated ringing as well as the introduction of a combined vector magnitude consisting of the filtered signals from three orthogonal leads, X, Y, and Z. The vector magnitude defined a QRS duration in which a significant number of patients without late potentials fell below 120 msec and those with ventricular tachycardia had filtered QRS durations > 120 msec. Furthermore, utilizing the root mean square of the voltage, he devised cut-off levels for late potential amplitudes (< 25 μV) in the last 40 msec which have gained wide acceptance in signal-averaged studies. The importance of these quantitative measures can readily be appreciated by noting the wide range of variability in the presentation of data in the earliest clinical studies which utilized high-resolution electrocardiography to detect late potentials.[45,49–51]

Within the last few years there has been a crescendo of clinical interest in high-resolution electrocardiography specifically for recording late potentials as a potent predictor of future arrhythmic events, i.e., sustained ventricular tachycardia, in the post-myocardial infarction patient.[52–66]

Future of High-Resolution Electrocardiography

Recently, two new directions have been undertaken in the clinical application of high-resolution electrocardiography to the study of late potentials. The first is the use of signal enhancement and noise reduction which provides beat-to-beat recordings of late potentials.[67–69] This approach would be advantageous in following dynamic changes in late potentials and associated arrhythmogenesis whereas signal averaging would not be appropriate under these conditions. The technology for beat-to-beat high-resolution ECG recordings has been quite variable and the technique has not, as yet, been widely implemented. Another area that has attracted interest is the study of late potentials in the frequency domain. Cain and his associates and Haberl et al have reported that in the last 40 msec of the QRS, frequency domain analysis with fast Fourier transform provides equal success as time domain analysis in separating patients with and without ventricular tachycardia.[70,71] Others have criticized this approach as not providing any significant advantage over time domain analysis[72] or find the frequency analysis fraught with technical drawbacks.[73]

There have also been attempts to analyze the initial portions of the QRS with signal averaging as a means of differentiating patients with and without ventricular tachycardia.[74] Another group has used signal averaging applied to high-frequency electrocardiograms, viz., QRS complex, to determine the presence of coronary artery disease.[75] Whether the clinical usefulness of high-resolution electrocardiography will continue to be limited to detection and pathologic evaluation of late potentials or whether it will be extended to other facets of cardiac disease can only be answered by future basic and clinical research.

Acknowledgment: We thank our many colleagues who graciously responded to our letters, calls, and interviews which aided substantially in this historical review: Drs. Edward J. Berbari, Nancy Flowers, Mariusz J. Stopczyk, Guy Fontaine, Andre Varenne, Michael A. Simson, and Vincenz Hombach. We also thank Pamela Tomey and LaVonna Blair for their help in the preparation of the manuscript.

References

1. Cranefield PF, Hoffman BF: The electrical activity of the heart and the electrocardiogram. J Electrocardiol 1:2, 1968.
2. Scherlag BJ, Helfant RH, Damato AN: A catheterization technique for His bundle stimulation and recording in the intact dog heart. J Applied Physiol 25:425, 1968.
3. Scherlag BJ, Lau SH, Helfant RH, Berkowitz WD, et al: Catheter techniques for recording His bundle activity in man. Circulation 39:13, 1969.
4. Perry NW, Childers DG: The Human Visual Evoked Response: Method and Theory. Springfield, IL: Charles C Thomas, 1969.
5. Hon EH, Lee ST: Noise reduction in fetal electrocardiography. Am J Obst & Gynec 87:1086, 1963.
6. Brody DA, Woolsey MD, Arzbaecher RC: Application of computer techniques to the detection and analysis of spontaneous P wave variation. Circulation 36:359, 1967.
7. Pryor TA, Ridges JG: A computer program for stress test data processing. Comput Biomed Res 7:360, 1974.

8. Berbari EJ: A non-invasive technique for recording the depolarization of the heart's electrical conduction system. Master's Thesis. University of Miami, Coral Gables, Florida, 1973.

9. Berbari EJ, Lazzara R, Samet P, Scherlag BJ: Non-invasive technique for detection of electrical activity during the P-R segment. Circulation 48:1005, 1973.

10. Berbari EJ, Lazzara R, El-Sherif N, Scherlag BJ: Extracardiac recordings of His-Purkinje activity during conduction disorders and junctional rhythms. Circulation 51:802, 1975.

11. Berbari EJ, Scherlag BJ, El-Sherif N, Befeler B, Aranda J, Lazzara R: The His-Purkinje electrocardiogram in man: An initial assessment of its uses and limitations. Circulation 54:219, 1976.

12. Langner PH: Further studies in high fidelity electrocardiography: myocardial infarction. Circulation 8:905, 1953.

13. Bass M: Sudden sniffing death. JAMA 212:2075, 1970.

14. Flowers NC, Horan LG: His-bundle and bundle branch recordings from the body surface. Circulation 48(Suppl IV):IV-102, 1973.

15. Flowers NC, Hand RC, Orander PC, Miller CB, Walden MO, Horan LG: Surface recording of electrical activity from the region of the bundle of His. Am J Cardiol 33:384, 1974.

16. Stopczyk MJ, Kopec J, Zochowski RJ, Pieniak M: Surface recording of electrical activity during the P-R segment in man by computer averaging technique. Int Res Com Syst (73-78) 11, 21, 2, 1973.

17. Stopczyk MJ, Wajszczuk WJ, Zochowski RJ, Rubenfire M: Pre-P (sinoatrial node region) activity recording from the right atrial cavity by signal averaging. PACE 2:156, 1979.

18. Wajszczuk WJ, Stopczyk MJ, Moskowitz MS, Zochowski RJ, Bauld T, Dabos PL, Rubenfire M: Non-invasive recording of His-Purkinje activity in man by QRS-triggered signal averaging. Circulation 58:95, 1978.

19. Varenne A: In: High Amplification Electrocardiography. First International Symposium on High Amplification Electrocardiography. Nice, 1980.

20. Stopczyk MJ, Palko T, Peczalski K, Wajszczuk W: Recording sino-atrial node activity by prememorized signal averaging. In Varenne A (ed): High Amplification Electrocardiography. Nice: JM Vidal, Crenaf, 1980.

21. Fontaine G, Gallais-Hamonno F, Frank R, Fillette F, Malkawi K, Grosgogeat Y: High amplification electrocardiography in cardiac arrhythmias and conduction defects. In Varenne A (ed): High Amplification Electrocardiography. Nice: JM Vidal, Crenaf, 1980.

22. Fontaine G, Guiraudon G, Frank R, Vedel J, Grosgogeat Y, Cabrol C, Facquet J: Stimulation studies and epicardial study of mechanisms and selection for surgery. In Kulbertus HE (ed): Reentrant Arrhythmias. Lancaster: MTP Pub, 1977, pp 334–350.

23. Han J: Mechanisms of ventricular arrhythmias associated with myocardial infarction. Am J Cardiol 24:800, 1969.

24. Durrer D, vanDam RT, Freud GE, Janse MJ: Re-entry and ventricular arrhythmias in local ischemia and infarction of the intact dog heart. Proc. K of Nedrl Akad van Wetensch. Amsterdam, Series C 73:321, 1971.

25. Boineau JP, Cox JL: Slow ventricular activation in acute myocardial infarction. A source of reentrant premature ventricular contractions. Circulation 48:702, 1973.
26. Waldo AL, Kaiser GA: Study of ventricular arrhythmias associated with acute myocardial infarction in the canine heart. Circulation 47:1222, 1973.
27. Scherlag BJ, El-Sherif N, Hope R, Lazzara R: Characterization and localization of ventricular arrhythmias resulting from myocardial ischemia and infarction. Circ Res 35:372, 1974.
28. Harris AS, Guevera-Rojas A: The initiation of ventricular fibrillation due to coronary occlusion. Experimental Medicine & Surgery 1:105, 1943.
29. Williams DO, Scherlag BJ, Hope R, El-Sherif N, Lazzara R: The pathophysiology of malignant ventricular arrhythmias during acute myocardial infarction. Circulation 50:1163, 1974.
30. Hope R, Williams DO, El-Sherif N, Lazzara R, Scherlag BJ. The efficacy of anti-arrhythmic agents during acute myocardial ischemia and the role of heart rate. Circulation 50:507, 1974.
31. Kaplinsky E, Ogawa S, Kmeto J, Balke CM, Dreifus LS: Intramyocardial activation in early ventricular arrhythmias following coronary artery ligation. J Electrocardiol 13:1, 1980.
32. Hope R, Scherlag BJ, El-Sherif N, Lazzara R: Ventricular arrhythmias in healing myocardial infarction: role of rhythm versus rate in reentrant activation. J Thorac Cardiovasc Surg 75:458, 1978.
33. Hope R, Scherlag BJ, El-Sherif N, Lazzara R: Continuous concealed ventricular arrhythmias. Am J Cardiol 40:733, 1977
34. El-Sherif N, Scherlag BJ, Lazzara R, Hope R: Reentrant ventricular arrhythmias in the late myocardial infarction period. I. Conduction characteristics in the infarction zone. Circulation 55:686, 1977.
35. El-Sherif N, Hope R, Scherlag BJ, Lazzara R: Reentrant ventricular arrhythmias in the late myocardial infarction period. II. Patterns of initiation and termination of reentry. Circulation 55:702, 1977.
36. El-Sherif N, Lazzara R, Hope R, Scherlag BJ: Reentrant ventricular arrhythmias in the late myocardial infarction period. III. Manifest and concealed extrasystolic grouping. Circulation 56:225, 1977.
37. Berbari EJ, Scherlag BJ, Hope R, Lazzara R: Recordings from the body surface of arrhythmogenic ventricular activity during the ST segment. Am J Cardiol 41:697, 1978.
38. Josephson ME, Horowitz LN, Farshidi A, Kastor JA: Recurrent sustained ventricular tachycardia. 1. Mechanisms. Circulation 57:431, 1978.
39. Josephson ME, Horowitz LN, Farshidi A, Spear JF, Kastor JA, Moore EN: Recurrent sustained ventricular tachycardia. 2. Endocardial mapping. Circulation 57:440, 1978.
40. Josephson ME, Horowitz LN, Farshidi A: Continuous local electrical activity. A mechanism of recurrent ventricular tachycardia. Circulation 57:659, 1978.
41. Josephson ME, Horowitz LN, Farshidi A, Spielman SR, Michelson EL, Greenspan AM: Recurrent ventricular tachycardia. 4. Pleomorphism. Circulation 59:459, 1979.

42. Berbari EJ, Scherlag BJ, El-Sherif N, Befeler B, Aranda JM, Lazzara R: The His-Purkinje electrocardiogram in man: an initial assessment of its' uses and limitations. Circulation 54:219, 1976.
43. Fontaine G, Fontaliran F, Linares-Cruz E, Chomette G: The arrhythmogenic right ventricle. In Iwa T, Fontaine G (eds): Cardiac Arrhythmias—Recent Progress in Investigation and Management. The Hague: Elsevier Science Publishing, 1988, pp 189–202.
44. Wit AL, Dillon S, Ursell PC: Influences of anisotropic tissue structure on reentrant ventricular tachycardia. In Brugada P, Wellens HJJ (eds): Cardiac Arrhythmias—Where To Go From Here? Mount Kisco, NY: Futura Publishing Co, 1987, pp 27–50.
45. Fontaine G, Pierfitte M, Tonet JL, Fillette F, Frank R, Grosgogeat Y: Interpretation of afterpotentials registered from epicardium, endocardium, and body surface in patients with chronic ventricular tachycardia. In Hombach V, Hilger HH (eds): Signal Averaging Technique in Clinical Cardiology. Stuttgart-New York: F.K. Schattauer Verlag Publ, 1981, p 177.
46. Varenne A (ed): Second Symposium on High Amplification Electrocardiography. (abstrs) OPFMN, Nice, France, 1981.
47. Hombach V, Hilger HH: International Symposium on Signal Averaging Technique in Clinical Cardiology. Stuttgart-New York: F.K. Schattauer Verlag Publ., 1981.
48. Simson MB: Use of signals in the terminal QRS complex to identify patients with ventricular tachycardia after myocardial infarction. Circulation 64:235, 1982.
49. Uther JB, Dennett CJ, Tan A: The detection of delayed activation signals of low amplitude in the vectorcardiogram of patients with recurrent ventricular tachycardia by signal averaging. In Sandoe E, Julian DG, Bell JW (eds): Management of Ventricular Tachycardia-Role of Mexiletine. Amsterdam-Oxford: Excerpta Medica, 1978.
50. Breithardt G, Boggrefe M, Schwarzmaier J, Karbenn U, Yeh HL, Seipel L: Clinical significance of ventricular late potentials. In Hombach V, Hilger HH (eds): Signal Averaging Technique In Clinical Cardiology. Stuttgart-New York: Schattauer Verlag Publ,: 1981, pp 219–232.
51. Rozanski JJ, Mortara D: Delayed depolarizations in patients with recurrent ventricular tachycardia and left ventricular aneurysm. In Hombach V, Hilger HH (eds): Signal Averaging Technique in Clinical Cardiology. Stuttgart-New York: F.K. Schattauer Verlag Publ, 1981, pp 205–218.
52. Breithardt G, Becker R, Seipel L, Abendroth RR, Ostermeyer J: Noninvasive detection of late potentials in man—A new marker for ventricular tachycardia. Eur Heart J 2:1, 1981.
53. Breithardt G, Borggrefe M, Karbenn U, Abendroth RR, Yeh HL, Seipel L: Prevalence of late potentials in patients with and without ventricular tachycardia: correlation with angiographic findings. Am J Cardiol 49:-1932, 1982.
54. Gomes JA, Mehra R, Barreca P, El-Sherif N, Hariman R, Holtzman R:

Quantitative analysis of the high-frequency components of signal-averaged QRS complex in patients with acute myocardial infarction: a prospective study. Circulation 72:105, 1985.

55. Breithardt G, Borggrefe M, Haerten K, Trampisch HJ: Prognostic significance of programmed ventricular stimulation and non-invasive detection of ventricular late potentials in the post-infarction period. Z Kardiol 74:389, 1985.

56. Breithardt G, Borggrefe M: Pathophysiology mechanisms and clinical significance of ventricular late potentials. Eur Heart J 7:364, 1986.

57. Denniss AR, Richard DA, Cody DV, Russell PA, Young AA, Cooper MJ, Ross DL, Uther JB: Prognostic significance of ventricular tachycardia and fibrillation induced at programmed stimulation and delayed potentials detected on the signal-averaged electrocardiograms of survivors of acute myocardial infarction. Circulation 74:731, 1986.

58. Gallagher JD, Fernandez J, Maranhao V, Gessman LJ: Simultaneous appearance of endocardial late potentials and ability to induce sustained ventricular tachycardia after procainamide administration. J Electrocardiol 19:197, 1986.

59. Cain ME: Predicting sustained VT by ECG signal averaging. Cardio: 54, 1986.

60. Kuchar DL, Thorburn CW, Sammel, NL: Late potentials detected after myocardial infarction: natural history and prognostic significance. Circulation 74:1280, 1986.

61. Denniss AR, Ross DL, Richards DA, Cody DV, Russell PA, Young AA, Uther JB: Effect of antiarrhythmic therapy on delayed potentials detected by the signal-averaged electrocardiogram in patients with ventricular tachycardia after acute myocardial infarction. Am J Cardiol 58:261, 1986.

62. Gomes JA, Winters SL, Stewart D, Horowitz S, Milner M, Barreca P: A new noninvasive index to predict sustained ventricular tachycardia and sudden death in the first year after myocardial infarction: based on signal-averaged electrocardiogram, radionuclide ejection fraction and Holter monitoring. J Am Coll Cardiol 10:349, 1987.

63. Denniss AR, Johnson DC, Richards DA, Ross DL, Uther JB: Effect of excision of ventricular myocardium on delayed potentials with ventricular tachycardia. Am J Cardiol 59:591, 1987.

64. Denniss AR, Richards DA, Cody DV, Russell PA, Young AA, Ross DL, Uther JB: Correlation between signal-averaged electrocardiogram and programmed stimulation in patients with and without spontaneous ventricular tachyarrhythmias. Am J Cardiol 59:586, 1987.

65. Nalos PC, Gang ES, Mandel WJ, Ladenheim ML, Lass Y, Peter T: The signal-averaged electrocardiogram as a screening test for inducibility of sustained ventricular tachycardia in high risk patients: a prospective study. J Am Coll Cardiol 9:539, 1987.

66. Buckingham TA, Ghosh S, Homan SM, Theesen CC, Redd RM, Stevens LL, Chaitman BR, Kennedy HL: Independent value of signal-averaged electrocardiography and left ventricular function in identifying pa-

tients with sustained ventricular tachycardia with coronary artery disease. Am J Cardiol 59:568, 1987.

67. Flowers NC, Shvartsman V, Kennelly BM, Sohi GS, Horan LG: Surface recordings of His-Purkinje activity on an every beat basis without digital averaging. Circulation 63:948, 1981.

68. El-Sherif N, Mehra R, Gomes JA, Kelen G: Appraisal of a low noise electrocardiogram. J Am Coll Cardiol 1:456, 1983.

69. Hombach V, Kebbel V, Hopp HW, Winter V, Hirche H: Noninvasive beat-by-beat registration of ventricular late potentials using high resolution electrocardiography. Int J Cardiol 6:167, 1984.

70. Cain ME, Ambos HD, Witkowski FX, Sobel BR: Fast-Fourier transform analysis of signal-averaged electrocardiograms for identification of patients prone to sustained ventricular tachycardia. Circulation 69:711, 1984.

71. Haberl R, Filge G, Pulter R, Steinbeck G: Comparison of frequency and time domain analysis of the signal-averaged electrocardiogram in patients with ventricular tachycardia and coronary artery disease: methodologic validation and clinical relevance. J Am Coll Cardiol 12:150, 1988.

72. Machac J, Weiss A, Winters SL, Barreca P, Gomes JA: A comparative study of frequency domain and time domain analysis of signal-averaged electrocardiograms in patients with ventricular tachycardia. J Am Coll Cardiol 11:284, 1988.

73. Kelen GJ, Henkin R, Fontaine JM, El-Sherif N: Effects of analyzed signal duration and phase on the results of fast-Fourier transform analysis of the surface electrocardiogram in subjects with and without late potentials. Am J Cardiol 60:1282, 1987.

74. Kienzle MG, Falcone RA, Simson MB: Alterations in the initial portion of the signal-averaged QRS complex in acute myocardial infarction with ventricular tachycardia. Am J Cardiol 61:99, 1988.

75. Abboud S, Belhassen B, Miller HI, Sadele D, Laniado S: High frequency electrocardiography using an advanced method of signal averaging for noninvasive detection of coronary artery disease in patients with normal conventional electrocardiograms. J Electrocardiol 19:371, 1986.

2

Techniques for Processing of Cardiac Signals: Fiducial Formulae for Fidelity

William Craelius, Mark Restivo, Nabil El-Sherif

Introduction

Precise timing of events within the cardiac cycle is an important task for any high-resolution electrocardiographic system. Electrocardiographic averaging systems, for example, require precise temporal alignment of successive ventricular activations prior to averaging in order to reliably detect signals such as late ventricular potentials and the bundle of His potential. Similarly, resolution of cardiac structures by magnetic resonance imaging depends to a large extent on the degree of synchrony that can be achieved between the scanning beam and constant phases of the cardiac cycle. Even the fundamental measurement of sinus heart rate demands increasingly precise and reliable estimates of sinus node activation times, because of the powerful new treatments, such as spectral

From El-Sherif N, Turitto G (eds): *High-Resolution Electrocardiography.* Mount Kisco, NY, Futura Publishing Co., Inc., ©, 1992.

analysis, being applied to it. Compounding the need for increased accuracy is the increasing demand on diagnostic systems to behave robustly under varied conditions of body position, activities, disease states, and cardiac stress.

This chapter presents signal processing options for determining fiducial points on cardiac signals. We outline the characteristics of signals relevant to ischemia and electrical instability, on the surface of the heart and on the body surface. Then, we present the theory of alignment of cardiac signals, with particular reference to signal averaging, and practical design and optimization procedures for signal averaging. For a general review of high-resolution signal averaging, the reader is referred to reference 1. Finally, we present a brief discussion of the more advanced signal processing methods that can be applied to cardiac timing measurements.

Properties of Cardiac Signals

General

Electrical signals emanating from the heart are not constant, predictable waveforms, but are rather arbitrary in shape, continually influenced not only by myocardial electrophysiology, but by body position, and bodily movements caused by respiration and speech. The signals vary from beat-to-beat, from subject to subject, and may be affected by certain diseases, drugs, or altered physiologic states. Locating a fiducial marker of the cardiac cycle is therefore an inherently empirical task, whose accuracy depends on the degree of signal variability, a quantity that is not fully controllable. The following sections will address the characteristics of signals present directly on the heart surface and on the body surface.

Heart Surface Signals

When the normally propagating wave of systolic depolarization encounters regions of diseased myocardium, propagation is slowed, and late ventricular potentials (LVPs) are produced. LVPs may be defined as electrical activations that occur or persist after the major portion of the ventricle has completed its activation. LVPs are usually generated by a small mass of ventricle within a diseased or ischemic region and are usually smaller in amplitude than the background noise of the electrocardiogram (ECG).

LVPs have been directly recorded by multiple site electrophysiologic recordings from infarcted dog ventricles,[2-4] as well as human ventricles.[5] The amount of propagation delay can range from a small fraction of the cardiac cycle to more than one cardiac cycle, depending on the nature of ischemia, and external influences such as heart rate and neurohormonal activities. While LVPs thus may occur at any time during the cardiac cycle, they most often appear during and shortly following the end of normal ventricular depolarization.

Since LVPs originate from ischemic areas, where physiologic conditions are unstable, they are inherently variable in terms of amplitude, bandwidth, and timing within the cardiac cycle.[4,6] Figure 1 shows recordings obtained from silver wires placed on an infarcted canine ventricle. The ECG and electrograms from a normal zone and two ischemic zones are shown for each of two successively paced beats in panels A, B, C, and D, respectively. Electrograms in B were recorded from a nonischemic site and typify the normal activation of myocardium that occurs regularly from beat-to-beat. Electrograms in C and D represent late potentials recorded from ischemic areas. Late potentials are smaller in amplitude, less sharp, and are more variable in timing with respect to the QRS, compared with potentials from normal areas. Late potentials may vary in timing from beat-to-beat, as seen in D, or may appear in alternate beats, as was the case for C. LVPs can thus be characterized as having variable latency with respect to the cardiac cycle, as well as variable amplitude and bandwidth.

The limited data available for human diseased hearts suggest that clinical LVPs are similar to those found in experimental canine hearts. Figure 2 shows electrograms recorded from a subendocardial slice taken from a patient undergoing surgery for recurrent ventricular tachycardia.[7] Electrophysiologic mapping prior to and during surgery had localized the site of earliest activation during ventricular tachycardia to regions within the resected tissue. The tissue was paced from a site located approximately 1 cm from sites 1 and 2, which were separated by approximately 1 cm. Pacing at a rate of 1.5

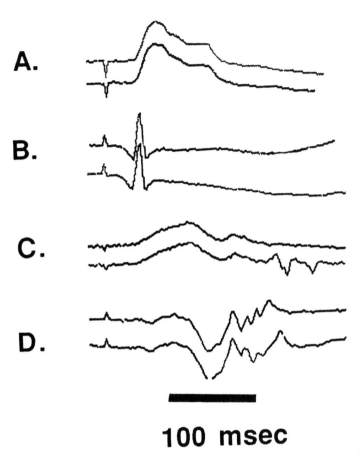

Figure 1. Ventricular potentials from an ischemic dog heart. Each panel shows two successive ventricular activations during ventricular pacing at 180 beats/min. Panel A shows ECG records. Panel B shows electrograms from nonischemic areas. Amplitude scale is approximately equal for all electrograms, which are about 1 mV peak-to-peak.

seconds resulted in a 1:1 capture of site 2, while site 1 experienced 2:1 block. Extremely prolonged functional refractory periods similar to that recorded in site 2 were consistently found in regions of other resected human tissue specimens. Thus, it appears that ischemic regions of human ventricle, similar to ischemic dog ventricles, experience 2:1 conduction block and related phenomena at slow sinus rates, due to highly prolonged refractoriness.

The inherent variability of LVPs is compounded by variations

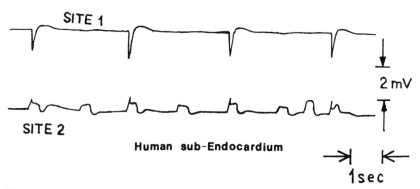

2:1 ENTRANCE BLOCK

Figure 2. Ventricular potentials from human endocardium. Tissue was removed from site located near point of origin of ventricular tachycardia. Pacing was at 1.5-second intervals from a site approximately 1 cm from sites 1 and 2.

in heart rate. Variations in heart rate as small as 20% can shift activation patterns on ischemic ventricles by as much as 10 msec.[4]

Body Surface Signals

Probably the most important and best known source of beat-to-beat variability in cardiac electrical signals is respiration. Expansion of the thorax during inspiration produces two main effects on the surface ECG. First, it induces a direct baseline shift mainly as a result of electrode impedance changes, and second it alters the electrical propagation of electrical signals from the heart to the body surface. Both artifacts can introduce significant timing errors that need to be considered.

A systematic study of 194 patients that was considered representative of those undergoing cardiac catheterization, quantified the degree of respiratory influence on the Frank ECG leads.[7] The most prominent influences of respiration on the Frank leads were found to be on QRS amplitude and azimuth. During deep inspiration, QRS amplitude declined by 25% and azimuth increased significantly (in 69 patients) by an average 11°. Respiration thus adversely influences the ability to align successive QRS complexes and to determine fiducial points.

The effect of respiration can be seen by simulating the ECG with the sinusoidal equation:

$$Y(t) = A [\sin (2 \Pi t/ T + \phi - \sin \phi], \qquad (1)$$

where A is amplitude of the QRS, T is QRS duration, and ϕ is the axis.

Two QRS complexes differing in axis by 11° are simulated by the above equation and shown in Figure 3. As can be seen, perfect alignment of these complexes is not possible, and hence any method, including cross correlation, will accumulate errors in estimating fiducial points.

The effects of respiration on small signals such as LVPs are also substantial. Using isopotential mapping and vectorcardiography, it was found that propagation from parts of the ventricle to the surface

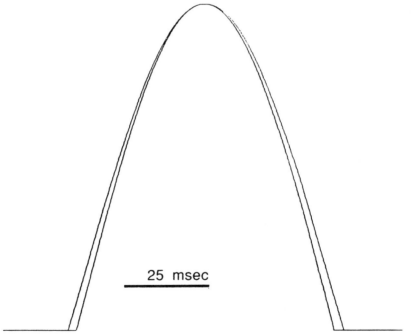

25 msec

Figure 3. Simulation of respiratory effects on QRS shape. The simulated QRS complexes differ in azimuth by 11°.

may be delayed by as much as 5 msec, compared to beats occurring at noninspiratory cycles.[8]

Baseline shifting of the ECG induced by breathing is a separate problem, and can be reduced by high-pass filtering. The drawback to this solution is the distortion produced by differentiating the QRS, whereby small variations are amplified, increasing the errors in alignment. A reasonable compromise is high-pass filtering with a cut-off frequency of about 1 Hz.

Fiducial Timing Theory

As already noted, it is not possible to find invariant fiducial points on waveforms generated by the heart because the waveforms continually vary. It is possible, however, to estimate the amount of variability in fiducial timing, as outlined below.

Temporal alignment of successive cardiac cycles can be modeled as a linear system with transfer function $h(t)$, input $a_i(t)$, and output $b(t)$, as shown in Figure 4 A.[9] To derive the transfer function, consider its response to the input shown in Figure 4 B. The alignment scheme has divided the input into a series of signals $a_i(t)$ of fixed period T, aligned with respect to the trigger point represented by the left-hand border. The fiducial point is defined as the peak of the triangle, and is invariant since all triangles are identical. Since an imperfect alignment system is assumed, the time between the fiducial point on the triangle and the trigger at time 0 is a variable t_f. The time between the fiducial point and the step signal is also a variable t_s. Both t_f and t_s are assumed to be random variables normally distributed, with variances σ_f and σ_s, respectively. The total time between the trigger point and the step signal can be defined as:

$$\tau = t_f + t_s \qquad (2)$$

with variance defined by:

$$\sigma_\tau{}^2 = \sigma_f{}^2 + \sigma_s{}^2 + \sigma_f \sigma_s r_{fs} \qquad (3)$$

where r_{fs} is the correlation coefficient between the variables t_f and t_s[10].

A.

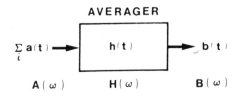

B.

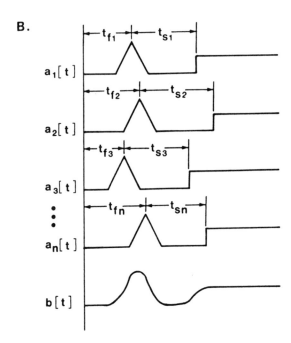

C.

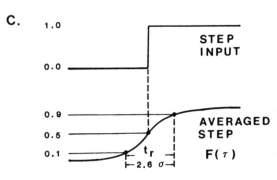

Figure 4. Theoretical model of cardiac alignment. (A) Linear model showing inputs, outputs, and transfer function. (B) Model inputs with QRS represented as an invariant triangle, followed by a step input. The items t_f and t_s are random variables. (C) The step input at top will resemble the sigmoid shape at bottom after averaging. Rise time as shown will have the value 2.6 σ.

The random variable τ represents the temporal misalignment of each step as it is summed. The total variance of alignment errors $\sigma_\tau{}^2$ can be used as a measure of misalignment and equation 3 states that it is dependent on the sum of the variances, σ_f and σ_s, and on their correlation. For convenience, the single parameter σ will be used to represent total temporal misalignment.

Note that if the two times t_f and t_s are not correlated, then the third term of equation 3 can be ignored. A perfect negative correlation between t_f and t_s, on the other hand, would minimize the total variance, and a positive correlation would maximize it. It can be seen that optimal alignment points for signal averaging are those that maximally correlate with the arrival of the signal. This implies that the goal of temporal alignment should be to establish a point that maximally correlates with the signal, if it can be found, and align all cycles with that point. Each $a_i(t)$ contains the unit step input $u(t)$ that occurs at time τ. The step input, $u(t)$, is defined as:

$$u(t) = 1 \text{ if } x(t) \geq \tau$$
$$u(t) = 0 \text{ if } x(t) < \tau \tag{4}$$

where:

$$x(t) = t - (i - 1)T \tag{5}$$

where i is the sequential average number and T is the period of averaged signal.

Using the general definition of time average,[11] time average of $u(t)$ can be written as:

$$\text{AVERAGE } \{u(t)\} = \lim \frac{1}{2T} \int_{-T}^{T} u(t) \, dt \tag{6}$$

and is shown to be equivalent to $F(\tau)$ where F is the probability distribution function.[11] Assuming a Gaussian distribution:

$$f(\tau) = \int_{-\infty}^{T} \frac{1}{2\Pi \sigma} e^{-(t^2/2\sigma^2)} \, dt. \tag{7}$$

Thus, the average response to a step input in the presence of temporal misalignment τ, a normally distributed random variable, is the normal distribution function shown in Figure 4 C. The rise time t_r of the step from 10% to 90% of its unit magnitude has the value

2.6 σ as can be verified from tabulated values of the distribution function.[10] The step response thus provides a way to directly measure σ, the temporal misalignment:

$$\sigma = 0.38t_r. \tag{8}$$

Frequency response as a function of rise time can be estimated by:

$$f_c = 135 / \sigma, \tag{9}$$

with σ measured in milliseconds, and f_c is the 3-dB cut-off frequency.

This model assumes that sufficient samples of the random variable τ have been taken such that a statistically accurate value of σ has been achieved. As a rule of thumb approximately 30 samples would be sufficient to obtain a reasonably confident estimate of τ and its variance.[10] It can be concluded that increasing the number of averages beyond 30 would not significantly affect σ and hence would not further alter the frequency response, assuming a normally distributed τ.

To derive the transfer function from the step response we recognize:

$$b(\tau) = \int_{-\infty}^{\tau} h(t)\, dt. \tag{10}$$

Recalling equation 7, it follows that:

$$h(t) = f(t), \tag{11}$$

where f is the probability density function. Assuming a Gaussian distribution, the frequency response $H(\omega)$ is given by the characteristic function:

$$H(\omega) = e^{-\sigma^2\omega^2/2} \tag{12}$$

and is plotted for various values of σ in Figure 5 A.

The response curves for averaging with varying degrees of temporal misalignment is shown in Figure 5 B. The agreement between the two estimates of frequency response, one based on the step response (equation 8) and the other on the transfer function (equation 12), is reasonable.

A.

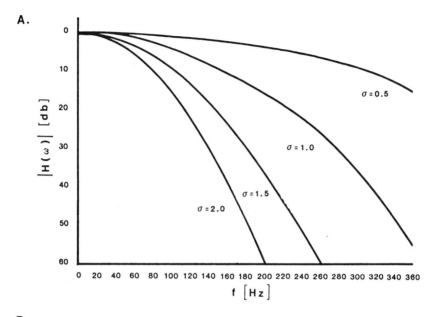

B.

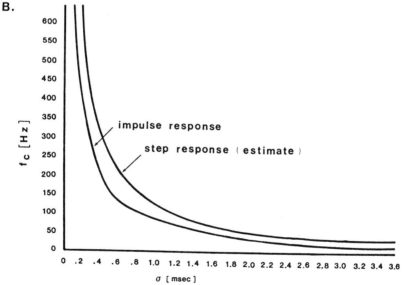

Figure 5. Effect of temporal misalignment on frequency response of averaging system. (A) Bode plot of equation 12 for selected values of σ. (B) Response curves showing the -3-dB frequency point as function of σ. Equation 12 was used to calculate the impulse response, and equation 8 was used for the step response.

Practical Averaging Systems

Requirements

A high-resolution ECG averaging system should be capable of:

1. low-noise amplification of 30,000–50,000;
2. precise detection of normal sinus beats and rejection of others;
3. evaluation of its own temporal alignment accuracy for any given ECG;
4. adjustment for temporal precision prior to averaging.

Low-Noise Design

One implementation of a precision low-noise amplifier is a standard three operational amplifier (op amp) design, based on the Precision Monolithic Instruments, OP227 (Santa Clara, CA), shown in Figure 6 A. The gain of the input stage is set at the maximum that can be tolerated without saturation, which is about 5000. Output gain is achieved at the isolation amplifier stage (Burr-Brown 3562-J (Tucson, AZ). This provides a gain of 10 and electrically isolates the input stage from the rest of the system. Final system gains of 30,000–50,000 are used.

Optimal gain settings were determined by measuring system noise, referred to the input, as defined in Figure 6 B and below.

$$N_s = \frac{N_1 A_1 A_2 A_3 + N_2 A_2 A_3 + N_3 A_3}{A_1 \ A_2 \ A_3} \tag{13}$$

where N_s represents total rms system noise, N_i represents the root mean square (rms) noise of each amplifier stage, and A_i is the gain of each stage. From equation 13 it is apparent that, assuming the noise is the same at each stage, system noise can be minimized by maximizing the gain of the first stage A_1. This prediction was empirically validated by varying A_1 with a 1000 Ω source impedance at the input. Figure 6 C shows that total rms noise referred to the input declines with increasing input gain. This point should be used in designing input amplifiers.

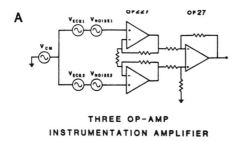

A

THREE OP-AMP
INSTRUMENTATION AMPLIFIER

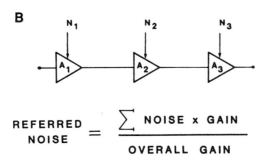

B

$$\text{REFERRED NOISE} = \frac{\sum \text{NOISE} \times \text{GAIN}}{\text{OVERALL GAIN}}$$

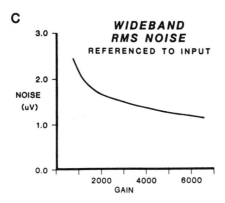

C

Figure 6. Design of input amplifier. (A) Schematic diagram showing common mode voltage, V_{cm} and inputs from surface ECG electrodes and noise. (B) Schema of gain relationships in the multistage amplifier. (C) Relationship between RMS noise, referred to the input, and total gain in a multistage amplifier. A 1000-Ω source impedance was applied to the input, and bandwidth was 1–500 Hz.

QRS Alignment

QRS Alignment by Hardware

Design

A real-time system for precision QRS alignment is schematized in Figure 7 A.[12] The system consists of two comparators, one based on amplitude, the other based on slope within a specified interval. The ECG signal is high-pass filtered at a cut-off of 1 Hz to reduce baseline drift, and low-pass filtered at a cut-off of 500 Hz. This signal is fed into two circuits: (1) an amplitude level detector, consisting of a comparator; and (2) a differentiator. The level detector triggers a timing circuit that sends a variable width pulse after a delay to an analog switch. The switch gates a selected portion of the differentiated signal and transmits this to a second comparator. If the slope is above the specified threshold, the final trigger pulse is generated. This final pulse is known as the "window trigger," since it is based on a windowed portion of the QRS slope. It is used as the QRS alignment point for signal averaging, has a duration set just below the expected minimum ST interval of 300 msec, and is nonretriggerable.

An important feature of the above scheme is that the rising phase of the QRS is used to trigger a square pulse that then enables a second trigger along a selected portion of the falling phase as illustrated in Figure 7 B. Note that the window pulse is synchronized to a point on the rising phase of the QRS, while the final trigger is synchronized to a point on the falling phase. Temporal variability in alignment of the window pulse with the trigger pulse can thus be used as a systematic measure of temporal accuracy, with the window pulse being equivalent to a step input, similar to the input of Figure 4 B.

Details of the circuit are shown in Figure 8. The timing of the pulses is precisely controlled by a 1-MHz crystal oscillator, with a selectable resolution of 0.1 msec. The timing, including the duration and delay of the window pulse, is controlled by thumbwheel switches. Threshold levels are controlled by 10-turn potentiometers.

Basic operation of the window trigger is shown in Figure 9A. The QRS from a normal human subject is shown at top, and the level trigger is seen in the trace below. When the QRS exceeds threshold

A.

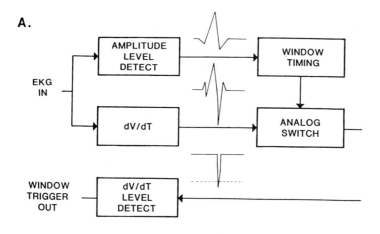

B.

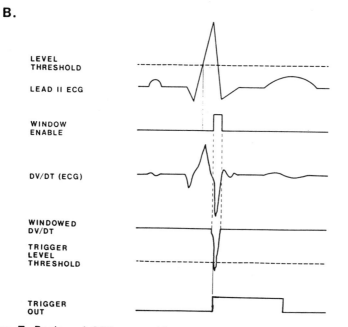

Figure 7. Design of QRS recognition system. (A) Schematic diagram. (B) Timing diagram.

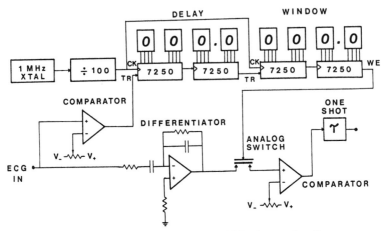

Figure 8. Circuit diagram of QRS trigger circuit.

Th_1 a window pulse is triggered following a preset delay. The window pulse occurs during a 30-msec period of the falling phase of the QRS. The delay and duration of the window for gating the dV/dt signal are both variable from 0.1 to 1000 msec. When the differentiated ECG signal in the bottom trace exceeds threshold Th_2 during the period when the window is high, the final trigger pulse is generated.

The QRS recognition system can be adjusted for rejection of premature ventricular contractions (PVCs), as shown in Figure 9B, the ECG signal from a patient showing a PVC in between two normal QRS complexes. Note that while the PVC is larger than the normal QRS in amplitude and peak dV/dt, its slope during the window period is below threshold, and it is rejected.

Figure 9C illustrates the superiority of the window trigger over a trigger based purely on QRS slope. The top trace is the ECG record from a normal subject who was asked to cough. The EMG noise generated by coughing can be seen as high-frequency deflections in the ECG trace at the top as well as the dV/dt trace at the bottom. Note that although the dV/dt amplitude of the noise exceeds that of the QRS, triggers are generated only for heart beats.

Discrimination ability of the system is related to the duration of the window pulse, as shown in Figure 10. With a window duration of 50 msec in (A), the system does not distinguish between normal beats and PVCs. Narrowing the window to 5 msec causes the dV/dt in the windowed segment of PVCs to be below threshold, and discrimination is achieved (Fig. 10B).

The results of the Figures 9 and 10 demonstrate that the R wave

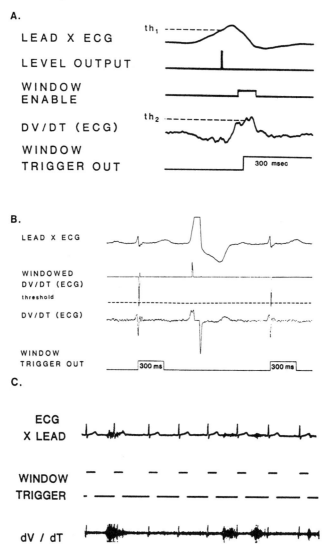

Figure 9. Operation of QRS recognition system. (A) At top, a QRS from the X lead of a human subject is shown. When the voltage level exceeds Th_1, a level output is triggered below. After a preset delay, the window enable pulse is triggered. The differentiated *(dV/dt)* QRS is shown below. When threshold Th_2 is reached, the final window trigger is initiated. (B) At top, an ECG record from a patient shows 2 sinus beats with a PVC interposed. The *dV/dt* of the top trace during the window enable periods is shown below, with the dotted line indicating threshold setting for *dV/dt*. The complete *dV/dt* of the ECG is shown in the next trace, and the window trigger is shown at bottom. (C) ECG record from a normal subject is shown in the top trace. Note the noise deflections, representing coughing, present in the ECG and its derivative in the bottom trace. The middle trace shows the window trigger for each QRS.

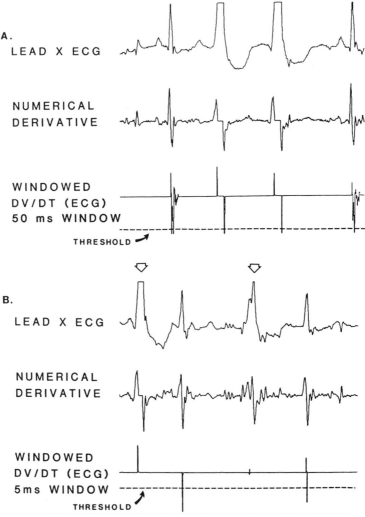

Figure 10. Effect of window duration on discrimination ability of QRS recognition system. (A) With window duration of 50 msec, *dV/dt* exceeds threshold for sinus beats and ventricular beats of the patient. (B) With window duration of 5 msec, ventricular beats are rejected.

slopes of PVCs as measured by their R wave derivatives, can be larger than those of sinus beats. R wave slope alone is thus an inadequate criterion for the separation of sinus beats from PVCs.

Optimizing Alignment

Typical beat-to-beat variability in QRS shape in a healthy subject is shown in Figure 11. The subject was lying down and breathing quietly. Seven superimposed QRS complexes recorded at a bandwidth of 1–300 Hz and sampled at random are shown in the top traces. Since they have been aligned using the window trigger, the falling phases are closely matched in time. The rising phases, however, have temporal disparities ranging from 0 to 3 msec at various portions of the waves. The middle trace displays the high-pass filtered QRS complexes that have even greater disparities than the wide-band records. The bottom trace shows the numerical derivatives of the QRS complexes that closely match the high-pass filtered traces, due to the differentiation effect of the filter. From these records, it can be seen that temporal alignment errors cannot be systematically evaluated from either the wide-band or filtered QRS complexes, due to irregularity in their shapes. It can also be concluded that temporal alignment errors can be greatly magnified by high-pass filtering.

Figure 12 shows the use of the window pulse to estimate temporal misalignment during averaging. The QRS wave from a normal subject shown at the top triggers the window pulse shown immediately below. After 20 averages, the pulse is no longer square, but has a sawtooth appearance on the rising and falling edges. This effect is due to the temporal misalignment occurring from beat-to-beat. After 51 averages, the edges are smoother, and after 266 averages, the rising and falling edges resemble sigmoid curves, as predicted by equation 7. The width of the pulse has broadened from its original 21-msec duration to 26 msec measured from the points at 10% of the peak. Averaging the window pulse is equivalent to the situation in Figure 4B, and the rise time can be used to compute temporal misalignment of the pulse. This measurement yields a value of 5 msec and from equation 7 a value for σ of 1.9 msec is obtained. The upper limit frequency response of approximately 45 Hz can be found from Figure 5B. Note that the rise time can be estimated roughly after 20 averages even though the edge is not smooth.

Use of the step response to optimize temporal alignment is shown in Figure 13. The trace in the upper left is the QRS from the

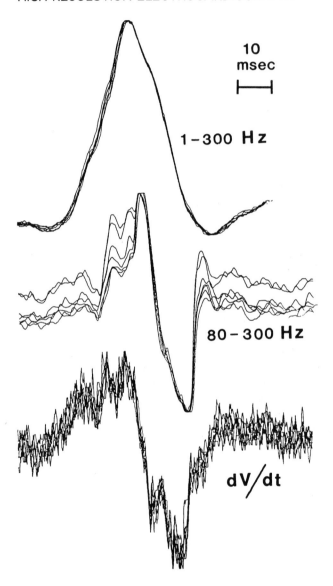

10
msec
⊢——⊣

1-300 Hz

80-300 Hz

dV/dt

Figure 11. Superimposed QRS. Variability in QRS shape in a healthy subject. At top, seven *QRS* complexes from the *X* lead with a bandwidth of 1–300 Hz are superimposed. Alignment of the traces was done using the window trigger method. The middle traces are high-pass filtered records of the top traces, and the bottom traces are the numerically differentiated records of the QRS complexes at the top.

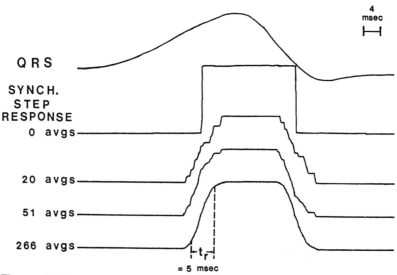

Figure 12. Averaged step responses. The top trace shows a single QRS complex that was used to synchronize the square wave shown immediately below. The next three traces below represent the square waves after 20, 51, and 266 averages, respectively.

Z lead of a patient after 375 averages, and the trace at right is the averaged step input. From the rise of 3.7 msec, a σ of 1.4 msec is obtained and a frequency response up to 70 Hz is determined. The trace at the bottom left represents an equal number of averages taken from the same patient after refining the QRS alignment by narrowing the window pulse. During this average due to the greater selectivity of the trigger, approximately every fifth beat was rejected. Note the high-frequency deflections of >10 µV that are evident in this QRS that are not visible in the top trace. The step response measured from the trace at right indicates that the alignment accuracy was improved to 0.3 msec, yielding a frequency response up to 340 Hz. The crucial importance of alignment in detection of high-frequency low level potentials is thus evident.

From Figure 13, it can be concluded that a substantial amount of information is present in the QRS above 70 Hz. This conclusion seems to conflict with reports that found no substantial energy above 50 Hz in the averaged QRS of normals as well as patients with ventricular arrhythmias.[13] Since these reports did not directly estimate the frequency response, their spectral analyses cannot be eval-

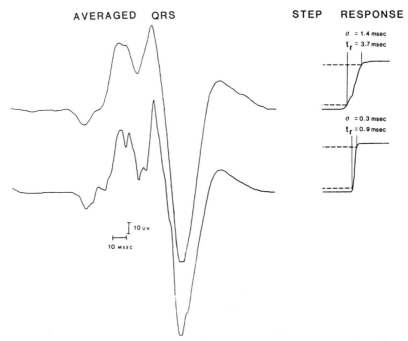

Figure 13. Optimizing average fidelity. The trace at top left is the QRS from the Z lead of a patient recorded at 25–500 Hz after 375 averages. At top right is the step response obtained from this average showing a temporal misalignment, σ, of 1.4 msec. The lower two traces were similarly obtained, after reducing temporal misalignment to 0.3 msec by adjusting the window trigger. Note the presence of rapid deflections in the lower QRS that are not present in the upper one.

uated. Regardless of their degree of accuracy, it is likely that spectral analyses would be relatively insensitive to the small notches seen in the lower trace of Figure 10, since their spectral energy is low. Thus, direct comparisons between time and frequency analyses of cardiac signals are not straightforward.

Alignment by Software

Cross correlation of QRS complexes is a convenient method for alignment of digitized ECG recordings using a software algorithm based on the equation below[14]:

$$r = \frac{\Sigma (X_i - X)(Y_i - Y)}{\Sigma (X_i - X)^2 \, \Sigma (Y_i - Y)^2} \tag{14}$$

where X_i and Y_i represent sampled points on two digitized waves, and r represents the linear correlation coefficient. The algorithm thus involves maximizing r, the correlation between each sampled QRS and a reference QRS. Cross correlation optimizes alignment by minimizing the temporal disparities between selected points on sampled QRS complexes.

The alignment accuracy of cross correlation is somewhat arbitrary, depending on the sampling rate as well as the underlying cardiac variability. The limitations of cross correlation can be appreciated by showing the alignment of simulated Gaussian waveforms, as depicted in Figure 14. A series of wave-pairs, whose correlation is > 95%, are shown. Panel A shows that cross correlation is not sensitive to amplitude differences, since two waves with identical standard deviation but widely different amplitudes have a correlation coefficient of 1. Panel B shows a Gaussian wave and a half-sine wave that differ by more than 20 msec in overall duration (assuming 1 msec per sample point) and are quite dissimilar in shape, nevertheless they correlate to within 96%. Panel C shows a Gaussian wave and a square wave whose correlation is 95%. These illustrations demonstrate that cross correlation is completely insensitive to amplitude variations among waves, and is relatively insensitive to vari-

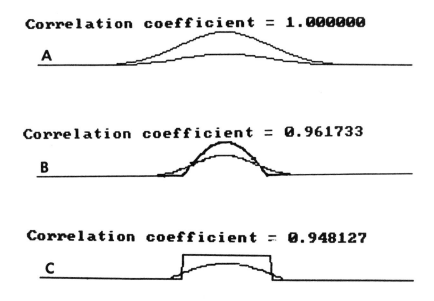

Figure 14. Cross correlation of simulated wave pairs.

ations in shape. Cross correlation thus must be used cautiously as a method of alignment.

Modern Signal Processing of the ECG

Periodicity Analysis of Ventricular Potentials

Given the variable nature of the heart, especially in the presence of ischemia, it would be advantageous for diagnostic systems to exploit the variability rather than be defeated by it. One such system is outlined here. From Figures 1 and 2, it is clear that the potentials from ischemic ventricular areas sometimes describe regular patterns such as 2:1 or higher degree of activation block. One powerful method that can detect such patterns is spectral analysis of the ECG,[15] as illustrated in Figure 15. The electrograms at top left were recorded from ischemic regions of a dog ventricle and show a 1:1 activation pattern during constant pacing at intervals of 400 msec. The power spectral density of ECG lead II during 512 seconds of pacing at this rate is shown below. Note that a single peak at the pacing rate of 2.5 Hz is seen. When stimulus interval was decreased to 350 msec, the electrograms all show a 2:1 pattern of activation. The corresponding spectrum below shows a peak at 2.8 Hz and a subharmonic peak at 1.4 Hz, indicative of an event in the ECG that occurred on alternate beats. The coincidence of 2:1 activation failure at several sites in the ventricle induced by increased pacing, with the appearance of the subharmonic suggests that spectral analysis may be fruitful in detecting variable LVPs. Studies on infarcted canine hearts have suggested that regions such as those represented in Figure 15 are prime substrates for reentrant arrhythmias. Thus, this method, called 'periodicity analysis', could be a useful diagnostic tool for arrhythmias.

Heart Rate Variability

Heart rate variability (HRV) is becoming an important indicator of cardiac-autonomic nervous interactions, and may be a useful prognosticator for patients with ischemic heart disease.[16–18] Considering the power and sensitivity of the signal processing analyses

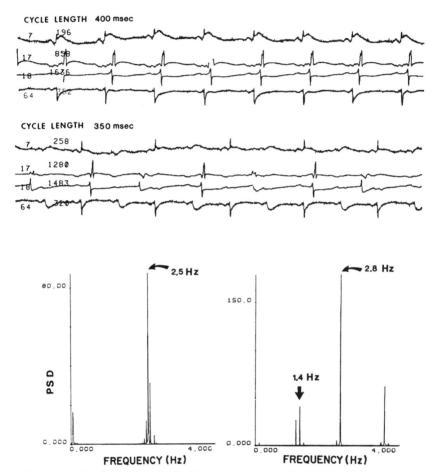

Figure 15. Periodicity analysis. Electrograms from four sites within the ischemic region of a 4-day post-LAD ligation dog heart are shown at top for two pacing rates. At a cycle length of 350 msec, the sites are blocked in a 2:1 pattern. The corresponding power spectral density analyses of ECG recorded during the two pacing periods are shown below. Note the appearance of the subharmonic at the faster (2.8 Hz) pacing rate.

that are involved in HRV, it is important to maximize the accuracy of the basic measurement, that of heart rate.

A heart rate measuring device ideally should detect sinus node activations, represented on the body surface by the P wave of the ECG. However, since reliable detection of the P wave is difficult due to its low amplitude, its occurrence can be estimated by the occurrence of the much larger R wave provided by ventricular activation, with the assumption that the interval between the P and R waves is constant from beat-to-beat. The first and most important step in the measurement of heart rate is thus accurate determination of fiducial points corresponding to activation.

Fiducial timing is particularly relevant to the measurement of respiratory sinus arrhythmia (RSA), a useful index of the parasympathetic nervous activity.[18] A system that is sensitive to the respiratory-induced amplitude variation in ECG does not measure pure variability in heart rate, but rather measures variation in ECG amplitude changes, along with heart rate. Since ECG-respiratory interactions are largest in the supine position, when RSA is presumed to be most prominent, serious RSA measurement errors are likely commonplace. Fiducial point selection should, therefore, be insensitive to R wave amplitude and low-frequency ECG variations. The QRS trigger system outlined in Figure 7, that is a pattern recognition algorithm implemented in hardware, has proven to be a stable and accurate rate meter.[17] Once the system is adjusted so that each sinus beat is reliably detected, the computer data acquisition system need only detect TTL pulses corresponding to each beat and can sample at high rates. The method is clearly superior to the simple R wave detectors coupled with an integrating capacitor that is provided as a tachometer on several commercial heart rate meters, and also has advantages over cross correlation.

Once an adequate series of raw heartbeat intervals is acquired by the computer, analysis of their variability is carried out in software. Premature ventricular contractions can be recognized and labeled by the hardware, but then the software must interpolate the missing sinus beats at points in time when they would be expected. This practice is required for further signal processing, but is only justified when PVCs appear rarely in the record. After the raw intervals are checked and corrected if necessary, a variety of time-domain and frequency-domain techniques can be used to provide HRV indices. Standard time-domain measurements include the mean and standard deviation of RR intervals over selected time segments, the

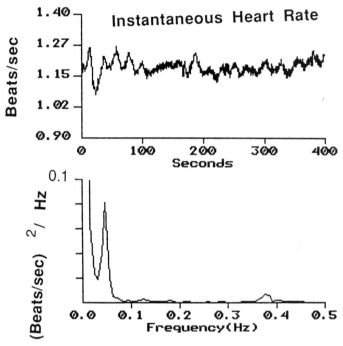

Figure 16. Heart rate variability analysis. Instantaneous heart rate function at top was derived from 10 minutes of patient ECG in supine position. Bottom trace is spectrum of the top function, showing a prominent peak at about 0.1 Hz, corresponding to mainly sympathetic influence.

standard deviation of mean RR intervals, and the average number of beat-to-beat differences in RR interval greater than specified values during segments of time.

Before frequency-domain analyses can be applied, a measure of the instantaneous heart rate must be derived. The simplest formula is: instantaneous rate = $1/RR_i$, where RR_i represents successive RR intervals. This function is not an accurate representation of heart rate, since it is a discrete function, whereas the output of the sinus node is a continuous function of time. Furthermore, the inverse RR equation can only provide one value of rate for each beat, representing the rate corresponding to the previous beat. For spectral analysis, a continuous time function is much preferable to a discrete one. A more ideal heart rate function, therefore, would provide an instantaneous rate function, that is smoothed and valid for all points in time. Such a smooth function, known as instantaneous heart rate, was derived by Berger et al.[19] Spectral estimation can then be usefully applied to heart rate, as illustrated in Figure 16.

Conclusion

Any system that depends on a fiducial reference point is subject to unavoidable errors due to the inherent variability of the cardiac signal. This chapter has reviewed some of the known characteristics of normal and ischemic signals and has outlined established, as well as newer, methods for understanding and minimizing fiducial timing errors.

Acknowledgment: This work was supported in part by National Institutes of Health, Grants R0731341 and 36680 and by the Coronary Heart Disease Research, a program of the American Health Assistance Foundation.

References

1. Berbari EJ: High-resolution electrocardiography. CRC Crit Rev Biomed Eng 16:67, 1988.
2. Berbari EJ, Scherlag BJ, Hope RR, Lazzara R: Recording from the body surface of arrhythmogenic ventricular activity during the S-T segment. Am J Cardiol 41:697, 1978.
3. Simson MB, Euler D, Michelson EL, Falcone RA, Spear JF, Moore EN: Detection of delayed ventricular activation on the body surface in dogs. Am J Physiol 24:H363, 1981.
4. Restivo M, El-Sherif N, Kelen GJ, Henkin R, Craelius W, Gough WB: Correlation of late potentials on the body surface and ventricular activation maps of reentrant circuits in the post-infarction dog heart. Circulation 72(Suppl II):2, 1985.
5. Josephson ME, Horowitz LN, Farshidi A: Continuous local electrical activity. A mechanism of recurrent ventricular tachycardia. Circulation 57:659, 1978.
6. Craelius W, Restivo M, El-Sherif N: Signal processing options for late potentials. J Electrocardiol 30:345, 1987.
7. Riekkinen H, Rautaharju P: Body position, electrode level, and respiration effects on the Frank lead electrocardiogram. Circulation 53:40, 1976.
8. Flaherty JT, Blumenschein SD, Alexander AW, Gentzler RD, Gallie TM, Boineau JP, Spach MS: Influence of respiration on recording cardiac potentials. Isopotential surface-mapping and vectorcardiographic studies. Am J Cardiol 20:21, 1967.

9. Craelius W, Restivo M, Assadi AA, El-Sherif N: Criteria for optimal averaging of cardiac signals. IEEE Trans Biomed Eng 33:957, 1986.
10. Mood AM, Graybill FA: Introduction to the Theory of Statistics. New York: McGraw-Hill, 1963.
11. Papoulis A: Probability Random Variable and Statistical Procedures. New York: McGraw-Hill, 1965.
12. Craelius W, Restivo R, Henkin E, Caref E, El-Sherif N: High resolution ECG amplifier for signal averaging. IEEE/Seventh Annual Conference of the Engineering in Medicine and Biology Society, 1985, p 860.
13. Cain ME, Ambos HD, Witkowski FX, Sobel BE: Fast Fourier transform analysis of signal averaged electrocardiograms for identification of patients prone to sustained ventricular tachycardia. Circulation 69:711, 1984.
14. Press WH, Flannery BP, Teukilsky SA, Vetterling WT: Numerical Recipes. Boston: Cambridge University Press, 1986.
15. Craelius W, Chen VK-H, Restivo M, El-Sherif N: Rhythm analysis of arterial blood pressure. IEEE Trans Biomed Eng 33:1166, 1986.
16. Myers GA, Martin GJ, Magid NM, Barnett PS, Schaad JW, Weiss JS, Lesch M, Singer DH: Power spectral analysis of heart rate variability in sudden cardiac death: comparison to other methods. IEEE Trans Biomed Eng 33:1149, 1986.
17. Bekheit S, Tangella M, El-Sakr A, Rasheed Q, Craelius W, El-Sherif N: Use of heart rate spectral analysis to study the effects of calcium channel blockers on sympathetic activity after myocardial infarction. Am Heart J 119:79, 1990.
18. Pomeranz B, Macaulay RJB, Caudill A, Kutz I, Adam D, Gordon D, Kilborn KM, Barger AG, Shannon DC, Cohen RJ, Benson H: Assessment of autonomic functions in humans by heart rate spectral analysis. Am J Physiol 248:H151, 1985.
19. Berger RD, Akselrod S, Gordon D, Cohen RJ: An efficient algorithm for spectral analysis of heart rate variability. IEEE Trans Biomed Eng 33:900, 1986.

3

Principles of Noise Reduction

Edward J. Berbari, Paul Lander

Introduction

High-resolution electrocardiography (HRECG) implies an increased time and voltage scale compared to standard ECG techniques. Increasing the time scale is as simple as turning a knob on an oscillographic recorder or increasing the sampling rate of a digital-based system. However, such simple means are not usually possible for the voltage scale because of the fact that many other signals are added to the cardiac signals. The typical 1-mV/cm scale of a standard ECG machine imposes a threshold for small amplitude signals (< 0.1 mV).

Typically, there are three sources of interfering signal which seem to confound an HRECG recording. These are: 1) system or electronic noise; 2) 60-Hz interference; 3) and unwanted physiologic signals. For the most part the first two sources are relatively small with modern preamplifiers. It is the latter source that is the limiting factor for recording cardiac signals < 100 μV.

Defining noise is much like gardening. It is a contextual problem. Weeds are things that grow where you don't want them to grow. Noise is a signal that interferes with a signal of interest. In order to eliminate either, it is essential to define the characteristics of the wanted and unwanted items. Therefore, analysis of low level cardiac signals will require definitions for the signal of interest and the

From El-Sherif N, Turitto G (eds): *High-Resolution Electrocardiography.* Mount Kisco, NY, Futura Publishing Co., Inc., ©, 1992.

interfering noise. After defining the problem it becomes important to describe methods to quantify both entities. Some examples will be given which demonstrate this quantification, but it also becomes imperative to offer suggestions and methods which will improve HRECG recordings. This latter step amounts to introducing some concepts of quality control in what is essentially a statistical estimation problem.

Definition of Noise and Signals

The simple definition of the ECG signal source is the potential which is generated by cardiac cells and the noise is simply all other potentials. However, the HRECG usually requires signal averaging to enhance the signal-to-noise ratio (SNR). [1,2] This digital procedure introduces many uncertainties which can form the basis of more complicated definitions of signal and noise. For example, a primary requisite of signal averaging is the proper identification and alignment of the cardiac signal of interest. Once this is done the computer sums subsequently occurring time aligned signals. For most problems, e.g., His-Purkinje or late potentials, the HRECG usually identifies signals that are temporally referenced to the QRS complex. Improper identification or poor alignment (jitter) of the QRS will result in signals being inappropriately identified even though they are of a cardiac origin. Hence, these improperly identified signals may also be considered as noise. The results of jitter on the signal averaging process have been examined [3,4] and when present it acts as a low-pass filter on the averaged waveform.

The realm of ECG processing is almost entirely digitally based. There are many well known problems associated with digital signal processing which can also be considered as a source of noise in the HRECG. Digitalization is an estimate of a signal during a short period of time. The estimate is limited to discrete values evenly spaced within the dynamic range of the A/D converter. With 12- to 16-bit A/D converters over a dynamic range of ± 10 mV (assuming a gain of 1000) this uncertainty is in the range of 5 to 0.3 µV. This quantization noise is not usually considered significant particularly when signal averaging is employed. In this case the quantization noise is reduced by averaging in a manner similar to other sources of noise. For instruments which employ an 8-bit A/D converter this noise is 0.078 mV and could be considered problematic in some cases.

A report by Gaumond [5] does demonstrate that signal averaging improves the dynamic range of low bit A/D converters.

The digitization process has two time components: 1) the time to digitize; and 2) the time between each digital sample. For typical A/D converters used for ECG signal processing, sampling time (or aperture time or dwell time) does not introduce significant uncertainties. The time between samples or the sampling rate can be of significance if improperly chosen. Theoretically the Sampling Theorem dictates a sampling rate *at least* twice the highest frequency of interest. When this rule is not observed then aliasing will occur. Aliasing defines the situation where signals which are greater than half the sampling rate will fold back and appear as signals of a lower frequency. For example, if one assumes no ECG signals of interest have a frequency > 300 Hz then the minimum sampling rate would be 600 Hz. If a 301-Hz signal is present it will alias and appear as an equal amplitude 299-Hz signal. An antialiasing low-pass filter is usually used. A fourth order, 300-Hz low-pass filter will only attenuate signals out to 600 Hz by 24 dB, at most. Thus, noise power in this range will only be minimally attenuated and will contaminate the entire signal spectrum. Increasing the sampling rate is recommended to increase the aesthetic view of the waveforms and to prevent signal contamination with aliased noise. A 2000-Hz sampling rate follows the rule of thumb to sample 5 to 10 times the highest frequency of interest and limits signal contamination. It does improve the SNR, in the bandwidth of interest, as a function of the roll off characteristics of the antialiasing filter.

Another example of altering the definition of noise is to include poorly identified or misaligned-aligned QRS complexes. If a premature ventricular beat or fusion beat is accepted into the average then the widened QRS will most likely add to the late potentials and cause a distortion. Similarly, a misaligned QRS complex can cause similar problems. Figure 1 demonstrates this point. Panel A shows the filtered vector magnitude, $\sqrt{X^2 + Y^2 + Z^2}$. This is a common format for displaying late potentials. This is a normal subject and the QRS duration is 98 msec. The shaded region represents the terminal 40 msec of the QRS and it has a root mean square (RMS) value of 13 μV. For the 40-Hz high-pass filter, QRS duration > 120 msec and RMS-40 < 20 μV are considered abnormal. There were 177 beats in the average and the average was terminated when the noise measurement reached 0.3 μV. Panels B, C, and D represent the same

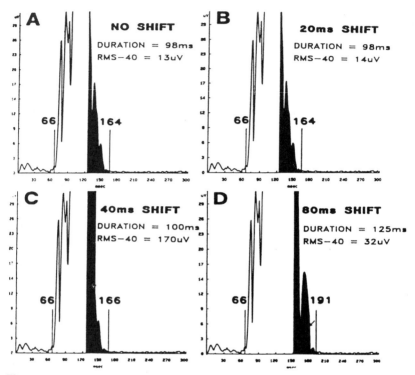

Figure 1. Demonstration of the effect of 1 misaligned beat in a 177-beat signal average. Panel A is the average with no misaligned beats. Panels B, C, and D have 1 misaligned beat with a shift of 20, 40 and 80 msec, respectively.

average with 1 additional beat added, but shifted by 20, 40 and 80 msec, respectively. The 20-msec shift did not cause a change in QRS duration and only a 1.0-µV increase in the RMS-40 value. The 40-msec shift, panel C, increased QRS duration by only 2 msec, but significantly increased RMS-40 to 170 µV. In panel D, the 80-msec shift of a single QRS caused an increase in QRS duration to 125 msec and the RMS-40 voltage to 32 µV. It can be deduced that such a shift if undetected can cause serious misinterpretation. One way to assure that this does not occur is to observe every accepted beat with respect to the chosen alignment or fiducial point. One may increase the acceptance threshold to eliminate false detection. Without this visual feedback it may not be possible to provide 100% quality control on the averaging process.

Thus, the simple definitions of the ECG signal and noise take on a much more complicated meaning when discussing the digitized ECG and the HRECG obtained via signal averaging. The newer definitions of signal and noise include more than just the signal sources as their primary descriptors and imply that the measuring devices (hardware and software) operate properly. It is not always possible to insure this so means must be employed to quantify both signal and noise.

Quantifying Noise and Signals

The above discussion was aimed at broadening the definition of noise in an HRECG. It is important to understand the digital processing methods which can introduce errors (or noise) in measuring latent cardiac signals. These methods also inject another constraint often overlooked in recording HRECGs. This constraint is that there is now a statistical element in analyzing the HRECG. For example, as signal averaging is used to enhance the SNR it only creates a statistical view of what is occurring. The driving force behind this is the statistical nature of the noise which interferes with the low level ECG signal sources and in some cases the nondeterministic nature of cardiac sources. In the latter case it has been demonstrated that under certain circumstances the low level cardiac sources, e.g., His-Purkinje system or late potential substrate, will vary on a beat-to-beat basis.[6,7] While not diminishing the possible importance of these signal variations they will not be the focus of this presentation and the cardiac signals of interest will be considered to be deterministic on a beat-to-beat basis over the period of time they are being studied.

Other simplifying assumptions are that the noise is purely additive and that it is uncorrelated with the signal of interest. Periodic, asynchronous noise, e.g., 60-Hz interference is a special case and will not be considered in this analysis.[8] Attention to proper lead attachment and good amplifier design will cure this problem at its source.[9] The most common source of noise that is in this category is electromyographic (EMG). All of the skeletal muscles generate ongoing electrical activity which is the primary interfering signal of the HRECG. Even simple breathing and the normal function of the intercostal muscles will cause significant noise contamination. The total EMG noise often reflects the physiologic and psychologic state of the subject.

The following is a statistical approach to quantifying the signal average and signal variance.[2] The latter is a measure of the contaminating noise power. The signal average is represented by a summation of n points.

$$\overline{X}_j = \frac{1}{n} \sum_{i=1}^{n} X_{ij} \tag{1}$$

where j is a particular point in the averaging window and i is the cardiac cycle number. X_{ij} is the sum of the signal of interest, S_{ij}, and the noise, N_{ij}. So equation 1 becomes:

$$\overline{X}_j = \frac{1}{n} \sum_{i=1}^{n} S_{ij} + \frac{1}{n} \sum_{i=1}^{n} N_{ij}. \tag{2}$$

The SNR can be defined as the magnitude of S_{ij} divided by the root mean square (RMS) value of the noise. The RMS represents the equivalent average voltage from which the power within a time varying signal can be computed.

$$SNR = \frac{|S_{ij}|}{(N_{ij})RMS} = \frac{|S_{ij}|}{\sqrt{E[N^2_j]}} = \frac{|S_{ij}|}{\sigma_{Nj}} \tag{3}$$

where σ_{Nj} is the standard deviation of the underlying noise process which has a zero mean. The cardiac signal repeats on a beat-to-beat basis so that $S_{ij} = S_j$. The noise is assumed to be uncorrelated but in practice this is not usually true. EMG noise and 60-Hz noise violate this assumption. But the noise is assumed to be independent of the signal, to have a zero mean, and to be stationary. Thus $\sigma_{Nj} = \sigma_N$.

Equation 2 can be rewritten:

$$\overline{X}_j = S_j + \overline{N}_j. \tag{4}$$

The expected value of X_j, the signal average, will yield the desired signal, S_j.

$$E[\overline{X}_j] = S_j + E[\overline{N}_j] = S_j. \tag{5}$$

Of particular importance in this development is the quantification of noise. The most common measurement of noise power within a signal is the variance of that signal.

$$\text{VAR}[X_j] = \text{VAR}[S_j + \overline{N}_j]$$
$$= \text{VAR}[S_j] + \text{VAR}[\overline{N}_j]$$
$$= 0 + E[\overline{N}_j{}^2] - E[\overline{N}_j]^2$$
$$= \sigma_N{}^2/n \qquad (6)$$

The SNR of the signal average can be directly calculated.

In this case the standard deviation is taken as the RMS value of the noise. The SNR of the signal average improves as the $\sqrt{n}$. Of more interest in this discussion is the quantification of the noise. There are two noise calculations in this presentation: (1) the variance of the underlying noise process, $\sigma_N{}^2$; and (2) the variance of the signal average, $\sigma_N{}^2/n$. Both of these are easily calculated during the averaging process and have been used in a number of studies to quantify physiologic noise in evoked response studies.[10,11] In particular this measure was used to evaluate esophageal lead systems for recording His-Purkinje potentials[12] and in late potential measurements.[2,13]

Of interest is the use of the signal variance to provide a measure of the noise present during signal averaging from a particular subject and to provide a measure of the quality of an average. A single noise measure is calculated by selecting a signal free portion of the averaging window, e.g., the latter portion of the ST segment, in the XYZ leads. The width of the window is somewhat arbitrary, but should be at least 5-msec long in order to exceed the time that the EMG exhibits nonwhite noise characteristics.[14] The following noise figure is defined.

$$\text{N.F.} = \left[\frac{1}{3m} \sum_{j=1}^{3} \sum_{k=1}^{m} \sigma_{Njk}{}^2\right]^{1/2} \qquad (7)$$

where j equals 1, 2, 3 for the X, Y, Z leads, respectively, and m equals the number of points in each lead from which the noise is calculated.

This is the average of the signal variance for n points in the noise window which is again averaged over the XYZ leads. The square root of this is the standard deviation of the noise process. Dividing the N.F. by $\sqrt{n}$ results in average measure of the standard deviation of the signal average. Both of these noise factors can be calculated after each new beat is added to the signal average. Figure 2 shows data for each noise factor in a dog recording obtained during general anesthesia before and after the administration of pancuronium bromide (0.08 mg/kg). This agent is a nondepolarizing neuromuscular blocking agent and will greatly reduce EMG activity as a source of noise. Panels A and B were obtained prior to drug administration. Panel A is the NF as a function of beats. Ideally this curve would show a convergence to a constant value. This constant value would be the estimate of the RMS voltage of the underlying noise from all sources. In panel A, even after 265 beats, an upward trend is still apparent at 4.8 µV. Dividing the values in panel A by the $\sqrt{n}$ yields the curve in panel B which is the estimate of the RMS value of noise remaining in the average. Theoretically this curve should approach 0 V. Panels C and D were obtained from the same dog after drug injection. Note that there is a rapid convergence after about 50 beats to a noise estimate of about 1.8 µV (panel C) and 0.1 µV for the average (panel D).

For a variety of reasons some subjects present with a poor SNR and at times a nonstationary event may occur to cause a burst of noise which heavily contaminates the average, e.g., a cough or other gross muscle movement. Ideally this should be detected prior to including the beat in the signal average. Figure 3 demonstrates the noise factor curve from a normal subject. After about 200 beats the subject was asked to briefly raise his arms as if reading a book. Note the large step change in the noise curve after which it continued its convergence path. Such nonstationary events can be readily detected and the noise curves provide a means of providing a quality control mechanism for the signal average.

There are other ways to estimate the noise. One is to take a signal average of a large number of beats and subtract from it one individual beat. The assumption is that there is only a signal present in the average, and the difference is composed primarily of noise. The disadvantage is that the estimate would only be based on one epoch of time. A more involved method is to calculate the alternate average.[15] This is done by adding even number beats and subtracting odd number beats. For an even number of these addition/subtraction operations the result is a continual estimate of the underlying noise process based upon all of the beats which comprise the traditional average. Further discussion of the use of these methods is beyond the scope of this chapter.

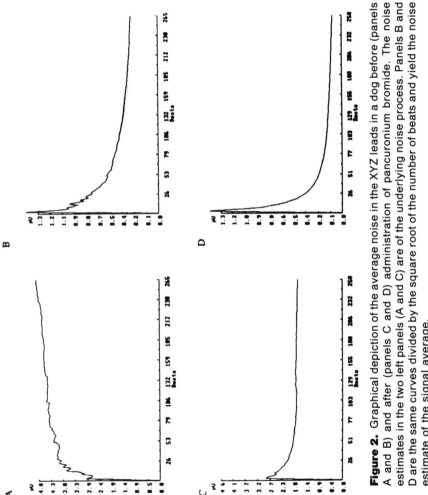

Figure 2. Graphical depiction of the average noise in the XYZ leads in a dog before (panels A and B) and after (panels C and D) administration of pancuronium bromide. The noise estimates in the two left panels (A and C) are of the underlying noise process. Panels B and D are the same curves divided by the square root of the number of beats and yield the noise estimate of the signal average.

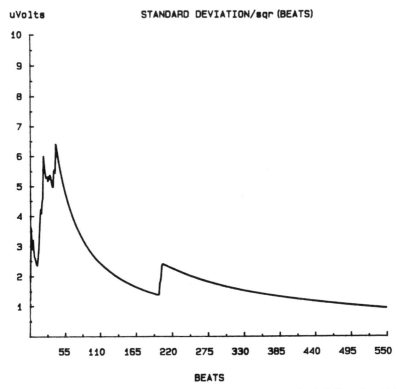

Figure 3. A noise estimate curve from a normal subject who briefly raised his arms at beat 200 to demonstrate the effect of small movements and the quality control function of these noise estimates.

Improving the Signal-to-Noise Ratio

Increasing the signal with respect to the noise or decreasing the noise with respect to the signal are the two most obvious ways to improve the SNR. Examining the SNR problem with respect to the HRECG and keeping in mind the various noise problems outlined above, there are several application specific methods that can be used to improve the SNR. However, prior to presenting these a common HRECG analysis method will be critically examined with respect to the SNR.

The vector magnitude derived from the orthogonal XYZ leads is defined as $VM = \sqrt{X^2 + Y^2 + Z^2}$. To determine the residual noise power in the VM it becomes considerably more complicated to calculate the expected value and the variance due to the nonlinear vector operation[16] and is beyond the scope of this chapter. However, the results of this derivation can be summarized. If one assumes that the signals in the XYZ leads are uncorrelated and that the noise components in each lead are also uncorrelated with each other and the signals in the XYZ lead, then it follows that the signal average of each lead may have significantly different SNRs. This is borne out by many observations of individual XYZ lead recordings. For example, the X lead may have a good SNR with a relatively small signal, the Y lead may have a marginal SNR, and the Z lead may have a poor SNR with a relatively large noise level. Combining these into a vector magnitude will only decrease the good SNR of the X lead. This is because in calculating the E[VM] and the VAR[VM], the absolute values of signal and noise will be used in the calculations and not the relative values used to express SNR. Thus one may argue that one way to improve the SNR of the HRECG is not to perform the VM operation. An example of detecting a late potential in an individual lead and not in the vector magnitude is shown in Figure 4. The top panel is the signal-averaged (200 beats) filtered vector magnitude. A 40-Hz bidirectional filter was used. The QRS onset and offset points are chosen by an algorithm (described below). The duration is 113 msec and the RMS of the last 40 msec (shaded region) is 36 µV. This does not meet the criteria for a positive late potential identification. The bottom panel has four traces, labeled Y1 + Y2 + Y3, Y1, Y2, and Y3. Each trace is a 200-beat, averaged Y lead, filtered with the 40-Hz bidirectional filter. The individual averages, Y1, Y2, and Y3 show a signal after the QRS complex with a poor SNR. These three averages are combined to obtain a 600-beat average (Y1 + Y2 + Y3). The late potential clearly emerges from the noise and the automatic algorithm selects an offset at 218 msec yielding a total QRS duration of 164 msec which is clearly abnormal. This patient had an inducible ventricular tachycardia during electrophysiologic testing.

Most approaches for analyzing the HRECG, particularly with respect to the late potentials, use algorithms to identify the onset and offset of the QRS complex. In the latter case this includes those signals usually identified as late potentials. These algorithms depend, implicitly and explicitly, on the SNR. For example, a method outlined by Simson[17] examines the filtered vector magnitude by retrospectively searching the ST segment for late potentials to

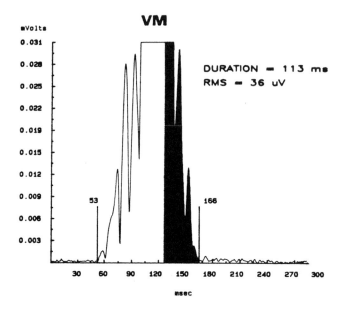

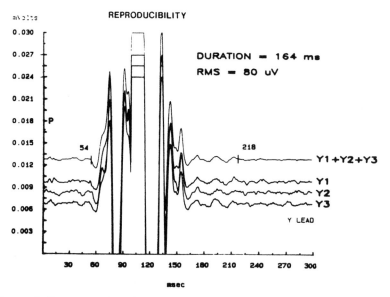

Figure 4. Demonstration of how the vector magnitude decreases the SNR. The top panel shows the vector magnitude of a subject with ventricular tachycardia, but no apparent late potentials. The bottom panel shows three successively averaged Y leads (Y1, Y2, Y3). Visual reproducibility strongly suggests the presence of late potentials. Combining these three leads (Y1 + Y2 + Y3) elucidates a late potential extending to 218 msec from the abscissa and total QRS duration of 164 msec.

emerge from the residual noise in the ST segment. The mean noise level is found by averaging the values in a 5-msec window at the end of the signal-averaged window. Shifting the window backwards in time, late potential activity is detected when the level of the waveform rises above the mean noise level by 3.5 standard deviations. One could define this as the SNR of the filtered vector magnitude, Θ, where:

$$\Theta = \sum_{m = X,Y,Z} \overline{S}_{k^2} \bigg/ \sum_{k = X,Y,Z} \overline{N}_{k^2}. \tag{8}$$

In practice this approach has the advantage of applying the same criteria to all subjects. However, because there is a large threshold for the SNR there are times when late potentials will go undetected. Visual inspection of repeated averages as shown in Figure 4 for individual leads often shows features which are reproducible and hence are cardiac late potentials but below the threshold of the automatic detector. Methods which rely on the SNR will fail to identify true cardiac signals with marginal SNRs.

Another common approach that will be challenged, if the improvement of the SNR is optimizing criteria, is the use of three XYZ leads. In another study[2,18] 24 precordial sites were signal averaged and compared to the individual XYZ leads. If one relies on the automatic methods of detection it was found that leads other than the XYZ leads showed the longest duration late potentials. Upon closer inspection, it was evident that the distribution of the SNR was not uniform, i.e., the automatic algorithm missed signals in the XYZ leads which were more prominent in some of the other precordial leads. Even if one argues that the XYZ leads are truly orthogonal and the late potential generator is a true dipole, late potential detection may be poor because of the unknown distribution of the noise on the body surface. Following this line of thought, the search for an optimal lead or leads may be defined as a search for the site which produces the highest SNR. The novel volume conductor electrode of Mehra et al[19] was an attempt to improve the SNR on a biophysical basis. In this case a thick, 2- to 3-inch conducting media was placed between the electrode and the skin. This produces a greater difference in the distance between the electrode and the EMG source but only marginally increases the distance between the electrode and the ECG source.

Physiologic noise is a function of the state of the patient. An excited or nervous patient will most likely have greater EMG activity. Without resorting to pharmacologic intervention to limit EMG activity, it is essential that patients remain calm and still during a study. Even then repeated studies often show evidence of varying SNR between averages. Studies by Vatterott et al[20] and Steinberg et al[21] have examined the effect of residual noise on the accuracy of late potential measurements. In the first study, repeated averages to a fixed number of beats were performed. The automatic measurement algorithm was used, but residual noise in the ST segment of the filtered vector magnitude was quantified. In the second study, averaging to a specific noise factor was performed. Late potential measurements were done with the automatic algorithm, but the accuracy of classification was judged with respect to different noise factors. Averaging to a noise factor of 0.3 μV was recommended in order to obtain optional classification of patients with and without ventricular tachycardia.

Conclusion

This has been a brief overview of some of the noise problems encountered in the HRECG. It was essential to go beyond the abstract definitions of signal and noise and to include errors in methodology in defining noise. Once defined it is possible to quantify these noise processes and to point out means of quality control. This is important because the HRECG depends heavily on signal averaging and hence reduces to a statistical estimation problems. Even after arriving at a presumed result, measurement methods and other forms of analysis also become statistically based as in choosing QRS onset and offset points as well as such operational methods like the vector magnitude calculation. More efforts are needed in advanced areas of signal and noise estimation but even simple practices like proper electrode attachment, lead selection, and a cooperative patient will greatly improve SNR from the outset.

Acknowledgment: We would like to thank Pamela Tomey for preparing the manuscript and John Dyer for preparing the figures. This work has been funded in part by grants from NIH (HL36625), the Whitaker Foundation, and the VA Merit Review Program.

References

1. Rhyne VT: Comparison of coherent averaging techniques for repetitive biological signals. Med Res Eng 9:22, 1969.
2. Berbari EJ: High-resolution electrocardiography. Crit Rev Biomed Eng 16:67, 1988.
3. Ros HH, Koelman SM, Akker TJVD: The technique of signal averaging and its practical application in the separation of atrial and His-Purkinje activity. In: Signal Averaging Technique in Clinical Cardiology. Stuttgart: Schatter Verlag, 1981.
4. Ishijima M: Noninvasive, real-time examination of atrio-ventricular conduction system. Ph.D. Thesis, Iowa State University, Ames, IA, 1977.
5. Gaumond RP: Roundoff errors in signal averaging systems. IEEE Trans Biomed Engr BMS-33:365, 1986.
6. Berbari EJ, Scherlag BJ: Recording from the ventricular conduction system. In Webster J (ed): Encyclopedia of Medical Devices and Instrumentation. New York: John Wiley & Sons (in press).
7. El-Sherif N, Mehra R, Gomes JAC, Kelen G: Appraisal of a low noise electrocardiogram. J Am Coll Cardiol 1:456, 1983.
8. Evanich MJ, Newberry O, Partridge LD: Some limitations on the removal of periodic noise by averaging. J Appl Physiol 33:536, 1972.
9. Huhta JC, Webster JG: 60 Hz interference in electrocardiography. IEEE Trans Biomed Eng 20:91, 1973.
10. Brian ERJ: Evoked potentials: Acquisition and analysis. In RF Thomson, MM Patterson (eds): Bioelectric Recordings Technique. New York: Academic, 1973.
11. Glaser EM, Ruchkin DS: Principals of Neurobiological Signal Analysis. New York: Academic, 1976.
12. Berbari EJ, DiCarlo L, Scherlag BJ, Lazzara R: Optimizing the signal averaging method for ventricular late potentials. In: Computers in Cardiology. Los Angeles: IEEE Computer Society Press, 1984.
13. Berbari EJ, Collins SM, Arzbaecher R: Evaluation of esophageal electrodes for recording His-Purkinje activity based upon signal variance. IEEE Trans Biomed Eng BME-33:922, 1986.
14. Santopietro RF: The origin and characterization of the primary signal, noise, and interference sources in the high frequency electrocardiogram. Proc IEEE 65:707, 1977.
15. Lander P: Computer processing methods for the recovery of low amplitude ECG signals. D. Phil. Thesis, University of Sussex, Brighton, United Kingdom, 1986.
16. Lander P, Deal RB, Berbari EJ: The analysis of ventricular late potentials using orthogonal recordings. IEEE Trans Biomed Eng (in press).
17. Simson MB: Use of signal in the terminal QRS complex to identify patients with ventricular tachycardia after myocardial infarction. Circulation 64:235, 1981.
18. Berbari EJ, Ozinga L, Albert D: Methods for analyzing cardiac late

potentials. In: Computers in Cardiology. Los Angeles: IEEE Computer Society Press, 1986.

19. Mehra R, Restivo M, El-Sherif N: Electromyographic noise reduction for high resolution electrocardiography. In: IEEE Frontiers of Engineering and Computing in Health Care. New York: IEEE, 1983, p. 298.

20. Vatterott P, Hammill S, Berbari EJ, Bailey K, Matheson S, Worley S: The effect of residual noise on the predictive accuracy of the signal averaged electrocardiogram. PACE 10:450, 1987.

21. Steinberg JS, Bigger JT Jr: Importance of the endpoint of noise reduction in analysis of the signal-averaged electrocardiogram. Am J Cardiol 63:556, 1989.

4

Role of Filtering in the Analysis of the Signal-Averaged Electrocardiogram

Edward B. Caref, Nabil El-Sherif

Introduction

It is often desirable to extract a bioelectric signal of interest from an environment which contains "noisy" or interfering signals. Special signal processing techniques are frequently employed to obtain an accurate recovery of the signal of interest. The signal-averaged electrocardiogram (SAECG) primarily uses two signal processing techniques to process the cardiac signal for late potential analysis: time-ensemble averaging; and filtering. Because the signal of interest (QRS complex) is repetitive while much of the interfering 'noise' is random, time-ensemble averaging is used to increase the signal-to-noise ratio. With this technique, the summation of the repetitive

From El-Sherif N, Turitto G (eds): *High-Resolution Electrocardiography*. Mount Kisco, NY, Futura Publishing Co., Inc., ©, 1992.

cardiac signal is additive while 'noise' elements get canceled. Ideally, the signal-to-noise ratio improves by the square root of the number of QRS beats averaged.

However, even after hundreds of averaged cardiac cycles, there remains some residual noise, typically measuring several microvolts in amplitude. Filters are now applied in an attempt to eliminate this remaining noise. Since much of the noise appears to contain frequencies that do not overlap those of late potentials, different filtering techniques, so long as they do not introduce distortions to our signal of interest, have proven to be fairly successful in eliminating nearly all residual noise. Filtering, therefore, plays a prominent role in the processing of the SAECG because the residual noise after averaging is still large enough to distort or conceal ventricular late potentials, which have been identified as a marker of ventricular arrhythmias.[1] In this chapter, we will give a review of filter characteristics, how filters are currently implemented in the analysis of the SAECG, and how significantly filters affect both the analysis of the SAECG and its predictive accuracy for life-threatening ventricular arrhythmias. In addition, some of the major technical limitations of filtering the SAECG will be presented.

Description of a Filter

A typical filter arrangement is shown in Figure 1. An unfiltered input signal x(t) is fed into a "black" box, which may be comprised of electronic circuitry, computer program, or both. The black box acts on x(t), changing it so that a new signal is created, the output

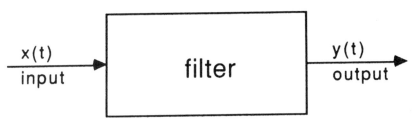

Figure 1. Box diagram of a filter, which acts on some input signal, x(t), to create a new signal, y(t), the output of the filter.

signal y(t). In the most general sense, any black box that changes an input signal x(t) into an output signal y(t) is called a filter.

Filters can come in many types and configurations.[2,3] Special purpose filters are available to perform operations on signals such as differentiation, integration, and summation. However, the most popular filters amplify only some portions of a signal while suppressing the rest. One important filter often used is the notch filter, where perhaps only a single frequency is filtered out, while frequencies above and below are passed. Elimination of 60-Hz noise is a common usage of a notch filter. These types of filters are designed to act on signals based in the frequency domain rather than in the time domain. Any time varying signal can be perfectly represented as a series of sine and cosine waves having different frequencies and amplitudes.[4] An example of a signal represented in the time and frequency domains is shown in Figure 2. Because filters which do their work in the frequency domain are so powerful in terms of their ability to modify and improve signals efficiently, frequency-domain analysis has become quite common. Filters convert the input signal into its frequency components, then either remove some of those components, or amplify other portions, or both. As shown in Figure 3, a low-pass filter passes undisturbed that portion of the input signal with frequency components below some cut-off, and then suppresses the signal with frequencies higher than the cut-off. Conversely, a high-pass filter suppresses frequencies below the chosen cut-off while passing frequencies higher than the cut-off. The combination of low-pass and high-pass filters, where only that portion of the input signal that lies between the two cut-offs is passed undisturbed, is called a bandpass filter. Filtering signals based on frequency-domain analysis is widespread in the biomedical field.

For the processing of the SAECG, filters are used after signal averaging surface ECG signals from three orthogonal bipolar leads (X, Y, and Z). The summed signal is then bandpassed filtered. The filtering is usually performed on the vector magnitude ($\sqrt{X^2 + Y^2 + Z^2}$), although it can be performed on individual leads as well. As will be shown, the choice of filter as well as the cut-off frequencies selected play a crucial role in the analysis of the SAECG.

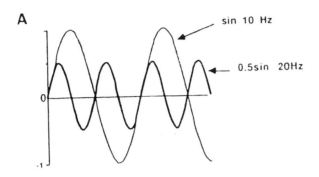

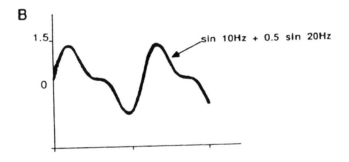

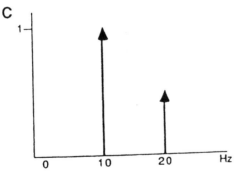

Figure 2. Idealized representations of signals in time and frequency domains. (A) Two time-varying signals; the sine 10-Hz waveform has twice the amplitude and is one-half the frequency of the 0.5-sin 20-Hz waveform. (B) The summation of waveforms in (A). (C) Representation of (B) in the frequency domain.

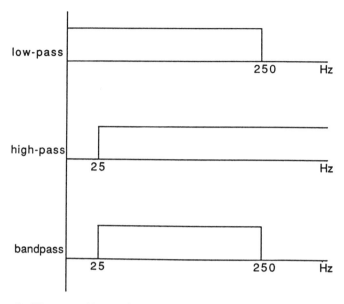

Figure 3. Diagram of low-, high-, and bandpass filters. Idealized here, showing sharp corners between the stop and passbands. For a low-pass filter, the signal is passed unchanged for frequencies ≤250 Hz. In high-pass filters, the frequencies <25 Hz are completely attenuated, while signals ≥25 Hz are passed undisturbed. Only signals ≥25 Hz and ≤250 Hz are allowed in the bandpass filter, the rest are totally filtered out.

Types and Classes of Filters

There are many classes of filters. Those that differentiate belong to the class of differentiable filters, while those that are frequency-selective form another important class. In reality, frequency-selective filters behave differently from the idealized version described in Figure 3, where the transition between the stopband and passband is sharp and discontinuous, with no distortion at the corners. Based on the characteristics of their behavior, several types and classes of frequency-selective filters are available. Nonrecursive filters are commonly used to smooth data, since there are no sharp transitions from the stopband to the passband. Recursive filters can have sharp transitions, limited by the order of the difference equations used to implement them. These are true digital filters, because unlike non-recursive filters, they must be implemented by a computer program. The order of a filter defines how sharp the transition from passband to stopband will be.

There are two main implementations of filters: analog and digital. For signals that are continuous in time, analog filters, built with operational amplifiers, resistors, and capacitors, are used to modify the signal. Digital filters act on digital data, which is obtained by sampling continuous signals at discrete times and assigning a discrete voltage level to each sample. Some early investigators relied on analog filtering for SAECG analysis,[5,6] but digital filters are now commonly used, since computers can perform many varied and powerful tasks on digital data efficiently.

The most commonly used filter for SAECG processing is the digitally implemented Butterworth filter, belonging to the class of recursive filters. Implemented as a fourth order (4-pole) difference equation, this filter has sharp transitions at the cut-off frequencies. For example, for a low-pass 4-pole cut-off of 50 Hz, the output gain at 60 Hz will be only 15% of the input signal. At input signals consisting of frequencies 70 and 100 Hz, the output gain will be 10% and 4%, respectively, of the input amplitude. For input frequencies < 50 Hz, the output of the Butterworth filter produces gains equal to the input, for a maximally flat response.

One problem with Butterworth filters and with other infinite impulse response filters is that small oscillations in the output can occur when the input is a steep step. The oscillations are called ringing, formally known as Gibb's phenomena. Ringing is a serious problem when analyzing for late potentials, because a sharp down-stroke in amplitude of the terminal QRS may cause filter ringing effects that could be confused as late potentials. To overcome this effect, Simson employed a bidirectional Butterworth filter, in which the first half of the QRS is bandpass filtered, and then the second half of the QRS as well as the ST segment are filtered in reverse time, starting from the end of the data and moving forward toward the middle of the QRS.[7] With this implementation, any ringing will lie in the region well inside the QRS complex, however, the morphology of the mid-QRS region may be distorted due to filter ringing effects.

Another solution to the problem of ringing is to use another type of filter. Analysis of digital, finite impulse response filters (FIR) shows that no ringing occurs.[2,3] Furthermore, FIRs have the advantage of providing a zero phase shift. Phase shifting implies that the filtered signal in the frequency domain shifts frequencies as a function of frequency. For example, with an ideal linear phase shift filter, the phase shift at the cut-off is zero, and then rises in direct proportion to frequencies above the cut-off, where the higher the frequency, the greater the phase shift. In the time domain, phase shifting produces a time shift of the output signal.

FIR filters are computationally efficient, and the fact that they can be implemented with no ringing or phase distortion makes them attractive for investigating their effects on the SAECG. However, one possible disadvantage of FIR filters, unlike Butterworth and other infinite impulse response filters, is that they generally do not have sharp transitions at the cut-off frequencies. In addition, other filter types such as the least squares fit filter may also prove beneficial in filtering the SAECG. Figure 4 shows an SAECG analyzed with four different filter types, and shows the large differences that filters can have on QRS morphology. Preliminary studies of the effects of phase shifting, ringing, and a comparison of different filter classes on the SAECG have been reported;[6,7] however, much more evaluation is required.

Implementation of Filters Used for Analysis of SAECG

Although some studies, especially in the early period of developing the SAECG as a diagnostic tool, provided data based on the implementation of customized filtering schemes, most authors reported studies employing one of several commercially available machines. The most frequent filter type used is the digitally implemented Butterworth filter, implemented bidirectionally. Table I compares commercial and custom filter implementations. Some units offer several filter types, filter implementations, and choice of cut-off frequencies. The nonstandard use of all these choices has led to a situation where studies may not be directly comparable because of the filtering scheme employed, because, among other things, different filters and filter settings have a marked effect on SAECG parameters.

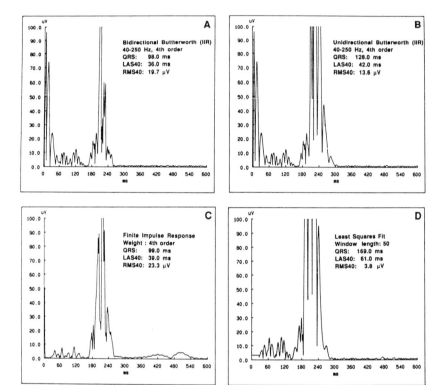

Figure 4. SAECG analyzed with four different filters. (A) Bidirectional Butterworth. (B) Unidirectional Butterworth. (C) Finite impulse response (FIR). (D) Least squares fit. Analysis of parameters was performed in the same manner in each instance. Note how the QRS duration ranges from 99.0–169 msec and RMS40 ranges from 3.8 µV to 23.3 µV depending on choice of filters. See text for more discussion.

There are a number of clinical studies in which the SAECG was analyzed at high-pass settings of 0.05 Hz, 30 Hz, 50 Hz, 60 Hz, 67 Hz, 80 Hz, 100 Hz, and 150 Hz, and implemented either in analog or digital format, varying from 1–4 poles.[8,10–14] However, most SAECG clinical studies in the literature used one of two high-pass settings, 25 Hz and/or 40 Hz, with the low-pass fixed at 250 Hz.

Table I

Characteristics of Filters Used in Signal Averaging Studies Using More Than One Filter Setting

Author	Filter Type	Bidirectional	Analog/Digital	Number of Poles	Low-pass Setting	High-pass Setting
Simson	Butterworth	Yes	Digital	4	250	25,40
Rozanski et al	Butterworth	Yes	Digital	4	250	0,20,40,80
Denes et al	Butterworth	Yes	Digital	4	250	25,40
Coto et al	Butterworth	Yes	Digital	3	250	25,50
Gomes et al	Butterworth	Yes	Digital	4	250	10,15,20,25,40,80,100
Nalos et al	?	No	Analog	1	400	67,100
Machac et al	Butterworth	Yes	Digital	4	250	25,40,80
Caref et al	Butterworth	Yes	Digital	4	250	10,20,25,30,40,50,60,70, 80,90,100

Effect of Bandpass Filters on SAECG Parameters in Normal Subjects

Several studies compared the effects of different bandpass filter settings of a digital Butterworth, bidirectional implementation on the SAECG. This filter, first introduced for SAECG analysis by Simson, will be the subject for the remaining discussion below. Direct comparisons of these studies are difficult to make for the following reasons: (1) template matching, alignment, and sampling frequency vary;[15] (2) the exact implementations of these filters vary slightly between the different machines used; (3) other portions of the algorithm used to analyze the SAECG, such as determination of the baseline noise level, and calculation of the QRS offset, vary such that significant differences between machines may exist; (4) the average number of QRS complexes averaged for each study vary, as well as other data acquisition specifics; (5) quantitative cut-off values of parameters characterizing normal and abnormal SAECGs are different; (6) different parameters or combinations of SAECG parameters are used to describe late potentials; and (7) there are differences in the patient populations and the number of subjects studied. However, despite these differences, a number of important observations regarding the effects of bandpass filters on the SAECG may be gleaned from these reports.

In early studies, the SAECG was analyzed by simple visual detection of low amplitude, delayed QRS waveforms. Soon, however, more precise quantitative analysis of the SAECG was devised. Most reports analyzed three SAECG parameters: (1) the filtered QRS duration; (2) the duration of low amplitude signals < 40 μV of the terminal QRS (LAS40); and (3) the root mean square voltage of the last 40 msec of the QRS complex (RMS40). Normal values for these three parameters were developed based on relatively small studies of SAECGs of normal subjects. The analysis of the SAECG at different filter settings created a set of normal values that varied slightly between investigators.

QRS Duration in Normal Subjects' SAECGs

Studies show that changing the high-pass filter cut-off changed the QRS duration significantly (Table II). Simson reported a slight

Table II

Comparison of Studies Analyzing Filtered QRS Duration Mean Values at More Than One Filter Setting in Different Population Groups

Author	Year	Population	Frequency(Hz)	0	10	15	20	25	30	40	50	60	70	80	90	100
Normal Subjects																
Denes et al	1983	42 normals		—	—	—	—	96	—	94	—	—	—	—	—	—
Coto et al	1985	50 athletes		—	—	—	—	97	—	—	95	—	—	—	—	—
Gomes et al	1987	25 normals		—	87	94	95	94	—	94	—	—	—	87	—	85
Machac et al	1988	11 normals		—	—	—	—	96	—	94	—	—	—	91	—	—
Simson	1988	42 normals		—	—	—	—	96	—	96	—	—	—	—	—	—
Caref et al	1989	100 normals		—	88	—	95	94	94	92	91	90	89	88	87	86
Patients With Organic Heart Disease Without Spontaneous or Inducible Sustained Ventricular Tachycardia																
Rozanski et al	1981	12 aneurysm, no VT		*	—	—	*	—	—	*	—	—	—	*	—	—
Coto et al	1985	11 NS-VT		—	—	—	*	—	—	—	—	—	—	—	—	—
Gomes et al	1987	29 organic heart disease		—	101	106	104	118	—	110	—	—	—	—	—	—
Nalos et al**	1987	56 NS-VT, not Ind		—	—	106	104	104	—	103	—	—	104***	—	—	—
Machac et al	1988	18 organic heart disease		—	—	—	—	101	—	98	—	—	—	94	—	—
Simson	1988	52 prior Q wave MI		—	—	—	—	98	—	97	—	—	—	—	—	—
Caref et al	1989	52 NS-VT, not Ind		—	98	—	103	102	101	100	99	98	97	96	95	94

Table II (Continued)

Patients With Spontaneous or Inducible Sustained Ventricular Tachycardia

Author	Year	Population	Frequency(Hz)	0	10	15	20	25	30	40	50	60	70	80	90	100
Rozanski et al	1981	16,8 with aneurysm, 8 without		*						*				*		
Denes et al	1983	12 sustained VT		—	—	—	—	117	—	117	—	—	—	—	—	—
Gomes et al	1987	33 sustained VT		—	108	121	123	123	—	121	—	—	—	116	—	114
Nalos et al**	1987	13 Ind sustained VT		—	—	—	—	—	—	—	—	—	138	—	—	141
Machac et al	1988	26 sustained VT		—	—	—	—	126	—	124	—	—	—	119	—	—
Simson	1988	82 sustained VT/VF, Ind VT		—	—	—	—	137	—	136	—	—	—	—	—	—
Caref et al	1989	28 Ind sustained VT		—	130	—	131	132	132	131	129	129	127	125	124	122

MI = myocardial infarction; NS-VT = nonsustained ventricular tachycardia; Ind = inducible; * = visual detection of delayed waveform activity was used; ** = measurements were made visually by two individuals; *** = high-pass setting was 67 Hz.

decrease in QRS duration from 96.4 msec at 25 Hz to 95.6 msec at 40 Hz.[16] Denes and coworkers, using a customized SAECG unit based on the Simson algorithm, showed a decrease in the QRS duration from 95.9 msec at 25 Hz to 93.7 msec at 40 Hz in 42 normal subjects.[17] A similar but smaller decrease in QRS duration was reported by Coto et al in their study of 50 athletes, from 96.9 msec at 25 Hz to 95.4 msec at 50 Hz.[18] Gomes and colleagues studied the effects of seven different high-pass filters (10, 15, 20, 25, 30, 40, 80, and 100 Hz) on 25 normal subjects and found an initial increase in QRS duration as the high-pass setting changed from 10 to 15 Hz, a plateau phase between 15–25 Hz, and a small decrease in duration at 40–100 Hz.[19] Caref et al, in their study of 100 normal subjects of changes produced by 11 different high-pass cut-offs (10, 20, 25, 30, 40, 50, 60, 70, 80, 90, and 100 Hz), also showed an initial increase in QRS duration at 10 to 20 Hz, followed by a small incremental decrease in duration between 20–100 Hz (Figure 5, group I).[20] These differences were shown to be statistically significant (p < 0.001), when comparing all neighboring filter pairs (10 with 20 Hz, 20 with 25 Hz, etc).

LAS40 Duration in Normal Subjects' SAECGs

Unlike the filtered QRS duration, which showed a decrease in duration as the high-pass filter setting increased, the LAS40 duration increased in duration as the high-pass filter setting increased. This was evident in all studies discussed above (Table III), and in fact, the reported figures at each filter setting for normal subjects are similar. The mean values at each setting were statistically significant when neighboring filter values were compared, with the exception of 80- to 90-Hz and 90- to 100-Hz comparisons.[20] The gradual, almost stepwise increase in LAS40 duration as the filter setting increased in normals is shown in the bottom curve of Figure 6 (group I).

RMS40 in Normal Subjects' SAECGs

Analysis of the effect of high-pass filters on the RMS40 voltage revealed a large exponential decrease in RMS40 amplitude as the high-pass filter setting increases (Figure 7, group I). In both the

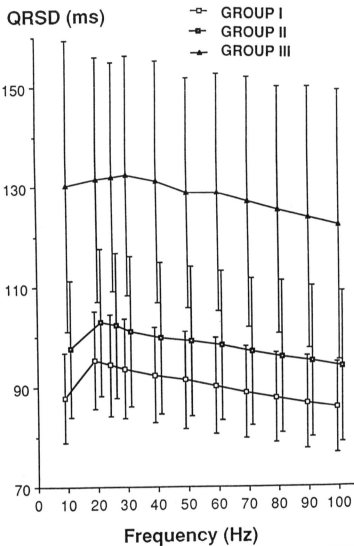

Figure 5. Mean ± standard deviation of filtered QRS duration (QRSD) for groups I, II and III at 11 high-pass filter settings. The low-pass filter was fixed at 250 Hz. Group I, 100 normals; group II, 52 patients with spontaneous nonsustained VT without inducible sustained-VT by programmed stimulation; and group III, 28 patients with inducible sustained-VT. (Reprinted with permission from Caref et al. Am J Cardiol 64:16, 1989.)

LAS40 (ms)

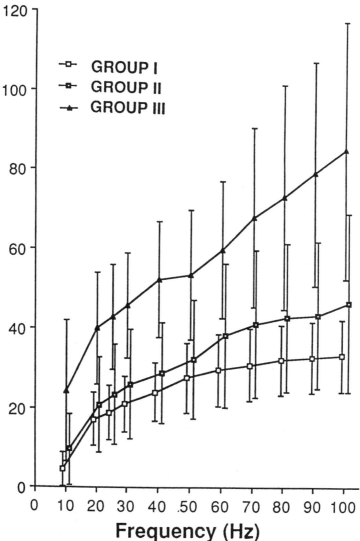

Figure 6. Mean ± standard deviation of low amplitude signals <40 μV (LAS40) for groups I, II and III at 11 high-pass filter settings. The low-pass filter was fixed at 250 Hz. Groups are the same as in Figure 5. (Reprinted with permission from Caref et al. Am J Cardiol 64:16, 1989.)

Table III

Comparison of Studies Analyzing LAS40 Duration Mean Values at More Than One Filter Setting in Different Population Groups

Author	Year	Population	Frequency(Hz)	0	10	15	20	25	30	40	50	60	70	80	90	100
Normal Subjects																
Denes et al	1983	42 normals		—	—	—	—	23	—	30	—	—	—	—	—	—
Coto et al	1985	50 athletes		—	—	—	—	21	—	—	28	—	—	—	—	—
Gomes et al	1987	25 normals		—	4	15	18	20	—	26	—	—	—	30	—	33
Machac et al	1988	11 normals		—	—	—	—	22	—	26	—	—	—	30	—	—
Simson	1988	42 normals		—	—	—	—	—	—	29	—	—	—	—	33	—
Caref et al	1989	100 normals		—	5	—	17	19	21	24	28	30	31	32	33	33
Patients With Organic Heart Disease Without Spontaneous or Inducible Sustained Ventricular Tachycardia																
Rozanski et al	1981	12 aneurysm, no VT		*	—	—	—	—	—	*	—	—	—	*	—	—
Coto et al	1985	11 NS-VT		—	—	—	*	34	—	—	50	—	—	—	—	—
Gomes et al	1987	29 organic heart disease		—	8	14	23	24	—	32	—	—	—	36	—	49
Nalos et al**	1987	56 NS-VT, not Ind		—	—	—	—	—	—	—	—	—	—	—	—	24
Machac et al	1988	18 organic heart disease		—	—	—	—	27	—	33	—	—	—	41	—	—
Simson	1988	52 prior Q wave MI		—	—	—	—	—	—	29	—	—	—	—	44	—
Caref et al	1989	52 NS-VT, not Ind		—	10	—	21	23	26	29	32	38	41	43	44	47

Table III (Continued)

Author	Year	Population	Frequency(Hz)	0	10	15	20	25	30	40	50	60	70	80	90	100
Patients With Spontaneous or Inducible Sustained Ventricular Tachycardia																
Rozanski et al	1981	16,8 with aneurysm, 8 without		*			*			*				*		
Denes et al	1983	12 sustained VT		—	—	—	—	33	—	46	—	—	—	—	—	—
Gomes et al	1987	33 sustained VT		—	7	22	30	36	—	44	—	—	—	66	—	73
Nalos et al	1987	13 Ind sustained VT		—	—	—	—	—	—	—	—	—	—	—	—	47
Machac et al	1988	26 sustained VT		—	—	—	—	38	—	47	—	—	—	69	—	—
Simson	1988	82 sustained VT/VF, Ind VT		—	—	—	—	—	46	57	53	—	—	—	—	—
Caref et al	1989	28 Ind sustained VT		—	24	—	40	43	46	52	53	60	68	73	79	85

MI = myocardial infarction; NS-VT = nonsustained ventricular tachycardia; Ind = inducible; * = visual detection of delayed waveform activity was used; ** = LAS20 duration was measured visually by two individuals.

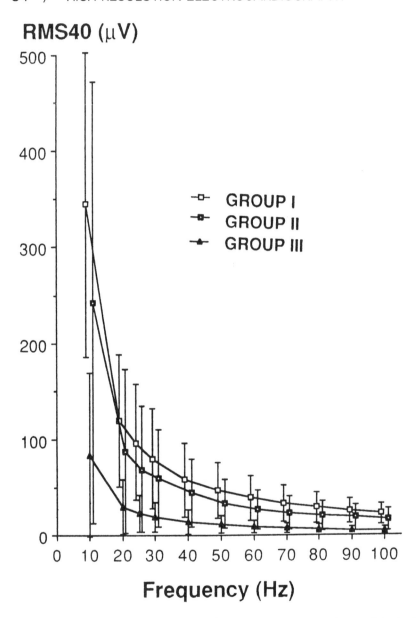

Figure 7. Mean ± standard deviation of root mean square voltage of the last 40 msec of the filtered QRS (RMS40) for groups I, II and III at 11 high-pass filter settings. The low-pass filter was fixed at 250 Hz. Groups are the same as in Figure 5. (Reprinted with permission from Caref et al. Am J Cardiol 64:16, 1989.)

Gomes[19] and Caref[20] reports, RMS40 mean values for normals at 10 Hz were in the range of hundreds of microvolts, whereas higher filter settings resulted in sharply decreasing RMS40 values (Table IV) and were shown to be statistically significant between all neighboring high-pass filter settings analyzed between 10–100 Hz. Two factors are believed to cause the exponential decline in RMS40 mean values: (1) the amount of energy in RMS40 is sharply reduced at higher frequencies. For example, the mean RMS40 voltage at 20 Hz decreases to one-half its voltage at the 40-Hz high-pass cut-off; and (2) the noise measurements at the 10-Hz setting are high, and the calculated QRS offset is, therefore, well within the QRS complex. This may argue for a narrower useful range for this parameter.

Normal Values of SAECG Parameters

Normal values for the QRS and LAS40 durations were obtained by most centers by including the mean +2 standard deviations and the mean −2 standard deviations, respectively. Because these parameters exhibit normal distributions (Figures 8A and 8B) the normal values include 95% of the normal population. In contrast, the RMS40 parameter has a large variability between normal subjects. In fact, the standard deviation is high in this group, making it impossible to select normal values based on the mean −2 standard deviations. Figure 8C shows a nonnormal distribution of RMS40 values from 100 normal subjects.[20] Thus, normal values for RMS40 were usually chosen empirically. In an alternate approach, Caref et al[20] took the natural logarithm of RMS40 values, which, when plotted and analyzed, showed a normal distribution (Figure 8D). With this transformation, the mean −2 standard deviations were used to calculate normal values, with the cut-off values at each filter setting exponentiated for clinical use. The normal values for the QRS and LAS40 durations, and the RMS40 voltage calculated by this method are displayed in Table V. The RMS40 normal cut-off value of 25 µV at the 25 Hz high-pass setting is similar to published studies where the normal values at that setting were chosen empirically; however, there are significant differences between these two methods at the other high-pass filter settings.

Table IV

Studies Analyzing RMS40 Mean Values at More Than One Filter Setting in Different Population Groups

Author	Year	Population	Frequency(Hz)	0	10	15	20	25	30	40	50	60	70	80	90	100
							Normal Subjects									
Denes et al	1983	42 normals		—	—	—	—	67	—	42	—	—	—	—	—	—
Coto et al	1985	50 athletes		—	—	—	—	76	—	41	—	—	—	—	—	—
Gomes et al	1987	25 normals		—	443	—	171	117	—	81	—	—	—	47	—	27
Machac et al	1988	11 normals		—	—	240	—	88	—	71	—	—	—	54	—	—
Simson	1988	42 normals		—	—	—	—	—	80	37	—	—	—	—	—	—
Caref et al	1989	100 normals		—	344	—	119	97	—	58	47	39	33	29	25	23

Patients With Organic Heart Disease Without Spontaneous or Inducible Sustained Ventricular Tachycardia

Author	Year	Population	Frequency(Hz)	0	10	15	20	25	30	40	50	60	70	80	90	100
Rozanski et al	1981	12 aneurysm, no VT		*	—	—	*	—	—	*	—	—	—	*	—	—
Coto et al	1985	11 NS-VT		—	—	—	—	46	—	—	20	—	—	—	—	—
Gomes et al	1987	29 organic heart disease		—	234	—	96	82	—	50	—	—	—	20	—	22
Nalos et al**	1987	56 NS-VT, not Ind		—	—	124	—	—	—	—	—	—	**	—	—	**
Machac et al	1988	18 organic heart disease		—	—	—	—	114	—	67	—	—	—	31	—	—
Simson	1988	52 prior Q wave MI		—	—	—	—	—	60	37	—	—	—	—	—	—
Caref et al	1989	52 NS-VT, not Ind		—	242	—	88	69	—	45	33	27	23	20	19	17

Table IV (Continued)

Patients With Spontaneous or Inducible Sustained Ventricular Tachycardia

Author	Year	Population	Frequency(Hz) →	0	10	15	20	25	30	40	50	60	70	80	90	100
Rozanski et al	1981	16,8 with aneurysm, 8 without		*			*			*			*			
Denes et al	1983	12 sustained VT		—	—	—	—	30	—	17	—	—	—	—	—	—
Gomes et al	1987	33 sustained VT		—	184	82	57	45	—	23	—	—	**	12	—	11
Nalos et al	1987	13 Ind sustained VT		—	—	—	—	—	—	—	—	—	—	—	—	**
Machac et al	1988	26 sustained VT		—	—	—	—	37	—	20	—	—	—	16	—	—
Simson	1988	82 sustained VT/VF, Ind VT		—	—	—	—	—	—	12	—	—	—	—	—	—
Caref et al	1989	28 Ind sustained VT		—	84	—	29	23	19	14	12	9	8	7	6	5

MI = myocardial infarction; NS-VT = nonsustained ventricular tachycardia; Ind = inducible; * = visual detection of delayed waveform activity was used and maximum amplitudes calculated; ** = the number of terminal deflections was reported at 67 Hz and 100 Hz.

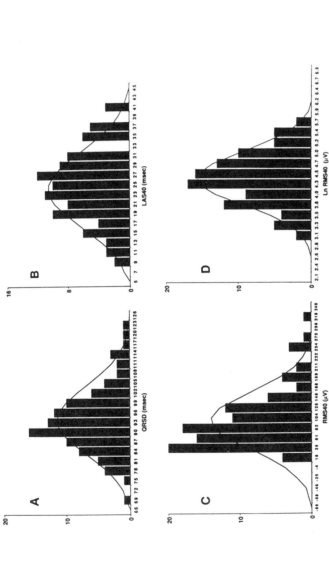

Figure 8. Histograms show observed distribution of SAECG parameters from 100 normal subjects at 40 Hz, with overlayed bell-shaped line curves representing their expected normal distribution. (A) Normal distribution for filtered QRS duration (QRSD). (B) Similar results for duration of low amplitude signals <40 µV (LAS40). (C) The distribution of root mean square voltage of the last 40 msec (RMS40) is significantly different from normal (p <0.002). (D) The transformation of each value of RMS40 into its natural logarithm (LnRMS40) results, however, in normal distribution. (Reprinted with permission from Caref et al. Am J Cardiol 64:16, 1989.)

Table V

Normal Values of Signal-Averaged Electrocardiogram Parameters at 11 High-Pass Filter Settings in 100 Normal Subjects

	Frequency (Hz)										
	10	20	25	30	40	50	60	70	80	90	100
QRS duration (≤) (msec)	106	115	115	113	111	111	109	107	106	105	104
LAS40 (≤) (msec)	13	31	32	35	39	45	48	49	50	50	51
RMS40 (≥) (μV)	103	32	25	21	16	13	11	10	9	8	7

Normal values for QRS duration and LAS40 were based on the mean +2 standard deviations. For RMS40, normal distribution was first obtained by taking the natural logarithm, then the mean −2 standard deviations was used to calculate the logarithmic normal value, which was finally exponentiated and tabulated for clinical use.

LAS40 = duration of low amplitude signals <40 μV; RMS40 = root mean square voltage of the terminal 40 msec of QRS.

Effect of Bandpass Filters on SAECG Parameters in Patients

The effects of high-pass filtering on QRS and LAS40 durations, and RMS40, in patients' SAECGs showed similar patterns to normals as the filter setting increased, although the absolute values for patient populations differ from normals significantly. The mean values reported by studies comparing three SAECG parameters at different filter settings are also presented in Tables II–IV, grouped by the presence or absence of spontaneous or induced (by programmed electrical stimulation) sustained ventricular tachycardia (VT). A typical effect of varying high-pass filter cut-offs from 10 to 100 Hz in a SAECG of a patient with inducible sustained VT is shown in Figure 9.

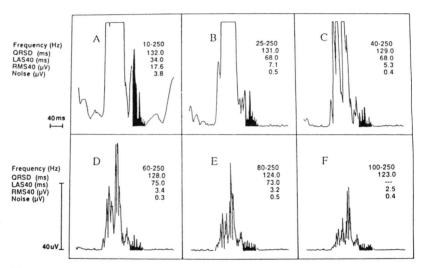

Figure 9. Typical effect of high-pass filters on SAECG parameters in a patient with inducible sustained monomorphic VT. The QRS duration (QRSD) shows slight gradual decrease at higher filter settings (A through F), whereas the RMS40 shows significant, nonlinear decrease. The LAS40 shows significant increase between 10 to 60 Hz (A through D) and then a slight decrease at 80 Hz (E). It could not be measured due to low amplitude of the filtered QRS at 100 Hz (F). The RMS40 is highlighted in each panel. Note the high noise level at 10 Hz (A), which significantly decreases and stabilizes at higher filter settings. (Reprinted with permission from Caref et al. Am J Cardiol 64:16, 1989.)

QRS Duration in Patients' SAECGs

The QRS duration is longest in patients with spontaneous or induced sustained VT at all filter settings compared to either normals or patients without sustained VT. Patients with organic heart disease but no inducible sustained VT as well as those with nonsustained VT but no inducible sustained VT are characterized by mean QRS values that lie in between normals and patients with sustained VT. In both the Gomes and Caref studies,[19,20] the QRS duration increases from 10 Hz to 20–25 Hz, then slowly decreases as the filter setting increases. Rozanski et al[10] in their study using visual detection of delayed waveform activity extending 70 msec beyond the signal-averaged QRS as a definition of abnormality, found eight patients with both sustained VT and aneurysm abnormal, and eight patients with sustained VT but no aneurysm with normal recordings.

Figure 5 shows the mean ± standard deviation plotted values of the QRS duration at 11 high-pass filter settings in three groups of subjects studied by Caref et al:[20] group I, 100 normals; group II, 52 patients with spontaneous nonsustained VT (≥ 3 premature ventricular contractions, at a rate > 100 beats/min, lasting < 30 sec) without inducible sustained VT by programmed stimulation; and group III, 28 patients with inducible sustained VT. The values between each group at each setting were statistically significant, and was also the case for Machac,[21] whereas in Gomes' study, QRS duration was significantly different at five of seven high-pass settings (excepting 10 and 20 Hz) when comparing 29 patients with organic heart disease and without VT to 33 patients with sustained VT.

LAS40 Duration in Patients' SAECGs

LAS40 duration showed a gradual, almost linear increase in duration between 20–100 Hz as the high-pass filter setting increased. The mean values for each group were most significantly different from neighboring filter settings in the 10- to 70-Hz range, whereas from 80–100 Hz, LAS40 parameters remained fairly stable.[20] Gomes and colleagues reported a large jump in LAS40 between 40 and 80 Hz in patients with sustained VT, however, the analysis did not include any filter settings between these two settings. In the Caref et al report, LAS40 differences between patients with inducible sustained VT and those without inducible sustained VT grew larger as the filter setting increased, due mainly to a proportionally greater LAS40 increase in sustained VT patients (Figure 6). Differences between each of the three groups were statistically significant at all 11 settings, while in the Gomes and Machac reports[19,21] five of seven (15, 25, 40, 80, and 100 Hz) and two of three (40 and 80 Hz) settings, respectively, achieved significance between the two groups analyzed.

An interesting phenomena, in which LAS40 duration can no longer be measured because no portion of the QRS reaches 40 µV was shown by Caref and coworkers.[20] This occurred in 24 of 180 (13%) of subjects analyzed at high-pass settings ≥ 60 Hz (Figure 10). The decrease of LAS40 duration and RMS40 voltage as high-pass filter settings increased was reflected in another parameter analyzed, the root mean square voltage of the QRS complex (RMSQRS). Figure 11

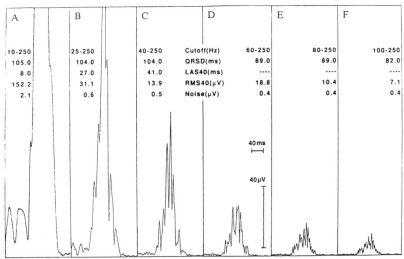

Figure 10. SAECG analyzed at six selected high-pass settings from a patient with nonsustained VT who was not inducible by programmed stimulation. The QRS duration (QRSD) was normal at all settings. The LAS40 was normal at 10 to 30 Hz (A,B), became abnormal at 40 and 50 Hz (C), and could not be analyzed at ≥ 60 Hz (D through F) because of the marked attenuation of the RMSQRS. The RMS40 was normal between 10 to 25 Hz (A,B), became abnormal at 40 Hz (C), and reverted back to normal at 60 to 100 Hz (D through F). (Reprinted with permission from Caref et al. Am J Cardiol 64:16, 1989.)

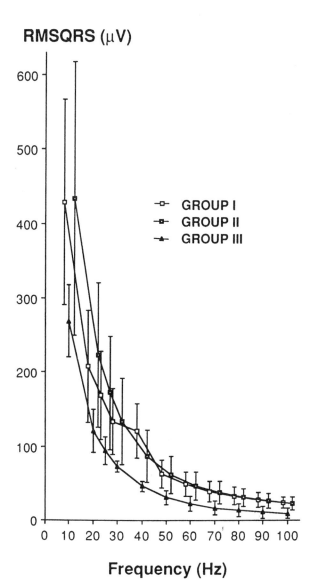

Figure 11. Mean ± standard deviation of root mean square voltage of the filtered QRS (RMSQRS) for groups I, II and III and 11 high-pass filter settings. The low-pass filter was fixed at 250 Hz. Groups are the same as in Figure 5. (Reprinted with permission from Caref et al. Am J Cardiol 64:16, 1989.)

shows the plot of mean values for the three analyzed groups, with an exponential decline in amplitude as the high-pass filter setting increases. The significance of this finding awaits further study, however, the figure suggests that using the RMSQRS parameter may be useful in quantitating the SAECG, particularly in the 30- to 60-Hz range, where there is little overlap between patients with and without inducible sustained VT.

RMS40 Parameter in Patients' SAECGs

The RMS40 voltage is relatively large at 10 Hz, and sharply declines between 10–20 Hz. Between 20–100 Hz, the decrease continues less rapidly (Figure 7), and closely parallels the curves of RMSQRS (Figure 11). Normal subjects have highest mean values than either patients with or without sustained VT or inducible sustained VT, patients with sustained VT or inducible sustained VT have the lowest mean values, and patients without spontaneous or inducible sustained VT lie in between, but closer to normal values. Between patient groups, Caref et al[20] report statistical significance between groups at all settings, while Gomes et al describe significance at five of seven settings (20–100 Hz),[19] and Machac et al at two of three settings (25 and 40 Hz).[21]

Effects of High-Pass Filtering on Noise

The signal averaging technique is employed to significantly reduce the amplitude of "noise," which arise from several sources. The primary component of noise is probably due to the asynchronous firing of skeletal muscle myopotentials.[1] While the frequency range of myopotentials overlaps late potentials, they tend to be averaged out since these myopotentials are asynchronous. Much of the residual noise is then filtered to achieve a basically noise-free signal. The selection of high-pass filters, therefore, plays a significant role in removing noise effects. Achieving a low-noise level is especially important since the analysis algorithm uses measurements of noise level to determine the QRS offset, which is used to define all three parameters.

Both the Gomes et al and Caref et al reports noted high-noise levels at the 10-Hz high-pass filter setting (range 3.3–6.0 μV for all groups studied). At 20 Hz, the noise levels fall dramatically (range 0.7–0.9 μV), then decreases slightly and stabilizes at higher settings. Gomes et al reports no change in noise levels in the high-pass interval 80–100 Hz (range 0.4–0.5 μV for all three groups), while in the Caref and coworkers' study, noise levels remained fairly stable (0.3–0.5 μV) between the 50- to 100-Hz interval for all groups. Despite the stability of noise levels at higher settings, the mean values between neighboring filter settings for most groups studied by Caref et al remained statistically significant until the 90- to 100-Hz comparison. These reports suggest that noise reduction above 50- to 80-Hz high-pass settings offer little improvement over what can be obtained at settings 25–50 Hz. The distortions of the QRS and LAS40 durations and RMS40 voltage due to noise level is highest at 10–15 Hz. All three parameters continue to have significantly different changes between neighboring high-pass filter settings as it increases, despite stabilizing noise levels at high-pass filter settings 50–100 Hz.[20] This suggests that in high-pass cut-offs 50–100 Hz, late potentials are more filtered than residual noise, and therefore may be less useful for analysis of the SAECG. Late potentials of low amplitude in the presence of residual noise continue to pose a problem in interpretation.[22] Figure 12 shows an SAECG of a patient without inducible sustained VT analyzed at four different high-pass settings. At the 40-Hz filter setting the terminal signal is small, and it is not recognized as part of the QRS by the algorithm. The electrophysiologic significance of these relatively broad, low amplitude, low-frequency signals remains unclear.

Low-Pass Filtering Versus Bandpass Filtering

The effect of low-pass filtering was examined in a study by Vacek et al where the SAECG parameters were analyzed and compared at 40- to 250-Hz bandpass to the 40-Hz high-pass filter alone in 18 patients.[23] No statistical significance was found. This should not be surprising given that the RMSQRS and RMS40 parameters already show small voltage levels at high-pass settings > 100 Hz. In addition, other studies analyzing the frequency characteristics of the QRS complex show little energy content at frequencies > 100 Hz.[24–26]

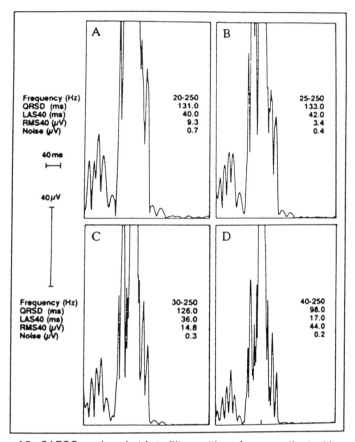

Figure 12. SAECG analyzed at four filter settings from a patient with nonsustained VT who was not inducible by programmed stimulation. Marked attenuation of a late potential is seen as the high-pass filter setting increases (A through C) and results in its annihilation (D). (Reprinted with permission from Caref et al. Am J Cardiol 64:16, 1989.)

Effect of Bandpass Filters on SAECG Prediction of Malignant Ventricular Tachyarrhythmias

While currently there are no studies which optimize the predictive accuracy of the SAECG analyzed at different filter settings to predict sudden cardiac electrical death, studies have attempted to test its accuracy using a surrogate endpoint, the inducibility of sustained monomorphic VT on programmed electrical stimulation. Simson[16] studied SAECG analysis at 25 and 40 Hz to optimize the scoring of the SAECG to correctly classify 82 patients with prior Q wave myocardial infarction with a history of spontaneous and inducible sustained VT from 52 patients with prior myocardial infarction but no sustained VT. The best total predictive accuracy of 89% was obtained at both high-pass filter settings.

Using an abnormal RMS40 as a definition of late potentials, Gomes and colleagues studied the sensitivity, specificity, and positive and negative predictive accuracy for optimal separation of 29 patients with organic heart disease without VT from 33 patients with sustained VT.[19] From the seven high-pass filter settings studied, they found that 80 Hz provided the best sensitivity (88%) but low specificity (69%), while at 25 Hz, the specificity was maximal (90%), but sensitivity was poor (42%). The 40 Hz setting provided the best combination of sensitivity and specificity values, 61% and 83%, respectively.

The finding that 40 Hz was a good high-pass filter setting for analyzing the SAECG confirmed results provided earlier in a study by Denes et al,[17] which found a sensitivity and specificity of 83% and 90%, respectively, for RMS40 at 40 Hz compared to 25-Hz values of 58% and 96%. Coto et al provided optimal sensitivity and specificity at 50 Hz as opposed to 25 Hz; however, the patient group used to discriminate from normals included nonsustained and sustained VT.[18] Nalos et al reported a sensitivity and specificity at 100 Hz of 93% and 94%, respectively, for the induction of sustained VT in 100 patients; however, measured values determining the presence of late potentials were obtained by visual inspection.[5]Machac et al reported a maximum sensitivity of 85% for RMS40 at 80 Hz and specificity of 88% for QRS duration at 25 Hz.[21]

In a study by our group, a computer program was written in Pascal in which the QRS and LAS40 durations and RMS40 voltage were analyzed at 11 high-pass filter settings and combined in 6017 combinations of singles, pairs, and triplets of parameters to optimize the prediction of the results of programmed stimulation in 80 patients presenting with spontaneous nonsustained VT, of whom 28 had inducible sustained VT and 52 did not. This approach allowed for the comparison of the three parameters across all high-pass filter settings. Analysis of each parameter taken alone showed maximal sensitivity of 82% at the 40-Hz high-pass filter setting (LAS40 or RMS40 at 40 Hz). The maximal specificity was 87% (RMS40). While

Table VI

Thirty-Two Combinations of Signal-Averaged Electrocardiogram Parameters with the Best Total Predictive Accuracy of 89%

	Sensitivity (%)	Specificity (%)	Positive Predictive Accuracy (%)	Negative Predictive Accuracy (%)	Total Predictive Accuracy (%)
RMS40(20Hz),RMS40(40Hz)	79	94	88	89	89
RMS40(25Hz),RMS40(40Hz)	79	94	88	89	89
LAS40 (30Hz),LAS40 (40Hz),LAS40 (50Hz)	75	96	91	88	89
LAS40 (25Hz),LAS40 (30Hz),RMS40(40Hz)	79	94	88	89	89
LAS40 (30Hz),LAS40 (40Hz),RMS40(60Hz)	79	94	88	89	89
LAS40 (30Hz),LAS40 (50Hz),RMS40(40Hz)	75	96	91	88	89
LAS40 (30Hz),LAS40 (50Hz),RMS40(60Hz)	75	96	91	88	89
LAS40 (40Hz),LAS40 (50Hz),RMS40(20Hz)	71	98	95	87	89
LAS40 (40Hz),LAS40 (50Hz),RMS40(25Hz)	71	98	95	87	89
LAS40 (40Hz),LAS40 (50Hz),RMS40(30Hz)	71	98	95	87	89
RMS40(20Hz),RMS40(40Hz),LAS40 (25Hz)	79	94	88	89	89
RMS40(20Hz),RMS40(40Hz),LAS40 (30Hz)	79	94	88	89	89
RMS40(20Hz),RMS40(40Hz),LAS40 (40Hz)	75	96	91	88	89
RMS40(20Hz),RMS40(40Hz),LAS40 (50Hz)	71	98	95	87	89
RMS40(20Hz),RMS40(50Hz),LAS40 (40Hz)	75	96	91	88	89
RMS40(20Hz),RMS40(60Hz),LAS40 (40Hz)	75	96	91	88	89

Table VI *(Continued)*

	Sensitivity (%)	Specificity (%)	Positive Predictive Accuracy (%)	Negative Predictive Accuracy (%)	Total Predictive Accuracy (%)
RMS40(20Hz),RMS40(60Hz),LAS40 (50Hz)	71	98	95	87	89
RMS40(25Hz),RMS40(40Hz),LAS40 (25Hz)	79	94	88	89	89
RMS40(25Hz),RMS40(40Hz),LAS40 (30Hz)	79	94	88	89	89
RMS40(25Hz),RMS40(40Hz),LAS40 (40Hz)	75	96	91	88	89
RMS40(25Hz),RMS40(40Hz),LAS40 (50Hz)	71	98	95	87	89
RMS40(25Hz),RMS40(50Hz),LAS40 (40Hz)	75	96	91	88	89
RMS40(25Hz),RMS40(60Hz),LAS40 (40Hz)	75	96	91	88	89
RMS40(25Hz),RMS40(60Hz),LAS40 (50Hz)	71	98	95	87	89
RMS40(30Hz),RMS40(40Hz),LAS40 (25Hz)	79	94	88	89	89
RMS40(30Hz),RMS40(40Hz),LAS40 (50Hz)	71	98	95	87	89
RMS40(30Hz),RMS40(50Hz),LAS40 (40Hz)	75	96	91	88	89
RMS40(30Hz),RMS40(60Hz),LAS40 (40Hz)	75	96	91	88	89
RMS40(30Hz),RMS40(60Hz),LAS40 (50Hz)	71	98	95	87	89
RMS40(20Hz),RMS40(25Hz),RMS40(40Hz)	79	94	88	89	89
RMS40(20Hz),RMS40(30Hz),RMS40(40Hz)	79	94	88	89	89
RMS40(25Hz),RMS40(30Hz),RMS40(40Hz)	79	94	88	89	89

Abbreviations as in Table V.

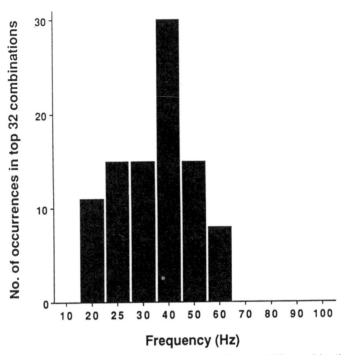

Figure 13. Distribution of high-pass filter settings of 32 combinations of SAECG parameters with 89% total predictive accuracy. The most represented filter setting was 40 Hz, whereas <20 Hz and >60 Hz were not represented. See text for details. (Reprinted with permission from Caref et al. Am J Cardiol 64:16, 1989.)

no combination of parameters could provide a greater sensitivity than single parameters of LAS40 or RMS40 at 40 Hz, there were 267 combinations that could improve the specificity to 98%.

When optimizing for total predictive accuracy, 32 combinations provided the highest total predictive accuracy of 89% (Table VI). The dominant filter setting of these 32 top combinations was 40 Hz, which was utilized in 28 of 32 (87%) combinations. In contrast, high-pass settings <20 Hz or >60 Hz were not represented (Figure 13). Only two combinations were pairs, RMS40 at 20 or 25 Hz combined with RMS40 at 40 Hz; the remaining 30 were composed of triplets. In addition, none of the top combinations included the QRS duration parameter.

Limitations of Filtering the SAECG

Filtering can do nothing about residual noise contained in the SAECG that has similar frequency characteristics of late potentials. Another major technical limitation of SAECG filtering are the undesirable filter-created changes in morphology seen in the time domain. Butterworth filters, while producing sharp transitions between the passband and stopbands, are prone to ringing effects and phase shifting. Even though bidirectional filters are used to divert ringing to the middle of the QRS complex, the morphology of that area may change dramatically. Other filters, such as FIR filters, are known to cause spreading of the signal.[2,3,8]

There are still questions regarding the optimal high-pass filter settings to use for filtering the SAECG that best separate unwanted frequencies in the terminal QRS from those of late potentials while retaining much of the late potential signal. While the useful range of high-pass filters appears to be 20–100 Hz (depending on the technique and filter type used), it may be that late potentials have varying frequency characteristics, so that optimal filtering will remain elusive until complete frequency characterization of late potentials and residual noise is undertaken. Several reports have examined frequency characteristics of late potentials[27–30]; however, the different frequency analysis techniques used remain to be validated.

Acknowledgment: This work was supported in part by grant HL 31341 from the National Institutes of Health and by medical research funds from the Veterans Administration, Washington, D.C.

References

1. El-Sherif N, Gomes JAC, Restivo M, Mehra R: Late potentials and arrhythmogenesis. PACE 8:440, 1985.
2. Oppenheim AV, Shafer RW: Digital signal processing. Englewood Cliffs, NJ: Prentice-Hall, 1975.
3. Jackson LB: Digital Filters and Signal Processing. Norwell, MA: Kluwer Academic Publishers, 1986.
4. Papoulis A: The Fourier Integral and its Applications. New York: McGraw-Hill, 1962.
5. Nalos PC, Gang ES, Mandel WJ, Ladenheim ML, Lass Y, Peter T: The signal-averaged electrocardiogram as a screening test for inducibility of

sustained ventricular tachycardia in high risk patients: a prospective study. J Am Coll Cardiol 9:539, 1987.

6. Stopczyk MJ, Kopec J, Zochowski RJ, Pieniak M: Surface recording of electrical heart activity during the P-R segment in man by a computer averaging technique. Int Res Com Syst 11:73, 1973.

7. Simson MB: Use of signals in the terminal QRS complex to identify patients with ventricular tachycardia after myocardial infarction. Circulation 61:235, 1981.

8. Lander P, Berbari EJ: Use of high-pass filtering to detect late potentials in the signal-averaged ECG. Electrocardiol 22(Suppl):7, 1990.

9. Christenson DW, Reddy BRS, Rowlandson GI: Evaluation of Fourier transform filter for high-resolution ECG. Electrocardiol 22(Suppl):33, 1990.

10. Rozanski JJ, Mortara D, Myerburg RJ, Castellanos A: Body surface detection of delayed depolarizations in patients with recurrent ventricular tachycardia and left ventricular aneurysm. Circulation 63:1172, 1981.

11. Berbari EJ, Scherlag BJ, Hope RR, Lazzara R: Recording from the body surface of arrhythmogenic ventricular activity during the S-T segment. Am J Cardiol 41:697, 1978.

12. Breithardt G, Borggrefe M, Karbenn U, Abendroth RR, Yeh HL, Seipel L: Prevalence of late potentials in patients with and without ventricular tachycardia: correlation with angiographic findings. Am J Cardiol 49:1932, 1982.

13. Denniss AR, Ross DL, Uther JB: Reproducibility of measurements of ventricular activation time using the signal-averaged Frank electrocardiogram. Am J Cardiol 57:156, 1986.

14. Abboud S, Belhassen B, Laniado S, Sadeh D: Non-invasive recording of late ventricular activity using an advanced method in patients with a damaged mass of ventricular tissue. J Electrocardiol 16:245, 1983.

15. Henkin R, Caref EB, Kelen GJ, El-Sherif N: The signal-averaged electrocardiogram and late potentials. A comparative analysis of commercial devices. J Electrocardiol 22 (Suppl):19, 1990.

16. Simson MB: Optimal identification of late potentials. In Santini M, Pistolese M, Alliegro A (eds): Progress in Clinical Pacing. Amsterdam: Excerpta Medica, 1988, pp 225–238.

17. Denes P, Santarelli P, Hauser RG, Uretz EF: Quantitative analysis of the high-frequency components of the terminal portion of the body surface QRS in normal subjects and in patients with ventricular tachycardia. Circulation 67:1129, 1983.

18. Coto H, Maldonado C, Palakurthy P, Flowers NC: Late potentials in normal subjects and in patients with ventricular tachycardia unrelated to myocardial infarction. Am J Cardiol 55:384, 1985.

19. Gomes JA, Winters SL, Stewart D, Targonski A, Barreca P: Optimal bandpass filters for time-domain analysis of the signal-averaged electrocardiogram as a predictor of the results of programmed stimulation. Am J Cardiol 64:16, 1989.

20. Caref EB, Turitto G, Ibrahim BB, Henkin R, El-Sherif N: Role of bandpass filters in optimizing the value of the signal-averaged electro-

cardiogram as a predictor of the results of programmed stimulation. Am J Cardiol 64:16, 1989.

21. Machac J, Weiss A, Winters SL, Barreca P, Gomes JA: A comparative study of frequency domain and time domain analysis of signal-averaged electrocardiograms in patients with ventricular tachycardia. J Am Coll Cardiol 11:284, 1988.

22. Steinberg JS, Bigger JT Jr: Importance of the endpoint of noise reduction in analysis to the signal averaged electrocardiogram. Am J Cardiol 63:556, 1989.

23. Vacek JL, Smith S, Dunn MI: Late potential parameter and noise level variability caused by bandpass versus high-pass filtering and type of signal averaging equipment used. J Electrophysiol 3:278, 1989.

24. Scher AM, Young AC: Frequency analysis of the electrocardiogram. Circ Res 8:344, 1960.

25. Golden DP, Wolthius RA, Hoffler GW: A spectral analysis of the normal resting electrocardiogram. IEEE Trans Biomed Eng 20:366, 1973.

26. Thakor NV, Webster JG, Tompkins WJ: Estimation of QRS complex power spectra for design of a QRS filter. IEEE Trans Biomed Eng BME-31, 11:702, 1984.

27. Cain ME, Ambos HD, Witkowski FX, Sobel BE: Fast Fourier transform analysis of signal-averaged ECGs for identification of patients prone to sustained ventricular tachycardia. Circulation 69:711, 1984.

28. Cain ME, Ambos HD, Markham J, Fischer AE, Sobel BE: Quantitation of differences in frequency content of signal-averaged ECGs in patients with compared to those without sustained ventricular tachycardia. Am J Cardiol 55:1500, 1985.

29. Kelen GJ, Henkin R, Fontaine JM, El-Sherif N: Effects of analyzed signal duration and phase on the results of fast Fourier transform analysis of the surface electrocardiogram in subjects with and without late potentials. Am J Cardiol 60:1282, 1987.

30. Haberl R, Jilge G, Pulter R, Steinbeck G: Comparison of frequency and time domain analysis of the signal-averaged electrocardiogram in patients with ventricular tachycardia and coronary artery disease. J Am Coll Cardiol 12:150, 1988.

5

Principles of
Frequency-Domain Analysis

Paul Lander, David Albert, Edward J. Berbari

Introduction

Modern spectral analysis has its roots in the Fourier transform, named after the French mathematician, Joseph Fourier. With the Fourier transform, it is possible to obtain a representation of signals using weighted integrals of sinusoids that are not harmonically related. This method of decomposition, or modeling, of signals has had a great impact on many areas in mathematics, science, and engineering. The tools of Fourier analysis have been prominent in studies on vibration, heat diffusion, alternating current, climate, radio, and television, to name but a few. The original mathematical development of Fourier methods took place for continuous-time signals. However, with the advent of digital computers, a discrete-time Fourier theory appeared for use with sampled signals. An important step in this development was the fast Fourier transform (FFT), an

From El-Sherif N, Turitto G (eds): *High-Resolution Electrocardiography*. Mount Kisco, NY, Futura Publishing Co., Inc., ©, 1992.

algorithm designed to efficiently compute the discrete Fourier transform (DFT). In general, the properties of the DFT are analogous to those of the continuous-time transform.

There are some theoretical and practical limitations to the application of spectral analysis techniques. This chapter will examine the most important of these limitations, as they apply to the analysis of the high-resolution electrocardiogram (ECG). Foremost, it should be recognized that the Fourier transform of the signal-averaged ECG is a transformation of the information in the signal average into another form. No new information is created in the process.

Cain et al [1,2] introduced spectral analysis of the high-resolution ECG in an attempt to take advantage of the idea that late potentials have a different spectral character to the QRS and ST segment waveforms. The prospective advantages of frequency-domain analysis are that it might obviate the needs for filtering and exact localization of the time-domain signal. Some of the difficulties involved in the frequency-domain approach have been discussed by Kelen et al, [3] Worley et al, [4] and Haberl et al. [5]

The first part of this chapter will introduce the basic concepts of Fourier analysis. The practical aspects of implementing the DFT and the issues of spectral resolution and time dependence of the spectrum will be discussed. In the second part, some approaches for addressing these problems will be considered. These involve the use of spectral smoothing and maximum entropy methods to enhance the spectrum. In an effort to extend the use of spectral analysis techniques for the high-resolution ECG, the concept of a combined time and frequency signal representation will be introduced.

Introduction to Frequency-Domain Representation of Signals

The high-resolution ECG is measured from the body surface as a continuous electrical waveform. To perform spectral analysis with a digital computer, this continuous signal must be digitized, that is sampled at discrete, evenly spaced intervals in time. The sampling rate has a theoretical lower limit, known as the Nyquist rate, equal to twice the expected bandwidth of the ECG signal. Assuming a frequency band of interest in the high-resolution ECG of approximately 0.05 to 250 Hz, this implies that a sampling rate of about 500 Hz is theoretically sufficient. However, in practice, a rate of between 5 and 10 times the Nyquist rate is chosen to avoid *aliasing* (to be discussed). Hence a sampling rate of 2000 samples per second can be expected to give a detailed reproduction of the continuous ECG waveform.

The following discussion of the discrete Fourier transform applies to deterministic, finite energy signals. The sampled—or discrete—waveform, x(n), for n = 0 to N−1, has a DFT defined by

$$X(k) = \sum_{n=0}^{N-1} x(n) \exp(-j2\pi nk/N) \tag{1}$$

where x(n) is the N-sample discrete waveform. The result of the discrete Fourier transform is the Fourier spectrum, X(k). This is defined for k = −N/2 to N/2 − 1. The value of X(k) at k = 0 is termed the dc component, or 0 Hz value. Values of X(k) for k = 0 to N/2 − 1 are termed the 'positive frequency' values; values of X(k) for k = −N/2 to −1 are termed the 'negative frequency' values. The negative frequency values are a mirror image of the positive frequencies, hence only the latter are generally analyzed. The exponential term in equation 1 includes the constant j $(=\sqrt{-1})$, which implies that X(k) is a complex entity. Equation 1 can be rewritten as:

$$X(k) = \sum_{n=0}^{N-1} x(n) (\cos(2\pi nk/N) - j \sin(2\pi nk/N)). \tag{2}$$

X(k) has a *real part,* consisting of the cosine terms, and an *imaginary part,* consisting of the sine terms. The inverse discrete Fourier transform of X(k) may be defined as:

$$x(n) = \sum_{k=0}^{N-1} X(k) \exp(j2\pi nk/N) \tag{3}$$

X(k) and x(n) are considered a Fourier transform pair because of this reciprocal relationship. From the complex Fourier spectrum, X(k), we can compute phase, amplitude, and power spectra. The phase spectrum, F(k), is defined as:

$$F(k) = \arctan(-\text{Im}\{X(k)\} / R\{X(k)\}) \tag{4}$$

where $\text{Im}\{X(k)\}$ and $R\{X(k)\}$ are the imaginary and real parts of $X(k)$, respectively. The amplitude—or magnitude—spectrum, A(k), is defined as:

$$A(k) = |X(k)| \tag{5}$$

where $||$ denotes the modulus, or absolute value. The complex entity, $X(k)$, has a modulus defined as:

$$|X(k)| = \sqrt{R\{X(k)\}^2 + \text{Im}\{X(k)\}^2}. \tag{6}$$

The power spectrum, P(k), is defined as:

$$P(k) = |X(k)|^2. \tag{7}$$

The units of P(k) are actually power per Hertz. Hence the actual power over any frequency band is found by rectangular integration of the area under P(k). For this reason P(k) is more properly called a *power density spectrum (PDS)*. The inverse discrete Fourier transform of the PDS is the autocorrelation function, r(n).

$$r(n) = \sum_{n=0}^{N-1} P(k) \exp(j2\pi nk/N). \tag{8}$$

It should be noted that in computing P(k) the modulus of the Fourier spectrum is taken (see equation 6). Hence the phase information (see equation 4) is lost and it is not possible to reconstruct X(k) or x(n) from the PDS. The autocorrelation function and the PDS constitute a Fourier transform pair.

Figure 1 graphically illustrates a sample spectral analysis of a sine wave of frequency 100 Hz. The complex output of the discrete Fourier transform is shown in Figure 1B. The power density spectrum (Figure 1C), plotted on a logarithmic scale, shows a single peak at 100 Hz. This spectrum is ideally an impulse: there are several factors contributing to its smeared appearance which will be discussed.

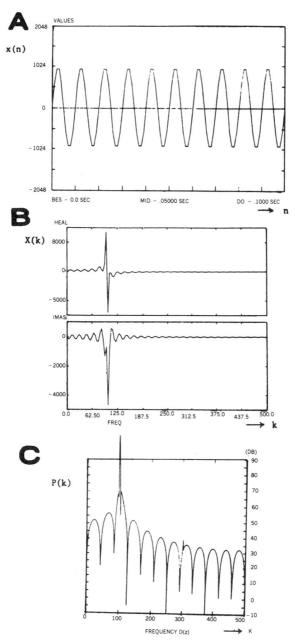

Figure 1. An example of spectral analysis. (A) A sine wave signal, x(n). (B) Its Fourier spectrum, X(k). (C) Its power spectrum, P(k).

Fourier Transform Properties

The relationships between x(n), X(k), F(k), A(k), P(k), and r(n) are illustrated in Figure 2. There are a number of important properties of the discrete Fourier transform. We will list two properties which are necessary to follow the discussions in this chapter.

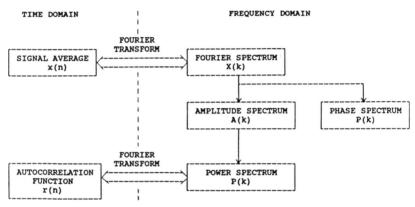

Figure 2. Fourier transform relationships between the time and frequency domains.

Linearity

If two signals, c(n) and d(n), are summed the Fourier transform is equal to the sum of the individual Fourier spectra of both.

$$\sum_{n=0}^{N-1} (c(n) + d(n)) \exp(-j2\pi nk/N) = C(k) + D(k). \qquad (9)$$

Multiplication/Convolution

A multiplication operation in the frequency domain is equivalent to a convolution in the time domain.

$$\sum_{n=0}^{N-1} (c(1) \, d(n+1)) \exp(-j2\pi nk/N)$$

$$= C(k) \cdot D(k) \text{ for } 1 = 0 \text{ to } N-1. \qquad (10)$$

For example, some types of digital filters are implemented by convolving the filter's impulse response with the signal in the time domain. This operation could be replaced by multiplying the Fourier spectra of the filter and the signal, and inverse transforming the product.

Often the quantities in the power spectrum are expressed on a decibel (dB) scale, as in Figure 1C. P(k) is given a value relative to $P_{max}(k)$ the maximum spectral value. This decibel value for each component of P(k) is given by:

$$\text{decibel value of } P(k) = 10 \log_{10} (P(k) / P_{max}(k)). \qquad (11)$$

Hence the decibel scale is a relative scale.

To summarize this introduction to Fourier analysis, it can be appreciated intuitively that a large number of different signals can be reconstructed using building blocks of sines and cosines. This finds a mathematical expression in the Fourier spectrum, which is found via the Fourier transform. From the Fourier transform result we can move to the power density spectrum and measure spectral power by summing the spectrum over the frequency interval of interest. For the reader who would like a more detailed introduction to the Fourier representation of signals, the introductory texts "Signals and Systems" by Oppenheim and Willsky[6] and "The FFT" by Ramirez[7] are recommended.

Fourier Analysis in Practice

Several issues which arise when performing Fourier analysis in practice will be introduced here. These are: windowing; dc removal; zero-padding; and spectral resolution.

The first step is to select a period of interest in the ECG to analyze. Figure 3 shows a signal-averaged ECG with evident ventricular late potentials. Assuming only the late potential period, T_2, is to be analyzed this section of the ECG is isolated by multiplying the ECG waveform with a window function. Just 'cutting out' the period of interest—i.e., not explicitly applying a window—is equivalent to multiplying the ECG waveform by the rectangular window, rect(n), of Figure 3. However, this abrupt truncation has undesirable side effects, as will be seen later, and so a smoother window function such as the Hamming or Blackman-Harris window, bh(n) of Figure 3, is generally used.

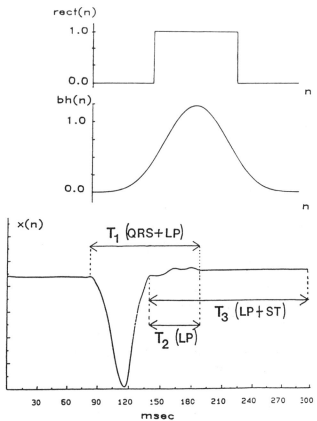

Figure 3. A signal-averaged ECG, with the rectangular (rect[n]) and Blackman-Harris (bh[n]) windows (inset).

The mean value of the ECG data in the time window to be transformed is usually not equal to zero. This mean value consists of two components. First, there is a dc component due to voltage drifts at the electrodes, or caused by the recording instrumentation. This is of no interest. Second, the ECG waveform itself has a non-zero mean value. This may be of interest. For example, a normal and a post-exercise ST segment waveform have different mean values. However, for consistency, the mean value in both cases should be referenced to the zero ECG value, i.e., the value in the TP interval which represents zero heart action. Because the first (dc) component often predominates over the two, it is usually advisable to subtract the mean value from the period of interest before Fourier transformation.

The discrete Fourier transform, X(k), is usually computed with a high speed computer algorithm known as the fast Fourier transform (FFT). The FFT requires that the number of samples making up the time-domain waveform be a power of two (32, 64, 128, etc.). This is accomplished by 'zero-padding,' i.e., the input data to the FFT is augmented with zeros placed after the ECG data points.

The mean value of the ECG data should be subtracted before windowing. This may leave a small residual dc component after windowing, but the ECG data is properly tapered to zero at the beginning and end of the window. However, if the windowed ECG data has a non-zero mean then subtracting this mean will create an abrupt transition between the first and last data points and the augmenting zeros. This is equivalent to superimposing upon the ECG data a rectangular pulse of the same length as the window, with a height equal to the subtracted mean value. The resulting spectrum will be the sum of the spectra due to the ECG data and the newly created pulse waveform.

Figure 4 illustrates the effects of dc removal, zero-padding, and interval selection on the power density spectrum of the signal-averaged ECG of Figure 3. Panel A shows the PDS, computed over interval T_2 (= 60 msec), without dc removal or zero-padding. Panel B shows the same spectrum with the dc component removed. Note that a fundamental harmonic component is always present. This is equal to the reciprocal of the observation interval, in this case, 1/60 msec = 16.7 Hz. This component must be taken into account when the spectrum is analyzed. Panel C shows the effect of zero-padding. The fundamental harmonic occurs at a lower frequency and the spectrum has a smooth appearance. However, zero-padding does not improve the resolution of the spectrum, an issue that will be considered in detail in the next section. Panel D shows the spectrum resulting from shifting the period T_2 6 msec back into the QRS complex. The shape of the spectrum is radically altered because of the prominence of QRS spectral characteristics. Panel E shows the spectrum resulting from the selection of interval T_3, i.e., the late potential waveform and the ST segment. The low-frequency characteristics of the ST segment are evident in this spectrum. However, the resolution of the late potential spectral components is not improved at all by this extension of the observation interval (as will be examined in the next section). In addition, the late potential spectrum is ob-

scured due to the superposition of the spectral components of the ST segment.

Spectral Resolution

The concept of spectral resolution is intimately bound up with the use of a window function. To investigate the meaning of spectral resolution, let us first consider the power density spectrum of a 40-msec time period from a time-domain waveform sampled at 2000 Hz. There are 80 samples input to the Fourier transform and the resulting power density spectrum has 41 samples evenly spaced between 0 and 1000 Hz. This implies that there is one sample every 25 Hz: thus 25 Hz may be termed the *nominal* spectral resolution.

However, the actual, or effective, spectral resolution is considerably worse because of the effect of applying a window function in the time domain. The concept of the *effective spectral resolution* is best developed by establishing the idea of a *time-bandwidth product* for window functions. Figure 5 illustrates a sine wave signal, of frequency 100 Hz, and its spectrum after windowing with the Blackman-Harris function, bh(n). Instead of an impulse at 100 Hz, the spectrum is in the form of the discrete Fourier transform of the Blackman-Harris window, BH(k). The spectral energy of the sine wave has been smeared due to the finite truncation and windowing in the time domain. This phenomenon is known as spectral leakage. To find the actual power of the sine wave, we must integrate the spectrum over all frequencies. This is because applying a window of finite duration in the time domain results in a spectrum of infinite length. In practice, however, we are interested in determining what frequency interval contains the essential part of the power spectrum: for example, the 95% power frequency interval. If the sine wave is observed for a longer time, i.e., a longer duration window is used, the mainlobe width of the window (Figure 5) narrows. Hence the time-bandwidth product of the window, K_w, which is a constant, may be defined as:

$$K_w = B_e \cdot T \qquad (12)$$

where T is the observation period in the time domain and B_e is the frequency interval which encompasses the significant (i.e., 95%) power of the window function in the frequency domain. The analytic approaches taken in defining K_w may be found in references 8 and 9.

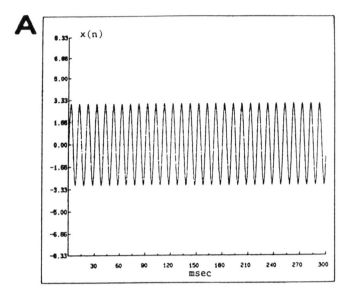

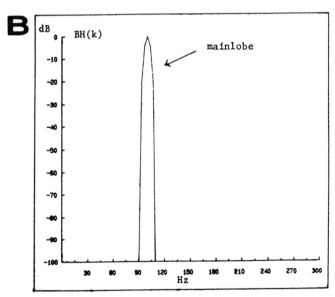

Figure 5. Spectral characteristics of the Blackman-Harris window. (A) A sine wave signal. (B) Its PDS after windowing with the Blackman-Harris window, revealing the PDS of the window function and illustrating the phenomenon of spectral leakage.

To resolve the power of a single sine wave it is not sufficient to be able to pinpoint the peak value of the spectrum, rather the spectrum must be integrated over a frequency interval decided by: (1) the absolute duration, T, of the time-domain waveform of interest included in the period for FFT analysis; and (2) the time-bandwidth product, K_w, of the window. Note that the peak value of the spectrum can be more accurately localized by zero-padding, but that the frequency interval, B_e, remains unchanged.

A formal approach to defining spectral resolution can be taken by asking what is the minimum frequency interval by which two sine waves must be separated in order that their spectral powers are distinct. A number of approaches to this problem have been taken.[10] The two most common measures are that the spectra be distinct up to 6 dB below the peak value, or that 95% of their powers are distinct. For the Blackman-Harris window, the 6 dB bandwidth criterion gives a value of K_w = 2.72,[10] and the 95% power criterion gives a value of K_w = 3.7.[8,11]

This discussion is exact for the idealized two-sinusoid case. The high-resolution ECG does not appear to exhibit distinct peaks, or strong sinusoidal components, but has a more continuous spectral appearance. As a result, the power of any spectral sample is inextricably smeared across adjacent samples. In this situation the definitions of spectral resolution taken above apply in principle. The exact spectral resolution is determined by two factors: (1) the absolute duration of the late potential waveform; and (2) the interaction between the second order statistics (i.e., the true power spectrum) of the signal and the mainlobe/sidelobe characteristics of the window used. (Note that the spectrum of the Blackman-Harris window (Figure 5) has no sidelobes extending beyond the mainlobe.)

As an example of typical spectral resolutions available, a 40-msec waveform, windowed with the Blackman-Harris function has a spectral resolution of 68 Hz by the 6 dB bandwidth criterion, and 90 Hz by the 95% power criterion. These figures give guidelines for the frequency intervals which should be integrated to obtain the power at a particular frequency, although power from neighboring frequencies is inseparably mixed due to the smearing discussed above.

In summary, spectral resolution cannot be improved by zero-padding the data before input to the FFT, or by sampling at a higher rate. The only improvement possible is achieved by taking a longer time period of interest, or by using a higher performance window (i.e., one with a lower value of K_w). Apart from the rectangular window, which is a poor performer, the other windows commonly considered, the Blackman-Harris, Kaiser-Bessel etc., are close in performance to the theoretical limit of K_w which is about 3.6 using the 95% power criterion.[8] A final point is that the period, T, cannot be arbitrarily increased to improve spectral resolution. For example, if period T_2 from Figure 2 is chosen for analysis, the resolution of the spectral components of the late potential waveform depends not on T_3 but on its own duration T_2. This follows from the DFT property of linearity, discussed above, where the ST segment and late potential waveforms may be considered as two distinct signals added together before input to the FFT. Extending the period for analysis in this way means that the late potential spectral energy is underestimated by a factor of T_2/T_3.

In conclusion, spectral resolution depends primarily on the absolute duration of *the waveform of interest,* and secondarily on the time-bandwidth characteristic of the window. The concept of spectral resolution is immanent in the properties of signals, as opposed to the techniques used to analyze them.

The material for this section has been taken from a broad range of sources dealing with the development of spectral analysis from the 1940s to the present. The interested reader will find a more in-depth discussion in a comparison of various window functions, performed by Harris,[10] a discussion of time-bandwidth product by de Weerd and coworker,[11] and a sophisticated treatise on spectral analysis methods by Marple.[9]

Aliasing

Aliasing occurs when the time-domain signal has energy at frequencies greater than half the sampling rate; this latter value being known as the Nyquist rate. The spectral components of the signal that exceed this limit are aliased: that is, they are represented in the Fourier spectrum at frequencies below the Nyquist frequency. An example of aliasing can be seen in Western movies, when the wheels of wagons supposedly moving at high speed appear to be turning backward. This phenomenon occurs because the camera is "sampling" the position of the wheels at a fixed rate, e.g., 25 frames/sec. If the wheels are moving at the Nyquist rate, i.e., 12½ revolution/ sec, they will appear completely stationary on film. If the frequency spectrum were plotted, the energy of the wheels would appear as the dc component, i.e., at 0 Hz. On the other hand, if the wheels are actually revolving at 24 resolutions/sec, they will appear to be revolving backwards at 1 revolution/sec on film. In practice, the true speed of the wheels will only appear on film at speeds somewhat less than the Nyquist rate, due to the phenomenon of spectral leakage. Hence it is customary to sample at rates between 5 and 10 times the highest expected signal frequency. Assuming late potentials to be nominally bandlimited to 250 Hz, a sampling rate of at least 1000 Hz, and preferably 2000 Hz, is necessary to completely avoid aliasing. It is also common practice to apply an electronic low-pass filter (an antialias filter) to the signal before sampling to attenuate frequencies outside the band of interest.

Spectral Smoothing

Applying a window in the time domain and computing the power density spectrum via the FFT produces only an *estimate* of the true spectrum. Because the act of windowing in the time domain, known as *tapering,* is equivalent to low-pass filtering the spectral waveform, this procedure is usually referred to as *smoothing.* The degree of smoothing obtained in this way cannot be varied. An added disadvantage of tapering is the arbitrary suppression of the waveform toward the ends of the window. This is an acute problem because of the timing of late potentials in the high-resolution ECG, i.e., their close proximity to the main QRS.

An alternative approach, known as spectral smoothing, is to low-pass filter—or smooth—the power density spectrum directly. Recall from Figure 2 that the complex Fourier spectrum, X(k), and the original time-domain signal, x(n), are a Fourier transform pair. That is, X(k) is the Fourier transform of x(n), and x(n) is the inverse Fourier transform of X(k). The original signal, x(n), cannot be recovered from the power density spectrum. The inverse Fourier transform of the PDS is the autocorrelation function, r(n). A smoothed estimate of the true power density spectrum can be achieved by windowing the autocorrelation function. The PDS is first computed via the FFT of the time series, x(n), with the rectangular window. This power spectrum, known as the *raw* spectral estimate, is then inverse Fourier transformed to obtain r(n). The autocorrelation function is then windowed and the windowed version of r(n) is then forward transformed to get the smoothed spectral estimate, $P^s(k)$, i.e.,

$$P^s(k) = \sum_{n=0}^{N-1} (r(n) \cdot w(n)) \exp(-j2\pi nk/N) \tag{13}$$

where w(n) is the window function used. The degree of smoothing can be varied by using a different window type or by altering the window length, T, between N samples and some fraction of N. In general the shorter the window, the greater the degree of smoothing and the poorer the spectral resolution. The spectral resolution is still given by equation 12, where T refers to the window length.

This method, spectral smoothing, is generally preferred to applying a window directly to the original time series because of the avoidance of arbitrarily reducing the information in the signal waveform, and the greater flexibility in smoothing that is obtainable. Choosing the appropriate degree of smoothing for a new class of signals, such as the signal-averaged ECG, is invariably an empirical procedure. It is usually performed by applying progressively heavier degrees of smoothing until spectral features of interest can be consistently reproduced with different waveforms.

Time-Varying Spectra

The above discussion has introduced the topic of spectral analysis and its practical considerations. An important question that is often overlooked is what interaction is there between the time- and frequency-domain representations of a signal? In other words, what happens if the signal spectrum to be measured is changing with time? In this case, the signal is said to have a time-varying spectrum. This issue is important in the analysis of the high-resolution ECG. The QRS, late potential, and ST segment waveforms have different spectral characteristics. When analyzing late potentials, the observation interval ideally should be increased to get higher spectral resolution, but this means including QRS and/or ST segment samples as well as the late potential waveform in the time period for spectral analysis. The result of attempting to measure this time-varying spectrum is that the power density spectrum obtained is an average of all the spectra that exist within the observation interval.

Figure 6 illustrates this concept, using a sine wave signal whose

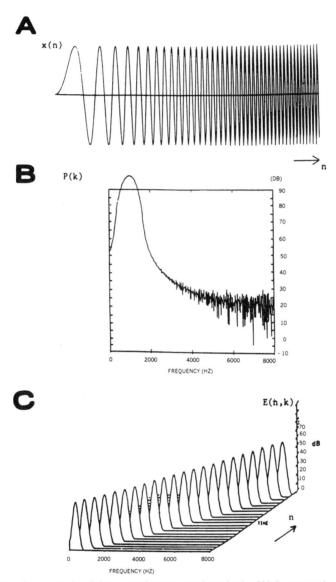

Figure 6. An example of time-varying spectral analysis. (A) A swept sine wave of linearly increasing frequency from 0 to 8000 Hz. (B) Its PDS. (C) Its time-varying spectrum, E(n,k). (See text for computational details.)

frequency increases continuously with time. This signal is called a swept sine wave. Figure 6A shows the test signal. Figure 6B is the power density spectrum of the complete time-domain waveform. The spectrum has no features that uniquely relate it to the swept sine wave. It is just the time average of all the frequency components of the signal. Note that increasingly higher frequencies are progressively underestimated due to the fact that, by definition, they exist for a shorter time period. Figure 6C shows the time-varying spectrum of the swept sine wave, or the variations of energy in time and frequency. This time-varying spectrum was obtained by placing a 'short-time' window, of duration T, at the start of the signal (Figure 6A), computing a power density spectrum, and plotting it on the time axis of Figure 6C. The window was then shifted in time by a small amount τ, and another spectrum was computed and plotted. This procedure is repeated throughout the time period of interest.

The ideal time-varying spectrum would be a continuous sequence of impulses along the diagonal in Figure 6C. However, the actual sequence of smeared spectra shown represents a compromise between the dynamic changes in time of the signal and the superior spectral resolution obtainable with longer observation periods. Dynamic changes in time of signal energy are better represented by a short window duration, whereas spectral resolution improves with a longer window duration. Formally, the spectral slice at time n_0 of the time-varying spectrum of Figure 6C, E(n,K), can be mathematically expressed as:

$$E(n_0,k) = \sum_{n=0}^{T-1} (x(n+n_0-T/2) \cdot w(n)) \exp(-j2\pi nk/N) \quad (14)$$

where w(n) is the window function, of length T samples, employed.

Figure 7 illustrates a time-varying spectrum of the signal-averaged ECG shown in Figure 3. For comparison, the power density spectrum of this signal-averaged waveform is that shown in Figure 4. The time-varying spectrum reveals the *spectro-temporal* variation in energy of the signal. Hence the term *Spectro-Temporal Map*—or STM—is an adequate description of the time-varying spectrum of the signal-averaged ECG. The STM illustrates late potential activity in this subject with accurate identification of the end of the QRS plus late potential waveform (i.e., the end of the period T_2 in Figure

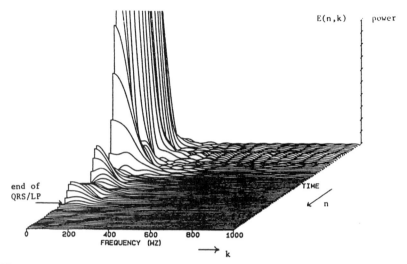

Figure 7. A time-varying spectrum—or spectro-temporal map—of the signal-averaged ECG of Figure 3. The STM is computed using a sequence of FFT derived power spectra. The end of the QRS/LP power is coincident with the end of period T_2 in Figure 3. The spectrum is plotted on a magnitude scale.

3), compared with the unfiltered signal average. Note that the terminal portion of the QRS (including the late potentials) appears to have low-level continuous variations in spectro-temporal energy.

This STM of the signal-averaged ECG was computed from the differenced waveform, y(n), which is defined by:

$$y(n) = x(n) - x(n-1) \tag{15}$$

where x(n) is the original ECG waveform. Simple differencing is an elementary form of high-pass filtering that is usually sufficient to substantially reduce the predominantly low-frequency energy of the ST segment waveform. The exact values of the parameters for computing the STM, i.e., the values of T and τ, are not of critical importance. For the STM of Figure 7, values of T = 16 msec and τ = 2 msec were used. The basic shape and outline of the spectro-temporal map did not change significantly in the ranges T = 12–24 msec and τ = 1–4 msec. The spectral resolution of each slice in the STM is poor: at T = 16 msec, the effective spectral resolution, B_e, is only 225 Hz (as defined by equation 12, using the 95% power criterion).

Autoregressive Models and Spectra

Use of the FFT is based on the idea that the signal under analysis is autoregressive in structure: i.e., each future value can be found from a linear combination of past values. From the discussion of spectral resolution and windowing above, it can be seen that the FFT gives only an *estimate* of the true power spectrum. The FFT uses a specific mathematical model to depict the spectrum, namely a *moving average model.* As discussed previously, FFT analysis runs into problems when high spectral resolution is required from short-time series. Another type of model, the *autoregressive or AR model,* is better suited to estimating power density spectra with sharp spectral features. This section will develop the basic ideas behind AR modeling on an intuitive basis, and illustrate their possible application to the signal-averaged ECG. (The properties of AR models are best explained using Z-transform mathematics, however, the topic is somewhat beyond the scope of this chapter. For the interested reader the subject is dealt with in a readable way in reference 12.)

An AR model is fitted not to the original signal, x(n), but to its autocorrelation function, r(n). (Recall that the autocorrelation function was introduced earlier and defined by equation 8.) The AR model has a number of terms or coefficients, M, usually referred to as its order. Mathematically, the AR model is related to the autocorrelation function with M coefficients, C_0 to C_m, attempting to model the autocorrelation function of the original signal.

Typically M is much smaller than the number of samples, N, of the original signal x(n). However, the M-term AR model can actually generate an *extrapolated* autocorrelation function of more than N samples in length. It can be shown that the extrapolation achieved gives a maximum entropy estimate of the autocorrelation function, in the sense understood by information theory. In other words, the AR model adds terms to the autocorrelation function that are not strictly measurable from the original N-sample signal. A number of computer algorithms exist to solve for the values of the AR model coefficients C_0 to C_m. The original algorithm was introduced by Burg in 1968 (see reference 9), and subsequent variations on this algorithm have since appeared for use with specific types of signals.

Once the AR model has been obtained it is used to generate the extrapolated autocorrelation function, which is then Fourier transformed to obtain the AR power spectral estimate. The extrapolated autocorrelation function gives a higher resolution power spectrum. Therefore, the power spectral estimate produced by the AR model would seem to be enhanced over the one given by the FFT. In practice, though, the apparent advantages of AR modeling via the maximum entropy method (MEM) are not always realized. From a historical perspective, MEM was developed to estimate the power spectra of sonar and speech waveforms. These are signals where sharp spectral peaks with a short frequency interval between them are anticipated. The main advantage of MEM is its ability to resolve sharp spectral features and to keep spectrally adjacent peaks distinct. Where narrowband signals, possibly in the presence of noise, must be identified, MEM gives superior spectral estimates, compared to the FFT approach. However, if no such distinctive spectral peaks are present, MEM offers no fundamental improvement over the FFT. In fact, MEM may likely introduce artifacts into the spectral estimate in the form of spurious peaks. No concrete guidelines are available to assist in the choice of the order, M, of the AR model. Consequently values of M must be developed empirically for the class of signal-averaged ECG waveforms. Using different choices of M can cause spectral estimates of the same time-domain signal to vary dramatically. Because of this the MEM approach to spectral analysis is inherently less stable than that of the FFT. In summary, MEM offers the prospect of reducing the spectral artifacts caused by windowing, but at the possible expense of destabilizing the estimated power spectrum.

Figure 8 illustrates the use of MEM to compute the spectro-temporal map of the signal-averaged ECG shown in Figures 3 and 7. Note that the MEM derived STM of Figure 8 is plotted on a logarithmic scale, while the FFT derived STM of Figure 7 is plotted on a magnitude scale. Both STMs have been scaled individually in order to optimally present their spectral features. The MEM STM was computed with parameter values of $T = 16$ msec and $\tau = 2$ msec (similarly to the FFT STM) and using a fourth order AR model ($M = 4$). The time-varying spectral features of the signal-averaged ECG are consistently reproduced by the FFT and MEM STMs. In both cases the end of the ventricular activity is readily identifiable and the essential form of the STMs are similar. The spectral edge frequencies (the highest frequency in each slice at which there is signal energy) are more clearly discernible in the MEM STM, due to the suppression of windowing artifacts.

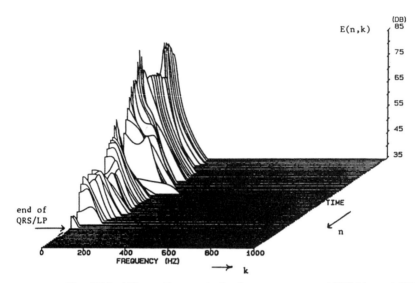

Figure 8. The STM of Figure 7 computed using a sequence of MEM-based AR models instead of the FFT. Note that the spectral slices appear more sharply defined than the FFT derived STM. The reproduction of spectro-temporal characteristics between this Figure and Figure 7 is generally good. This spectrum is plotted on a logarithmic scale.

Conclusions

The primary difficulties with frequency-domain analysis of the high-resolution ECG are concerned with the question of spectro-temporal resolution. This is a direct consequence of the signal-averaged ECG having a time-varying spectrum. Spectro-temporal mapping suggests that the QRS/late potential waveforms have a time-varying spectrum which could be consistently represented using FFT and MEM approaches to power spectrum computation. If the signal under analysis has a time-varying spectrum, the time window chosen should be short in order to resolve temporal changes in signal energy. However, this accommodation of temporal changes results in a poor spectral resolution. Using approximate figures, the frequency band of late potentials is about 0.05–250 Hz, while their duration is of the order of 20–100msec. Using equation 12, assuming a window constant of $K_w = 3.6$ which is essentially optimal, analysis of a 40-msec waveform implies a spectral resolution of $B_e = 90$ Hz, using the 95% power criterion. Analysis of a 100-msec waveform implies a spectral resolution of 36 Hz. In the case of a 40-msec waveform, area measurements of the power density spectrum made over frequency intervals of < 90 Hz would be subject to variability. There would also be significant interaction between spectral components spaced at < 90 Hz apart. Because late potentials have a time-varying spectrum, either moving the location of the time window, or making measurements in arbitrarily narrow frequency intervals will both make the measured spectral energy subject to variability. Improving spectral resolution using modern spectral analysis techniques, such as MEM, is a possibility if these techniques can be consistently implemented for the class of signal-averaged ECG waveforms. However, the potential improvement offered by MEM is limited in that the spectra of late potentials do not consist of isolated peaks but have a more continuous appearance.

In conclusion, the applicability of frequency-domain analysis must be judged on its clinical utility. A consideration of the properties of the signal-averaged ECG suggests that considerable difficulties in implementing a spectral analysis technique must be overcome. However, the usefulness of spectral analysis in specific circumstances, such as serial ECG analysis for testing drug efficacy, and recognition of bundle branch block, has not yet been widely investigated. Hence there may emerge an identifiable role for spectral, or spectro-temporal, analysis of the high-resolution ECG.

Acknowledgment: Portions of this research have been funded by grants from the National Institutes of Health (HL 36625), the Whitaker Foundation, and the Veterans Administration Merit Review Program.

References

1. Cain ME, Ambos HD, Witkowsi FX, Sobel BE: Fast Fourier transform analysis of signal-averaged electrocardiograms for identification of patients prone to sustained ventricular tachycardia. Circulation 69:711, 1984.
2. Lindsay BD, Ambos HD, Schechtman KB, Cain ME: Improved selection of patients for programmed ventricular stimulation by frequency analysis of signal-averaged electrocardiograms. Circulation 73:675, 1986.
3. Kelen GJ, Henkin R, Fontaine JM, El-Sherif N: Effects of analyzed signal duration and phase on the results of fast Fourier transform analysis of the surface electrocardiogram in subjects with and without late potentials. Am J Cardiol 60:1282, 1987.

4. Worley SJ, Mark DB, Smith WM, Wolf P, Califf RM, Strauss HC, Manwaring MG, Ideker RE: Comparison of time domain and frequency domain variables from the signal-averaged electrocardiogram: A multivariable analysis. J Am Coll Cardiol 11:1041, 1988.

5. Haberl R, Jilge G, Pulter R, Steinbeck G: Comparison of frequency and time domain analysis of the signal-averaged electrocardiogram in patients with ventricular tachycardia and coronary artery disease: methodologic validation and clinical relevance. J Am Coll Cardiol 12:150, 1988.

6. Oppenheim AV, Willsky AS: Signals and Systems. Englewood Cliffs, NJ: Prentice-Hall, 1983.

7. Ramirez RW: The FFT Fundamentals and Concepts. Englewood Cliffs, NJ: Prentice-Hall, 1985.

8. Gabor D: Theory of communication. J IEE 93:429, 1946.

9. Marple SL Jr: Digital Spectral Analysis—With Applications. Englewood Cliffs, NJ: Prentice-Hall, 1987.

10. Harris FJ: On the use of windows for harmonic analysis with the discrete Fourier transform. Proc IEEE 66:51, 1978.

11. de Weerd JPC, Kap JI: Spectro-temporal representations and time-varying spectra of evoked potentials. Biol Cybern 41:101, 1981.

12. Press WH, Flannery BP, Teukolsky SA, Vetterling WT: Numerical Recipes: The Art of Scientific Computing. Cambridge/London/New York/New Rochelle/Melbourne/Sydney: Cambridge University Press, 1987.

6

Techniques for Detection of His Bundle Potential in the Wolff-Parkinson-White Syndrome

Shimon Abboud, Bernard Belhassen

Introduction

High-resolution electrocardiography has been applied to record the electrical activity of the His-Purkinje system from the body surface. Studies[1-19] from different groups using various techniques of signal averaging have shown that a reliable His bundle activity can be identified in 30% to 100% of the subjects investigated and satisfactorily correlated with the His bundle activity determined by intracardiac recordings. However, three conditions have been recognized as major obstacles for easy recording of His-Purkinje activity from the body surface: (1) a short atrio-His (AH) interval or a prolonged atrial conduction time resulting in inability to separate atrial from His bundle activity; (2) a low signal-to-noise ratio that results from an excessive noise level; and (3) the location of the optimal recording lead site. In patients with Wolff-Parkinson-White syndrome (WPW), the external recording of the His bundle activity

From El-Sherif N, Turitto G (eds): *High-Resolution Electrocardiography*. Mount Kisco, NY, Futura Publishing Co., Inc., ©, 1992.

is apparently even more difficult since the His bundle activity is usually buried within the delta wave reflecting the ventricular pre-excitation. However, since the delta wave has a rising slope lower than that of the QRS complex in the absence of ventricular pre-excitation, we speculated that the electrical activity that resulted from the delta wave has frequency components lower than those of the His bundle and the QRS complex. Therefore, we used a special filtering process which reduces the electrical activity of the delta wave and presents the His bundle signal on an isoelectric line. We present here our experience with this signal averaging system which enables us to record the His bundle activity from the body surface in patients with WPW syndrome.

The Signal Averaging Technique

The externally recorded signal from the His bundle is relatively small, ranging from 1 to 10 μV, whereas the noise level of most amplifiers and electrical activity of the skeletal muscles is above these levels. High-gain amplification, signal filtering, and averaging are therefore necessary in order to improve the signal-to-noise ratio of the output signal. N waveforms are aligned in time and then summed point by point to obtain an average waveform. Assuming the noise to be random and perfect alignment of the sum waveforms to be achieved, this process increases the output signal-to-noise ratio by a factor of $\sqrt{N}$.

External Recording Instrumentation

Three unipolar precordial leads are positioned as follows: lead I at the third intercostal space and the right sternal border; lead II at the third intercostal space and the left sternal border; and lead III at the fifth intercostal space and the left sternal border. The electrocardiogram (ECG) from these leads is simultaneously recorded (with an HP 3964A recorder; bandpass filter of DC to 2500 Hz) and digitized by a 10-bit analog to digital converter with a sampling rate of 1.28 kHz. The digitized data are stored on a magnetic tape and are processed with a CDC-6600 computer. A block diagram of the instruments arrangement is given in Figure 1.

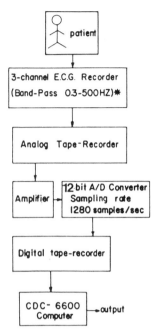

Figure 1. A block diagram representing the arrangement for data collection and processing for noninvasive recording of His bundle activity.

The Averaging Process

The ECG waveforms are averaged together to reduce the relative contribution of noise in order to obtain the His bundle activity. During the averaging process highly accurate waveform alignment and total elimination of artifacts (e.g., extrasystoles) are required. When a measurement of the similarity or the relative time delay between two ECG waveforms is necessary, correlation techniques can be used.[20–22] Therefore, the cross correlation function is a useful measurement procedure for extrasystole's rejection and for obtaining the fiducial synchronizing marks in the averaging process of ECG waveforms.[16,20,21]

The Cross Correlation Procedure

Let us assume that x(t) and y(t) are two ECG waveforms over interval T. The cross correlation function between x and y is given by the following expression:

$$Ryx(\tau) = \int_0^T y(t)x(t + \tau)dt$$

where Ryx is the averaged product of y(t) lagged with respect to x(t). When the value of the cross correlation is high for some value of the lag τ, it can be said that x(t) and y(t) are similar at this lag value. [22]

The cross correlation is normalized by dividing by the geometric mean of x(t) and y(t) mean square value, giving:

$$\Phi yx(\tau) = \frac{Ryx(\tau)}{\sqrt{Rxx(0)Ryy(0)}}$$

where Φyx is the normalized cross correlation and Rxx(0) and Ryy(0) are the autocorrelation functions of x(t) and y(t) for zero lag. When the normalized cross correlation is +1.0 for lag τ, x, and y are identical for that value of lag.

The cross correlation function is calculated by means of the cross spectrum, which is the Fourier transform of the cross correlation function:

$$Pyx = F\{Ryx\}.$$

The cross spectrum is calculated using the Fourier transform of x(t) and y(t):

$$Sx = F\{x(t)\}$$
$$Sy = F\{y(t)\}.$$

The cross spectrum is defined as:

$$Pyx = SySx^*$$

where the asterisk indicates a complex conjugate.

Figure 2 shows the recorded ECG waveforms (a,b,c) from a patient with idiopathic premature ventricular contractions (PVCs). Waveforms a and b are normal sinus beats and waveform c is a PVC. Prior to the averaging, the candidate waveforms are first passed through a nonrecursive digital bandpass filter with low-frequency cut-off at 30 Hz and high-frequency cut-off at 250 Hz, and subsequently cross correlated with a reference template. Figure 3 shows the normalized cross correlation between waveforms a and b. The maximum value is 0.924814 at time lag of 5 digitization points. Fig-

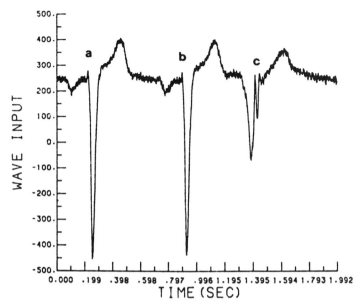

Figure 2. Recorded ECG waveforms from a patient with idiopathic premature ventricular complexes. Waveform c is a premature ventricular complex.

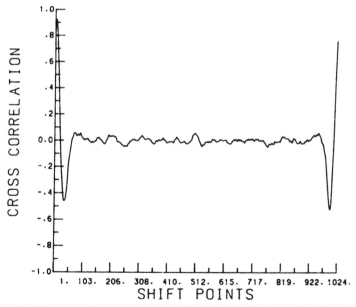

Figure 3. The normalized cross correlation function between the filtered ECG waveforms a and b shown in Figure 2. The maximum value was 0.924814 at time lag of 5 digitization points.

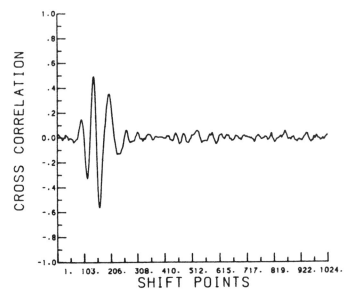

Figure 4. The normalized cross correlation function between the filtered ECG waveforms a and c shown in Figure 2. Curve c is a premature ventricular complex. The maximum value was 0.493181 at time lag of 140 digitization points.

ure 4 shows the normalized cross correlation function between waveforms a and c (a PVC). The maximum value is 0.493181 at time lag of 140 digitization points. As can be seen the maximum value of the normalized cross correlation function can be used to achieve accurate waveform alignment in the averaging process. This value decreases as an extrasystole (which is not correlated with the reference waveform) appears thus enabling the identification of artifacts.

The Filtering Process

Prior to the correlation procedure, each of the ECG waveforms is passed through a nonrecursive digital bandpass filter.[23] The filtering process takes place in the frequency (Fourier) domain using the fast Fourier transform algorithm.

Let the response of a nonrecursive digital filter, h(t), to an excitation x(t) (the ECG waveform) be z(t). This response of the filter can be computed by using the following procedure:

1. Compute H(s) and X(s) which is the Fourier transform of h(t) and x(t), respectively.
2. Compute the product Z(s) = H(s)X(s).
3. Compute the inverse Fourier transform of Z(s) which is equal to z(t).

The frequency response, H(s), of the nonrecursive digital band-pass filter which is used is represented by the following equation:

$$H(s) = [1/\sqrt{1+(S_L/s)^{2n}}][1 - 1/\sqrt{1+(S_H/s)^{2m}}]$$

where S_L is the low frequency for which $H(S_L) = 1/\sqrt{2}$ and S_H is the high frequency for which $H(S_H) = 1 - (1/\sqrt{2})$. n and m are the orders of the filter (higher n or m result in a steeper filter cut-off).

Using this filter with S_L = 30 Hz and S_H = 250 Hz appears to maintain the high-frequency components in the QRS complex while reducing interference from the noise of the equipment and low-frequency noise as the effects of respiratory variations. Figure 5 shows the frequency response of the filter. Using this filter gives more accurate results for the fiducial synchronizing marks during the correlation procedure. The fiducial points are used to align the original (unfiltered) waveforms for averaging. The averaged waveform can then be bandpass filtered to obtain the His bundle activity.

In patients without the WPW syndrome[16] where no overlap of the atrial activity over the His bundle signal occurs, various low-frequency cut-off (S_L) between 30–100 Hz can be used. The external recording of the His bundle activity from a patient without the WPW syndrome is shown in Figure 6. The upper trace is the PR interval from an averaged waveform without any digital filter but with an analog filter with a 500-Hz upper frequency cut-off and a 0.3-Hz lower frequency cut-off. From this curve, which includes the P wave, PR segment, and the beginning of the QRS complex, we can determine the time of onset of the QRS complex (Q). In the lower trace the averaged ECG waveform is bandpassed with the filter shown in Figure 5. Both curves are fully synchronized. As can be seen the averaged and filtered curve contains in the P-QRS interval a clear deflection (HQ = 47 msec) which is significantly greater than the random noise level. This deflection represents the electrical activity of the His bundle (H). The intracardiac electrogram shows an HV interval of 45 msec.

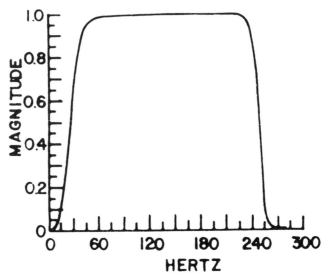

Figure 5. Frequency response of digital filter with the parameters S_L = 30 Hz, n = 2, S_H = 250 Hz, and m = 50.

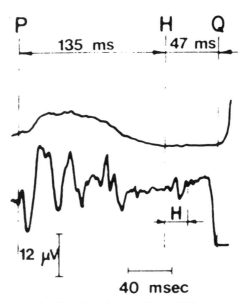

Figure 6. An example of external recording of His bundle activity from a patient without the WPW syndrome. Upper trace is the PR interval from the average of ECG waveforms without digital filtering. The lower trace is the averaged and filtered curve using digital filter with low- and high- cut-off frequencies at 30 Hz and 250 Hz, respectively. The HQ interval is 47 msec. The vertical scale applies only to the lower trace.

External His Bundle Recording in WPW Patients

In the WPW syndrome the His bundle activity is usually buried in the deflection of the delta wave which results from the ventricular pre-excitation.[24] This prevents the external recording of the His bundle activity using filters with low-frequency cut-off ranging from 30 Hz to 100 Hz. Using a bandpass digital filter with low-frequency cut-off of 150 Hz (n = 20) and high-frequency cut-off of 250 Hz (m = 50) enables the recording of the His bundle activity in patients with WPW syndrome. The frequency response of the filter is shown in Figure 7. The external recording of the His bundle activity from a patient with WPW syndrome is shown in Figure 8. Trace a is the average of the nonfiltered ECG waveforms. The three characteristic electrocardiographic features of the WPW syndrome: a delta wave; a short PR interval; and a wide QRS complex are present. Trace b is the average of the same ECG waveforms passed through a digital

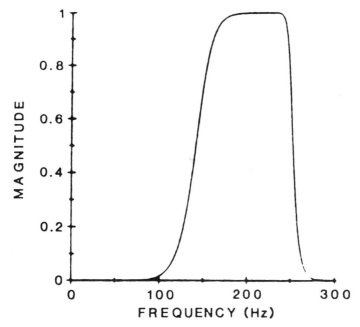

Figure 7. Frequency response of digital filter with the parameters S_L = 150 Hz, n = 10, S_H = 250 Hz, and m = 50. This filter is used for external His bundle recording in patients with WPW syndrome.

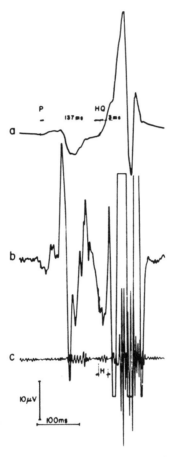

Figure 8. External recording of the His bundle activity from a patient with WPW syndrome. Trace a is the average of nonfiltered ECG waveforms; traces b and c are the average of the same ECG waveforms passed through a digital filter with low-frequency cut-off at 30 Hz (n = 2) and 150 Hz (n = 10), respectively. The His bundle activity which is masked by the delta wave cannot be recognized in trace b. Using low-frequency cut-off at 150 Hz (trace c) enables recording of the His bundle activity (HQ = +3 msec). The μV scale relates to traces b and c.

filter with low-frequency cut-off of 30 Hz. The His bundle activity which is masked by the delta wave cannot be recognized. Trace c is the average waveform passed through a digital filter with low-frequency cut-off of 150 Hz. The use of this filter reduces the electrical activity of the delta wave and presents the His bundle signal (H) on an isoelectric line (HQ = +3 msec). It seems that the electrical

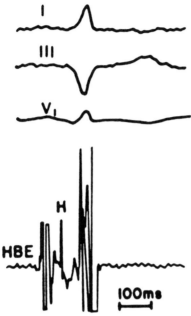

Figure 9. Intracardiac His bundle recording from the same patient shown in Figure 8. Shown are recording of ECG leads I, III, and V_1 as well as the intracardiac His bundle electrogram (HBE). HV interval is +10 msec similar to the HQ interval shown in Figure 8.

activity that results from the ventricular pre-excitation (delta wave) has frequency components up to 150 Hz, whereas the electrical activity of the His bundle has frequency components up to 250 Hz. Intracardiac His bundle recording from the same patient is shown in Figure 9. The HV interval is +10 msec similar to the HQ interval.

Effects of Ajmaline

External recording of the His bundle activity can be carried out in patients before and after the intravenous administration of ajmaline chlorhydrate (50 mg over 1 minute). The intravenous administration of ajmaline frequently abolishes the pre-excitation or lessens its degree,[25] enabling the recording of the His bundle activity while using digital filter with low-frequency cut-off of 30 Hz. External recording of the His bundle activity from a patient with WPW syndrome can be seen in Figure 10. Trace a is the average nonfiltered ECG waveforms and traces b and c are the average of the same ECG waveforms passed through a digital filter with low-frequency cut-off of 30 Hz and 150 Hz, respectively. The His bundle activity cannot be recognized in trace b. The use of a low-frequency cut-off of 150 Hz (trace c) enables recording of the His bundle activity within the QRS complex (HQ = −19 msec). The intracardiac His bundle recording is shown in Figure 11. The His bundle activity merges with the ventricular activity and the HV interval of −20 msec is similar to the HQ interval. Averaged waveforms from the same patient after the administration of ajmaline which abolishes the pre-excitation pattern can be seen in Figure 12. The His bundle activity can be recorded while using low-frequency cut-off of 30 Hz (trace b) or 150 Hz (trace c). HQ interval is 49 msec. Data obtained from the same patient during electrophysiologic study after the administration of ajmaline can be seen in Figure 13. The HV interval of 50 msec is similar to HQ interval. Results[26] which were obtained using the above described method of signal averaging on ten patients with the WPW syndrome are summarized in Table I.

Discussion

The WPW syndrome is an electrocardiographic phenomena, which denotes pre-excitation of part of the ventricles by an anomalous accessory pathway which bypasses the normal atrioventricular conduction system. The three electrocardiographic features of the WPW syndrome are: (A) a delta wave; (B) a short PR interval; and (C) a wide QRS complex.[24] In the WPW syndrome the His bundle activity may be recorded at a short interval preceding (HQ = 10–30 msec) or simultaneous with the onset of the QRS complex (HQ = 0 msec) or within the QRS complex (negative HQ interval).[24]

Many investigators have attempted to record the electrical activity of the His bundle from the body surface in patients without the WPW syndrome. Almost all the previously described methods have used analog bandpass filters with low-frequency cut-off ranging from 10 to 80 Hz. These filters are incapable of performing a total rejection of artifacts (i.e., extrasystoles) and cause temporal distortion of the electrical events along the ECG waveforms. In order to avoid the use of analog filters, McKenna et al,[14] employed a three pole Butterworth digital filter with corner frequencies of 20, 40, and 80 Hz.

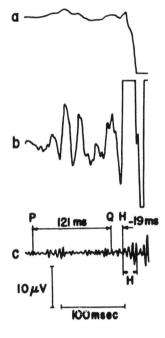

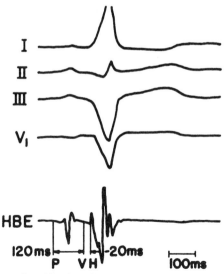

Figure 10. A second example of the external recording from another patient with WPW syndrome. The His bundle activity can be recognized only in trace c (S_L = 150 Hz, n = 10) at an HQ interval of −19 msec.

Figure 11. Intracardiac His bundle recording from the same patient as in Figure 10. The His bundle signal merges with the ventricular activity and the HV interval of −20 msec is similar to HQ interval shown in Figure 10.

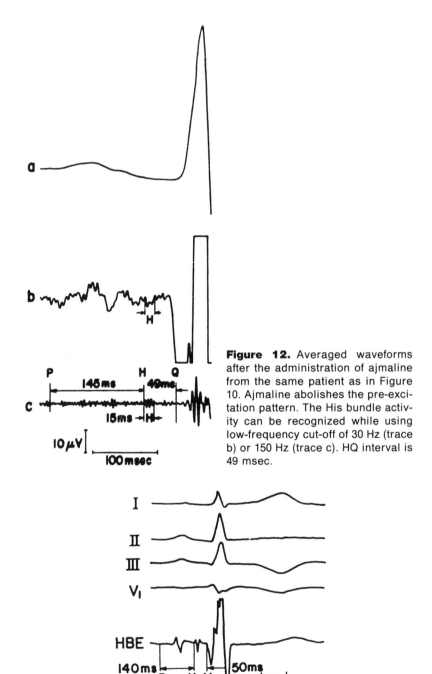

Figure 12. Averaged waveforms after the administration of ajmaline from the same patient as in Figure 10. Ajmaline abolishes the pre-excitation pattern. The His bundle activity can be recognized while using low-frequency cut-off of 30 Hz (trace b) or 150 Hz (trace c). HQ interval is 49 msec.

Figure 13. Data obtained from the same patient as in Figure 12 during electrophysiologic study after the administration of ajmaline. The HV interval of 50 msec is similar to HQ interval shown in Figure 12.

Table I
Patient Data

Patient	Sex/ Age	WPW Type	Control		After Ajmaline	
			HV	HQ	HV	HQ
1	M/36	A	+ 30	+ 28	—	—
2	M/34	B	—	+ 10	—	+ 48
3	F/28	B	—	− 33*	—	—
				+ 37**		
4	F/70	A	0	− 20	—	—
5	F/16	B	− 20	− 19	+ 50	+ 49
6	M/22	A	0	− 10	—	—
7	M/41	A	− 15	− 13	—	—
8	F/20	A	0	—	—	+ 25
9	M/48	A	0	− 10	—	+ 44
10	M/50	A	+ 10	+ 3	—	+ 40

M = Male; F = Female; HV and HQ values are in msec; * = with pre-excitation; ** = without pre-excitation.

While the use of the filter with low corner frequencies of 20 or 40 Hz causes ringing in the PR interval which overlaps the His bundle activity, the use of 80 Hz as a corner frequency, minimizes the ringing effect. In addition, during the averaging process an accurate waveform alignment is necessary. Goovaerts et al[27] count three common causes for jittered triggering which interfere with correct alignment of successive ECG waveforms: (1) low-frequency components and baseline shift (DC shift); (2) variations in the steepness of the signal; and (3) variations in the steepness as a result of variations in amplitude. When using these signal averaging techniques, with analog or recursive digital filters, recording the His bundle activity in patients with WPW syndrome may be difficult, even impossible because of sizable overlapping by the electrical activity resulting from the delta wave. Indeed, analog or recursive digital filters with frequency response similar to that used in our method will be difficult to obtain without phase shift and ringing effects. The nonrecursive digital filters using the fast Fourier transform algorithm have absolutely constant bandpass limits and gain, and thus, the error which is introduced with gain changes of the analog filters is avoided. The nonrecursive filter with low-frequency cut-off of 150 Hz reduces the electrical activity of the delta wave and presents the His bundle signal on an isoelectric line. Cross correlation function is used to achieve highly accurate waveform alignment during the averaging process and enables the total elimination of artifacts (e.g., extrasystoles).

Our data confirm our speculation that the electrical activity resulting from the ventricular pre-excitation has frequency components lower than those of the electrical activity of the His bundle. Thus, the use of nonrecursive bandpass digital filter with low-frequency cut-off of 150 Hz and high-frequency cut-off of 250 Hz separates the His bundle signal from that of the delta wave. In addition, a drug known to affect ventricular pre-excitation, can be used to separate the His bundle activity from that of the delta wave. Ajmaline abolishes conduction in the accessory pathway or lessens the degree of pre-excitation that enables recording of the His bundle while using a digital filter with a low-frequency cut-off of 30 Hz. Following the administration of ajmaline, the deflection of the His bundle activity has a low amplitude. This is most probably due to the fact that the minimal number of cycles which have to be averaged (250–300) are recorded at a time when the electrophysiologic effects of ajmaline on the conduction system show slight, but continuous, change.

Based on the results of our previous studies we found a good correlation between the HV and the HQ intervals measured invasively and noninvasively, respectively.[16] The discrepancy of a few milliseconds, which was noted between these two values, might be explained in part by the difficulties in determining accurately the onset of the delta wave in the internal His bundle recording. However, this discrepancy is within the uncertainty of the measurements and we believe that it does not have any clinical significance.

In conclusion, the use of a computerized cross correlation method which employed nonrecursive digital filters with the fast Fourier transform algorithm enables the external accurate recording of the His bundle activity in patients with the WPW syndrome.

References

1. Berbari EJ, Lazzara R, Samet P, Scherlag BJ: Noninvasive technique for detection of electrical activity during the P-R segment. Circulation 48:-1005, 1973.
2. Flowers NC, Hand RC, Orander PC, Miller CB, Walden MO, Horan LG: Surface recording of electrical activity from the region of the bundle of His. Am J Cardiol 33:384, 1974.
3. Hishimoto Y, Sawayama T: Noninvasive recording of His bundle potential in man: simplified method. Br Heart J 37:635, 1975.
4. Berbari EJ, Scherlag BJ, El-Sherif N, Befeler B, Aranda JM, Lazzara R: The His-Purkinje electrocardiogram in man. An initial assessment of its uses and limitations. Circulation 54:219, 1976.
5. Vincent R, Stroud NP, Jenner R, English MJ, Woollons DJ, Chamberlain DA: Noninvasive recording of electrical activity in the PR segment in man. Br Heart J 40:124, 1978.
6. Wajszczuk WJ, Stopczyk MJ, Moskowitz MS, Zochowski RJ, Bauld T, Dabos PL, Rubenfire M: Noninvasive recording of His-Purkinje activity in man by QRS-triggered signal averaging. Circulation 58:95, 1978.
7. Berbari EJ, Lazzara R, El-Sherif N, Scherlag BJ: Extracardiac-recording of His-Purkinje activity during conduction disorders and junctional rhythms. Circulation 51:802, 1975.
8. Furness A, Sharratt GP, Carson P: The feasibility of detecting His-bundle activity from the body surface. Cardiovasc Res 9:390, 1975.
9. Van den Akker TJ, Ros HH, Goovaerts HG, Schneider H: Real-time method for noninvasive recording of His bundle activity of the electrocardiogram. Com Biomed Res 9:559, 1976.
10. Takeda H, Kitamura K, Takanaski T, Tokuoka T, Hamamoto H, Katoh T, Niki I, Hishimoto Y: Noninvasive recording of His-Purkinje activity in patients with complete atrioventricular block. Clinical application of an automated discrimination circuit. Circulation 60:421, 1979.
11. Rozanski JJ, Castellanos A: Clinical evaluation of an improved high resolution ECG cart for recording the His bundle electrogram noninvasively. PACE 3:479, 1980.
12. deFeyter PJ, Ros HH, Majid PA, van Eenige MJ, Karreman J, Roos JP: Clinical evaluation of His bundle electrogram recorded from the body surface. Clin Cardiol 4:80, 1981.
13. Mohammad Djafari A, Heron F, Duperdu R, Perrin J: Noninvasive recording of the His Purkinje system electrical activity by a digital system design. J Biomed Eng 3:147, 1981.
14. McKenna WJ, Rowland E, Mortara D, Divers T, Krikler DM: Noninvasive recording of the His bundle electrogram: value of supplementary verapamil. PACE 4:281, 1981.
15. Mehra R, Kelen GJ, Zeiler R, Zephiran D, Fried P, Gomes JA, El-Sherif N: Noninvasive His bundle electrogram: value of three vector lead recordings. Am J Cardiol 49:344, 1982.

16. Abboud S, Belhassen B, Pelleg A, Laniado S, Sadeh D: An advanced noninvasive technique for the recording of His bundle potential in man. J Electrocardiol 16:397, 1983.
17. Nathan AW, Bexton RS, Levy AM, Parmar N, Camm AJ: Noninvasive recording of the His bundle electrogram in neonates. Pediatr Cardiol 5:7, 1984.
18. Ward DE, Makinen L, Jones S, Carter S, Shinebourne E: Signal averaged electrocardiography in infants and children with congenital heart disease. Int J Cardiol 6:699, 1984.
19. Otsuka K, Otsuka K, Nojima K, Saito H, Seto K, Ozawa T: The applicability of noninvasive His bundle electrogram to assessing the effect of digitalis on atrioventricular conduction. Clin Cardiol 9:203, 1986.
20. Abboud S, Sadeh D: The waveform's alignment procedure in the averaging process for external recording of the His bundle activity. Com Biomed Res 15:212, 1982.
21. Abboud S, Sadeh D: The use of cross-correlation function for the alignment of ECG waveforms and rejection of extrasystoles. Com Biomed Res 17:258, 1984.
22. Roth PR: Effective measurements using digital signal analysis. IEEE Spectrum 8:62, 1971.
23. Abboud S, Sadeh D: The digital filtering process in the external recording of the His bundle activity. Com Biomed Res 15:418, 1982.
24. Narula OS: Wolff-Parkinson-White syndrome. A review. Circulation 47:872, 1973.
25. Eschchar Y, Belhassen B, Laniado S: Comparison of exercise and ajmaline test with electrophysiologic study in the Wolff-Parkinson-White syndrome. Am J Cardiol 57:782, 1986.
26. Abboud S, Belhassen B, Pelleg A, Laniado S, Sadeh D: Noninvasive recording of His bundle activity in patients with Wolff-Parkinson-White syndrome. PACE 7:40, 1984.
27. Goovaerts HG, Ros HH, Van den Akker TJ, Schneider H: A digital QRS detector based on the principle of contour limiting. IEEE Trans Biomed Eng 23:154, 1976.

7

High-Resolution Electrocardiography and Magnetocardiography

Riccardo R. Fenici, Mariella Masselli,
Luisa Lopez, Guido Melillo

Introduction

The noninvasive study of cardiac electrogenesis is an intriguing problem which has challenged the electrophysiologist and clinical cardiologist since almost 100 years ago. So far, all the investigation methods have been variants of potential measurements at the body surface. Therefore, although the advent of vectorcardiography and body surface mapping has improved the time resolution and sensitivity of the electric measurements for specific diagnosis, still all these methods suffer from the limitations intrinsic to all surface potential recordings. First of all, the surface potential is only indirectly linked to the primary intracellular electrogenetic phenomena (the action currents), as it is a representation of the extracellular potential changes induced by the intracellular primary sources.[1,2,3] Moreover the flux of the volume currents, which carries the potential difference at the surface of the torso, is significantly affected by the conductivity of the different tissues, which generates secondary

From El-Sherif N, Turitto G (eds): *High-Resolution Electrocardiography*. Mount Kisco, NY, Futura Publishing Co., Inc., ©, 1992.

sources and somehow distorts the potential distribution at the body surface. Taking into account the effects of the different boundaries, an inverse solution could be attempted to reconstruct from surface recordings the potential distribution at the epicardial level.[4] However, even so, the information is still limited at the extracellular level.

In theory, the major advantage in measuring magnetic fields is that the normal component of the magnetic field is directly linked to the intracellular action current of fibers tangential to the chest surface[2] and only partially affected by the volume currents (secondary sources).[3,5] The magnetocardiogram (MCG) therefore, should provide more direct information about the cardiac generators in respect to the electrocardiogram (ECG), which is significantly affected by inhomogeneity of tissue conductivity. Although there is a partial loss of information about fibers which are perpendicular to the chest, the field generated by the tangential component of oblique fibers will maintain a symmetric pattern. This means that the major advantage of MCG is to localize, by a simple mapping on the anterior chest wall, cardiac sources which would not be electrically localized.[1]

The amplitudes of the magnetic fields generated by bioelectric sources, quantified during the last 10 years, range between $10°$ and 10^{-15} femtoteslas ($1fT = 10^{-15}$ Tesla). The earth magnetic field micropulsations, line frequency and harmonics, or other instrumentations located in proximity of the biomagnetic sensor can generate "noise" in the frequency range of the bioelectric signals (0.01–1 KHz), which can be orders of magnitude stronger than the biomagnetic fields themselves. The "noise" therefore, can be defined as any kind of unwanted magnetic field of intensity strong enough to impede an adequate detection of the signal of interest. This means that in order to detect the biomagnetic fields we need sensors of sufficient sensitivity and method to reduce the ambient noise.[1,6–9] The technology for magnetic studies has greatly advanced since 1963 when an MCG was recorded for the first time by means of induction coils.[10] Subsequently a fundamental progress was achieved when, in 1970, a superconducting instrumentation was used to record the MCG in the magnetically shielded room of the MIT.[11,12] The Superconducting Quantum Interference Devices (SQUID) has the necessary sensitivity to investigate all kinds of biomagnetic fields. However, measurements of the magnetic field associated with bioelectric activity of the human heart in a clinical setting requires a higher level of performance from the instrumentation than the one generally needed for laboratory researches.[13,14] The development of gradiometric detection coils was a significant step forward to improve the sensitivity of biomagnetic instrumentations which allowed first magnetocardiographic recording in unshielded laboratories[13,15-18] and the introduction of biomagnetism in the hospital environment.[14,19-35] An additional help to reduce environmental noise to levels comparable with, or even smaller than, the amplitude of the signals to be measured, can be the use of electromagnetic shielding.[1,3,8,9,11,36,37] The latter method, initially too expensive for a widespread application in hospital laboratories, has been significantly improved during the last few years. With present technology reasonably large (about 30 m) shielded rooms, with an effective depletion of line frequency noise larger than 90 dB, and weight adequate for clinical setting, can be purchased at relatively low prices.[1,9]

As mentioned above, the most significant advantage of biomagnetic recordings is the capability to localize, in the three dimensions, bioelectric sources with an uncertainty of only few millimeters.[28,34,38,39] During the last few years the biomagnetic method has given important results in the field of neurophysiology, such as the experimental demonstration of the tonotopic organization of the auditory cortex, the identification of epileptic foci in partial epilepsy and the study of spontaneous brain activity.[1,40-42]

Concerning the heart, although the analysis of MCGs at a resolution comparable with that of standard ECGs has improved the diagnostic sensitivity in specific pathology[43-51] this would probably not justify enough the use of such an expensive method at clinical level. However, during the last 5 years computer processing of magnetocardiographic maps has been demonstrated to be effective in giving three-dimensional images of the depolarization pathways of the His-Purkinje system[15,16,19,21,23-25,38,52-54] and of the Kent bundles.[26,29,31,32,34,35,38,39] More recently, three-dimensional localization of the site of origin of ventricular tachycardia and focal atrial tachycardia have been attempted as well.[33-35] This "functional" localization capability, based on the development of a relatively simple mathematical model of the cardiac sources to confront the "inverse problem",[55,56] has been used since the early 1980s to give images of physiologic and pathologic phenomena in the human heart. Erroneously this MCG localization method has maintained the original denomination of "high-resolution magnetocardiography," used by some authors when attempting first high-resolution analysis of the

MCG waveform in order to recruit low amplitude signals in the PR interval. [16,19] Indeed it is evident that its "functional localization" capability provides unrivaled resolution for the study of cardiac electrophysiology, and has allowed the interpretation of highly amplified ECG waveforms whose electrogenesis was unclear. [27,57] However, it is our opinion that the term "high resolution," as conventionally used in electrocardiography, is misleading and should not be used for magnetocardiography, which should be considered only one of the applications of the "biomagnetic imaging" method.

In spite of the strong evidence that the biomagnetic imaging could be useful for the noninvasive study of cardiac electrophysiology, still there are difficulties for the biomagnetic method to enter in the clinical arsenal, mostly because of technological limitations. Indeed, there are some points which require deeper experience to define, for example, the optimal instrumental configuration, the recording protocols, the data analysis, and presentation which could be appropriate for clinical work. [1,9,17,58]

In this chapter we will mainly describe the results of cardiac studies which can trace a perspective for the potential application of magnetocardiography at a diagnostic level. However, a brief summary of the "state of art" of instrumentation and a simple outline of the problem of modeling biomagnetic sources will be given, as well as an introduction for the clinical cardiologist into the world of biomagnetism.

Instrumentation

When dealing with magnetic heart signals, the amplitude of the magnetic fields generated by the ventricles (in the order of several picotesla [pT]) is sufficiently high, so that it would not be necessary to use a SQUID for all kinds of measurements. [59]

However, dealing with smaller fields, like those generated by atrial activity or His-Purkinje system, a superconducting sensor is mandatory. Schematically, a superconducting instrumentation consists of a cryogenic part contained in a superinsulated fiberglass Dewar filled with liquid helium to keep the temperature as low as 4.2 kelvin. At that temperature, the detection coil becomes intrinsically noise free. The magnetic field sensed by the detection coil generates a proportional current in the superconducting flux transporter which, by means of an input coil, imposes a magnetic flux to the

SQUID that converts it into a voltage. The output voltage is proportional to the magnetic field over a frequency range between 0 and 10 kHz. At first radiofrequency-biased SQUIDs have been used, being that these devices are reliable and sufficiently stable in their performance. More recently, microfabricated ultra-low noise dcSQUIDs are replacing radiofrequency SQUIDs, being that the former was more reliable for the development of integrated multisensor devices.

Although it is well demonstrated that the SQUID has sufficient sensitivity to investigate all cardiac magnetic fields, indeed their field sensitivity is not particularly high. Therefore, it is necessary to couple the SQUID to an external detection coil, whose shape can be adjusted to achieve the best reduction of ambient noise and improve spatial discrimination. For a detailed description of the instrumental problems, the interested reader is addressed to recent exhaustive review articles.[1,3,7,9] Here we will only mention that the gradiometric geometries so far used for magnetocardiographic recordings have the common feature of a vertical symmetry axis. A more recent approach consists of using a planar configuration and integrating the gradiometer directly in the same chip that contains the planar SQUID.[1,40,42,60] The interest in using planar first-order or higher order gradiometers is to improve the spatial resolution because the net magnetic flux from a more distant source is reduced in favor of the closest sources. Moreover, microfabricated planar gradiometers should simplify the integration of a large number of magnetic sensors in a complex multichannel system in respect of accurate balancing of each channel. To summarize, the advantages of the use of planar gradiometers would be: (1) higher rejection factor of the "noise"; (2) larger sensitivity to higher spatial frequency[60]; and (3) better "intrinsic" balancing. However, as planar gradiometers measure field differences, the detected patterns are more complex and do not show the symmetry for different orientation of the source. This implies different computer processing.[42]

Mathematical Models

In cardiomagnetism, interesting results have been obtained in the localization of equivalent sources during the activation of the heart conduction system, as well as during ventricular pre-excitation, using the Equivalent Current Dipole (ECD) model for the expansion of the primary source density.[22,38,61-63] However, this first-order approximation model works well when the active tissue is relatively small.[64] On the contrary, when a larger mass of myocardium or different areas of the heart are simultaneously activated, the ECD model represents only the major part (around 80%) of the measured field, but some contribution due to other dipolar sources, or to higher order terms of the current multipole would be erroneously neglected with consequent errors in the localization procedures.[39,61,62,64] For this reason, during the last 7 years there has been a growing interest in the use of multipole expansions of primary sources for the study of cardiac magnetic fields.[39,61,62,65,66] Localization procedures based on these more sophisticated mathematical models require more computer work and time. However, they are probably mandatory when source localization is attempted in specific cardiac pathology which implies pathologic anisotropic myocardium,[67] like for instance in the arrhythmogenic myocardial infarction.

Clinical Applications

First, high-resolution magnetocardiographic recordings in our unshielded hospital laboratory were carried out at the beginning of 1982.[14,21,24] Since then more than 100 patients affected by different kinds of cardiac pathology were studied.[30,35] Since the beginning our approach was to introduce magnetocardiography in the hospital and to define its potentiality as a diagnostic tool. In theory, the method had the potentiality to provide information about the three-dimensional spread of myocardial activation currents, thus resulting in "functional" imaging of electrophysiologic phenomena. However, in order to validate this hypothesis it became necessary to compare MCG data with other electrophysiologic parameters and even perform MCG mapping during cardiac pacing. This was apparently impossible taking into account the natural electromagnetic noise of a catheterization laboratory and the artifacts induced by ferromagnetic material usually present in commercial electrocatheters.[28] Therefore, the experimental measurements here reported became possible only after the set up of our laboratory, which satisfies the needs of a biomagnetic facility and a cardiac catheterization room.

The Magnetocardiographic Mapping has been performed with the prototype of a commercial biomagnetic instrumentation (BIO-

MAG I, Elettronica S.p.A., Rome, Italy) which is based on a single channel radiofrequency SQUID. In order to reduce the ambient noise, working in an unshielded room, a vertical second-order gradiometer is used, shaped in such a way as to be insensitive to fields generated by sources far and different from the patient's heart.[1,6,14]

Two different symmetric second-order gradiometers have been subsequently used in our laboratory, the diameter of the pick-up coil being 3 or 1.5 cm, respectively. In both gradiometers a baseline of 5 cm was adopted as the best compromise between optimal sensitivity to the investigated field and rejection of the environmental noise.[34,35,58]

The output of the SQUID is preamplified and coupled to a COMB filter to reject power line interferences (50 Hz) and harmonics. The final amplification and filtering before A/D conversion is provided by a custom made four-channel signal conditioning unit for the magnetocardiographic and three surface electric signals. This system consists of three optically isolated preamplifiers coupled to high-pass RC filters with a time constant of 10 seconds, intermediate adjustable gain amplifiers, and final low-pass filters (eight poles Bessel type). The three preamplified channels are used for surface electrical recordings. The input to the electric channels are three couples of Ag/AgCl surface chest electrodes. Their outputs can be electronically added to obtain a single, spatially averaged, high-resolution bipolar ECG (HR ECG). The fourth channel is used to handle the magnetic signal in the same way (bandwidth 0.016–250 Hz).

Magnetocardiographic recordings are performed in supine position, mapping the signal sequentially from 36 positions over the anterior chest wall according to the standard grid proposed by Karp et al[46] (Figure 1A), which is normalized to the size of the subject's chest. However, the recording grid can be shifted or reduced to obtain a more appropriate window for the study of specific pathology. Intraindividual reproducibility of MCG measurements has been tested by repeating MCG mapping in different recording sessions (Figures 2 and 3), with the same and/or different gradiometers, and with different extension of the recording grid.

Magnetocardiographic computer processing is performed, after 12-bit resolution A/D conversion, with an HP A700 minicomputer. The software programs, previously described in detail,[36,38,55] allow analysis of the recordings in the time domain at various levels of resolution, isofield contour map drawing, and automatic computa-

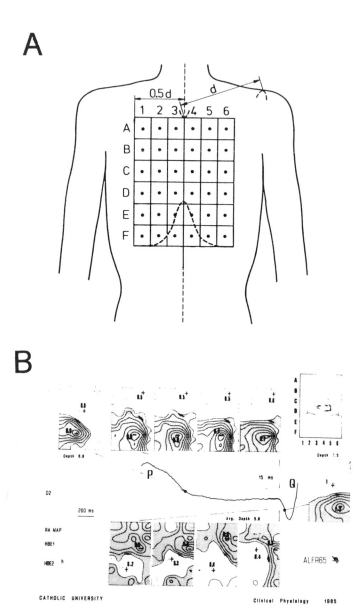

Figure 1. (A) Standard recording grid for MCG mapping.[46] A seventh column could substitute column 1 when studying left-sided abnormalities. (B) Magnetic field distribution patterns and ECD localization during the PR interval of a normal subject: typical atrial repolarization field pattern (upper maps), septal depolarization field (middle), and His-Purkinje system activation pattern after subtraction of atrial repolarization (bottom maps). By comparison with catheter recording of the HV interval (bottom left) it is evident that the MCG is sensitive, in this case, only to the last 15 msec of the His-Purkinje system activity.

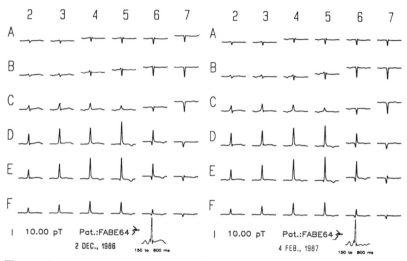

Figure 2. Intraindividual reproducibility of the MCG waveforms, mapped 2 months apart, in a patient with a left posterolateral Kent bundle.

tion of the ECD parameters when a magnetic field distribution of dipolar configuration is experimentally found.[22,38,39] Further offline processing provides bidimensional as well as three-dimensional displays of cardiac activation pathways, given by the movement of the ECD, in function of time, within the patient's heart silhouette (Figure 1B).

Validation of Magnetocardiographic Localization Accuracy

Mapping of the magnetic field distribution, automatic computation of the intensity, and three-dimensional localization of the equivalent cardiac sources, which have been successful even with the obvious limitations of sequential mapping carried out with a single channel, represent an important step forward to obtain, noninvasively, a functional imaging of cardiac electrogenesis. However, a validation of the MCG method is necessary. In our laboratory it has been performed by: (1) testing the intraindividual reproducibility of the measurements; (2) testing the accuracy of the MCG localization by comparison with invasive (endocardial and/or epicardial) map-

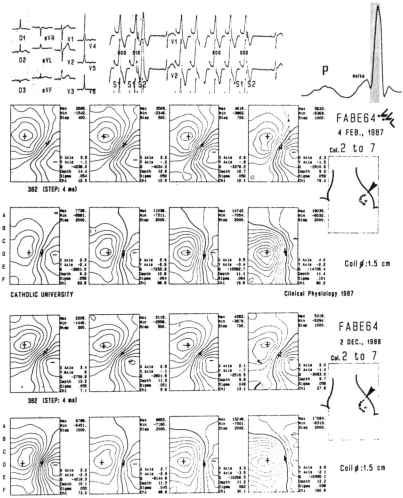

Figure 3. Same patient as in Figure 2. Reproducibility of the field distribution and ECD localization which fairly depicts a left posterolateral pre-excitation pathway. The site of onset of pre-excitation is marked by the arrow.

ping; and (3) inversely localizing an artificial dipolar source, that is, a catheter pacing the heart independently localized by three-dimensional fluoroscopy.

Clinical Measurements

His-Purkinje System

First high amplification analysis of the magnetic PR segment was reported by Farrell and coworkers in 1978,[15] who described a small "bump" superimposed to the slow varying waveform after the end of the P wave. In 1980 a "ramp" pattern, changing polarity more or less symmetrically across the longitudinal axis of the heart, was found mapping the signal systematically over the anterior chest wall.[16,19,22] Immediately the question arose whether the "bump" or the "ramp" should be interpreted as related to the His-Purkinje activation.[15,16,19-21,68] In order to clarify this problem, both experimental animal studies[68] and mathematical modeling were used.[22,38,52,53,56] Unfortunately, the results of such investigations were partially contradictory. Therefore, a definitive interpretation of the magnetic waveform in the time domain was impossible. In fact, despite the satisfactory agreement between theoretical predictions on the basis of mathematical models of the His-Purkinje system[22,55,56,69] and the measured patterns, the stronger field generated by atrial repolarization which overlaps the His-Purkinje activity could significantly affect the measurements. This point has been long debated.[53,68,69] Only recently, by analyzing the field distribution patterns, it has been demonstrated that whereas the contribution of atrial repolarization is properly subtracted, a remaining field is reproducibly measurable in the last part of the PR interval, whose duration can be in agreement with the duration of the simultaneously recorded HV interval.[25,28] In other cases, like the one shown in Figure 1B, the His-Purkinje system field can be detected only in the terminal part of the PR interval. This could be due to excessive background noise, or to individual variants in the geometry of the system with a common His bundle perpendicular to the anterior chest wall. However, although the MCG "functional" localization method has given images of cardiac activation pathway during the PR interval, well in agreement with the anatomy of the conduction system (Figure 1B),[23,24,30] further experimental work is needed in this field to ascertain whether or not the MCG method could provide information of potential diagnostic use.

Wolff-Parkinson-White Syndrome

First MCG recording in one patient with Wolff-Parkinson-White syndrome has been reported by Erne' and Fenici in 1984.[38] Since then several preliminary measurements but no systematic perspective work have been published.[7,26,30,32,33,39]

In our laboratory, 21 patients with stable ventricular pre-excitation on the surface 12-lead ECG were magnetically studied during spontaneous sinus rhythm. An example of MCG waveforms mapping is given in Figure 2, where the similarity between magnetocardiographic and electrocardiographic waveforms is appreciable, as well as the intraindividual reproducibility of the magnetic measurements. In figure 3, the isofield contour maps are shown, computed in time coincidence with the delta wave and QRS of the same patient. Again the reproducibility of magnetic field distribution and three-dimensional localization of the left-sided pre-excitation pathway are striking, in spite of a time lag of about 2 months between the two recording sessions. Four different patterns of cardiac pre-excitation were reproducibly found in the 21 investigated patients (Figure 4). Eleven patients had paraseptal accessory pathways, all of them magnetically localized at the right side of the interventricular septum.[32] Significant interindividual reproducibility of the MCG pattern was found in all patients with similar Kent bundle localizations. Ajmaline and/or flecainide induced normalization of atrio-ventricular conduction provided additional information about the respective three-dimensional localization of normal and abnormal atrio-ventricular activation pathways and was helpful to evaluate the locations of the accessory pathways with respect to the interventricular septum. An example of pharmacologic validation of the right insertion of a paraseptal Kent bundle is given in Figure 5. All symptomatic patients were invasively investigated. Therefore validation of MCG localization of the pre-excited areas was possible by comparison with conventional endocardial mapping or direct catheter recording of the Kent bundle electrogram.[26,29] In one case surgical interruption was necessary, because of drug resistant paroxysmal atrial fibrillation, inducing syncopal attacks with ventricular rates

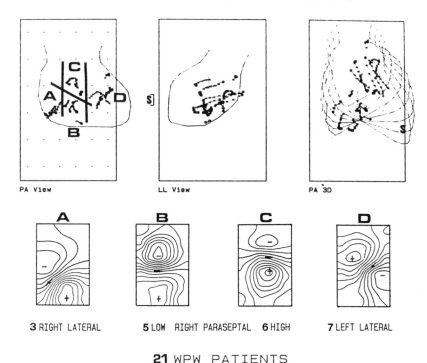

PA View   LL View   PA 3D

A   B   C   D

3 RIGHT LATERAL   **5** LOW RIGHT PARASEPTAL **6** HIGH   **7** LEFT LATERAL

21 WPW PATIENTS

Figure 4. Twenty-one Wolff-Parkinson-White patients: MCG imaging of pre-excitation pathways. Four different localizations (A–D) are clearly defined on the posteroanterior (PA) view (top left). The respective magnetic field distributions are shown at the bottom. All paraseptal tracts are right sided. Five low are more posterior (B), six high are more anterior (C). All localizations have been normalized to the center of the 36-point grid. The heart silhouette is an average of the different individual hearts.

as high as 300 beats/min. In this patient a comparison was possible between MCG localization of the pre-excited area, catheter mapping, epicardial mapping, and the anatomic location of the Kent bundle. The average three-dimensional localization uncertainty was expressed by a sphere, being the diameter equal to the distance found, in the three dimensions, between the position of the mapping catheter (or epicardial probe) closer to the pre-excited area, and the magnetic reconstruction of the pre-excitation pathways (Figures 2, 3, and 6). The anatomic location of the left Kent bundle was fluoroscopically identifiable, after surgery, by localizing several hemostatic radiopaque clips placed in the area of successful cryoablation.

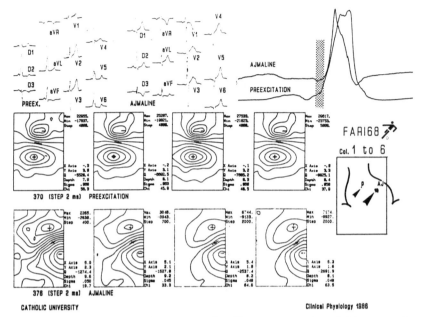

Figure 5. Right paraseptal Kent bundle. The pre-excitation field pattern is shown (upper maps). The localization of the pre-excited area is marked by the smaller arrow in the heart silhouette. After ajmaline-induced block of the accessory pathway, normal septal activation pattern is observed (bottom maps). The site of normal depolarization of the interventricular septum is indicated by the bigger arrow (Aj). It is immediately evident that the pre-excitation initiates at the right of the interventricular septum.

It has been indicated, in Figure 6, by an open square in the patient's heart silhouette together with the results of the MCG localization. The average three-dimensional uncertainty was 10 mm (range 3–26 mm). The minimal error was observed when it was assumed that the ECD calculated in time coincidence with the transition between the delta wave and the R wave was representative of the Kent bundle localization. In the same case the reproducibility and accuracy of source localization was also tested as a function of the number of mapped grid points. By decreasing the number of recording points from 36 to 16 the average three-dimensional localization accuracy didn't change significantly, the average three-dimensional uncertainty being 11 mm (range: 7–19 mm).

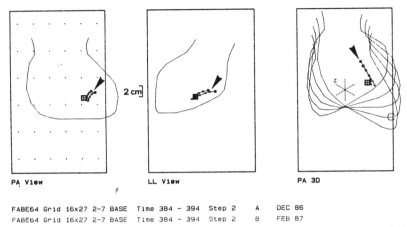

PA View   LL View   PA 3D

FABE64 Grid 16x27 2-7 BASE   Time 384 - 394   Step 2   A   DEC 86
FABE64 Grid 16x27 2-7 BASE   Time 384 - 394   Step 2   B   FEB 87

Figure 6. Left posterolateral Kent bundle (same case as in Figures 2 and 3). The anatomic location of the accessory pathway, inferred by epicardial mapping, is marked by the open square. The MCG imaging of the pre-excitation pathway starts with the onset of the delta wave (arrow). The minimal divergence between MCG and surgical localization was obtained with ECD computation at the transition between delta and R waves.

Localization of Ventricular Arrhythmias

First localization of the site of origin of a ventricular tachycardia has been reported by Fenici et al in a patient affected by arrhythmogenic right ventricular dysplasia.[35] Since then, magnetic localization of ventricular arrhythmias has been attempted in several patients with stable ventricular bigeminy and in two other patients with iterative ventricular tachycardia. The major problem to face when studying ventricular arrhythmias is that sequential mapping with a single sensor is too long lasting for the study of risk patients. Nevertheless, we have recently had the opportunity to investigate one patient with stable and well tolerated post-myocardial infarction ventricular tachycardia. In Figure 7 magnetic reconstruction of ventricular depolarization pathway during the arrhythmia is shown. The onset of ventricular depolarization (marked by the arrow) is localized in the postero-infero-lateral wall of the left ventricle, where a dyskinetic area was documented with two-dimensional echocardiography and phase analysis of gated pool scintigraphic images. Fragmented and continuous activity were found, with endo-

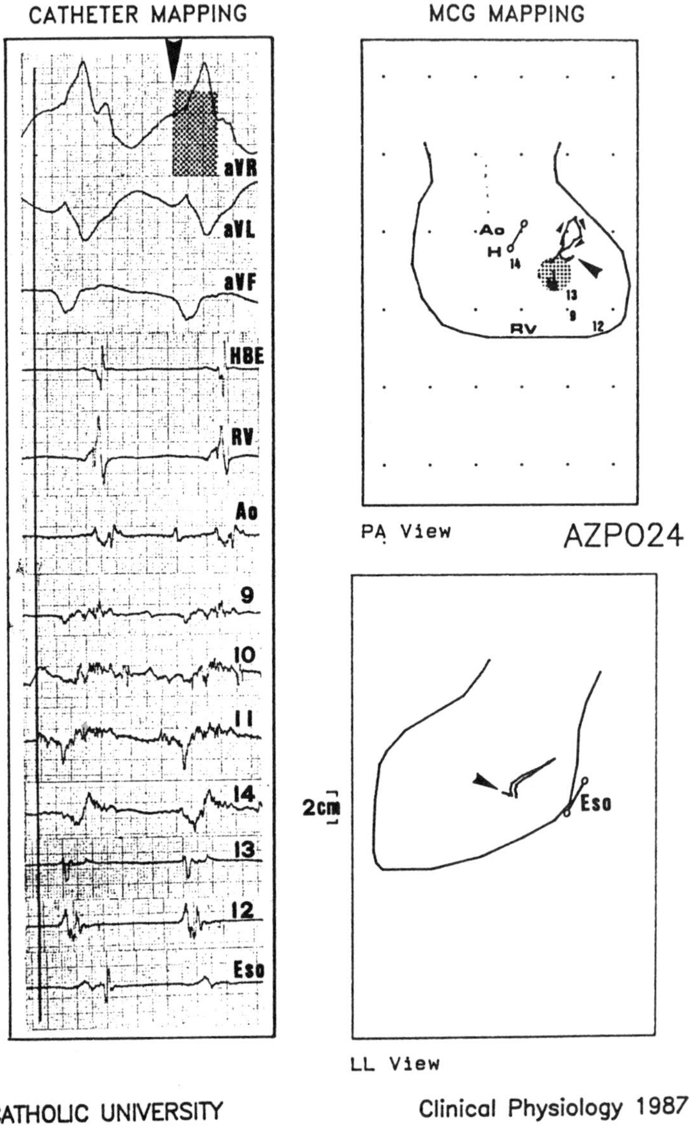
CATHETER MAPPING
MCG MAPPING
aVR
aVL
aVF
HBE
RV
Ao
9
10
11
14
13
12
Eso
Ao
H
14
13
9
RV
12
PA View
AZPO24
2cm
Eso
LL View
CATHOLIC UNIVERSITY
Clinical Physiology 1987

Figure 7. MCG localization of a sustained ventricular tachycardia. The onset of ventricular depolarization (marked by the arrow) is magnetically localized in the postero-infero-lateral wall of the left ventricle (right column), well in agreement with the results of catheter mapping (left column).

cardial catheter mapping during ventricular tachycardia (Figure 7), in proximity of the area of the left ventricle properly identified by the MCG as the site of origin of the arrhythmia. Obviously, few successful observations are insufficient to define the reliability of the MCG method for ventricular tachycardia localization, taking into account that pathologic anisotropy could, in other cases, generate magnetic field of nondipolar configuration and prevent a correct MCG localization of the arrhythmogenic area with a first-order inverse solution like the ECD presently used in our laboratory. However in such situations, as well as in the case of multiple accessory pathways, other kinds of inverse solution, like current multipole expansion, could be effective.[46,61,62,65-67]

Localization of a Pacing Catheter

Magnetocardiographic mapping during cardiac pacing was initially attempted by us, in patients undergoing invasive electrophysiology for clinical reasons, in order to quantify the accuracy of the biomagnetic method in localizing a dipolar source placed in the human heart. When performing MCG mapping under cardiac pacing, commercial intracardiac electrocatheters induced rhythmic, rate-dependent artifacts, due to the presence of ferromagnetic material. This drawback, which obviously prevented the recording of good quality MCGs, was overcome by manufacturing custom nonferromagnetic electrocatheters differently designed for pacing or monophasic action potential recordings (CNR Patent procedure n.47702A88). Fluoroscopic imaging of the position of the pacing dipole in the patient's heart was independently obtained with digital processing of orthogonal X-ray projections. Radiopaque references were placed on the chest surface as well as in the esophagus to define, in individual patients, the position and size of the heart as well as that of the catheters, with respect to the MCG recording grid.[32,35] The MCG three-dimensional localization of the pacing catheter was successful in all the ten investigated cases, being the average localization error 10 ±5 mm in the three dimensions. Best accuracy was found when pacing the apex of the right ventricle (Figure 8). Similar quantitative results have been recently reported by other authors both with an experimental animal study[70] and in two patients with implanted cardiac pacemakers.[71]

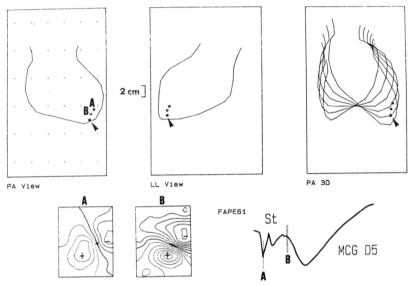

Figure 8. Magnetocardiographic localization of a pacing catheter. The fluoroscopic position of the catheter (right ventricular apex) is indicated by the black arrow. Point A is the MCG localization computed in time coincidence with the peak of the pacing field (three-dimensional error: 18 mm). Point B is the MCG localization computed at the onset of the evoked myocardial response (three-dimensional error: 9 mm).

Perspectives

So far almost all currently used cardiologic methods have been used to attempt a noninvasive localization of arrhythmogenic tissue expecially in patients with cardiac pre-excitation.[72-75] However, as recently pointed out by Gallagher,[76] the problem remains as to what the "gold standard" is to test their accuracy.

The results of our perspective work on patients with Wolff-Parkinson-White Syndrome demonstrate that magnetocardiography is highly effective in reproducibly localizing different pre-excitation pathways in patients with this syndrome. The above mentioned difficulties have been encountered to define the localization accuracy of the biomagnetic method. In fact, in spite of the promising results of preliminary research work,[30,34,38,52] the accuracy of the biomagnetic method to localize human cardiac sources has not so far been quantitatively determined.

The localization error of Kent-type accessory pathways found in our laboratory is satisfactory low, if the results of epicardial mapping and surgery are assumed as gold standard for validation. In the operated patient in fact the average three-dimensional localization error was 10 mm (Figure 6). Unfortunately, so far, the comparison in surgically treated patients is limited to this single case, only recently confirmed by a similar unpublished measurement carried out by other authors.[77] However, it is suggestive that the estimation error found is close to the one experimentally obtained with the localization of a pacing catheter (average three-dimensional uncertainty = 15 mm).[32]

One limitation in testing the accuracy of MCG localization procedure is that the three-dimensional reconstruction of the heart on the basis of orthogonal X-ray projections is obviously approximate. A more precise estimation could be obtained by combining magnetic resonance imaging of cardiac anatomy with MCG functional localization of the accessory pathways. This would be invaluable for a more accurate preoperatory study of Wolff-Parkinson-White patients, especially those with obliquely oriented accessory pathways,[78] or unidirectional retrograde pre-excitation which may reserve bad surprises for the surgeon if reentry is not reinducible during intraoperative mapping.[79,80] Another difficulty encountered in validating the MCG localization accuracy was the intrinsic limitation of catheter mapping as a "gold standard" for quantitative three-dimensional localization. In fact, although we have observed a clearcut qualitative coincidence between MCG and catheter mapping localization of Kent bundles in all patients, catheter fluctuations with respect to the recording grid, due to heart and respiratory movements, prevented a quantitative estimation of the localization differences. Probably the use of new catheter techniques would allow a more precise comparison with the two methods.[78] Finally, in patients with septal accessory pathways, it can be somehow difficult to establish the side of ventricular insertion of the accessory pathway with catheter endocardial mapping. On the contrary, the MCG method seems to be intrinsically more accurate to provide information on the direction of septal depolarization (Figure 5).

Conclusions

In spite of the primitive instrumentation used and the experimental character of the measurements reported so far, indeed the uncertainty of magnetic localization of cardiac sources seems to be acceptable and well within the resolution needed for the noninvasive preoperative study of candidates to antiarrhythmic surgery.[79,80] However, a real application of the method at a clinical level will be possible only when a medically oriented multichannel system will be available, capable to provide real-time images of the target tissue. This would enlarge the range of application of the biomagnetic functional imaging, to study transient, beat-to-beat, changes of the cardiac magnetic field, as in paroxysmal arrhythmias or acute myocardial ischemia, without artifacts due to sequential measurements with a single channel. Moreover, as the biomagnetic imaging can be used to localize a pacing catheter with a three-dimensional uncertainty of only few millimeters,[28,32,70] it could be used complementary to fluoroscopy, to drive an ablation catheter[32,65,81,82] as close as possible to an arrhythmogenic target by monitoring the catheter's and target's magnetic fields until matching. In order to reach this goal, a low-noise multichannel system is necessary, operating in the catheterization room, with high speed computer processing and real-time presentation of the localization procedures. Unfortunately, the majority of research groups and industries have been concentrated up to now to design and produce equipments appropriate for brain measurements.[1,9,40,42] A multichannel system, therefore optimal for magnetocardiography is not yet commercially available.

Acknowledgments: The authors are grateful to R. Frattin and C. Gobbi for their efficient technical and professional assistance. The work was partially supported by National Research Council (CNR) contracts N. PF 85.01473.57, 85.00462.04, 86.00062.04, 88.00503.04 and by grants 1986–88 (60%) from the Italian Ministry of Education.

References

1. Romani GL, Narici L: Principles and clinical validity of the biomagnetic method. In: Medical Progress through Technology. 11, 123–159, The Netherlands: Martinus Nijhoff Publ, 1986.
2. Wikswo JP Jr: Cellular action currents. In Williamson SJ, Romani G, Kaufman L, Modena I (eds): Biomagnetism. An Interdisciplinary Approach. NATO ASI Series A: Life Sciences, Vol. 66. Plenum Press, 1983, pp. 173–207.
3. Williamson SJ, Romani GL, Kaufman L, Modena I (eds): Biomagnetism: An Interdisciplinary Approach. New York-London: Plenum Press, 1983.
4. Taccardi B: Electrophysiology of excitable cells and tissue, with special consideration of the heart muscle. In Williamson SJ, Romani G, Kaufman

L, Modena I (eds): Biomagnetism. An Interdisciplinary Approach. NATO ASI Series A: Life Sciences, Vol. 66. Plenum Press, 1983, pp 141–171.

5. Horacek BM, Purcell C, Lamothe R, Merrit R, Kafer C, Periyalwar S, Dey S, Leon LJ, Stroink G: The effect of torso geometry on magnetocardiographic isofield maps. Phys Med Biol 32:121, 1987.

6. Romani GL: Biomagnetism: an application of SQUID sensors to medicine and physiology. Physica 126B:70, 1984.

7. Weinberg H, Stroink G, Katila T (eds); Biomagnetism: Applications and Theory. New York-Toronto: Pergamon Press, 1985.

8. Williamson SJ, Kaufman L: Biomagnetism. J Magn Mat 22:129, 1981.

9. Williamson SJ, Robinson SE, Kaufman L: Methods and instrumentation for biomagnetism. In Atsumi K, Katila T, Kotani M, Williamson SJ, Ueno S (eds): Biomagnetism 1987: Proceedings of the 6th International Conference on Biomagnetism. Tokyo: Denki University Press, 1987.

10. Baule GM, McFee R: Detection of the magnetic field of the heart. Am Heart J 66:95, 1963.

11. Cohen D, Edelsack EA, Zimmerman JE: Magnetocardiograms taken inside a shielded room with a superconducting point-contact magnetometer. Appl Phys Lett 16:278, 1970.

12. Cohen D, Lepeschkin E, Hosaka H, Massell B, Myers G: Abnormal patterns and physiological variations in magnetocardiograms. J Electrocardiol 9:398, 1976.

13. Barbanera S, Carelli P, Leoni R, Romani GL, Bordoni F, Modena I, Fenici RR, Zeppilli P: Biomagnetic measurements in unshielded, normally noisy environments. In Erne' SN, Hahlbohm HD, Lubbig H (eds): Biomagnetism. Berlin-New York: Walter de Gruyter, 1981, pp 139–149.

14. Barbanera S, Carelli P, Fenici RR, Leoni R, Modena I, Romani GL: Use of superconducting instrumentation for biomagnetic measurements performed in a hospital. IEEE Trans Magn MAG-17:849, 1981.

15. Farrell DE, Tripp J, Norgren R: Non-invasive information on the PR segment of the cardiac cycle: an assessment of the clinical potential of the electric and magnetic methods. Proc SPIE 167:173, 1978.

16. Farrell DE, Tripp JH, Van Doren CL: High resolution cardiomagnetism. In Erne' SN, Hahlbhom HD, Lubbig H (eds): Biomagnetism. Berlin-New York: Walter De Gruyter, 1981, pp. 273–282.

17. Opfer JE, Yeo YK, Pierce JM, Rorden LH: A superconducting second-derivative gradiometer. IEEE Trans Mag MAG-9:536, 1974.

18. Saarinen M, Karp PJ, Katila TE, Siltanen P: The magnetocardiogram in cardiac disorders. Cardiovasc Res 8:820, 1974.

19. Fenici RR, Romani GL, Barbanera S, Zeppilli P, Carelli P, Modena I: High resolution magnetocardiography: non-invasive investigation of His-Purkinje system activity in man. G Ital Cardiol 10:1366, 1980.

20. Fenici RR, Romani GL, Leoni R, Masselli M, Modena I: Magnetocardiographic recording of the His-Purkinje system activity in man. Jpn Heart J 23(Suppl 1):728, 1982.

21. Fenici RR: Clinical assessment of the magnetocardiogram. In Williamson SJ, Romani GL, Kaufman L, Modena I (eds): Biomagnetism. An Interdisciplinary Approach. NATO ASI series vol 66, 1982, pp 287–298.

22. Fenici RR, Romani GL, Leoni R: Magnetic measurements and modelling for the investigation of the human heart conduction system. In: Il nuovo cimento vol 2D, n 2, 1983, pp 280–290.

23. Fenici RR, Masselli M, Erne' SN, Hahlbohm HD: Magnetocardiographic mapping of the PR interval phenomena in an unshielded laboratory. In Weinberg H, Stroink G, Katila T (eds): Biomagnetism: Applications and Theory. New York-Toronto: Pergamon Press, 1985, pp 137–141.

24. Fenici RR, Masselli M, Lopez L, Sabetta F: High resolution magnetocardiography: electrophysiological and clinical findings. In: Proc of the XIV ICMBE and VII ICMP. Espoo, Finland: 1985, pp 1475–1478.

25. Fenici RR, Masselli M, Lopez L, Sabetta F: First simultaneous magnetocardiographic and invasive recordings of the PR interval electrophysiological phenomena in man. In: Proc of the XIV ICMBE and VII ICMP. Espoo, Finland: 1985, pp 1483–1484.

26. Fenici RR, Masselli M, Lopez L, Sabetta F: First simultaneous MCG and invasive Kent bundle localization in man. New Trends in Arrhythmias 1:455, 1985.

27. Fenici RR, Masselli M: Metodologia dello studio dell' attivita' elettrica cardiaca in atleti. Rev Lat Cardiol 6:133, 1985.

28. Fenici RR, Masselli M, Lopez L, Sabetta F: Simultaneous MCG mapping and invasive electrophysiology to evaluate the accuracy of the equivalent current dipole inverse solution for the localization of human cardiac sources. New Trends in Arrhythmias 2:357, 1986.

29. Fenici RR, Masselli M: Magnetocardiography: localization of accessory pathways (WPW). In: Proc of the IEEE Engineering in Medicine and Biology Society 8th Annual Conference. Dallas, Nov. 7–10, 1986, pp 437–438.

30. Fenici RR, Masselli M: Magnetocardiography: perspectives in clinical application. In: Proc of the IEEE Engineering in Medicine and Biology Society 8th Annual Conference. Dallas, Nov 7–10, 1986, pp 439–440.

31. Fenici RR, Masselli M, Lopez L, Melillo G: Clinical Magnetocardiography. Localization of arrhythmogenic structures. In Erne' SN, Romani GL (eds): Proceedings of Workshop on "Functional Localization, a Challenge for Biomagnetism." 1986.

32. Fenici RR, Masselli M, Lopez L, Melillo G: Catheter ablation of cardiac arrhythmias: magnetocardiographic localization of electrocatheters and arrhythmogenic foci. New Trends in Arrhythmias 3:723, 1987.

33. Fenici RR, Masselli M, Lopez L: Magnetocardiographic localization of arrhythmogenic sources. PACE 10:600, 1987.

34. Fenici RR, Masselli M, Lopez L, Melillo G: Magnetocardiographic localization of arrhythmogenic tissue. In Atsumi K, Katila T, Kotani M, Williamson SJ, Ueno S (eds): Biomagnetism 1987. Proceedings of the 6th International Conference on Biomagnetism. Tokyo:Denki University Press, 1987.

35. Fenici RR, Masselli M, Lopez L, Melillo G: Clinical value of magnetocardiography. In Hombach V, Hilger HH (eds): What's New in Electrocardiography and Drug Therapy. Boston: Martinus Nijhoff Publishers, 1989.

36. Erne' SN, Fenici RR, Hahlbohm HD, Jaszczuk W, Lehmann HP, Mas-

selli M: High resolution isofield mapping in magnetocardiography. In: Il nuovo cimento, vol 2D, 1983, pp 291–300.

37. Lepeschkin E: Tentative analysis of the normal magnetocardiogram. Adv Cardiol 10:325, 1974.

38. Erne' SN, Fenici RR: The present state of magnetocardiography. In Collan H, Berglund P, Krusius M (eds): Proc of the Tenth International Cryogenic Engineering Conference. Helsinki: Butterworth, Westbury House, 1984, pp 329–338.

39. Katila T, Maniewski R, Marijarvi M, Nenonen J, Siltanen P: On the accuracy of localization in cardiac measurements. Phys Med Biol 32:125, 1987.

40. Buchanan DS, Paulson D, Williamson SJ: Instrumentation for clinical application of neuromagnetism. Advances in Cryogenic Engineering. New York: Plenum Press, vol. 33, 1987, pp 97–106.

41. Ilmoniemi RJ, Williamson SJ, Hostetler WE: New method for the study of spontaneous brain activity. In Atsumi K, Katila T, Kotani M, Williamson SJ, Ueno S (eds): Biomagnetism 1987. Proceedings of the 6th International Conference on Biomagnetism. Tokyo: Denki University Press, 1987.

42. Romani GL: The use of the SQUIDS in the study of biomagnetic fields. In: Weinstock H, Nisenhoff M: Superconducting Electronics. Berlin, Springer-Verlay, 1989, pp 149–174.

43. Awano N, Owada K, Machip K, Kariyone S, Awano I: A study on magnetocardiograms of normal subjects. Jpn Circ J 46:870, 1982.

44. Barry WH, Fairbank WM, Harrison DC, Lehrman KL, Malmivuo JAV, Wikswo JP: Measurements of the human magnetic heart vector. Science 198:1159, 1977.

45. Fujino K, Sumi M, Saito K, Murakami M, Higuchi T, Nakaya Y, Mori H: Magnetocardiograms of patients with left ventricular overloading recorded with a second-derivative SQUID gradiometer. J Electrocardiol 17:219, 1984.

46. Karp PJ, Katila TE, Saarinen M, Siltanen P, Varpula TT: Etude comparative de magnetocardiogrammes normaux et pathologiques. Ann Cardiol Angeiol 27:65, 1978.

47. Malmivuo JAV, Wikswo JP Jr: A new practical lead system for vector magnetocardiography. Proceedings of the IEEE, May 1977, pp 810–811.

48. Nakaya Y, Takeuchi A, Nii H, Katayama M, Nomura M, Fujino K, Saito K, Mori H: Isomagnetic maps in right ventricular overloading. J Electrocardiol 21:168, 1988.

49. Nomura M, Fujino K, Katayama M, Takeuchi A, Fukuda Y, Sumi M, Murakami M, Nakaya Y, Mori H: Analysis of the T wave of the magnetocardiogram in patients with essential hypertension by means of isomagnetic and vector arrow maps. J Electrocardiol 21:174, 1988.

50. Sumi M, Takeuchi A, Katayama M, Fukuda Y, Nomura M, Fujino K, Murakami M, Nakaya Y, Mori H: Magnetocardiographic P waves in normal subjects and patients with mitral stenosis. Jpn Heart J 27:621, 1986.

51. Takeuchi A, Watanabe K, Nomura M, Ishihara S, Sumi M, Murakami

M, Saito K, Nakaya Y, Mori H: The P wave in the magnetocardiogram. J Electrocardiol 21:161, 1988.

52. Erne' SN, Fenici RR, Hahlbhom HD, Korsukewitz HP, Lehmann HP, Uchigawa Y: Magnetocardiographic study of the PR segment of normals. In Weinberg H, Stroink G, Katila T (eds): Biomagnetism, Application and Theory. New York: Pergamon Press, 1985, p 132.

53. Lorenzana HE, Pipes PB, Zaitlin MP, James D: Structures in the PR interval of the human magnetocardiogram. In Weinberg H, Stroink G, Katila T (eds): Biomagnetism: Applications and Theory. New York: Pergamon Press, 1985, p 142.

54. Makijarvi M, Maniewski R, Derka I, Puurtinen J, Katila T, Siltanen P: High resolution MCG study on heart conduction system. In: Proc of the XIV ICMBE and VII ICMP. Espoo, Finland: 1985, pp 1485–1486.

55. Erne' SN: High resolution magnetocardiography: modelling and sources localization. In: Proc of the XIV ICMBE and VII ICMP. Espoo, Finland: 1985.

56. Erne' SN, Lehmann HP, Masselli M, Uchigawa Y: Modelling of the His-Purkinje heart conduction system. In Weinberg H, Stroink G, Katila T (eds): Biomagnetism, Application and Theory. New York: Pergamon Press, 1985, p 126.

57. Erne' SN, Hahlbhom HD, Korsukewitz J, Lehmann HP: Late potential-like deflections in the ST segment of normal subjects. J Electrocardiol 18:315, 1985.

58. Abraham-Fuchs K, Schneider S, Reichenberger H: MCG inverse solution: influence of coil size, grid size, number of coils and SNR. IEEE Trans Bio Med Eng 35, 1988.

59. Denis B, Matelin D, Favier Ch, Tanche M, Martin-Noel P: L'enregistrement du champ magnetique cardiaque. Considerations techniques et premiers resultats en milieu hospitalier. Arch Mal Coeur 69:299, 1976.

60. Erne' SN, Romani GL: Performances of higher order planar gradiometers for biomagnetic source localization. In Hahlbhom HD, Lubbig H (eds): SQUID 85: Superconducting Quantum Interference Devices and their Applications. Berlin, New York: Walter de Gruyter, 1985, pp 951–961.

61. Gonnelli R, Sicuro M: Use of the current multipole model for cardiac source localization in normal subjects. In Atsumi K, Katila T, Kotani M, Williamson SJ, Ueno S (eds): Biomagnetism 1987, Proceedings of the 6th International Conference on Biomagnetism. Tokyo: Denki University Press, 1987.

62. Gonnelli R, Agnello M: Inverse problem in cardiomagnetism using a current multipole expansion of the primary sources. Phys Med Biol 2:133, 1987.

63. Uchikawa Y, Erne' SN: Modelling of the Wolff-Parkinson-White with magnetocardiography. In Atsumi K, Katila T, Kotani M, Williamson SJ, Ueno S (eds): Biomagnetism 1987: Proceedings of the 6th International Conference on Biomagnetism. Tokyo: Denki University Press, 1987.

64. Cuffin BN, Katila TE, Wikswo JP Jr: Theoretical models for sources localization. In Weinberg H., Stroink G., Katila T, (eds): Biomagnetism: Applications and Theory. Oxford: Pergamon Press 1985, pp 9–18.

65. Nenonen J, Salkola M, Katila T: On the current multipole expansion of biomagnetic fields. In: Proc of the XIV ICMBE and VII ICMP. Espoo, Finland: 1985, pp 20–21.
66. Erne' SN, Trahms L, Trontelj Z: Current multipoles as sources of biomagnetic and bioelectric fields. In Atsumi K, Katila T, Kotani M, Williamson SJ, Ueno S (eds): Biomagnetism 1987. Proceedings of the 6th International Conference on Biomagnetism. Tokyo: Denki University Press, 1987.
67. Gonnelli R, Agnello M: Simulation of an excitation wavefront spreading through an anysotropic myocardium: an analytical model study. In Atsumi K, Katila T, Kotani M, Williamson SJ, Ueno S (eds): Biomagnetism 1987. Proceedings of the 6th International Conference on Biomagnetism. Tokyo: Denki University Press, 1987.
68. Leifer M, Capos N, Griffin J, Wikswo J: Atrial activity during the P-R segment of the MCG. Nuvoo Cimento D:266, 1983.
69. Leoni R, Romani GL: Computer simulation of magnetic field patterns from the human cardiac conduction system. Nuovo Cimento ID:737, 1982.
70. Costa Monteiro E, Bruno AC, Louro SRW, Costa Ribeiro P, Fonseca C: Magnetic localization of a current dipole implanted in dogs. Phys Med Biol 32:65, 1987.
71. Schmitz L: Magnetocardiography: the clinician's point of view. In Atsumi K, Katila T, Kotani M, Williamson SJ, Ueno S (eds): Biomagnetism 1987. Proceedings of the 6th International Conference on Biomagnetism. Tokyo: Denki University Press, 1987.
72. Gulrajani RM, Pham-Huy H, Nadeau RA, Savard R, De Guise J, Primeau RE, Roberge FA: Application of the single moving dipole inverse solution to the study of the Wolff-Parkinson-White syndrome in man. J Electrocardiol 17:271, 1984.
73. Johnson LL, Seldin DW, Yeh HL, Sponitz HM, Reiffel JA: Phase analysis of gated blood pool scintigraphic images to localize bypass tracts in Wolff-Parkinson-White syndrome. J Am Coll Cardiol 8:67, 1986.
74. Kamakura S, Shimomura K, Ohe T, Matsuhisa M, Toyoshima H: The role of initial minimum potentials on body surface maps in predicting the site of accessory pathways in patients with Wolff-Parkinson-White syndrome. Circulation 74:89, 1986.
75. Windle JR, Armstrong WF, Feigenbaum H, Miles WM, Prystowsky EN: Determination of the earliest site of ventricular activation in Wolff-Parkinson-White syndrome: application of digital continuous loop two-dimensional echocardiography. J Am Coll Cardiol 7:1286, 1986.
76. Gallagher JJ: Localization of accessory atrioventricular pathways: What's the gold standard. PACE 10:503, 1987.
77. Novak H, Albrecht G, Burghoff M, Kirsch G: MCG measurements in WPW patients. (personal communication.)
78. Jackman WM, Friday KJ, Yeung-Lai-Wah JA, Fitzgerald DM, Beck B, Bowman AJ, Stelzer P, Harrison L, Lazzara R: New catheter technique for recording left free-wall accessory atrioventricular pathway activation. Circulation 78:598, 1988.

79. Guiraudon GM, Klein GJ, Sharma A, Jones D, McLellan D: Surgery for Wolff-Parkinson-White syndrome: further experience with an epicardial approach. Circulation 74:525, 1986.
80. Klein GJ, Guiraudon GM, Perkins DG, Jones DL, Yee R, Jarvis E: Surgical correction of the Wolff-Parkinson-White syndrome in the closed heart using cryosurgery: a simplified approach. J Am Coll Cardiol 3:405, 1984.
81. Narula OS, Bharati S, Chan MC, et al: Microtransection of the His bundle with laser radiation through a pervenous catheter: correlation of histologic and electrophysiologic data. Am J Cardiol 54:186, 1984.
82. Huang SKS: Use of radiofrequency energy for catheter ablation of the endomyocardium: a prospective energy source. J Electrophysiol 1:78, 1987.

8

A Comparative Analysis of Commercial Signal-Averaged Electrocardiogram Devices

Raphael Henkin, Edward B. Caref,
George J. Kelen, Nabil El-Sherif

Introduction

The signal-averaged electrocardiogram (SAECG) has become a widely accepted technique for risk stratification of patients with potential malignant reentrant arrhythmias. Late potentials (LPs) in the SAECG have been correlated with spontaneous sustained ventricular tachycardia,[1-3] the inducibility of monomorphic sustained ventricular tachycardia at electrophysiologic study,[4,5] and prediction of serious arrhythmic events post-myocardial infarction.[6-10] Presently, six devices are commercially available in the United States for identification of late potentials. They all employ a signal averaging algorithm for the reduction of random noise, thus improving the signal-to-noise ratio. They also use filtering techniques to further reduce the presence of baseline noise. All devices claim to analyze the filtered QRS vector sum by the method of Simson.[1] Although these devices employ a generally similar approach, totally standardized methods and criteria have not yet been developed for

From El-Sherif N, Turitto G (eds): *High-Resolution Electrocardiography*. Mount Kisco, NY, Futura Publishing Co., Inc., ©, 1992.

this technique. From the scientific and clinical standpoints it is imperative that the data obtained from these various devices be reproducible and comparable.

There are several studies which made comparisons of SAECG devices. The earliest report was from Oeff and coworkers, who in 1983 compared the results of four SAECG systems used on 109 patients.[11] Two of the systems were modified versions of the Princeton Signal Averager Model 4202, which is no longer commercially available. The third system was a MAC I (Marquette Electronics, Milwaukee, WI), and while still available, the hardware and software has been completely redesigned. The fourth system was a customized version based on Simson's described hardware and software,[1] and was the only system in this study which gave automatic, quantitative interpretation of each SAECG. Interpretation of the other three systems was performed by visual inspection. Oeff et al concluded that while significant differences among the four systems in the detection of LPs existed, this was due mainly to the different methods of interpretation employed (visual inspection versus automatic interpretation). Also, the fact that each system used a different lead system probably contributed to the disparate results.

In another study by Vacek and associates,[12] tests were performed on two of the devices currently available, the Corazonix Predictor (COR, Corazonix Corporation, Oklahoma City, OK) and the 1200EPX High Resolution Electrocardiograph (ART, Arrhythmia Research Technology Inc., Austin, Tx). Analyzing the SAECGs of 18 patients, they found significant differences between devices in both the quantitative parameters measured as well differences in the classification of patients having LPs (2 out of 3 parameters considered abnormal), in which 3 of 18 patients had differing classifications between the two devices. In addition, Vacek et al described significant differences in noise level (0.33 μV for COR vs 0.28 for ART), however, this may have been due to the large difference in the number of QRS complexes averaged by each system (300 for COR vs 126 for ART).

To evaluate possible differences among the devices, our laboratory recently conducted two comparative study protocols[13]:

1. We compared the results obtained from the same subjects upon sequential analyses by the different systems.
2. We compared the effects of the slightly differing analysis algorithms used by the various devices for determining noise and

QRS onset and offset on the clinical numeric data used to evaluate the presence or absence of late potentials.

Methods of Procedure

One hundred and twelve subjects (61 patients with known organic heart disease and 51 normal volunteers) were studied as part of two separate protocols.

Study Protocol 1

Sequential recordings of the SAECG were obtained in 32 subjects (21 patients with organic heart disease and 11 normal volunteers). Data were acquired from the same orthogonal bipolar X, Y, and Z leads. The four devices used for this study were the:

1. ART;
2. COR;
3. Fidelity Medical LP-3000 (FID, Fidelity Medical Systems, Inc., Milburn, NJ);
4. Custom designed (CUS)—this personal computer-based unit was the forerunner of the Cardiac Early Warning System, Model 183 (Del Mar Avionics, Irvine, CA).

Analysis using each device was performed in a randomized order, taking about 40 minutes in all. Sampling frequency was set at 1000 Hz for each device, and in each case 500 cycles were averaged. Late potential analyses were calculated using each device's own implementation of a 4-pole bidirectional Butterworth filter with a passband of 25–250 Hz. Vector sums of the three filtered leads were calculated and the root mean square voltage of the terminal 40 msec of the QRS (RMS40), duration of low amplitude signals in the terminal QRS below 40 µV (LAS40), and total filtered QRS duration (QRSD) were calculated. The scoring criteria for abnormal SAECG parameters at 25- to 250-Hz bandpass filtering were: RMS40 < 25 µV, LAS40 > 32 msec, and QRSD > 115 msec. These values were based upon data obtained from a large cohort of normal subjects.[14]

Study Protocol 2

The patient group was comprised of 80 subjects (40 patients with known organic heart disease and 40 normal volunteers). Data were acquired using the ART 1200 EPX from orthogonal bipolar X, Y, and Z leads. The files of raw signal-averaged data were analyzed and numeric data calculated as for study protocol 1. The original, unprocessed data files were then converted into a suitable format and submitted to analysis by the COR and CUS devices, as though the data had been acquired by the latter two. Thus the identical averaged data was submitted to analysis by all three systems. Differences in derived numeric output could result only from algorithmic differences in the analysis of each SAECG, rather than from different raw patient signals or techniques associated with data acquisition and averaging.

Statistics

All data are expressed as the mean ± SD. An analysis of variance with repeated measures (ANOVA) was used to evaluate interdevice and intradevice differences. A p value < 0.05 was considered significant.

Results

Study Protocol 1

Analysis of the data disclosed that significant discordances do indeed exist between devices. A discordant result was defined as any subject who was deemed to have late potentials by at least one but not all devices. Table I illustrates variability in the "detection" of late potentials depending on the number of abnormal parameters needed for classification as positive. For example, when only one SAECG parameter had to be positive for late potentials to be considered present (Column 1), 13 out of 32 subjects (41%) had late potentials using all devices, 14 (43%) had no LPs on any device, while 5 (16%) had LPs on 3 out of 4 devices. There were no subjects in whom

Table I
Parameter Variability

	Abnormal Parameters					
	≥ 1		≥ 2		3	
	No.	%	No.	%	No.	%
Late potentials	13	41%	11	34%	7	22%
No late potentials	14	43%	15	47%	21	66%
Discordant	5	16%	6	19%	4	12%

two devices indicated presence of late potentials while two indicated absence. Discordances ranged between 12%–19%, the largest occurring when a minimum of two criteria were required for LPs to be assessed.

In an attempt to identify reasons for this variability, we categorized the discordances by parameter and device. Table II indicates that a total of ten discordances were found, of which six were related to RMS40, three to LAS40, and one to QRSD. The RMS40 was by far the most variable of the parameters, consistent with its greater sensitivity relative to the other two parameters of the precise calculated position of QRS offset. Figure 1 is a composite of the vector magnitudes and the accompanying numeric parameters from the four devices, recorded from a normal subject. The general morphologies are similar except for different time and voltage scales used by each system for presentation. The differences in the numeric param-

Table II
Comparison of Discordancy

	QRSD	RMS40	LAS40
COR	—	—	—
ART	—	2	—
CUS	1	—	—
FID	—	4	3
Total	1	6	3

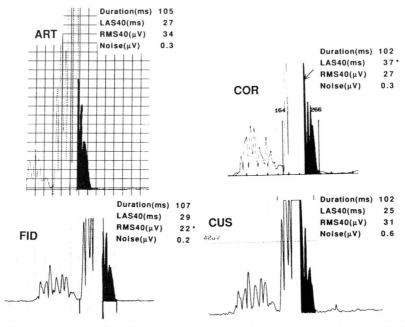

Figure 1. Composite of the vector magnitudes from the four devices and their associated numeric parameters. Note the morphologic similarities and yet the differences between parameter values. The asterisk identifies a discordant parameter value. (Reprinted with permission from Henkin R et al, J Electrocardiol 22 (Suppl):19, 1990.)

eters, although small, illustrate how sensitive the numbers are to small differences in the precise determined position of QRS offset. The RMS40 is presented as the shaded areas on the vector plots. The calculated values for the RMS40 are normal in all cases except in the FID device where a value of 22 μV would be considered abnormal.

Study Protocol 2

Although in the first protocol we attempted to standardize the acquisition process between the devices and assumed that sequential averaging would not in itself affect our results, the second protocol was specifically designed to identify differences that could result only from different algorithm implementations in the various devices by using identical averaged input data, thus isolating the analysis process from data acquisition and averaging variables.

Figures 2 and 3 graphically depict the results of an ANOVA test for QRSD and LAS40, indicating that there were no significant differences between the analyses of the three devices in either the normal or abnormal groups. However, when the analysis of RMS40 was compared, there were significant differences among the devices in the normal and abnormal groups (Figure 4). Thus, RMS40 was the most sensitive of the numeric parameters to device idiosyncrasies. To further characterize parameter variability, we compiled the number of normal, abnormal, and discordant results for QRSD, RMS40, and LAS40. A discordance was defined here as any value which crossed the boundary of normalcy when compared with the values from the other devices. Table III summarizes these results indicating that 23% of RMS40 values were discordant (18 of the 80 analyses performed). The QRSD and LAS40 were discordant in 11% and 15% of analyses, respectively. The differences between the morphologies of the vector magnitudes were negligible, yet wide variations in the values of the numeric parameters were evident even in cases where discordances were not found. Figure 5 is a composite of the vector magnitudes from a normal subject analyzed by the 3 devices. The

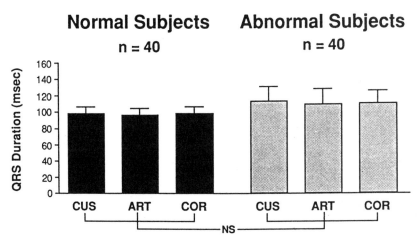

Figure 2. The graphs depict the mean QRS duration inclusive of late potentials if they exist. Analysis of variance revealed no statistically significant differences between devices. (Reprinted with permission from Henkin R et al, J Electrocardiol 22 (Suppl):19, 1990.)

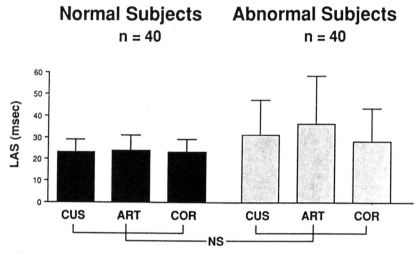

Figure 3. The graphs depict the mean durations of low amplitude signals < 40 µV for the three systems being compared. Analysis of variance revealed no statistically significant differences between devices. (Reprinted with permission from Henkin R et al, J Electrocardiol 22 (Suppl):19, 1990.)

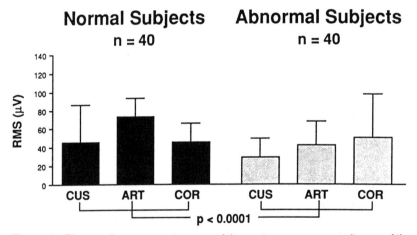

Figure 4. The graphs represent means of the root mean square voltages of the terminal 40 msec of the QRS. Analysis of variance revealed significant differences (p < 0.0001) between devices. (Reprinted with permission from Henkin R et al, J Electrocardiol 22 (Suppl):19, 1990.)

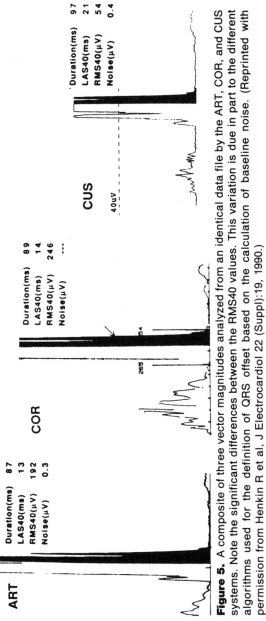

Figure 5. A composite of three vector magnitudes analyzed from an identical data file by the ART, COR, and CUS systems. Note the significant differences between the RMS40 values. This variation is due in part to the different algorithms used for the definition of QRS offset based on the calculation of baseline noise. (Reprinted with permission from Henkin R et al, J Electrocardiol 22 (Suppl):19, 1990.)

Table III
Parameter Variability

	QRSD		RMS40		LAS40	
	No.	%	No.	%	No.	%
Normal	39	49%	35	44%	36	45%
Abnormal	32	40%	27	33%	32	40%
Discordant	9	11%	18	23%	12	15%

RMS40 values are significantly different, although negative in each case—192, 246, and 54 µV for the ART, COR, and CUS, respectively. Notice that the RMS40 value for COR is approximately five times greater than the value calculated from the CUS device.

Discussion

The recording of low amplitude fractionated electrical activity at the terminal QRS/early ST segment from the body surface provides a feasible noninvasive means of identifying patients with a propensity for developing reentrant ventricular tachyarrhythmias. The signal averaging technique by reducing random noise and enhancing the signal-to-noise ratio makes visualization of these low amplitude late potentials possible. Various custom devices using a variety of lead configurations, amplification and filtering techniques, as well as multiple analysis schemes have been employed over the years. Yet, to date no 'gold standard' for the evaluation of late potentials has been accepted.

The simplicity of the technique has made its clinical utility attractive and its commercialization potentially financially lucrative. All commercial devices can analyze the SAECG using the Simson method for evaluation of late potentials. The Simson parameters are exquisitely sensitive to the precise QRS offset location. Commercial devices vary in the precise way in which they determine QRS onset and offset. There is no industry standard for exact and reproducible definition of this critical landmark, as well as a uniform definition of "noise" amplitude.

We found that sequential evaluations of the same subject yielded significant discordances between devices. Variability in the presence of late potentials was as much as 19% between devices. Upon further analysis it became evident that the major source of discordance was the RMS40 parameter, accounting for 60% of all deviations in study protocol 1 described above. This finding also held true for study protocol 2 which exclusively compared the analysis algorithms of the ART, COR, and CUS devices on identical averaged unfiltered data files. Inter- and intragroup variability measured by the ANOVA technique revealed statistically significant differences in the RMS40 parameter only. The RMS40 discrepancies amounted to 23% (18/80) of the entire study population and to 46% (18/39) of all discordances. All calculated SAECG parameters are dependent upon the definition of QRS offset which in turn is evaluated from an algorithm for the calculation of baseline noise. Since the commercial devices appear to use different algorithms for the calculation of baseline noise (at least their reported noise values vary widely), the three calculated SAECG parameters from each device are vulnerable to interdevice differences. It is important to note that only morphologically the vector magnitudes were similar yet the derived numerical parameters differed even without necessarily being discordant. At the sampling interval commonly used, 1000 Hz, each real data point is 1 msec from the next. A QRS offset defined by different noise algorithms may range over only a few milliseconds yet translate into significantly different values for RMS40.

Conclusion

The results of these studies suggest that numeric criteria be used with caution in the evaluation of patients for the presence of late potentials, especially when the numbers are "borderline," knowing that results may not be identical with other devices. Furthermore, caution should be exercised in comparing or pooling the results of clinical studies using different devices. Finally, there is a pressing need for devices that claim to perform a "standard" task to do so in a "standard" fashion, especially with respect to noise calculation and QRS limit delineation.

References

1. Simson MB: Use of signals in the terminal QRS complex to identify patients with ventricular tachycardia after myocardial infarction. Circulation 64:235, 1981.
2. Breithardt G, Borggrefe M, Karbenn U, Abendroth R-R, Yeh H-L, Seipel L: Prevalence of late potentials in patients with and without ventricular tachycardia: correlation with angiographic findings. Am J Cardiol 49:-1932, 1982.
3. Kanovsky MS, Falcone RA, Dresden CA, Josephson ME, Simson MB: Identification of patients with ventricular tachycardia after myocardial infarction: signal-averaged electrocardiogram, Holter monitoring, and cardiac catheterization. Circulation 70:264, 1984.
4. Turitto G, Fontaine JM, Ursell SN, Caref EB, Henkin R, El-Sherif N: Value of the signal-averaged electrocardiogram as a predictor of the results of programmed stimulation in non-sustained ventricular tachycardia. Am J Cardiol 61:1272, 1988.
5. Winters SL, Stewart D, Targonski A, Gomes JA: Role of signal averaging of the surface QRS complex in selecting patients with nonsustained ventricular tachycardia and high grade ventricular arrhythmias for programmed ventricular stimulation. J Am Coll Cardiol 12:1481, 1988.
6. Breithardt G, Schwarzmaier J, Borggrefe M, Haerten K, Seipel L: Prognostic significance of late ventricular potentials after acute myocardial infarction. Eur Heart J 4:487, 1983.
7. Denniss A, Richards D, Cody D, Russell PA, Young AA, Cooper MJ, Ross DL, Uther JB: Prognostic significance of ventricular tachycardia and fibrillation induced at programmed stimulation and delayed potentials detected on the signal-averaged electrocardiograms of survivors of acute myocardial infarction. Circulation 74:731, 1986.
8. Gomes JA, Winters SL, Stewart D, Horowitz S, Milner M, Barreca P: A new non-invasive index to predict sustained ventricular tachycardia and sudden death in the first year after myocardial infarction: based on signal-averaged electrocardiogram, radionuclide ejection fraction and Holter monitoring. J Am Coll Cardiol 10:349, 1987.
9. Kuchar D, Thorburn C, Sammel N: Prediction of serious arrhythmic events after myocardial infarction: signal-averaged electrocardiogram: Holter monitoring and radionuclide ventriculography. J Am Coll Cardiol 9:531, 1987.
10. El-Sherif N, Ursell SN, Bekheit S, Fontaine J, Turitto G, Henkin R, Caref EB: Prognostic significance of the signal-averaged electrocardiogram depends on the time of recording in the post-infarction period. Am Heart J 118:256, 1989.
11. Oeff M, Leitner RV, Sthapit R, Breithardt G, Borggrefe M, Karbenn U, Meinertz T, Zutz R, Clas W, Hombach V, Hopp H-W: Methods for non-invasive detection of ventricular late potentials: a comparative multicenter study. Eur Heart J 7:25, 1986.
12. Vacek JL, Smith S, Dunn MI: Late potential parameter and noise level

variability caused by bandpass versus high-pass filtering and type of signal averaging equipment used. J Electrophysiol 3:278, 1989.

13. Henkin R, Caref EB, Kelen GJ, El-Sherif N: The signal-averaged electrocardiogram and late potentials: a comparative analysis of commercial devices. J Electrocardiol 22(Suppl):19, 1990.

14. Caref EB, Turitto G, Ibrahim B, Henkin R, El-Sherif N: Role of bandpass in optimizing the value of the signal-averaged electrocardiogram as a predictor of the results of programmed stimulation. Am J Cardiol 64:16, 1989.

Section II.

Techniques and Clinical Application of Beat-to-Beat Recordings

Beat-to-Beat Recording of a High-Resolution Electrocardiogram: Technical and Clinical Aspects

Nabil El-Sherif, Rahul Mehra, Mark Restivo

Introduction

There are several low level electrocardiographic (ECG) potentials whose manifestations on the body surface are too small to be detected by routine measurement techniques. These include the potentials produced by the His-Purkinje system and by slow and inhomogeneous conduction in diseased ventricular myocardium (usually called *late potentials*). These potentials are small because the activation front is slow and fractionated or the mass of tissue undergoing depolarization is small, or both. However, the measurement of the bioelectric potentials produced by these tissues is important for diagnostic purposes. Identification of the His-Purkinje potential can localize the site of atrioventricular conduction disorders, and the detection of late potentials may identify patients at high risk for malignant ventricular tachyarrhythmias. The problem in identify-

From El-Sherif N, Turitto G (eds): *High-Resolution Electrocardiography*. Mount Kisco, NY, Futura Publishing Co., Inc., ©, 1992.

ing these potentials is that the signal is smaller than the electrical noise produced by various sources.

Different techniques have been utilized to improve signal-to-noise (S/N) ratio. A commonly used technique is ensemble or temporal averaging (usually referred to as *signal averaging*).[1-3] Temporal averaging is a process whereby fixed intervals of a noisy signal are aligned temporally with respect to a reference point and then summed. A signal averaging system stores the information of a designated interval of the ECG and sums the information received from successive intervals. Division of the sum of stored information by the number of cycles yields an ensemble average. In this average, the components of the information arising from the noise sources diminish because they are random, and the desired repetitive signal is accentuated, thus resulting in an improved S/N ratio. In fact, the averaging process reduces to a simple summation, with the signal present in the summations building up linearly owing to the coherent timings with which the samples were taken. The noise, if it is random, adds up in a root mean square sense with the net result that after X signal repetitions have been combined, the S/N ratio has been improved by $\sqrt{X}$.

There are two major limitations for recording the His-Purkinje signals and late potentials by the temporal averaging technique[4,5]: (1) it will not be able to detect dynamic (beat-to-beat) changes in the signal during sinus rhythm; and (2) the signal-averaged (SA) ECG cannot be recorded during complex cardiac arrhythmias.

The clinical advantage of identifying the His-Purkinje signal on a beat-to-beat basis is obvious when there is a dynamic change of the temporal relation between the atrial and ventricular potentials. On the other hand, late potentials may vary from beat-to-beat. Electrophysiologic observations in the canine post-infarction model of reentry suggest that spontaneous reentrant arrhythmias may be associated with a Wenckebach-like conduction pattern in a potentially reentrant pathway.[6-9] Recording of late potentials on a beat-to-beat basis has the potential of directly identifying reentrant "malignant" versus focal "benign" ventricular rhythms.[4,5] Several investigators have utilized different techniques to reduce the S/N ratio and to record His-Purkinje potentials or late potentials beat-to-beat basis.[10-26] These techniques as well as the clinical application of beat-to-beat high-resolution ECG will be discussed in this chapter.

Noise Sources in Electrophysiologic Signal Measurements

There are four primary noise sources in electrophysiologic signal measurements[24]: (1) power frequency; (2) electrode-tissue interface; (3) amplifier; and (4) electromyographic potentials.

Power Frequency Noise

A major source of artifact when one is recording physiologic signals is the electrical power system. Power lines are connected to other pieces of equipment in the typical hospital environment. Electrical field and magnetic field coupling can both give rise to power interference. A typical monitoring configuration uses two active electrodes as differential inputs to an amplifier and a third common electrode. This technique is used almost universally because differential amplifiers can be designed to give a high common mode rejection ratio and input impedance, both of which reduce interference. However, one has the choice of grounding the common or using different configurations of two electrode recording systems. A theoretical analysis of the problem reveals that least interference would be expected with an ungrounded three lead system. Lowering skin-electrode impedance and minimizing the difference between the two skin-electrode impedances is also important. Shielding the input cables and twisting them to reduce magnetic induction can further lower the interference. Power spectra of the ECG in a hospital environment show that sharp impulses occur not only at 60 Hz (50 Hz in Europe) but at many harmonics of the fundamental frequency. Although the higher harmonics are lower in magnitude, frequencies as high as 1500 Hz can sometimes be observed. One of the best ways to reduce interference is to enclose the patient and the recording system in a Faraday cage. Since this cage is grounded, most of the displacement currents are shunted. This technique, however, sacrifices the mobility of the measuring system. Low-noise electrophysiologic signal measurements such as evoked responses are frequently done in shielded rooms. A shielded room was also used by some investigators for their high-resolution ECG measurements.[26] Notch filters for 60 Hz and its harmonics can further reduce noise from the output signal.

Electrode-Tissue Interface Noise

The primary function of an electrode is to convert ionic conduction in tissue to electronic conduction in the measuring system. Silver-silver chloride electrodes are the least polarizable, and they result in a low impedance, low offset potential interface. The electrical stability of the electrode is considerably enhanced by mechanical stabilization of the electrode-tissue interface by interposing an electrolyte between the electrode and the tissue. Most commercial ECG electrodes are of this indirect contact design. In addition to their nonpolarizable behavior, the silver-silver chloride electrode exhibits less electrical noise than other metal electrodes. It has also been observed that newly prepared electrodes are often noisy; however, with the passage of time the noise decreases. Electrodes with a peak-to-peak noise of about 1 µV (measured in 0.9% saline) at a bandwidth of 0.1 to 1000 Hz can be commercially purchased with a minimal amount of electrode "popping." Typical offset voltages range between 0 and 4 µV.[27] Sanding of the skin lightly with fine sandpaper (3M Type 220) and wiping with alcohol can significantly reduce electrode impedance, resulting in recordings with less interference.

Amplifier Noise

The noise associated with a differential amplifier stage is the result of Schottky, or shot noise; Johnson, or thermal noise and flicker; or low-frequency ($1/f$) noise.[28] Shot noise is due to the discrete particle nature of current carriers in semiconductors; the origin of the $1/f$ noise is not well understood. Representation of all the noise sources by equivalent noise generators results in an equivalent input noise voltage and current with thermal noise of source resistance. All these noise sources are proportional to the square root of the bandwidth considered. Typically, with bipolar devices the input noise voltage is lower and the noise current higher than in field-effect transistor devices. In most applications, since the source resistances are low, the current noise figure does not add appreciably to the total noise as compared to the thermal noise of the source resistances. Most semiconductor devices have specified noise figures. As the technology changes, manufacturers continually introduce devices with lower input voltage and current noise specifications.

Electromyographic Potentials (EMG)

Physiologic signals recorded via body surface electrodes reflect the asynchronous firing at motor units that are dispersed temporally and spatially with a superimposed ECG signal. Attempts have been made to separate the two by optimal bandpass filtering but significant overlap exists between the power spectra of the two signals. About 95% of the EMG power is between 25 and 250 Hz, with the remaining 5% above this frequency.[29] Most of the spectral power of the ECG lies below 40 Hz, although small amounts of power have been measured in some patients at frequencies up to 500 Hz.[30] A spectral analysis of the His bundle electrogram recorded from the body surface indicates that most of the power spectrum is below 100 Hz.[26] Due to this overlap of spectral components, it becomes difficult to measure the electrical activity of the heart independent of skeletal muscle activity. The latter can be reduced by relaxing the patient or by the use of muscle relaxants. Significant variations can exist between muscle tone of patients during relaxation. Cyclic variation in EMG noise can also be observed with respiration. Administration of succinylcholine chloride during anesthesia virtually eliminates skeletal muscle activity, and heart activity up to 300 to 400 Hz can be measured.[30] This technique is obviously not applicable to routine clinical measurements.

Electromyographic noise could be reduced in relation to the ECG signal by the use of the spatial averaging technique. This technique could be utilized alone or in combination with other noise reducing measures. Two of the techniques that have been utilized in conjunction with spatial averaging are digital logic circuits to detect and attenuate undesirable noise signals[10,31] and the volume conductor electrode that attenuates EMG noise relative to ECG signal.[4,32] All of the above techniques will also help to attenuate other noise sources besides EMG noise.

Spatial Averaging

To enhance the S/N ratio in a beat-to-beat recording, a spatial averaging technique is frequently employed. In this technique, potentials recorded from multiple pairs of electrodes are averaged. The averaging reinforces the identical signals and attenuates the uncorrelated potentials. If the distance between pairs of surface electrodes is small, the EMG noise as well as the ECG signal from each pair would be correlated and spatial averaging would not enhance the S/N ratio. However, since the EMG potential source consists of multiple muscle units distributed proximal to the skin surface, and because the ECG biogenerator is more distal to the recording electrodes, increasing the distance between the pairs of electrodes should improve the S/N ratio, as the EMG signal would be less correlated compared with the ECG potential. ·

In order to optimize the distance between pairs of electrodes for spatial averaging, it is important to measure the spatial coherence of potentials associated with cardiac and skeletal muscle activity.[30] The magnitude squared coherence function defined below is a useful parameter for examining the improvement one would obtain by spatial averaging when electrodes are spaced at various distances. The magnitude squared coherence function is always normalized to values between 0 and 1 and is defined as[33]:

$$|Kvx(f)|^2 = \frac{|G\overline{vx}(f)|^2}{G\overline{vv}(f)\ G\overline{xx}(f)}$$

where v(t) and x(t) are two continuous, real wide-sense random processes and $G\overline{vv}(f)$ is the averaged auto power spectral density of v(t): $G\overline{xx}$ (f) is the averaged auto power spectral density of x(t); and $G\overline{vx}$ (f) is the averaged cross power spectral density function.

To determine the coherence between a pair of ECG leads, we built a two channel differential amplifier each equipped with a bandpass filter between 0.1 Hz and 1000 Hz (36 dB/octave) (Figure 1).[32] After amplification and filtering, the data was fed into a two channel spectrum analyzer (Wavetek/Rockland 5830A) which digitized the data at a sampling rate > 20000 samples per second. The sampling of the two channels of data was triggered by an external QRS detector unit. The variable delay on the trigger unit permitted sampling of the QRS complex or the TP segment of the ECG during which the EMG potentials are dominant. Since the EMG potentials present in the TP segment were significantly smaller, different gain settings were used for the analysis of QRS and EMG potentials. The magnitude squared coherence function of the QRS potentials and the EMG potentials was calculated at variable distances between pairs of

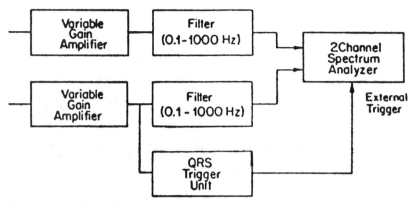

Figure 1. A block diagram of the system used for measuring the coherence function. (Reproduced with permission from Mehra et al, IEEE Frontiers of Engineering and Computing in Health Care, New York, 1983.)

surface leads. The stability of the spectral estimates was increased by averaging 64 beats. All recordings were made with the patients lying comfortably in the supine position. The first pair of electrodes were attached on the left and the right midaxillary line at the level of the V_4 electrode. Additional electrodes were attached below the first pair at a distance of 1, 2, 4, and 6 inches from it.

Figure 2 shows the results from one of the six patients in whom such measurements were made. In all the illustrations, the data up to 250 Hz has been presented because of the low S/N ratio at higher frequencies. The coherence function of EMG potentials from pairs of electrodes spaced 1 inch apart is nearly equal to unity at low frequencies and between 0.9 and 1.0 in the remaining frequencies except for the dip at 60 Hz and at its 180 Hz harmonic (Figure 2A). For purposes of comparison, the mean coherence function of the six patients was measured at two representative frequencies of 20 and 80 Hz and it was 0.93 and 0.90, respectively. When the distance between the electrode pair was increased to 2 inches, the coherence function of the EMG potentials decreased at all frequencies. It had a minima in the 30- to 50-Hz range. This characteristic minima was observed in all patients and was present even when the distance between the electrode pairs was increased. At 2 inches, the mean coherence function at 20 and 80 Hz was 0.72 and 0.62. At 4 inches, a more dramatic decrease in coherence was observed. In this patient it became almost zero in the 30- to 50-Hz range and the sharp peak thereafter corre-

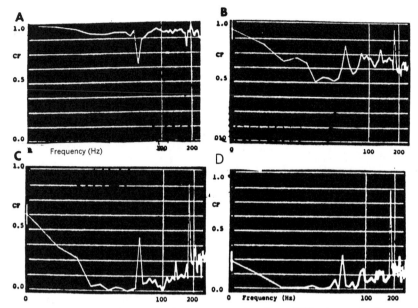

Figure 2. Magnitude squared coherence function (CF) of an electromyographic potential measured at a distance of 1 (A), 2 (B), 4 (C), and 6 inches (D) between electrode pairs in a resting subject. (Reproduced with permission from Mehra et al, IEEE Frontiers of Engineering and Computing in Health Care, New York, 1983.)

sponded to the 60-Hz interference noise. The mean coherence at 20 and 80 Hz was now 0.30 and 0.33. Increasing the electrode pair distance to 6 inches decreased the coherence function further and the mean values at 20 and 80 Hz were 0.17 and 0.20, respectively. It is interesting to note that if the patient performed an isometric exercise such as holding his breath following complete expiration, the EMG signals were of greater magnitude but the coherence function was lower than during the relaxed state. Similar observations have been reported previously.[30]

The results of the coherence function of the QRS signal were significantly different from those for the EMG potentials. The coherence function was between 0.9 and 1.0 at all electrode pair distances up to 6 inches. For the patient discussed previously, the coherence function of the QRS at 4 inches is shown in Figure 3.

It is evident from all these results that for spatial averaging, significant improvement in signal to EMG noise ratio can be ob-

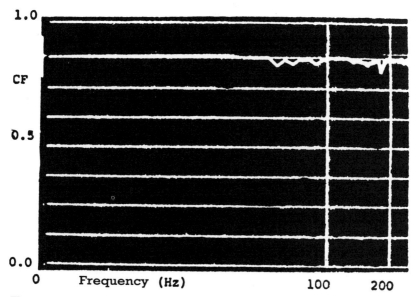

Figure 3. Magnitude squared coherence function (CF) of QRS potentials measured at a distance of 4 inches between electrode pairs in the same patient as illustrated in Figure 2. (Reproduced with permission from Mehra et al, IEEE Frontiers of Engineering and Computing in Health Care, New York, 1983.)

tained by spacing the electrode pairs up to 6 inches from each other. It is important to note that the optimum number of electrodes for spatial averaging depends not only on the reduction of EMG noise, which is the primary noise source, but also on the other random noise sources such as amplifier and electrode noise. The latter noise sources would undergo maximal reduction when the number of electrode pairs are increased as the noise between the various channels would be uncorrelated. Therefore, due to this need to spatially average from maximum number of electrodes and yet the limited surface available for electrode placement, an electrode pair separation of between 2 and 4 inches may be desirable.[32]

Digital Logic Circuits

The resolution of spatial averaging is limited by the size of the torso, the perimeters of the positive and negative fields on the chest, and the size of electrodes. Therefore, additional measures to improve the S/N ratio have been suggested. Shvartsman and associates[31] were the first to combine the spatial averaging technique with an algorithm for coincidence detection in order to enhance the ECG signal and suppress noise. A digital logic circuit based on the concept of double threshold detection, coincidence detection, or binary integration[33-35] examines phase coherence from multiple channels. If phase coherence exists in all channels, data is accepted, summed, and averaged. On the other hand, if one of the channels shows noncoherent data, the latter is markedly attenuated prior to summation and averaging. Although this technique can reduce electrode and amplifier noise, it will be less helpful in reducing synchronous EMG potentials from closely spaced electrodes.

Volume Conductor Electrode

An improvement in ECG signal to EMG noise can be obtained by recording signals not from the precordial surface but a certain distance away from it with the help of a column conductor electrode.[4,32] When an electrode is placed directly on the chest surface, the potential recorded can be expressed by the solid angle model.[36] It is directly proportional to the product of the potential difference of the activating biogenerator, the solid angle subtended by it, and a constant incorporating the conductivity of the medium. It is evident that if other variables do not alter and if the electrode was to be moved distal to the chest surface with a conducting medium in between, the reduction in the solid angle of the cardiac generator would be less than for the EMG generator. This is because the ECG biogenerator is more distal to the skin surface than the EMG biogenerator. Hence, an improvement in S/N ratio would occur even though both signals undergo attenuation.

In order to test this concept in our laboratory, two types of experiments were conducted.[32] For the first experiment, a volume conductor electrode was made which consisted of a large indirect electrode with a conductive sponge placed between the skin and the recording electrode. The electrode was housed in a cylindrical tube 8 cm in length. A cylindrical sponge, the length of the tube, was placed inside it and injected with electrode gel solution to make it slightly conductive. On the distal end of the tube, a silver-silver chloride electrode was attached. The complete electrode was placed on the belly of the thenar muscle of the right hand and potentials were recorded with respect to a standard ECG electrode placed on the left arm. Reproducible EMG potentials could be produced by stimulation of the median nerve at a rate of 1 stimulus every 2 seconds using 2-msec pulses. In ten volunteers, the EMG potentials during median nerve stimulation and the QRS potentials were recorded using volume conductor electrodes. The volume conductor electrode was then replaced by a standard surface ECG electrode and similar measurements were made again. It was observed that the peak-to-peak EMG potential from the volume conductor electrode was 11.7 ±3.8 mV and significantly smaller than that from the standard ECG electrode (15.6 ±4.4 mV; p <0.05). There was no statistical variation in the peak-to-peak QRS magnitude with either electrode. The results from one of the experiments are shown in Figure 4. It was evident from this study that significant improvement in

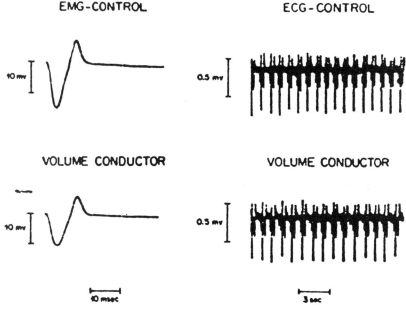

Figure 4. Electromyographic (EMG) potentials recorded from the belly of the thenar muscle during maximal stimulation of the median nerve. The EMG response has a peak-to-peak amplitude of 22 mV with the standard electrode and 16 mV with the volume conductor electrode (left panel). The QRS amplitudes (right panel) with the two electrodes are similar. (Reproduced with permission from Mehra et al, IEEE Frontiers of Engineering and Computing in Health Care, New York, 1983.)

S/N ratio could be obtained by the use of the volume conductor electrode.

In order to test this concept in a more physiologic situation, the second experimental protocol attempted to measure the reduction in S/N ratio produced by a volume conductor electrode during normal respiration. A large volume electrode housing (8" × 3" × 2") was filled with a sponge of equivalent dimensions. A recording electrode was attached to the back of this housing and a sponge moistened with diluted electrode gel was placed inside it. A pair of standard ECG electrodes were placed on the left and right midaxillary line at the level of the V_4 electrode and connected to an amplifier and filter (bandwidth, 0.1 to 1000 Hz). Immediately over each of these electrodes, a volume conductor electrode was placed and connected to a second amplification and filtering channel. During normal respiration these two signals from a pair of standard and volume conductor electrodes were recorded simultaneously and stored on the Norland 3001 Digital Oscilloscope. Such recordings were made in six volunteers. Although significant variation was observed from subject to subject, the volume conductor electrode reduced the EMG potentials in five of six patients. The greatest attenuation was observed during maximal EMG activity in the respiration cycle. The mean reduction of the maximum peak-to-peak amplitude of the EMG potential was 31.5 ± 10.2% (reduction in RMS 24.3 ± 4.2%) whereas the reduction of the peak-to-peak QRS potential was only 8.2 ± 4.7%. This data indicates that a 20%–30% improvement in S/N ratio can be obtained by this technique. The results from one of the subjects are shown in Figures 5 and 6. The EMG potentials from the standard electrode pair and the volume conductor in Figure 5A show a 24% reduction in the maximum peak-to-peak EMG potential. The corresponding reduction in power spectral density function is illustrated in Figure 5B. In the same patient, the reduction in the peak-to-peak QRS amplitude is only 6% (Figure 6).

Clinical Application of Beat-to-Beat High-Resolution ECG (HRECG)

In our laboratory the spatial averaging technique was utilized to record His-Purkinje potentials and late potentials on a beat-to-beat basis.[4,16] Recordings were obtained from 16 pairs of electrodes

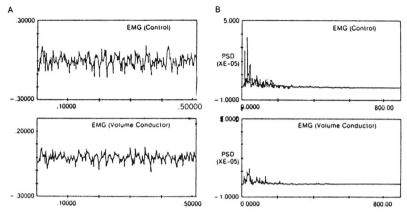

Figure 5. (A) Simultaneous electromyographic (EMG) potentials recorded from the skin surface with a standard ECG electrode (top) and with a "volume conductor" electrode (bottom). Note the significant reduction in EMG potentials with the "volume conductor" electrode. (Horizontal axis: seconds.) (B) The corresponding power spectral density function at frequencies up to 800 Hz. (Horizontal axis: Hertz.) (Reproduced with permission from Mehra et al, IEEE Frontiers of Engineering and Computing in Health Care, New York, 1983.)

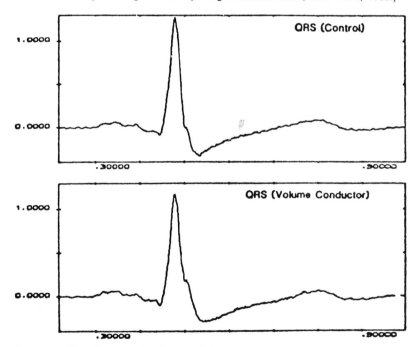

Figure 6. Simultaneous QRS potentials recorded with a standard ECG electrode (top) and with a volume conductor electrode (bottom). A 6% reduction in the peak-to-peak amplitude of QRS potential occurs with the volume conductor electrode. (Reproduced with permission from Mehra et al, IEEE Frontiers of Engineering and Computing in Health Care, New York, 1983.)

and the distance between electrodes was approximately 2.5 cm. A variable gain amplifier and variable low-pass and high-pass filters were used. The input leads were connected to a pair of specially designed volume conductor electrodes. The patient was asked to lie comfortably in the supine position. The room was electrically quiet but not shielded. Frequently, 10 to 15 minutes were required before the patient relaxed and reduced the noise potentials from EMG sources.

Recording of His-Purkinje Potentials on a Beat-to-Beat Basis by the HRECG

A HRECG was obtained in 14 patients. A His bundle potential could be identified in six patients (43%) (Figure 7). A deflection in the PR segment was considered a His bundle potential if it satisfied two criteria. First, it had to be at least 2 μV in amplitude. This ensured a minimal S/N ratio of 2, because the noise signal as measured from the late ST interval was typically 1 to 1.5 μV in cycles not contaminated by EMG potentials. Second, a relatively isoelectric segment of at least 10 msec was required between the terminal atrial activity and the deflection. This prevented late atrial potentials from being considered of His bundle origin. The HV interval in the six patients ranged from 35 to 60 msec. The His bundle potential and the HV interval were validated in all patients by signal averaging. Intracardiac His bundle recordings were also obtained in two patients. The His bundle potential in the HRECG was remarkably similar in configuration to the potential recorded in the SAECG from the X lead (Figure 7). In three patients, the His bundle potential was a biphasic or triphasic deflection, 15 to 20 msec in duration, and 2 to 6 μV in amplitude. In three other patients, an additional preventricular deflection (15 to 25 msec preceding the ventricular potential) was recorded in the HRECG and the SAECG. This deflection may represent bundle branch-His-Purkinje activation.

The HV intervals measured from the HRECG and the SAECG were remarkably similar (correlation coefficient [r] = 0.97, probability [p] <0.001). The HV interval of the HRECG also correlated well (within 5 msec) with that measured from the intracardiac His bundle electrogram in two patients. A major source of noise during the recording of the HRECG was potentials generated during respira-

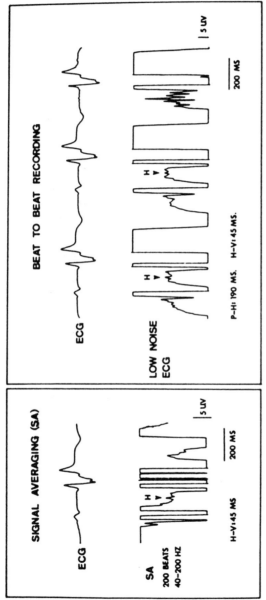

Figure 7. A beat-to-beat high-resolution electrocardiogram (HRECG) from a 76-year-old man. The 12-lead ECG showed sinus rhythm with first-degree atrio-ventricular block and right bundle branch block. Signal averaging (SA) of 500 beats in the X lead (left panel) shows a discrete triphasic His bundle potential (H) with an HV interval of 45 msec. The HRECG (right panel) reveals a remarkably similar H potential with an HV interval of 45 msec. Of the three consecutive beat-to-beat recordings, the third is a supraventricular premature beat. The preventricular segment of this beat is obscured by potentials originating from an ectopic P wave with a short PR interval. The possibility of electromyographic noise contributing to the preventricular potential cannot be excluded. (Reproduced with permission from El-Sherif et al, J Am Coll Cardiol 1:456, 1983.)

tion. This varied among patients, but could usually be diminished by teaching the patient to relax and breathe quietly. Although periodic contamination of the ECG with EMG potentials could obscure the His bundle potential, two or more successive cycles with minimal EMG potentials could be obtained in all patients.

The His bundle potential was identified in the X lead of the SAECG in 8 of 14 patients (56%) and in at least one of the three vectorial leads of the SAECG in 10 of 14 patients (71%). This was consistent with the observation that multiple spatial leads are more successful than a single lead in identifying the His-Purkinje potential because of the vectorial nature of the signal.[37] Thus in four patients, the SAECG was able to identify the His bundle potential while the HRECG was not. In two of these patients, the amplitude of the His bundle potential in the SAECG was 1 to 1.5 μV compared with 2 to 6 μV in the six patients in whom the His potential was recorded by both techniques. This suggests that the failure of the HRECG to identify a His potential may be a result of a low S/N ratio (the averaged noise signal in the SAECG was typically 0.2 μV[37] compared with 1 to 1.5 μV recorded in the HRECG). Another factor for the low success rate of the HRECG in identifying a His potential may be a short PR segment (there is a poor correlation between the PR segment and the PR interval).[37] Of the 14 patients, 9 had a PR segment >65 msec in the X lead. The HRECG was able to identify the His potential in five of the nine patients. In the remaining five patients with a PR segment of <65 msec, a His bundle potential was recorded in only one patient using the HRECG. Thus, the problem of the late atrial deflections obscuring the His bundle potential in patients with a short PR segment seems to apply to the HRECG and the SAECG.[37]

Recording of Late Potentials on a Beat-to-Beat Basis by the HRECG

The HRECG was recorded in 18 normal volunteers and in 20 other patients with various disorders of the cardiac rhythm.[16] None of the patients had acute myocardial infarction in the past year. Late potentials were recorded in only two patients (7%). On the other hand, late potentials in the HRECG were recorded in 15 of 21 patients within the first 3 weeks following acute myocardial infarction

(71%) (Figure 8). Twelve of the 15 patients had episodes of ventricular tachycardia and/or ventricular fibrillation either spontaneously or on programmed electrical stimulation. Only one of the remaining six patients who had no late potentials had spontaneous episodes of ventricular tachycardia. The HRECG had a sensitivity, specificity, and positive predictive accuracy of 80%, 83%, and 81%, respectively. The late potentials varied in amplitude between 2 and 25 μV and were continuous with high amplitude, high-frequency components in the late QRS complex. Late potentials extended up to 280 msec from the onset of the QRS complex (20 to 190 msec from the end of the QRS complex; the latter was approximately defined from normal standard leads I, AVF, and V, that were recorded simultaneously with the HRECG). Late potentials remained constant in successive sinus beats in nine patients, probably reflecting a 1:1 conduction pattern in ischemic myocardium. In six patients, late potentials varied in configuration and timing in successive sinus beats, probably reflecting a Wenckebach-type conduction pattern. In such patients HRECG was usually superior to the SAECG. Similar observations were reported by Hombach et al.[15] In four patients, late potentials were recorded during spontaneous ventricular premature beats. In two patients, late potentials were reproducible only in the ST segment preceding a ventricular premature complex (Figure 9). Multiform ventricular premature complexes recorded in two other patients did not appear to be related to the late potentials. An HRECG was not recorded during ventricular tachycardia in any of the patients.

The HRECG and the SAECG were compared in 20 patients. The SAECG was recorded in nine patients in whom an HRECG did not reveal late potentials. In two patients, late potentials, 2–5 μV in amplitude and 20–40 msec in duration, were recorded. On the other hand, in 11 patients in whom an HRECG revealed late potentials, an SAECG showed late potentials of similar duration in 8 patients (Figure 8) but failed to show consistent late potentials in 3 patients. In two of these three patients, the late potentials in the HRECG varied from beat-to-beat. No SAECG was recorded when late potentials and spontaneous ventricular arrhythmias in the HRECG were present. The data suggests that beat-to-beat HRECG recordings may provide complimentary data to the SAECG in some patients, particularly when there is a beat-to-beat variation of the signal and/or in the presence of spontaneous ventricular arrhythmias.

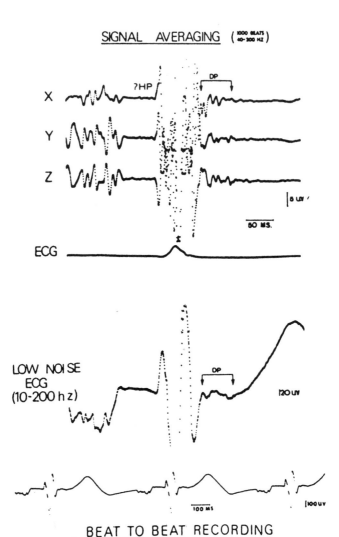

Figure 8. A beat-to-beat high-resolution electrocardiogram (HRECG) from a 51-year-old man 1 week after inferior wall myocardial infarction. The patient had transient complete atrio-ventricular dissociation and several runs of ventricular tachycardia during the first week after infarction. Signal averaging of sinus beats in the X, Y, and Z leads (upper panel) shows multiphasic diastolic potentials (DP) in the early part of the ST-T segment that extends for 150 msec from the onset of the QRS complex. An HRECG with the same time scale as that of the signal-averaged leads (middle panel) shows the presence of diastolic potentials up to 25 µV in amplitude in the early part of the ST segment that corresponded in duration to the diastolic potentials in the signal-averaged leads. A continuous recording of the low-noise electrocardiogram is shown (bottom). The His-Purkinje potential (HP) seen in the signal-averaged recording is labeled ? because the amplitude of the signal is <2.5 times the average noise signal as measured from the late ST-T segment. (Reproduced with permission from El-Sherif et al, J Am Coll Cardiol 1:456, 1983.)

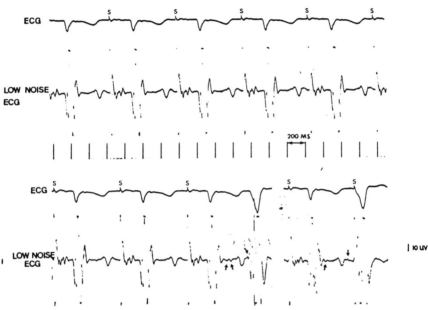

Figure 9. A beat-to-beat high-resolution electrocardiogram (HRECG) from a 59-year-old man with a 3-week-old inferoposterior wall myocardial infarction. The patient had frequent ventricular premature complexes and runs of nonsustained ventricular tachycardia. During electrophysiologic study, ventricular tachycardia that degenerated into ventricular fibrillation was induced by programmed stimulation. A continuous HRECG was obtained during atrial pacing (S) (upper panel) and shows no late diastolic potentials during paced beats. However, late potentials were consistently seen in the diastolic interval preceding spontaneous ventricular premature complexes in the early and late part of the ST segment (arrows, lower panel). Note that the diastolic potentials are unrelated to the coupling interval of the ventricular premature complexes. (Reproduced with permission from El-Sherif et al, J Am Coll Cardiol 1:456, 1983.)

Conclusions

The recording of microvolt ECG potentials (His-Purkinje potential and late potentials) on the body surface on a beat-to-beat basis is feasible and highly desirable. Spatial averaging as well as a number of other measures have been utilized to reduce the S/N ratio sufficiently to be able to retrieve these signals. However, more technical improvement of noise reduction are required, besides some efforts toward standardization of the recording and analysis of the signal before widespread clinical application is expected.

Acknowledgment: This study was supported by National Institutes of Health Grants HL36680 and HL31341 and the Veterans Administration Medical Research Funds.

References

1. Berbari EJ, Lazzara R, Samet P, Scherlag BJ: Noninvasive technique for detection of electrical activity during the P-R segment. Circulation 48:-1005, 1973.
2. Flowers NC, Hand RC, Orander PC, Miller KB, Walden MO, Horan LG: Surface recording of electrical activity from the region of the bundle of His. Am J Cardiol 33:384, 1974.
3. Stopczyk MJ, Kopec J, Zochowski RJ, Pieniak M: Surface recording of electrical activity during the P-R segment in man by computer averaging technique. Int Res Comm Systems (73–78), 11, 21, 2, 1973.
4. El-Sherif N, Mehra R, Gomes JAC, Kelen G: Appraisal of a low noise electrocardiogram. J Am Coll Cardiol 1:456, 1983.
5. El-Sherif N: The low noise (high resolution) electrocardiogram. Int J Cardiol 6:185, 1984.
6. El-Sherif N, Scherlag BJ, Lazzara R: Electrode catheter recordings during malignant ventricular arrhythmias following experimental acute myocardial ischemia. Circulation 51:1003, 1975.
7. El-Sherif N, Scherlag BJ, Lazzara R, Hope RR: Reentrant ventricular arrhythmias in the late myocardial infarction period. I. Conduction characteristics in the infarction zone. Circulation 55:586, 1977.
8. El-Sherif N, Lazzara R, Hope RR, Scherlag BJ: Reentrant arrhythmias in the late myocardial infarction period. 3. Manifest and concealed extrasystolic grouping. Circulation 56:225, 1977.
9. El-Sherif N, Gough WB, Zeiler RH, Hariman R: Reentrant ventricular arrhythmias in the late myocardial infarction period. 12. Spontaneous versus induced reentry and intramural versus epicardial circuits. J Am Coll Cardiol 6:124, 1985.
10. Flowers NC, Shvartsman V, Kennelly BM, Sohi GS, Horan LG: Surface recordings of His-Purkinje activity on an every beat basis without digital averaging. Circulation 63:948, 1981.
11. Kepski R, Plucinski Z, Walczak F: Noninvasive recording of His-Purkinje system (HPS) activity in man on beat-to-beat basis. PACE 5:506, 1982.
12. Oeff M, von Leitner ER, Erne SN, Hahlbohm HD, Lehmann HP, Schroder R: Einzelschlag-Registrierung Ventrikularer Spartdepolaisationen von der Korperoberflache Koronarkranker Patienten (abstr). Z Kardiol 71:627, 1982.
13. Erne SN, Fenici RR, Hahlbohm HE, Lehmann HP, Trontelj Z: Beat to beat surface recording and averaging of His-Purkinje activity in man. J Electrocardiol 16:355, 1983.
14. Flowers NC, Schvartsman V, Horan LG, Palakurthy P, Sohi GS, Sridharan MR: Analysis of the PR subintervals in normal subjects and early

studies in patients with abnormalities of the conduction system using surface His bundle recordings. J Am Coll Cardiol 2:939, 1983.

15. Hombach V, Kebbel U, Hopp H-W, Winter V, Hirche H: Noninvasive beat by beat registration of ventricular late potentials using high resolution electrocardiography. Int J Cardiol 6:167, 1984.

16. El-Sherif N, Gomes JAC, Restivo M, Mehra R: Late potentials and arrhythmogenesis. PACE 8:440, 1985.

17. Haberl R, Hengstenberg E, Steinbeck G: Single beat analysis of frequency content in the surface ECG for identification of patients with ventricular tachycardia (abstr). Circulation 72(Suppl III):III-433, 1985.

18. Hombach V, Hopp H-W, Kebbel U, Treis I, Osterpey A, Eggeling T, Winter V, Hirche H, Hilger HH: Recovery of ventricular late potentials from body surface using the signal averaging and high resolution ECG techniques. Clin Cardiol 9:361, 1986.

19. Chen WC, Zeng ZR, Chow C, Xine QZ, Kou LC: Application of a new spatial signal-averaging device for the beat-to-beat detection of cardiac late potentials. Clin Cardiol 9:263, 1986.

20. Ishijima M, Kimata S, Kasanuki H, Sakurai Y: The feasibility of beat-to-beat detection of His-Purkinje activity by finite element method. PACE 10:1107, 1987.

21. Adamec R, Zimmermann M, Richez J, Simonin P: A comparative study between non invasive registration of ventricular late potentials using beat-to-beat high-resolution electrocardiography and using signal-averaging technique. In Belhassen B, Feldman S, Copperman Y (eds): Cardiac Pacing and Electrophysiology: Proceedings of the VIIth World Symposium on Cardiac Pacing and Electrophysiology. Tel Aviv; R and L Creative Communications, 1987, p 309.

22. Lewis SL, Lander PT, Taylor PA, Chamberlain DA, Vincent R: Identification of ventricular late potential activity in single cardiac cycles using spatial averaging and advanced filtering techniques (abstr). J Am Coll Cardiol 11:183A, 1988.

23. Jesus S, Rix H: High resolution ECG analysis by an improved signal averaging method and comparison with a beat-to-beat approach. J Biomed Eng 10:25, 1988.

24. Mehra R, El-Sherif N: Signal averaging of electrocardiographic potentials. A review. Acupuncture and Electrotherapeutics Res Int J 7:133, 1982.

25. El-Sherif N, Restivo M, Craelius W, Mehra R, Henkin R, Caref EB, Kelen G: The high resolution electrocardiogram. Technical and basic aspects. In El-Sherif N, Samet P (eds): Cardiac Pacing and Electrophysiology. Philadelphia; WB Saunders, 1990, pp 349–371.

26. Berbari EJ, Scherlag BJ, Lazzara R: A computerized technique to record new components of the electrocardiogram. IEEE Trans Biomed Eng 65:799, 1977.

27. Patterson S: The electrical characteristics of some commercial ECG electrodes. J Electrocardiol 11:23, 1978.

28. Tobey GE, Graeme G, Huelsman LP: Operational Amplifiers: Design and Applications. New York, NY; McGraw Hill Co, 1971, pp 51–89.

29. Schweitzer TW, Fitzgerald JW, Bowden JA, Lynne-Davies P: Spectral

analysis of human inspiratory diaphragmatic electromyograms. J Appl Physiol 46:152, 1979.

30. Santipetro RF: The origin and characterization of the primary signal, noise and interference sources in the high frequency electrocardiogram. IEEE Proc 65:707, 1977.

31. Shvartsman V, Barnes GR, Schvartsman L, Flowers N: Multi-channel signal processing based on logic averaging. IEEE Trans Biomed Eng 29:531, 1982.

32. Mehra R, Restivo M, El-Sherif N: Electromyographic noise reduction for high resolution electrocardiography. In: IEEE Frontiers of Engineering and Computing in Health Care. New York; IEEE 1983, p 298.

33. Bendat JS, Piersol AG: Measurement and Analysis of Random Data. New York: John Wiley & Sons, 1966.

34. Worley R: Optimum threshold for binary integration. IEEE Trans Inform Theory IT-14:349, 1968.

35. Walker JF: Performance data for a double-threshold detector radar. IEEE Trans Aerosp Electron Syst AES-9:142, 1971.

36. Holland RP, Arnsdorf MF: Solid angle theory and the electrocardiogram: physiologic and quantitative interpretations. Prog Cardiovasc Dis 19:431, 1977.

37. Mehra R, Kelen GJ, Zeiler R, Zephiran D, Fried P, Gomes JAC, El-Sherif N: Noninvasive His bundle electrogram: value of three vector lead recordings. Am J Cardiol 49:344, 1982.

10

The High-Resolution Electrocardiogram: Clinical Aspects

Vinzenz Hombach

Introduction

The conventional surface electrocardiogram (ECG) provides information on atrial and ventricular depolarization, atrio-ventricular conduction, and ventricular repolarization.[1] Abnormalities of sinus node function can only be derived from short- and long-term (Holter) electrocardiograms (ECGs), whereas the exact electrophysiologic mechanisms (e.g., sinoatrial block, sinus node standstill) remain undetected from the body surface, because the low-voltage sinus node depolarization (in the range of 10–30 μV) will be buried in the baseline noise of conventional ECG amplifiers. The same holds true for atrio-ventricular conduction blocks, the site of which (e.g., supra- and infra-His) cannot be exactly localized by the normal ECG. Prolongation of intraventricular conduction of larger myocardial areas due to bundle branch block can be recognized in the conventional ECG from the typical hemiblock or bundle branch block patterns of the QRS complex. However, delayed activation of smaller areas of damaged myocardium in patients with acute or chronic

From El-Sherif N, Turitto G (eds): *High-Resolution Electrocardiography*. Mount Kisco, NY, Futura Publishing Co., Inc., ©, 1992.

myocardial infarction or with right ventricular dysplasia will be invisible on the surface ECG, due to the small amplitudes of the signals in the microvolt range.[2]

Some of these special electrophysiologic problems can be solved by direct intracardiac catheter recordings in the laboratory or by direct hand-held electrode mapping during open-heart surgery.[3] However, for routine detailed studies of the electrical behavior of the heart, noninvasive surface recordings would be highly desirable. The history of surface high-resolution electrocardiography began in 1973 with the attempt of the three groups to record His bundle potentials, using the signal averaging technique.[4-6] Since that time, different types of signal averaging computers have been designed, and many investigators have reported on recordings of sinus node ECG,[7-10] His bundle potentials,[11-15] and ventricular late potentials.[4,12,16-20]

In the following chapters, the spectrum of clinical application of the high-resolution ECG technique will be described, and the diagnostic and prognostic significance of the signals recorded with this technique will be described.

Preatrial Activity (Sinus Node Potentials)

From animal experiments it is well known that the depolarization of sinus node pacemaker cells resembles a slowly up- or down-sloping wave or ramp, both in transmembrane and in extracellular recordings, which precedes atrial depolarization by 30 to 40 msec.[10,21-23] Such preatrial depolarizations have also been found in humans, using intracardiac catheter electrode recordings from the endocardial surface of the sinus node area.[24-26] In these studies, the time interval from the beginning of preatrial to atrial depolarization was found to be 40 to 80 msec in normal subjects, and more than 100 msec in patients with sinus node disease.

From these results it seems clear that such preatrial activity may represent sinus node depolarization and may be retrieved from the body surface by high-resolution electrocardiography if the following conditions are met: (1) no cut-off of lower frequencies; that is, DC 0.05-Hz high-pass filtering must be used; (2) the signals of interest should resemble slowly depolarizing ramp- or wavelike depolarizations, which are separated from or merging into the P wave; and (3) the range of presumed sinoatrial conduction times should be 40 to 80 msec in normal individuals.

Using these criteria, several groups reported successful ECG recordings of preatrial activity in humans by means of the signal averaging technique.[7,10,27] In the study by Wajszczuk et al[10] of 40 consecutive patients, successful noise-free recordings were obtained in 36 individuals, and in 32, low-voltage deflections were seen before the onset of the P wave in the reference lead (highly filtered bipolar surface lead) and before the onset of the first large voltage deflection of atrial activity in the averaged leads. Using bandpass filtering of 30 to 300 Hz, these potentials preceded the onset of atrial activity by 24 to 40 msec, and their voltage varied from 4 to 15 μV. Ten patients from this study were additionally investigated with 0.1-Hz high-pass filtering, which revealed recordings with a long diastolic depolarization slope, followed by a steeper upstroke that made a transition into the P wave. Obviously, all these recordings were performed in patients with normal sinus rhythm, and none of them had evidence of overt sinus node disease.

Various precordial and transthoracic leads were tested for their efficacy in representing preatrial activity best with the longest intervals to the P wave. The transthoracic Z lead appeared to detect the most and the earliest activity of the sinus node region. Our group studied a total of 37 patients by averaging three bipolar precordial leads; the one from the second right intercostal space (ICS) to the fourth left ICS was the most effective for retrieving clear and reproducible preatrial signals in 23 of 37 patients.

In principle, two types of preatrial signals can be observed: one type has a small base width, rapid upstroke, and higher frequency components that are still visible with 50-Hz high-pass filtering, and with intervals to the atrial deflection of 30 to 45 ms; and the second type is characterized by a wider base width, a more wavelike structure (mono- or biphasic), with lower frequency components that are lost with 50-Hz high-pass filtering, and with intervals to the atrial depolarization of 50 to 165 msec. Drug testing with intravenous atropine decreased the interval of the preatrial to atrial depolarization in two patients (Figure 1), whereas this interval was prolonged after beta blockade with pindolol. From this study it was concluded that only the second type of preatrial depolarizations met the characteristics of sinus node depolarization (as described above) and thus could represent true sinus node activity in the averaged low-noise ECG.

In a second study by our group, the efficacy of the beat-to-beat resolution ECG technique was tested for continuous recording of preatrial activity.[19] Preatrial potentials were not reproducibly

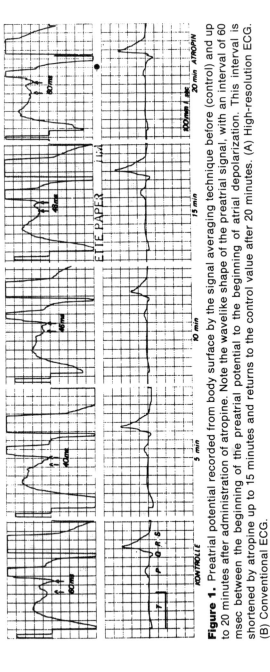

Figure 1. Preatrial potential recorded from body surface by the signal averaging technique before (control) and up to 20 minutes after administration of atropine. Note the wavelike shape of the preatrial signal, with an interval of 60 msec between the beginning of the preatrial potential to the beginning of atrial depolarization. This interval is shortened by atropine up to 15 minutes and returns to the control value after 20 minutes. (A) High-resolution ECG. (B) Conventional ECG.

found in any of eight normal subjects, whereas such signals were seen in two of five patients with coronary heart disease (Figure 2). By comparison, preatrial activity was detected in seven of 12 patients, using the signal-averaged surface ECG. Based on these preliminary reports, the high-resolution technique seems to be less efficient for noninvasive retrieval of sinus node depolarizations in humans. Moreover, no systematic studies have been conducted as yet in patients with normal and disturbed sinus node function, in

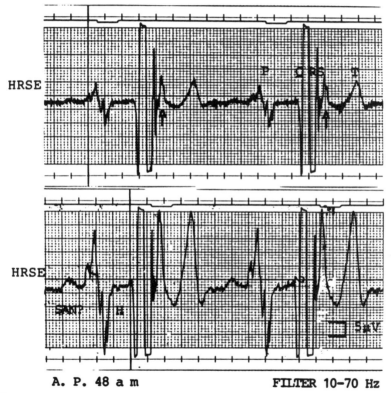

A. P. 48 a m   FILTER 10-70 Hz

Figure 2. Preatrial potential (SAN?) recorded beat-by-beat with the high-resolution real-time technique in a patient with a left ventricular aneurysm. Note the wavelike preatrial signal that merges into the rapid upstroke of atrial depolarization. The interval from the beginning of the preatrial signal to the beginning of atrial depolarization is 60 msec. HRSE = high resolution surface ECG; SAN? = possible sinus node potential; H = His bundle depolarization. Arrows = ventricular late potential.

whom the underlying pathophysiologic mechanisms of sinus node dysfunction could be documented with the low-noise ECG.

Summary and Conclusions

Successful surface ECG recordings of preatrial activity are feasible by means of the signal averaging and the high-resolution beat-to-beat techniques.

The success rates for recording preatrial potentials seem to be higher with the signal averaging than with the beat-to-beat high-resolution technique.

With the signal averaging technique, preatrial potentials can only be recorded in patients with regular sinus rhythm, whereas dynamic changes of these potentials, which are lost by the signal averaging process, may only be recorded by the beat-to-beat high-resolution technique.

No systematic studies have been published directly validating externally recorded preatrial potentials as true sinus node depolarizations by simultaneous intracardiac catheter recordings from the sinus node area.

Based on the presently available data, the clinical value of noninvasive recordings of preatrial activity is extremely limited. This holds particularly true for its contribution to clinical decision making (e.g., whether a patient should receive a cardiac pacemaker) and its prognostic significance for detecting high-risk patients prone to syncope or severe bradyarrhythmias.

Recording of His Bundle Potentials

Surface recordings of His bundle activity represented the first clinical application of the signal averaging technique.[4,5,28] Since these initial reports, numerous studies have been published dealing with surface His bundle recordings, which have been performed with different kinds of signal averaging computers.[11–15,29–32] In the earlier reports, successful His bundle recordings were made in 30% to 50% of cases, depending on the limited recording technology at that time and on problems with instability of the trigger mechanism. Reasons for failure to record His bundle activity included excessive trigger jitter and/or slight variations of the conduction velocity within the His-Purkinje system, as shown by Tonkin et al.[33] In more recent studies, the success rates for recording His bundle potentials were reported to be in the range of 50% to 75%, mostly due to better hardware and software technology. Some groups tried to confirm their surface His bundle electrograms by offline intracardiac catheter recordings.[30,34-37]

In most of these studies, good to excellent correlations were found, with correlation coefficients well beyond 0.90 (Figure 3). However, in none of these evaluation studies were direct online recordings performed, which may be a general limitation, since intraindividual variations of the atrio-ventricular conduction intervals are well known, depending on physical exercise or emotional stress during daily life.[33] His bundle spikes can be evaluated semidirectly in the signal-averaged ECG by administration of drugs that change the atrio-ventricular nodal conduction velocity, such as catechola-

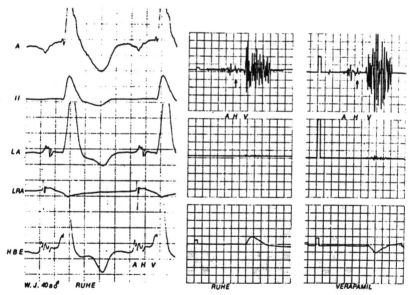

Figure 3. His bundle ECG obtained by intracardiac catheter recording (left panel) and by signal averaging of the high-gain amplified surface ECG at control (RUHE) and following intravenous administration of 10 mg of verapamil. Note the relatively short AH interval. The His bundle spike (arrows) is somewhat more separated from atrial depolarization after administration of verapamil. A = surface ECG lead A according to Trethewie; II = Einthoven lead II; LA = left atrial ECG; LRA = low right atrial ECG; HBE = His bundle ECG.

mines, oxyfedrine, or atropine for accelerating conduction (shortening of the PH interval), and beta blockers or verapamil for slowing conduction (prolongation of the PH interval). In a pilot study performed by our group (unpublished data), in a series of 15 patients with bradyarrhythmias during sinus rhythm, the effect of oxyfedrine (96 mg/day), on heart rate and cardiac conduction was evaluated, using the MAC-I averaging computer. In 11 of 15 patients a relatively stable and reproducible His bundle spike with an isoelectric interval to the preceding atrial complex was recorded, whereas in the remaining four patients the His bundle potential was obscure. In eight of 15 patients the PH interval decreased significantly (Figure 4); it remained unchanged in three of 15 patients, and in the remain-

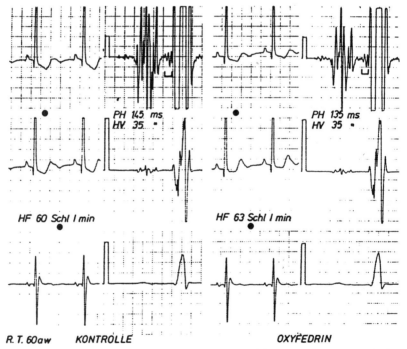

Figure 4. Signal-averaged surface His-bundle ECG before (control) and after administration of 96 mg of oxyfedrine. Note two cycles of the conventional ECG on the left and one cycle of the signal averaged high-gain amplified surface ECG on the right of each half of the figure. The heart rate (HF) increased slightly and the PH interval was shortened by the administration of oxyfedrine. HF = heart rate (beats per minute); PH = PH interval; HV = HV interval.

ing four patients the PH interval increased by the effect of oxyfedrine. In the whole group the PP interval decreased from 131.5 ± 38.0 msec before to 123.3 ± 40.2 msec after administration of oxyfedrine (statistically not significant), whereas the HV interval remained virtually unchanged (41.3 ± 5.2 msec before and 42.0 ± 4.9 msec after oxyfedrine). The observations on apparent prolongations of the PH interval in four patients of the latter group may be explained by the fact that in these individuals the His bundle spike could not be exactly separated from atrial depolarization and/or from background noise; thus the supposed negative dromotropic effect of oxyfedrine may be mimicked by the poor technical quality of the signal-averaged surface ECG. Nevertheless, these results show that with success rates of 60% to 80% of surface His bundle recordings, the influence of cardioactive drugs on the atrio-ventricular node and His-Purkinje system may be tested noninvasively by the signal-averaged high-resolution ECG. This may be particularly helpful in screening the effect of new cardiovascular drugs in the preclinical phase of evaluation, as well as for monitoring possible side effects of clinically used drugs in patients on oral maintenance therapy. The latter may be particularly important in patients receiving antiarrhythmic drugs, and the side effects of these drugs can be documented when the patient is in regular sinus rhythm. Two severe limitations of surface His bundle electrocardiography with the averaging technique have to be mentioned: (1) overlap of the His bundle potential by atrial activity; and (2) failure to document second- or third-degree atrio-ventricular blocks beat-by-beat.

Atrial overlapping of His bundle spikes may be observed in 20% to 40% of cases. In a study performed by McKenna et al,[35] of 70 individuals (five normal subjects, 21 patients with arrhythmias, and 44 patients with surgically corrected tetralogy of Fallot), a clear His bundle potential was seen in 31 of the 70 subjects (44%). Atrial overlap was observed in 25 individuals; in 10 patients no His bundle spike was present, and in the remaining four patients electrical interference prevented successful His bundle recordings. Intravenous administration of verapamil prolonged the PH interval, and in 48 individuals (69%) a His bundle potential of good quality was recorded, mainly due to the fact that in 23 of 25 individuals with atrial overlap, verapamil separated the end of atrial depolarization from the beginning of His bundle activation. These results show that the problem of atrial overlap in surface His bundle recordings may be overcome by administration of verapamil or by beta blocking drugs, and the success rates of His bundle recordings may be improved by 40% to 60%. This may be particularly helpful in patients with PQ intervals of 160 msec (see Figure 3) who have relatively short PH intervals (i.e., faster nodal conduction, in which atrial overlap is likely to occur).

The second problem, failure to document the site of atrio-ventricular block, may be overcome by selective triggering on blocked P and R waves, using the so-called automated discrimination circuit.[38,39] By means of this technique, superimposed P and R wave segments can be excluded, and signal averaging of the post-P intervals makes it possible to determine whether a His bundle potential exists (infra-His block) or not (supra-His block). In their recent study, Takeda et al[39] described the results in ten patients with a complete atrio-ventricular block, six of whom had supra-His blocks, and four infra-His blocks. In the selectively triggered and signal-averaged electrograms, five patients had no His spike in the post-P interval but did have a His bundle potential preceding the averaged pre-R interval. Four patients had no His bundle activity prior to the QRS complex but had consistent His spikes following the blocked P waves. Thus, in nine of ten patients, the site of complete atrio-ventricular block could be localized by an intelligent surface ECG signal averaging method, the results of which corresponded perfectly to catheter recordings from the His bundle area. However, in one patient with block proximal to the His bundle, the correct diagnosis could not be achieved by the surface averaging method.

In this special study, an esophageal atrial electrogram was taken for triggering the averager on the P wave, because its amplitude was much higher than that of the conventional bipolar surface ECG. This is a serious limitation of a "completely noninvasive" method, because many patients may feel much discomfort when swallowing a catheter electrode for recording the esophageal ECG. In addition, because the technical requirements are demanding, and the signal averaging process is complicated, methodology may not receive widespread application. Ultimately, the clinical information on the site of atrio-ventricular block seems to be rather limited, because, for example, patients with a complete block are absolute candidates for pacemaker implantation (with the exception of congenital complete heart block). In some patients with a second-degree block, the localization of the site of block might be helpful; for example, a Wenckebach supra-His block may be more benign than an infra-His block, which may also hold true for the Mobitz-type of second-degree block. However, the full dynamic behavior of atrio-ventricular conduction under various physiologic conditions can be documented more precisely by Holter long-term ECG monitoring, and the decision on pacemaker implantation will be made primarily by the patient's symptoms and the results of the Holter ECG, rather than by a short-term signal-averaged surface His bundle ECG.

One last peculiarity of surface His bundle electrocardiography with the signal averaging technique should be mentioned. In about 20% to 50%, the His bundle potential may appear bi, tri-, or quadriphasic (see Figure 4). It has been supposed that at least quadriphasic complexes might represent delayed intra-His activation (so-called split-His) or depolarization of the His bundle and its branches. The clinical and prognostic significance of such findings remains unclear because corresponding correlative studies with intracardiac catheter recordings and follow-up of these patients have not yet been conducted.

Since the introduction of spatial averaging technology the low-noise ECG can be recorded from the body surface on a beat-to-beat basis, and the first applications of this technique were again recordings of His bundle potentials.[6,40] In the study of Flowers et al,[6] 25 healthy individuals were investigated and their His bundle potentials were recorded. The mean PH interval values were 115.0 ±12.3 msec and the HV intervals were 40.5 ±3.5 msec. Owing to special computer algorithms and filtering procedures, relatively sharp spikelike His potentials were described. Occasional reports on continuous His bundle recordings from body surface have been published. El-Sherif and colleagues[41] reported recording rates of His bundle potentials of 43% using high-resolution beat-to-beat output compared with a 71% recording rate when using the signal averaging technique. Our group reported successful His bundle recordings with the beat-to-beat technique in nine of 14 subjects,[42] in whom His bundle potentials were found to be spikelike in two individuals (Figure 5), and ramplike in seven patients.

In all of these studies the surface beat-to-beat ECG recordings of His-Purkinje activity were not validated by intracardiac catheter studies. Moreover, although experiences with this new technique in patients with higher degree atrio-ventricular blocks have not been published as yet, theoretically real-time electrocardiography represents the most promising noninvasive technique for the detection of the site of block (e.g., second-degree block of Wenckebach-type or Mobitz-type and complete atrio-ventricular block). The presently

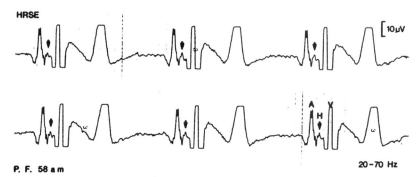

Figure 5. High-resolution real-time surface ECG (continuous strip) showing a spikelike His bundle potential (arrows). HRSE = high resolution surface ECG; A = atrial depolarization; H = His bundle deflection; V = ventricular depolarization.

available real-time ECG recording equipment apparently does not have enough noise reduction capabilities to retrieve His-Purkinje activity from baseline noise in a high, and for clinical purposes, sufficient percentage of cases. Thus, improvements in recording technology are necessary, before the high-resolution beat-to-beat technique will become a routine measure to study and screen larger patient populations with normal and disturbed atrio-ventricular conduction.

Summary and Conclusions

His bundle potentials can be recorded from the body surface by both the signal averaging and the high-resolution real-time techniques.

The recovery rates of His bundle potentials are presently higher with the signal averaging (60% to 80%) than with the real-time technique (40% to 60%).

The site of atrio-ventricular block (supra-His, infra-His) may be differentiated by a special averaging procedure (the application of the so-called automated discrimination circuit), but the beat-to-beat real-time technique is superior as an approach to this problem. However, the present experience with both techniques in larger patient groups with various types of atrio-ventricular blocks is greatly limited.

In 20% to 40% of cases, the signal-averaged His bundle potential appears tri- or quadriphasic, which may possibly indicate intra-His conduction disturbances (so-called split-His) or may represent both His bundle and bundle branch depolarization.

The knowledge of the atrio-ventricular conduction subintervals (PH and HV intervals) through noninvasive electrocardiography seems to be limited, so far as decisions from these values for treatment (e.g., pacemaker implantations) are concerned. More important information will be derived from the patient's symptoms and from the results of 24-hour ambulatory ECG monitoring.

His bundle electrocardiography with the signal averaging and the high-resolution real-time techniques may be useful for noninvasive screening of new cardiovascular drugs that influence atrio-ventricular conduction and for monitoring the effect of clinically established drugs during chronic maintenance therapy. The latter will be of particular importance for monitoring the effect of antiarrhythmic drugs that exert negative dromotropic effects mainly on intraventricular conduction (prolongation of the HV interval).

Recordings of Atrio-Ventricular Nodal Potentials

Attempts to record nodal activity itself by the extracellular route date back to 1907.[43] Since that time several groups have described nodal potentials by direct needle or catheter recordings; however, much controversy existed about the true waveform and the validation of these so-called nodal potentials in dogs by means of the signal averaging technique, the data of which was updated and reviewed in 1981 during the International Symposium on the Signal Averaging Technique in Cologne.[44]

In 15 dogs, high-gain amplified electrograms from catheter recordings, obtained from the His bundle region, were analyzed by signal averaging during junctional rhythms. One or more low-frequency wavelike potentials, with a duration of 26 to 47 msec and amplitudes of 1 to 15 μV, were observed, which preceded the His bundle deflection. These potentials were characterized and discussed as nodal potentials, and the underlying rhythm was confirmed as a true atrio-ventricular nodal rhythm rather than a His bundle rhythm. Similar results were obtained by our group from 1979 to 1981 in patients by signal averaging His bundle ECGs obtained by conventional catheter techniques. In 15 of 20 patients, reproducibly low-frequency wavelike potentials were recorded, which preceded the His bundle deflections by 20 to 106 msec. The amplitude of these potentials ranged from 1 to 12 μV, and their ratio to the amplitude of the His bundle potentials was 4:1 to 32:1. During sinus rhythm, 10 of 15 patients were studied with the MAC-I computer, and the following conduction times of the subintervals were recorded: A-H = 114 ±30 msec; A-N = 85 ±18 msec; and N-H = 29 ±17 msec. During atrial pacing, atrio-ventricular nodal conduction was considerably prolonged, as indicated by the prolonged N-H intervals: A-H = 133 ±38 msec; A-N = 85 ±18 msec; and N-H = 45 ±21 msec (Figure 6). In two patients atrio-ventricular nodal tachycardias were initiated by programmed atrial pacing, and the antegrade conduction intervals were considerably prolonged: A-H = 240 msec and 260 msec; A-N = 95 msec and 80 msec; and N-H = 145 msec and 160 msec. From this study it was concluded that additional potentials can be retrieved between the end of atrial depolarization and the beginning of His bundle activation by averaging high-gain amplified His bundle ECGs from catheter recordings, and that these potentials may reveal functional characteristics of nodal cells (i.e., low amplitude wavelike potentials and slowing of nodal conduction velocity during atrial pacing and during phases of nodal tachycardias).

Since the publication of these two reports, no further similar investigations have been conducted, although it might be of some clinical and theoretical interest to study the behavior of nodal conduction in humans under various physiologic and pathophysiologic conditions (e.g., exercise, drug administration).

Summary and Conclusions

Extracellular recordings of nodal potentials in animals and in humans are feasible by signal averaging high-gain amplified intracardiac catheter recordings from the His bundle region.

Validation of these potentials as being true nodal activity is crucial, at least in humans. This problem may be approached by testing the behavior of these "nodal" potentials during atrial pacing or following intravenous administration of drugs that are known to delay nodal conduction.

Atrio-ventricular nodal recordings in man may be of some theoretical and clinical interest in order to test the influence of various physiologic conditions and pharmacologic interventions on atrio-

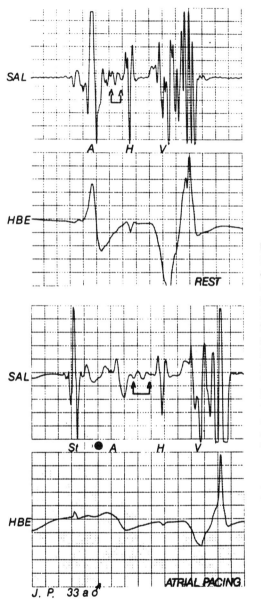

Figure 6. Signal-averaged high-gain amplified His bundle ECG. During sinus rhythm at resting conditions (REST) there are additional low amplitude signals between the end of atrial (A) and the beginning of His bundle (H) depolarizations, possibly indicating atrio-ventricular nodal activity. During atrial pacing (bottom) the interval from the end of atrial (A) and the beginning of His bundle (H) depolarizations is considerably prolonged, possibly indicating a rate-dependent conduction delay within the atrio-ventricular node. SAL = signal-averaged lead; HBE = intracardiac catheter His bundle ECG; ST = stimulus artifact; A = atrial depolarization; H = His bundle deflection; V = ventricular depolarization.

ventricular nodal conduction by means of a direct recording technology.

The true practical value of this technique may be limited. Because an invasive approach is required it cannot be performed in larger groups of patients for screening purposes, and the results of nodal recordings cannot support in any way the clinical decision of what type of treatment should be applied in an individual patient.

Recordings of Ventricular Late Potentials

Experimental and clinical data have convincingly shown that reentry plays a major role in the genesis of ventricular tachyarrhythmias. Prerequesites of reentry are unindirectional block, slow conduction, and recovery of excitability of the tissue ahead of the excitation wave front. As an expression of slow conduction, delayed, and fractionated electrical activity during diastole has been documented in experimental infarction and in the border zones of infarcted human myocardium. [17,45–48] Such late diastolic activity, commonly called "ventricular late potentials," may be recorded by direct intraoperative mapping during open-heart surgery, by intracardiac catheter mapping, and noninvasively from the body surface by high-resolution electrocardiography (signal averaging technique and beat-to-beat high-resolution technique). [20,49,50]

Larger studies of the diagnostic and prognostic significance of ventricular late potentials have been performed almost exclusively with the signal averaging technique. Several investigators have studied different patient groups according to the type of underlying heart disease and/or the prevailing type of ventricular arrhythmias. Our own group found that ventricular late potentials are an extremely rare finding in patients with congestive cardiomyopathy, aortic stenosis, and the so-called small vessel disease-type of coronary heart disease, irrespective of whether the patients were suffering from potentially dangerous repetitive ventricular ectopic activity. [51,52] Thus, ventricular late potentials seem to occur most frequently in patients with coronary heart disease, particularly in those with "regional" myocardial damage.

In a study of 50 patients with acute myocardial infarction, the spectrum of ventricular arrhythmias and the presence of ventricular late potentials was investigated, starting from the first day of illness, and the patients were followed for a mean of 30 ±6 months. [51] Seven patients died within 3 to 6 days after myocardial infarction, and six of these patients had ventricular late potentials. In the total group of myocardial infarction patients, ventricular late potentials were relatively rare during the acute phase (17 of 50 = 34%), and this finding has been corroborated by subsequent studies.[53,54] The predictive power of ventricular late potentials in the acute phase of myocardial infarction was evaluated only in the study of Hopp et al,[51] and the predictive value of ventricular late potentials for in hospital sudden cardiac death was 67%. In contrast, ventricular late potentials recorded in the acute phase of illness were not helpful in predicting an increased risk in the post-hospital period (predictive value for sudden cardiac death, 17%). The predischarge prevalence of ventricular late potentials post-infarction is in the range of 21% to 55%; that is, within the healing and reparative phase of infarction, delayed activation of circumscribed myocardial areas is more common than in the first hours of coronary artery occlusion.

Many prospective studies have been conducted to evaluate the long-term predictive power of ventricular late potentials post-infarction.[55-63] The mean follow-up periods in these studies varied from 6 to 30 months. In two studies the occurrence of new attacks of ventricular tachycardias could be predicted by the presence of ventricular late potentials (predictive value of 24%). In two further studies the risk of sudden cardiac death and/or ventricular tachycardia could be prognosticated by ventricular late potentials, with a predictive value of 50%.[60] In the study by our own group, sudden cardiac death was predictable by ventricular late potentials in 30% of cases.[52] By combining both variables (i.e., the presence of late potentials and the occurrence of repetitive forms of ventricular arrhythmias), the predictive value could be improved to 40%, but the sensitivity decreased from 88% to 50%.

Several reports have been published regarding the prevalence and prognostic significance of ventricular late potentials in patients with chronic coronary heart disease. In the study by Breithardt et al,[16] 146 patients (20 without coronary heart disease, 126 with coronary heart disease, and 16 with dilatative cardiomyopathy) were prospectively followed: 49 patients had ventricular late potentials, with a mean duration of 31 ±15.3 msec in patients without documented ventricular tachycardia, and of 51 ±31.5 msec in those with documented ventricular tachycardia. The predictive value for sudden cardiac death was not reported in this study.

In another study by our group, 200 patients with chronic coronary heart disease were investigated prospectively.[52] In 108 patients (54%), ventricular late potentials were found at entry into the study. After a follow-up period of 32 ±8 months, 25 patients died (18 from sudden cardiac death). The predictive value of ventricular late potentials for this event was 16%, and their sensitivity was 94%. The predictive value of spontaneous ventricular tachycardia (VT) and ventricular fibrillation (VF) attacks was 8%, and their sensitivity was 7%; the predictive value of left ventricular dysfunction (ejection fraction <40%) for sudden cardiac death was 21%, and its sensitivity was 72%. When combining the criteria of reduced ejection fraction and the presence of ventricular late potentials, the sensitivity for predicting sudden cardiac death was 67%, and the predictive value was 21%. Thus, the sensitivity of ventricular late potentials in the diagnosis of patients prone to sudden cardiac death was relatively high, whereas the predictive value was disappointingly low, due to the large number of false-positive late potential recordings.

Similar results were obtained by Zimmermann et al,[64] who found ventricular late potentials in 32 of 92 (35%) patients with coronary heart disease. For predicting sudden cardiac death, the detection of ventricular late potentials revealed a high sensitivity (100%) and a predictive value of 19%. The corresponding values of ventricular late potentials for predicting the occurrence of VT/VF were: sensitivity = 90%; predictive value = 31%.

Patients with spontaneous, documented VT/VF and those resuscitated from VF represent a special group of high-risk individuals. Ventricular late potentials were detected in 16 of 20 patients with coronary heart disease and documented VT/VF (Figure 7). During the follow-up period of 26 ±5 months, six patients died (five from sudden cardiac death). The sensitivity of ventricular late potentials for predicting sudden cardiac death was 100%, and the predictive value was 31%. Reduced ejection fraction (<40%) revealed a sensitivity of 80% and a predictive value of 44% for sudden cardiac death. A combination of three parameters (ventricular late potentials, plus VT/VF during Holter monitoring, plus reduced ejection fraction) showed the highest prognostic accuracy: sensitivity = 80%; and predictive value = 67%.[52] In a further group of 22 patients with coronary heart disease, who were resuscitated from VF, 15 (68%) had ventricular late potentials on the signal-averaged ECG. During a follow-up period of 29 ±8 months, eight patients died (six from sudden cardiac death). The prognostic power of ventricular late potentials for predicting the recurrence of sudden cardiac death

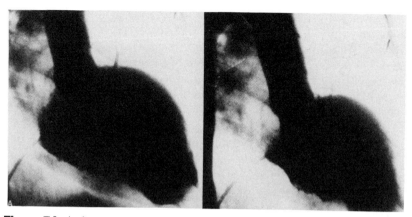

Figure 7A. Left ventricular angiogram in a 46-year-old man with large anterior wall myocardial infarction, showing left ventricular silhouette in diastole (top) and in systole (bottom). Note the large aneurysm of the whole anterior wall and of the left ventricular apex.

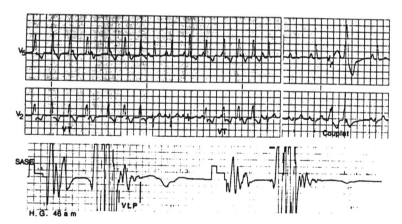

Figure 7B. Holter ECG (top) and signal-averaged surface ECG (bottom) in the same patient as in A. Note short runs of ventricular tachycardias (top left) and a ventricular couplet (top right) and a large ventricular late potential (VLP) at the end of the QRS complex (bottom). V_5 = thoracic bipolar lead V_5; V_2 = thoracic bipolar lead V_2; T = ventricular tachycardia; SASE = signal-averaged surface ECG.

was: sensitivity = 100%; and predictive value = 40%. The corresponding values for a reduced ejection fraction (<40%) were: sensitivity = 67%; and predictive value = 50%. The highest diagnostic accuracy was found by a combination of the presence of ventricular late potentials, reduced ejection fraction, and a repetitive ventricular response on programmed ventricular stimulation: sensitivity = 50%; and predictive value = 100%.

The disappointingly low predictive power of static ventricular late potentials obtained by the signal averaging technique have stimulated several groups to develop high-resolution ECG equipment that permits continuous recording of ventricular late potentials and, thus, the study of the dynamic properties of ventricular late potentials. El-Sherif et al[48] have pointed out that a Wenckebach conduction pattern in the peri-infarct zone may be the mechanism for initiating reentrant VT/VF. Such dynamic conduction implies a continuously increasing length of post-QRS activation (i.e., of ventricular late potentials that can only be detected by dynamic high-resolution surface ECG technology). Therefore, it is most important to investigate the transition of the last normal ventricular beat to the following single or repetitive ventricular ectopic beat, and to detect the functional role of ventricular late potentials between both. Using a special high-resolution ECG unit, El-Sherif et al[41] reported the following recovery rates of ventricular late potentials: in none of 18 healthy volunteers; in two of 20 patients with various cardiac disorders; and in 15 of 21 patients within the first three weeks following acute myocardial infarction. Twelve of 15 patients in the last group had episodes of VT/VF, either spontaneously or induced by programmed ventricular stimulation. Ventricular late potentials remained constant in successive sinus beats in nine of 15 patients, indicating a 1:1 conduction pattern in the ischemic myocardium, and varied in configuration and timing in successive sinus beats in six of 15 patients, probably reflecting a Wenckebach conduction pattern.

In our initial study in 1984, we found ventricular late potentials in 12 of 30 patients with cardiac disease, using our own high-resolution ECG equipment (Figure 8), and in five of 12 patients, ventricular late potentials occurred intermittently (Figure 9).[42]

In a further expanded series of 44 patients, the incidence and dynamicity of ventricular late potentials was studied by our group.[49] Ventricular late potentials were found in 27 patients within the ST segment and in 21 patients following the T wave. Ventricular late

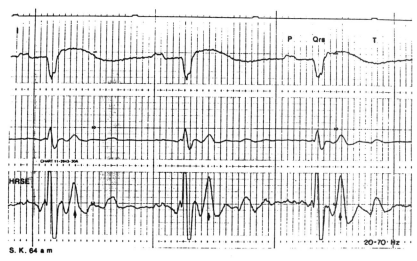

Figure 8. Continuous recording of the low-noise ECG in a patient with a large anterior wall aneurysm and repetitive attacks of sustained ventricular tachycardias. Note persistent ST segment elevations in Einthoven's lead I (top) as the electrocardiographic sign of aneurysm, and the large ventricular late potentials (arrows) extending to the entire ST segment of the low-noise real-time ECG (bottom). HRSE = high-resolution surface ECG.

potentials occurred intermittently in 11 of 27 patients within the ST segment, and in five of 21 individuals after the T wave. In one of 22 patients with single ventricular ectopic beats, a Wenckebach conduction pattern of ventricular late potentials was found (Figure 10), whereas a "focal" type of late potential-ectopic beat interaction was seen in 13 of 22 patients (Figure 11). During episodes of VT, slowly depolarizing diastolic potentials prior to each VT-QRS complex were seen in three of four patients, and "stressing" of ventricular late potentials by high ventricular rate or programmed pacing was achieved in nine of 15 patients.

These studies show that ventricular late potentials may reveal dynamic properties during spontaneous sinus rhythm, during episodes of single or repetitive ventricular ectopic activity, and during programmed ventricular stimulation. However, up to now the prognostic significance of such findings has not been studied, although long-term recordings of the high-resolution ECG are now feasible which allow a more comprehensive documentation of the dynamic behavior of ventricular late potentials. [65]

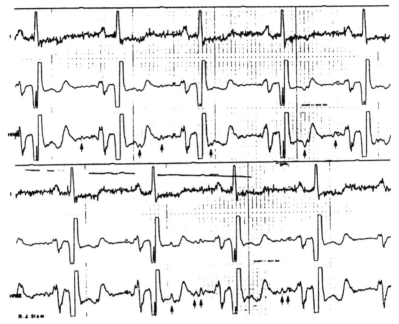

Figure 9. Einthoven's lead I and the low-noise electrocardiogram (HRSE) in a patient with left ventricular aneurysm and repetitive attacks of ventricular tachycardias. Note the intermittent occurrence of ventricular late potentials with varying timing to the preceding QRS complex and the T wave (arrows). For comparison the last ventricular depolarization (bottom right) does not show any abnormal depolarization within the ST and post-T segment. I = Einthoven lead I; HRSE = high-resolution surface ECG.

It should be mentioned that, mostly due to dynamic properties of ventricular late potentials, the beat-to-beat technique provides higher detection rates of these potentials than does the signal averaging technique.[2,49] This holds particularly true for patients with the congenital long QT syndrome.

Eggeling et al[66] found ventricular late potentials in six of seven patients with the congenital long QT syndrome, by means of the high-resolution beat-to-beat technique, but in only three of seven patients with the signal averaging technique. It is interesting that patients with the long QT syndrome reveal ventricular late potentials not only within the ST segment but also following the T wave and that these potentials are extremely variable with respect to timing to the QRS complex or to the T wave, amplitudes, and their

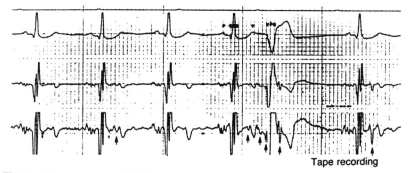

Tape recording

Figure 10. Low-noise ECG in real-time of a 66-year-old patient with coronary heart disease and single and repetitive ventricular ectopic activity. Note the intermittent, variable occurrence of ventricular late potential (arrows). Following the fourth normal ventricular complex, fractionated activity is seen within the ST and post-T segment, and this fractionation merges into the ventricular ectopic beat, indicating a Wenckebach-type of slowed ventricular conduction with one reentrant cycle. I = Einthoven lead I; HRSE = high-resolution surface ECG; VPB = ventricular premature beat.

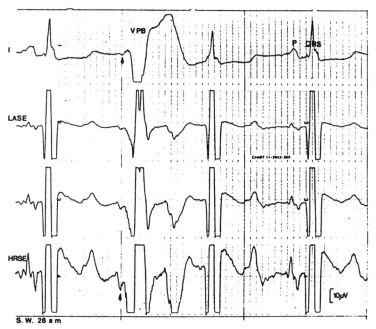

Figure 11. Low-noise ECG of a 28-year-old man with dilatative cardiomyopathy and repetitive attacks of sustained ventricular tachycardia. Note a single slowly depolarizing potential (arrow) that precedes and merges into the ventricular ectopic beat (VPB), indicating an ectopic type of ventricular premature depolarization. I = Einthoven lead I; LASE = low amplified surface ECG; HRSE = high-resolution surface ECG.

appearance per se. These parameters may show hour-to-hour, day-to-night, or day-to-day variability, depending on the level of sympathetic activity of the individual patient. Moreover, the amplitudes of the post-T wave late potentials in those patients can be enhanced by intravenous administration of catecholamines and can be diminished by intravenous beta blockade (unpublished observations). In our experience, in patients with the long QT syndrome the detection of ventricular late potentials by high-resolution electrocardiography proved to be the most accurate indicator of increased ventricular vulnerability, compared to the spontaneous occurrence of VT during exercise or emotional stress, the spontaneous occurrence of VT during Holter ECG monitoring, and the response to programmed ventricular stimulation.

Ventricular late potentials may also be found in patients with right ventricular outflow tract obstructions, particularly in those with corrected Fallot's tetralogy. In a preliminary study by our group, ventricular late potentials were detected in 26 of 29 patients who were corrected for right ventricular outflow tract obstructions plus ventriculotomy, using the high-resolution surface ECG method. Twenty-three patients were studied by endocardial right ventricular catheter mapping and by high-resolution electrocardiography; in 21 of these patients, catheter electrograms revealed clear to massive fractionated late potentials within the ST segment and after the T wave, whereas in 22 patients similar fractionated late potentials were seen within the ST segment and the post-T segment of the low-noise ECG. These late potentials correlated well with the spontaneous occurrence of VT in this special group of patients, in whom the prevalence of VT was known to be high. Thus, ventricular late potentials seem to be a valuable noninvasive marker of right ventricular electrical instability in those patients with surgically corrected right ventricular outflow tract obstructions.

A separate technique has been devised to discover abnormal electrical activity within the ST segment, based on the analysis in the frequency domain by means of the fast Fourier transform analysis (FFTA). Ventricular late potentials within the ST segment represent electrical signals with high-frequency components than are usually encountered in the normal ST segment. High-gain amplified signal-averaged or single-beat low-noise ECGs may be analyzed by FFTA, using special window functions (e.g., Blackman-Harris window).

Cain et al[67] described a device that performs FFTA of high-gain amplified signal-averaged X/Y/Z leads for noise reduction. For each ECG segment (e.g., QRS complex, terminal 40 msec of QRS/ST segment, T wave) spectral curves of the X/Y/Z leads are generated, and for quantitative comparison the energy spectra are calculated. Among three parameters of abnormal FFTA findings, the ratio of the area under the curve between 20 Hz and 50 Hz to the area under curve between 0 and 20 Hz was used for defining normal or abnormal frequency contents of the ST segment. In a group of 20 patients with spontaneous VT, this criterion was compared with the results of programmed ventricular stimulation. A logistic regression, with inducibility of VT as the dependent variable, was used to help define area ratio values > 20 as abnormal. Sustained monomorphic VT was induced in 18 patients, each with an area ratio value > 20. Sustained VT was not induced in two patients, each with an area ratio value < 20. In a group of 38 patients (12 with nonsustained VT and 26 with syncope), FFTA data were compared prospectively with the results of programmed ventricular stimulation. VT was not inducible in any of the 26 patients in this group with normal FFTA values. Sustained monomorphic VT was induced in five of 12 patients with abnormal FFTA values. Thus, the results of FFTA correctly predicted the results of programmed ventricular stimulation in 88% of patients studied and in 82% of patients with syncope or nonsustained VT.[68]

FFTA of single-beat high-resolution ECGs has been reported by Haberl et al[69] and by Oeff[70] with results similar to those of Cain et al.[67] A similar technique has been described by our own group,[49] using FFTA of the ST segment in single-beat low-noise ECGs. In a preliminary pilot study on 14 patients with coronary heart disease, three patients with sustained VT, one patient with VF, and four healthy individuals, FFTA revealed higher frequency components of the ST segment in the range of 0 to 100 Hz in the three VT patients, compared to the coronary disease patients without VT. Completely concordant results with the three methods (signal-averaged ECG, low-noise real-time ECG, and FFTA) were obtained in 11 of 14 patients (three patients with VT and late potentials had abnormal FFT results, and eight patients without VT had negative results with all three methods). Thus, preliminary data on FFTA of the ST segment suggest that patients prone to VT may be identified by certain characteristics of the frequency components of the ST segment. The prognostic significance of these FFTA findings has not yet been investigated.

Summary and Conclusions

Recordings of ventricular late potentials from body surface represent the most important and clinically relevant application of high-resolution electrocardiography.

Animal experiments have shown that ventricular late potentials represent slowed conduction within an area of depressed myocardium (mostly following myocardial infarction), thus representing one determinant of a reentrant circuit at the level of ventricular myocardium.

Ventricular late potentials as the electrical sign of slowed conduction may be detected in humans not only by intracardiac catheter mapping or direct intraoperative mapping but also noninvasively from the body surface by means of the high-resolution ECG technique.

The prevalence of late potentials is considerably different in patients with various cardiac disorders (e.g., coronary heart disease, dilated cardiomyopathy, hypertrophic obstructive cardiomyopathy, aortic stenosis, long QT syndrome, and surgically corrected Fallot's tetralogy).

Based on numerous correlative clinical studies, ventricular late potentials may be considered a parameter of increased ventricular electrical instability.

The prognostic power of ventricular late potentials, as detected by the signal averaging technique, for predicting episodes of VT/VF or sudden cardiac death, seems to be limited.

The prognostic significance of late potentials may be enhanced if a dynamic Wenckebach conduction pattern can be demonstrated.

Dynamic properties of ventricular late potentials can only be detected by the low-noise real-time ECG technique. Mainly due to the variability of timing and amplitudes of ventricular late potentials, the detection rates are higher with the beat-to-beat than with the signal averaging technique.

Dynamic changes of ventricular late potentials such as intermittent occurrence and variations in amplitude and timing to the QRS complex or to the T wave may occur during spontaneous sinus rhythm, during episodes of single or repetitive ventricular ectopic beats, and following programmed ventricular stimulation.

Ventricular late potentials are extremely variable in patients with the congenital long QT syndrome. In these patients, late potentials seem to be the most sensitive parameter of ventricular vulnerability.

The prognostic significance of the dynamic properties of late potentials, particularly the Wenckebach-type of slowed conduction, is as yet unknown.

Abnormal diastolic electrical activity may also be retrieved by FFTA, which detects higher frequency components within the ST segment than are usually encountered in normal individuals.

Abnormal results of the FFT analysis seem to correlate well with increased ventricular electrical instability, as documented by spontaneous or induced VT. However, the prognostic significance of abnormal FFT results in predicting sudden cardiac death is as yet unknown.

References

1. Heinecker R: Klinische Elektrokardiographic. Stuttgart: Thieme Publishers, 1986.
2. El-Sherif N, Restivo M, Craelius W, et al: High resolution electrocardiography—Basic and clinical aspects. In Hombach V, Hilger HH, Kennedy HL (eds): Electrocardiography and Cardiac Drug Therapy. Dordecht: Kluwer Academic Publishers, 1988, pp 395-410.
3. Josephson ME, Horowitz, LN, Spielman SR, et al: Role of catheter mapping in the preoperative evaluation of ventricular tachycardia. Am J Cardiol 49:207, 1982.
4. Berbari EJ, Lazzara R, Samet P, et al: Noninvasive technique for detection of electrical activity during the P-R segment. Circulation 48:1005, 1973.
5. Stopczyk MJ, Kopec J, Zochowski RJ, et al: Surface recording of electrical heart activity during the P-R segment in man by a computer averaging technique. Int Res Com Syst 73-8, 11, 21-2, 1973.
6. Flowers NC, Shvartsman V, Sohi GS, et al: Signal averaged versus beat-by-beat recording of surface His-Purkinje potentials. In Hombach V, Hilger HH (eds): Signal Averaging Technique in Clinical Cardiology. Stuttgart: Schattauer Publishers, 1981, pp 329–349.
7. Braun V, Hombach V, Hopp HW, et al: Preatrial activity recorded from intracardiac and surface leads by signal averaging. In Hombach V, Hilger HH (eds): Signal Averaging Technique in Clinical Cardiology. Stuttgart: Schattauer Publishers, 1981, pp 81–94.
8. Hombach V, Hopp HW, Brau V, et al: Pre-P potentials in the conventional body surface ECG. Dtsch Med Wochenschr 106:771, 1981.
9. Mackintosh AF, English MJ, Vincent R, et al: Low-voltage electrical activity preceding right atrial depolarization in man. Br Heart J 42:117, 1979.
10. Wajszczuk WJ, Palko T, Przybylski J, et al: External recording of sinus node region activity in animals and in man. In Hombach V, Hilger HH (eds): Signal Averaging Technique in Clinical Cardiology. Stuttgart: Schattauer Publishers, 1981, pp 65–79.

11. Hishimoto Y, Sawayama T: Non-invasive recording of His bundle potential in man—simplified method. Brt Heart J 37:635, 1975.
12. Hombach V, Brau V, Hopp HW, et al: Recordings of A-V nodal potentials in man using the signal averaging technique. In Hombach V, Hilger HH (eds): Signal Averaging Technique in Clinical Cardiology. Stuttgart: Schattauer Publishers, 1981, pp 131–144.
13. Honda N, Ianaka S, Kohno N, et al: Clinical studies on noninvasive investigation of the His bundle electrogram. Proc VIth Int Symp Card Pac. Amsterdam: Excerpta Medica, 1977, pp 19–25.
14. Van den Akker TJ, Goovaerts HG, Schneider H: Realtime method for noninvasive recording of His bundle activity of the electrocardiogram. Comp Biomed Res 9:559, 1976.
15. Vincent R, Stroud NP, Jenner R, et al: Noninvasive recording of electrical activity in the PR segment in man. Br Heart J 40:124, 1978.
16. Breithardt G, Becker R, Seipel L, et al: Noninvasive detection of late potentials in man—a new marker for ventricular tachycardias. Eur Heart J 2:1, 1981.
17. Fontaine G, Guiraudon G, Frank R: Intramyocardial conduction defects in patients prone to ventricular tachycardia. III. The post-excitation syndrome and ventricular tachycardia. In Sandoe E, Julian DG, Bell JW (eds): Management of Ventricular Tachycardia—Role of Mexiletine. Amsterdam: Excerpta Medica, 1978, pp 67–69.
18. Hombach V, Hopp HW, Braun V, et al: Significance of post-excitation potentials within the ST segment in the surface ECG of patients with coronary heart disease. Dtsch Med Wochenschr 105:1457, 1980.
19. Hombach V, Kebbel U, Hopp HW, et al: Continuous registration of micropotentials of the human heart: preliminary results with a new high resolution ECG-amplifier system. Dtsch Med Wochenschr 107:1951, 1982.
20. Simson MB: Identification of patients with ventricular tachycardia after myocardial infarction from signals in the terminal QRS complex. Circulation 64:235, 1981.
21. Bonke FIM: Electrophysiology of the sinus node. In Hombach V, Hilger HH (eds): Signal Averaging Technique in Clinical Cardiology. Stuttgart: Schattauer Publishers, 1981, pp 23–32.
22. Steinbeck G, Haberl R, Luderitz B, et al: Comparison of true and calculated sinoatrial conduction time by atrial pacing in the isolated rabbit heart. In Hombach V, Hilger HH (eds): Signal Averaging Technique in Clinical Cardiology. Stuttgart: Schattauer Publishers, 1981, pp 33–39.
23. Stopcyk MJ, Pieniak M, Wajszcuk W, et al: Sinus node activity in man and animal studies recorded intraatrially by online pre-memorized averaging technique. Proc Vth Int Symp Card Pac. Amsterdam: Excerpta Medica, 1976, pp 13–18.
24. Gebhardt-Seehausen U, Bethge C, Bonke FIM, et al: Continuous recordings of sinus nodal potentials. In Hombach V, Hilger HH (eds): Signal Averaging Technique in Clinical Cardiology. Stuttgart: Schattauer Publishers, 1981, pp 41–52.
25. Hombach V, Zanker R, Behrenbeck DW, et al: Recording of sinus node potentials in man. Z Kardiol 67:155, 1978.

26. Hombach V, Gil-Sanchez D, Zanker R, et al: An approach to direct detection of sinus nodal activity in man. J Electrocardiol 12:343, 1979.
27. Hombach V, Braun V, Hopp HW, et al: The applicability of the signal averaging technique in clinical cardiology. Clin Cardiol 5:107, 1982.
28. Flowers NC, Horan LG: His bundle and bundle-branch recordings from the body surface (abstr). Circulation 48:IV-102, 1973.
29. Furness A, Sharratt GP, Carson P: The feasibility of detecting His bundle activity from the body surface. Cardiovasc Res 9:390, 1975.
30. Hombach V, Braun V, Hopp HW, et al: Noninvasive detection of potentials of the bundle of His from the body surface. Munch Med Wochenschr 123:173, 1981.
31. Tournoux B, Poindessault JP, Gargouil YM, et al: Interet et limites de l'enregistrement des potentiels du fasceau de His par voie externe chez l'homme. Ann Cardiol Angeiol 29:327, 1980.
32. Wajszczuk WJ, Stopczyk MJ, Moskowitz MS, et al: Noninvasive recording of His-Purkinje activity in man by QRS-triggered signal averaging. Circulation 58:25, 1978.
33. Tonkin AM, Blood RJ, Riggs AR, et al: Non-invasive recording of His-bundle potentials: limitations of existing signal averaging techniques. In Hombach V, Hilger HH (eds): Signal Averaging Technique in Clinical Cardiology. Stuttgart: Schattauer Publishers, 1981, pp 291–299.
34. Berbari EJ, Scherlag BJ, Lazzara R: Recordings of A-V nodal potentials during junctional rhythms utilizing signal averaging. Am J Physiol 235:110, 1978.
35. McKenna WJ, Rowland E, Mortara D, et al: Non-invasive recording of the His bundle electrogram: Evaluation of the Marquette high resolution MAC unit. In Hombach V, Hilger HH (eds): Signal Averaging Technique in Clinical Cardiology. Stuttgart: Schattauer Publishers, 1981, pp 301–310.
36. Pernod J, Court L, Duret JC, et al: Possibilité de detection des potentiels hisiens a partir d'electrodes thoraciques de surface. Nouv Presse Med 6:2963, 1977.
37. Vincent R, English MJ, Woollons DJ, et al: Surface His bundle potentials and other low amplitude cardiac signals by signal averaging. In Hombach V, Hilger HH (eds): Signal Averaging Technique in Clinical Cardiology. Stuttgart: Schattauer Publishers, 1981, pp 351–362.
38. Takeda H, Kitamura K, Takamashi T, et al: Non-invasive recording of His-Purkinje activity in patients with complete atrioventricular block. Clinical application of an "automated discrimination circuit." Circulation 60:421, 1979.
39. Takeda H, Kitamura K, Tsujmura T, et al: Non-invasive localization of A-V block by an "automated discrimination circuit." In Hombach V, Hilger HH (eds): Signal Averaging Technique in Clinical Cardiology. Stuttgart: Schattauer Publishers, 1981, pp 311–327.
40. Stopczk MJ, Walcak F, Kepski R, et al: The history of noninvasive His-bundle recording: from averaging to continuous record. In Hombach V, Hilger HH (eds): Signal Averaging Technique in Clinical Cardiology. Stuttgart: Schattauer Publishers, 1981, pp 283–289.

41. El-Sherif N, Mehra R, Gomes JAC, et al: Appraisal of a low noise electrocardiogram. J Am Coll Cardiol 1:456, 1983.
42. Hombach V, Kebbel U, Hopp HW, et al: Noninvasive beat-by-beat registration of ventricular late potentials using high resolution electrocardiography. Int Cardiol 6:167, 1984.
43. Erlanger J, Blackman JR: A study of the relative rhythmicity and conductivity in various regions of the auricles of the mammalian heart. Am J Physiol 19:125, 1907.
44. Berbari EJ, Scherlag BJ, Lazzara R: Recordings of A-V nodal potentials in dogs with junctional rhythms. In Hombach V, Hilger HH (eds): Signal Averaging Technique in Clinical Cardiology. Stuttgart: Schattauer Publishers, 1981, pp 1121–1130.
45. Berbari EJ, Scherlag BJ, Hope R, et al: Recordings from body surface of arrhythmogenic ventricular activity during the ST segment. Am J Cardiol 41:697, 1978.
46. Boineau JP, Cox JL: Slow ventricular activation in acute myocardial infarction. A source of reentrant premature ventricular contractions. Circulation 48:702, 1973.
47. Durrer D, Van Lier A, Buller J: Epicardial and intramural excitation in chronic myocardial infarction. Am Heart J 68:765, 1964.
48. El-Sherif N, Gomes JAC, Restivo M, et al: Late potentials and arrhythmogenesis. PACE 8:440, 1985.
49. Hombach V, Eggeling T, Hoher M, et al: Methods for detection of ventricular late potentials-high resolution ECG, signal averaging technique, frequency analysis, intracardiac mapping. Herz 13:147, 1988.
50. Simson MB: Signalmittelung des oberflachen-elektrokardiogramms zur erkennung von spatpotentialen. In Steinbeck G (ed): Lebensbedrohliche ventrikulare herzhythmusstorugen. Darmstadt: Steinkopff Publishers, 1987, pp 85–92.
51. Hopp HW, Hombach V, Braun V, et al: Ventricular delayed depolarizations in patients with chronic stable coronary heart disease and with acute myocardial infarction. In Hombach V, Hilger HH (eds): Signal Averaging Technique in Clinical Cardiology. Stuttgart: Schattauer Publishers, 1981, pp 233–252.
52. Hopp HW: Der Plotzliche Herztod-Pathophysiologic und Klinik bei koronarer Herzerkankung. Stuttgart: Schattauer Publishers, 1987.
53. Goedel-Meinen L, Schmidt G, Jahns G, et al: Spapotentiale in den ersten 10 Tagen nach Myokardinfarkt. Z Kardiol 75:121, 1986.
54. Potratz J, Djonlagic H, Mentzel H, et al: Verlaufbeobachtung von spatpotentialen bei akuten infarktpatienten innerhalb der ersten drei wochen. Herz/Kreisl 8:397, 1985.
55. Billhardt RA, Mayerhofer KE, Uretz EF, et al: Serial signal averaged ECGs in acute myocardial infarction patients. Circulation 72:III-213, 1985.
56. Breithardt G, Boggrefe M: Pathophysiological mechanisms and clinical significance of ventricular late potentials. Eur Heart J 7:364, 1986.
57. Breithardt G, Boggrefe M, Haerten K, et al: Prognostische Bedeutung ventrikularer Spatpotentiale bei Postinfarktpatienten und Patienten mit stabiler koronarer Herzkarnkheit. In Steinbeck G (ed): Lebensbe-

drohliche Ventrikulare Herzrhythmusstorungen. Darmstadt: Steinkopff Publishers, 1987, pp 93–99.

58. Denniss A, Richards D, Cody D, et al: Prognostic significance of ventricular tachycardia and fibrillation induced at programmed stimulation and delayed potentials detected on signal-averaged electrocardiograms of survivors of acute myocardial infarction. Circulation 74:731, 1986.

59. El-Sherif N, Ursell SN, Bekheit S, et al: Prognostic significance of the signal-averaged ECG depends on the time of recording in the post infarction period. Am Heart J 118:256, 1989.

60. Gomes J, Winters, Stewart D, et al: A new noninvasive index to predict sustained ventricular tachycardia and sudden death in the first year after myocardial infarction based on signal-averaged electrocardiogram, radionuclide ejection fraction and Holter monitoring. J Am Coll Cardiol 2:349, 1987.

61. Grigg LE, Chan W, Hamer A, et al: Correlation between electrophysiological studies, Holter recordings, and signal averaged ECGs in the post-infarction period (abstr). Circulation 76:IV-32, 1987.

62. Hopp HW, Treis-Muller I, Osterspey A, et al: Ventricular late potentials in acute myocardial infarction. Herz 13:169, 1988.

63. Kuchar D, Thorburn C, Sammel N: Late potentials after myocardial infarction: natural history and prognostic significance. Circulation 74:1280, 1986.

64. Zimmermann M, Adamec R, Simonin P, et al: Prognostic significance of ventricular late potentials in coronary artery disease. Am Heart J 109:725, 1985.

65. Hombach V, Kebbel U, Hopp HW, et al: Longterm recording of the low noise ECG from body surface-technical development and clinical significance. Herz/Kreisl 112:621, 1984.

66. Eggeling T, Hopp HW, Schickendantz S, et al: Diostolic microvolt potentials within the high resolution surface ECG in long QT syndrome. Z Kardiol 75:410, 1986.

67. Cain ME, Ambos HD, Witkowski FX, et al: Fast-Fourier transform analysis of signal-averaged electrocardiograms for identification of patients prone to sustained ventricular tachycardia. Circulation 69:711, 1984.

68. Lindsay BD, Ambos HD, Schechtman KB, et al: Improved selection of patients for programmed ventricular stimulation by frequency analysis of signal-averaged electrocardiograms. Circulation 73:675, 1986.

69. Haberl R, Pulter R, Steinbeck G: Einzelschlaganalyse des Frequenzinhaltes von Spatpotentialen von der Korperoberfiache bei Patienten mit koronarer Herzkrankheit. Z Kardiol 75:98, 1986.

70. Oeff M: Einzelschlagregistrierung verspateter ventrikularer depolarisationen und ihre frequenzanalyse mit der Fast-Fourier-transformation-methodische aspekte. In Steinbeck G (ed): Lebensbedronliche ventrikulare herzhythmusstorugen. Darmstadt: Steinkopff Publishers, 1987, pp. 129–135.

11

Surface Recognition of His-Purkinje Activity on an Every Beat Basis

Nancy C. Flowers, Michael B. Simson,
Anita C. Wylds, Weiqun Yang,
Leo G. Horan

Introduction

Shortly after Scherlag et al reported a catheterization technique for recording electrical activity from the His bundle in the intact dog[1] and man,[2] investigators from three laboratories began to examine and report the feasibility of identifying His-Purkinje signals from the body surface.[3-10] The early work using temporal averaging will not be reviewed here except where pertinent, since the present work specifically addresses beat-by-beat recording of His-Purkinje activity.

Significant is the fact that the earliest recognition of His-Purkinje activity from the body surface was, in reality, on an every beat basis and occurred in the course of our pursuing another line of research entirely. As early as 1974 an illustration of a beat-by-beat recording of His-Purkinje activity was published from our laborato-

From El-Sherif N, Turitto G (eds): *High-Resolution Electrocardiography*. Mount Kisco, NY, Futura Publishing Co., Inc., ©, 1992.

ry.[10] From this set of experiments, we obtained a record of highly amplified and filtered recordings (Figure 1), one from across the tricuspid valve and the other from the body surface of an animal. Electrical activity from skeletal muscle was virtually nonexistent because of paralysis induced when the animals were exposed to varying concentrations of halogenated hydrocarbons in studies of the sudden sniffing death syndrome. Unwittingly, we had eliminated one of the major obstacles to ease of recording His-Purkinje activity from the surface, that is, the confounding electrical activity from myopotentials. In Figure 1 the His bundle electrogram (HBE) reflects loss of amplitude and diminution of rate of upstroke secondary to conduction system toxicity from the experimental agents; nevertheless, coincident deflections, B_1 and B_2, regularly occurred in the baseline of the surface HBE after the prolonged, electrically silent interval between atrial and ventricular activity. Further, the fact that 2:1 atrio-ventricular block above the level of the bundle of His had been induced made it possible to compare the absence of His bundle activity following each nonconducted impulse from the

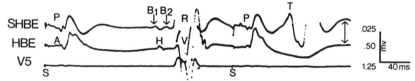

Figure 1. Surface and intracardiac recordings obtained from a dog exposed to high levels of halogenated hydrocarbons, Freon 11 and Freon 12, with development of 2:1 block above the level of the bundle of His. The top channel illustrates electrical activity arising from the His-Purkinje system recorded from the surface (SHBE), amplified and filtered at 30–600 Hz. The middle channel is an intracardiac record of His bundle activity (HBE). The bottom channel is a surface recorded conventional but inverted V_5 lead. Stimulus artifact is reflected in all three channels, indicated by the location of S. Gain settings for each channel and sweep speed are indicated at the far right. Note the coincidence of the B_1, B_2 deflections in the SHBE and the HBE. The arrows to the right indicate the expected location for the subsequent electrical activity from His bundle which is noticeably absent in both leads. This was a stable conduction defect that repeated in this fixed 2:1 fashion for many minutes. In each conducted cycle the His deflection from the HBE recording was invariably associated with deflections labeled B_1 and B_2 in the SHBE recording. P = Surface P wave; A = endocardial atrial activity; H = endocardial His bundle activity; R = surface ventricular activity; V = endocardial ventricular activity; T = surface T wave. (Modified and reproduced with permission from Flowers NC et al. Am J Cardiol 33:384, 1974.)

atrium with the presence of His deflections after each conducted impulse. Another obstacle to recording low level signals was unwittingly circumvented by the fact that this particular animal was studied late in the evening, at a time that an ordinarily electrically quiet laboratory was even quieter; it can be appreciated that baseline noise of the 60 Hz or 60-Hz harmonics variety is not detectable in these recordings.

Optimistically, we embarked on a search for surface His bundle activity, resulting alternately in discouragement and hope, leading ultimately to the focus on beat-by-beat recording.

Methodology with Comments

Table I lists problems identified in early efforts to record surface His-Purkinje activity. The following is a discussion of some of the techniques employed to overcome these obstacles in obtaining a favorable signal-to-noise ratio.

Noise from 60 Hz or the Harmonics of 60 Hz

In our early beat-by-beat work we resorted to a cumbersome but effective means of dealing with power frequency noise.[11–13] A cubicle was built from which cables were led out to the recording equipment. This cubicle, battery-lighted and magnetically as well as electrically shielded, consisted of a wooden frame around which an external layer of copper screen was placed after which a silicon-iron layer of high saturation, middle permeability shielding was placed (500–7000 μ). Additionally, 60-Hz notch filters were used in the instrumentation.

Table I
Problems in Recording His-Purkinje Activity

Noise from 60-Hz sources (or harmonics)
Amplifier noise/electrode-skin interface noise
Confounding signal from the atrium
Myopotentials
Low amplitude of signal of interest

Amplifier Noise/Electrode–Skin Interface Noise

Amplifier noise offers considerable interference, although low-noise amplifiers are more available commercially than they were 10 years ago. This problem becomes less with the years. (Our current system utilizes low-noise amplifiers from Analog Devices [Norwood, Massachusetts].) The electrode-skin interface is a source of troublesome noise and suggests the need for careful preparation and elimination of skin oils. Light abrasion of the skin after oil is removed and final preparation with acetone or alcohol is helpful. Most recently we have used silver-silver chloride electrodes, although we have tried other materials including gold. The use of any good quality silver-silver chloride electrode, as those used for ambulatory monitoring or in intensive care areas, diminishes skin electrode interference. The original channel selection algorithm [12,13] or recently developed alternatives (to be discussed later) further results in elimination of spurious noise.

Confounding Signal from the Atrium

Even atrial signals of average amplitude are 40–60 times the amplitude of surface His bundle signals. Atrial waveforms also contain a greater representation of the lower frequencies. A high-pass filter of 30 Hz or more addresses the issue of low-frequency interference arising from late atrial depolarization, and more predominantly, atrial repolarization. Although it is true that the atrial signal contains a greater representation of lower frequencies than the His bundle signal, it is also true that some portion of His-Purkinje signal is eliminated with high-pass filters. The higher amplitude, lower frequency components of the atrial signal, however, are relatively more suppressed, enhancing detection of the remaining higher frequency components contained in the His bundle signal. On the other hand, analog filters may produce a phase shift of atrial signals, resulting in a superposition of atrial signals on the His bundle signals in the atrio-ventricular segment. Some high-pass filters with a higher order of cut-off frequency may cause ringing at the end of the atrial waveform. Selection of the right type filter as well as an optimal frequency is crucial to the detection of His bundle potentials.

With our present system, there are five parallel channels for acquisition of His bundle signals. Each channel has an adjustable gain of 5000, 10000, or 50000 and a frequency range of 30–200 Hz. The analog high-pass and low-pass filters are used to eliminate DC offset and aliasing. The analog signals are then converted to digital signals by a 12-bit A/D converter at a sampling rate of 1 kHz or 2 kHz and are stored in a Hewlett-Packard 310 computer. The digital signals are further processed by a digital high-pass filter to eliminate low-frequency components contained in the atrio-ventricular segment; this generates a "flat" baseline, which ensures the best effect of the signal enhancing algorithm (discussed in the following section). A digital low-pass filter is also used to suppress the high-frequency noise. Digital implementation of filters provides great flexibility and the best effects for the detection of His bundle potentials.

Myopotentials

Human subjects vary greatly in the degree to which myopotentials arising from the intercostal muscles interfere with efforts to record surface His bundle activity. In the worst case, myopotentials are overwhelming, while in the best case they are hardly a problem at all. The degree of difficulty usually is somewhere between those extremes. Over the years, we have developed, improved, and drastically altered channel selection algorithms that are helpful in optimizing data from multiple simultaneous inputs. Certain channel selection algorithms are applicable to coping with myopotentials, but are also applicable to coping with transient noise, electrode-skin motion artifacts, or a combination of gaiting variables and ionic current.

In earlier work, we combined a spatial averaging technique with an algorithm for coincidence detection in order to enhance signal and suppress noise.[12,13] This approach falls into the category that has been referred to as a double threshold detector or coincidence detector or binary integrator.[14-19] The method employed is a nonparametric, constant false alarm rate principle which uses simultaneous closely spaced inputs. The goal is to reduce burst interference by attenuating a channel identified as noisy. The likelihood of detection of true signal depends on the signal-to-noise ratio at input and the specified threshold level, whereas the likelihood of false detection of noise as signal is a function of the threshold level.

Our goal was the recognition of the presence of signal in noise rather than the preservation of full fidelity of the transmitted signal.

Although we apply other signal enhancing algorithms as well, currently we employ a digital modification as well as logic modification of the early channel selection algorithm. First, data from the five channels are compared to a preset threshold every millisecond. If the data from the five channels exceed the threshold at the same time, that is, phase coherence exists in all channels, the data is accepted as true and the mean of the five is calculated as an output. When there is phase coherence in four of five channels, the noncoherent channel is rejected as noise, and the remaining channels are averaged. Similarly, if any two channels are out of phase with the other channels, three channels account for the output data. Phase coherence may also exist among noise from different channels. However, the duration of phase coherent noise is much shorter than that of the signal of interest.[13] Pulses <2 msec are rejected as coherent noise. Additional algorithms that can identify maximal "outlier" channels may also be applied which allow elimination of unhelpful input. Signal-to-noise ratio can be increased significantly by these algorithms.

The selection of lead sites is important in optimizing signal and attenuating myopotentials. Some degree of exploration is necessary in most patients for optimizing phase coherence. We attempt to select distances that will allow perception of the waveform as maximally similar from each of the sampling sites. Therefore, ideally the electrodes should be as close together as possible. However, proximity of electrodes for His bundle detection has to be balanced against the need to minimize confounding myopotential. This potential is best diminished by allowing maximal interpolar distance so that the sampling electrodes perceive myopotential as minimally coincident from each of the sampling sites. Having tried several lead sites, we are presently utilizing two configurations of bipolar leads (a cluster of five leads per pole): a V_1 position to a site near the apex of the heart; and a site between V_1 and V_2 to a corresponding left paraspinal site.

To some extent Santopietro's work[20] provides insights that are helpful, although this author did not specify minimal critical distances between sampling sites. The common poles of sampling sites must remain in the same electrical field as far as voltage polarity goes during the PR segment. They should be oriented approximately along an electrical lead axis (not necessarily the exact anatomic axis) of the His bundle. Electrode distances to optimize signal and to attenuate myopotential range from 0.5 to 2 cm and are usually between 1 and 1.5 cm.

If not clinically contraindicated and if myopotentials remain a problem, a carefully administered intravenous or oral dose of diazepam 2.5–5.0 mg in select patients can further attenuate myopotentials.

Low Amplitude of Signal of Interest

The magnitude of a His bundle signal from the surface generally falls between 3–5 µV. The magnitudes of the other components of the bundle branch system are even less. Only on rare occasions have His signals of amplitudes larger than 5 µV been recorded. Noise from cumulative sources in even quiet hospital environments frequently exceeds the magnitude of His signal by a factor of 10 or more. Thus, we originally adapted techniques already in daily use in our laboratory of serial signal averaging for purposes of noise reduction. However, since one of the primary values of detection of His bundle activity is to make diagnostic and therapeutic judgments based on an evaluation of the integrity of conduction from atrium to His bundle and His bundle to ventricles, the efficacy of temporal or serial signal averaging is limited. The ability not only to make baseline measurements of the subintervals of the PR segment, but to detect cycle-by-cycle changes in relationship between atrial, His bundle, and ventricular signals relative to each other is necessary for optimal utility. Further, serial signal averaging tends to eventually blunt deflections, even with the most precise fiducial point designated for ensemble averaging. Diminishing the sharpness of the signal becomes important if discrete measurements are to be made. For example, if the deflection of interest has frequencies of 100 Hz and the interval from the fiducial point to the signal of interest varies by even ±0.45 msec, amplitudes of averaged signals may be reduced by half from the single original signal, even if we otherwise assume no noise contamination.[13] With spatial averaging, the problems with serial signal averaging are avoided. It is appropriate when the goal is to record online. Because the ensemble is limited in spatial averaging by the size of the torso, perimeters of the positive and negative fields on the chest, and size of the electrodes, the noise reducing capacity with spatial averaging is considerably less than that of temporal averaging with infinite potential for ensemble size. Therefore, other signal enhancing approaches must be simultaneously applied, including the amplification and filtering described above as well as the signal enhancing algorithms.

To direct our site selection, in previous studies[10] we internally paced the His bundle in dogs, performed body surface mapping, and defined regions of maximum positivity and negativity, thus approximating what we hoped to be the approximate electrical axis of the His bundle. Signals thus recorded are summed electronically so that noise may be increased by the square root of n (n = number of original input signals) while signal is increased by a factor of n.

Results and Discussion

In some of our first attempts at beat-by-beat data acquisition logarithmic amplifiers were used. Figure 2 is an example of a beat-by-beat record using logarithmic amplifiers in the circuitry. Note the small deflections preceding each QRS complex in a subject with a high degree of atrio-ventricular block and junctional rhythm. Logarithmic amplifiers are theoretically an excellent idea in that they logarithmically amplify low level signals more than they amplify large signals such as the major deflections of P, QRS, and T wave. However, we abandoned this approach because it is effective only in extremely quiet circumstances and in instances in which myopotentials are inapparent. Thus, we elected to combine a shielded environment, spatial averaging, coincidence detection with amplification, and filtering for optimum signal-to-noise ratio.

Figure 3 is an example of the optimal situation in the presence of normal sinus rhythm for beat-by-beat recording in a highly shielded room using a third modification of the instrumental design. Instrumentation utilized included 30- to 300-Hz instrumentation amplifiers from which signals were recorded from five bipolar inputs. Notch filters of 60 Hz were introduced as well as a decision circuit described above. An automatic gain control amplifier followed by a low-pass filter immediately preceded the output signals.

Figure 4 is an example from a patient, also recorded in the shielded environment, with a permanent ventricular demand pacemaker at the right ventricular apex. Note the dissociated P wave and the signal following the atrial deflection representing His bundle activity (labeled "H"). This patient's electrophysiologic study

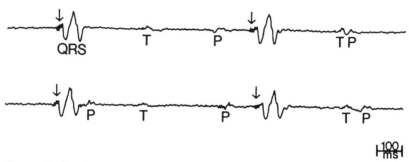

Figure 2. Continuous surface recording from a patient with complete heart block. In addition to preamplification, logarithmic amplifiers were used in this series of experiments. Notice the preventricular activity (indicated by arrows) associated with the QRS complex and unassociated with the P wave. This activity is believed to represent His-Purkinje signal recorded on a beat-by-beat basis. The key to this recording was the logarithmic amplification and filtering between 40–300 Hz.

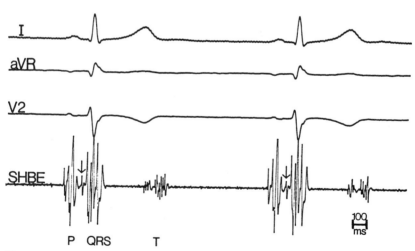

Figure 3. Surface leads I, aVR, V₂, and surface His bundle electrocardiogram (SHBE) from a healthy female subject. This is an example of the optimal recording obtained in the shielded environment, using amplification, spatial averaging, high-pass filtering, coincidence detection, and final low-pass filtering just prior to output. His bundle deflections are indicated by arrows.

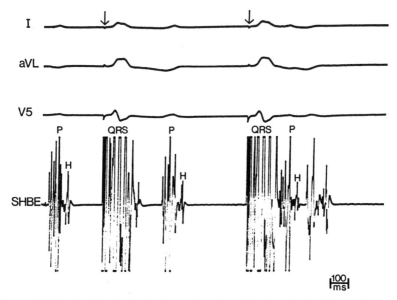

Figure 4. Surface leads I, aVL, V₅, and surface His bundle electrocardiogram (SHBE) from a human subject with a right ventricular endocardial permanent demand pacemaker. The block was below the level of the bundle of His in this patient. Note the association of the His bundle deflection (H) with each P wave and atrial deflection and its dissociation from the ventricular complex arising from the artificial pacemaker. The pacing artifact is indicated by the arrows.

confirmed the fact he had a block below the level of the bundle of His.

Following publications from our laboratory on beat-by-beat recording of surface His bundle electrograms (SHBE), other confirming reports have appeared.[21-26] In some of the examples, the signals probably originate from the His-Purkinje area[21,22]; in some of the illustrations, it is unclear that the activity being presented as from the His bundle is always from that source.

Although suggestive, the fact that SHBE and internal HBE coincide temporally does not necessarily prove that the SHBE deflection arises from the His bundle as the electronic processing of the two recordings is quite different. Additionally, there should be some break or clear baseline between the end of atrial activity and the origin of His bundle activity; otherwise, one can only guess as to the nature of a deflection that immediately abuts the electrical activity from the atrium. Likewise, if the magnitude of the His deflection and its morphology are no different from the magnitude and the morphology of baseline noise, it is difficult to be certain that the signal of question is, indeed, from the His bundle.

Current System in Use

Our most recent efforts have been to record SHBE on a beat-by-beat basis *entirely* outside a shielded environment. Since the magnetic field of 60 Hz and its harmonics is the primary source of interference noise, such noise is not noticeable in the recording if the magnetic flux density is < 10 milligauss.[27] When surface His bundle signals are being recorded, the magnetic field is measured by a magnetic field monitor developed in our laboratory. Digital implementation utilizes the Hewlett-Packard 310 computer system that allows the simultaneous acquisition of three surface ECGs and five parallel SHBEs. We have the option of displaying any combination of up to eight channels of data. Figure 5 is an example of a recording from a subject using the anterior-posterior lead configuration. With the lead II ECG as a reference, panels A, B, and C illustrate the SHBEs. Panel A is the output of the digital high-pass and low-pass filters from one of the five parallel channels. The His bundle signals have almost the same amplitude of noise. Panel B is the result of spatial averaging of the five channels. The signal-to-noise ratio is improved by 2.24 (square root of 5). Panel C is the final output after using the signal enhancing algorithms. Note that the signal-to-noise ratio has been greatly increased and the amplitude of the His bundle signal is about 2 µV. Figure 6 shows a recording on the same subject, but on an expanded scale, enables more accurate measurement of intervals. This is the early phase of this generation of equipment; software development and modifications are being constantly employed.

Insights Beyond Simple Recognition

Figure 7 illustrates a comparison of SHBEs in 41 asymptomatic normal volunteers and 47 patients referred for electrophysiologic study for symptoms of syncope or tachycardia, but who were demonstrated to be normal electrophysiologically.[28] Age and sex matched normal pairs were compared. In another group, data from patients

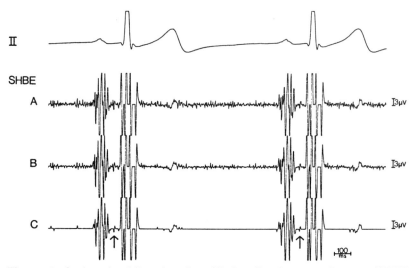

Figure 5. Surface lead II and surface His bundle electrocardiogram (SHBE) recorded from outside the shielded environment using the most recent digital implementation on the Hewlett-Packard 310 system. Panel A is the output of the digital high-pass and low-pass filters from one of the five parallel channels. Panel B is the result of spatial averaging of the five channels. Panel C illustrates the final output after using the signal enhancing algorithm. (See text for discussion.) His bundle deflections are indicated by arrows.

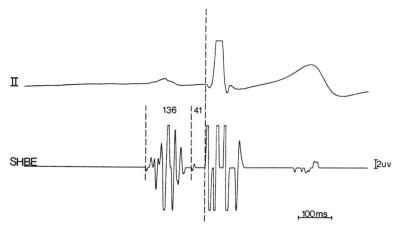

Figure 6. Expanded plot of the second cycle of the SHBE recording illustrated in Figure 5 C. Note the AH (136 msec) and HV (41 msec) intervals and the amplitude of the His bundle signal (1.9 µV).

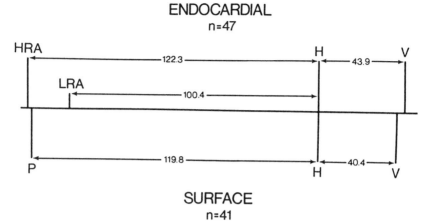

Figure 7. Comparison of endocardial and surface subintervals of the PR segment in normal subjects. Note that the high right atrial (HRA) to His (H) duration is somewhat longer than the low right atrial (LRA)-H duration, as is expected. Further note that the surface PH interval is slightly shorter than the HRA-H and longer than the LRA-H. No statistical difference was found between the HRA-H and PH intervals. Likewise, no statistical difference was found between the HV intervals recorded at the time of electrophysiologic study and from the body surface.

with conduction system abnormalities who had SHBE recordings as well as endocardially recorded HBEs were analyzed.[28,29] Onset of earliest atrial activity recognized in orthogonal leads in the standard ECG with 0.05-Hz high-pass filter usually slightly precedes the onset of surface P from the SHBE. This was in part due to the frequency limitation of the SHBE which attenuated the lower frequencies (high-pass filter 30 Hz). In part it may be that the SHBE was not necessarily at optimal vectorial advantage to record earliest atrial activity, while one of three vectorial leads should be. In the groups and in individuals studied by both methods, the SHBE consistently reflected atrial activity earlier than atrial activity was recorded in the HBE. This is logical since the electrode used for endocardial HBE is positioned relatively low, at the tricuspid valve level, and has small interpolar distances which record local activity. However, the fact that the SHBE recognizes atrial activity relatively early and only slightly after onset of atrial activity is recorded in the high right atrial (HRA) electrogram is reflected by the fact that the HRA-H duration and PH duration in the SHBE are not statistically different. The slight delay of P onset in the SHBE is due to the difference in proximity of the sampling sites and the fact that the HRA recording electrode is nearer the sinus node.

The PH interval in the SHBE is slightly longer than the AH interval seen in the HBE (p <0.05). Filtering is not a factor here, since filter settings are identical or nearly identical. The likely cause, as indicated above, is the earlier perception of atrial activity by the SHBE compared with the HBE.

Usually T waves can be distinguished from P waves even in complex arrhythmias in which atrio-ventricular dissociation is present. Although occasionally the two are similar in routine ECGs, their morphologies are rarely similar in the SHBE. This is partly because of a basically different frequency context and partly because of the difference in amplitudes. Also, they can be distinguished by the association of the T wave with a QRS. In instances of 2:1 or higher degrees of atrio-ventricular block, such as often occurs in atrial flutter and tachycardia, there are always more P waves than QRS and T deflections. The distinction, then, of P and T are rarely a problem in the SHBE.

Table II summarizes certain features which distinguished patients in whom His-Purkinje activity was recordable from those in whom it was difficult or impossible. The thinner the chest wall, the flatter the chest, the slower the heart rate, and the longer the AH component and HV components of the PR segment, the more likely His activity is to be isolated and recognized.

There is no question that surface His bundle activity can

Table II
Features Associated with Success in Recording
Surface Activity from the Bundle of His

Slight stature
Decreased anteroposterior dimension of the chest
Rapid upstroke of QRS
Intervals:
  RR ≥ 800 msec
  PH ≥ 140 msec
  HV ≥ 40 msec
  P wave ≤ 100 msec

---

become a part of the routine ECG, bringing to that dimension easy-to-acquire, low-cost information about the integrity of the atrio-ventricular conduction system. However, continued technical re-finement is mandatory before that goal is achieved. In summary, in the case of normal subjects, there was no statistical difference between the HV intervals recorded from the SHBE and the HV intervals measured at electrophysiologic study. We further conclude that the HRA-H interval is slightly longer than the PH interval in the SHBE, although not different statistically. The PH interval in the SHBE differs from the AH interval measured in the HBE, just as the HRA-H interval differs from the AH interval.

References

1. Scherlag BJ, Helfant RH, Damato AN: A catheterization technique for His bundle stimulation and recording in the intact dog. J Appl Physiol 25:425, 1968.
2. Scherlag BJ, Lau SH, Helfant RH, et al: Catheter technique for recording His bundle activity in man. Circulation 39:13, 1969.
3. Berbari EJ: A noninvasive technique for recording the depolarization potentials of the heart's electrical conduction system. (Masters Thesis) 1973.
4. Berbari EJ, Lazzara R, Scherlag BJ: Surface recording techniques for detecting electrical activity during the P-R segment (abstr). Am J Cardiol 31:120, 1973.
5. Flowers NC, Hand RC, Orander PC: Surface recording of electrical activity from the His bundle area (abstr). Proceedings of the Cardiac Electrophysiologic Group, Atlantic City, NJ, 1973.
6. Stopczyk MJ, Kopee J, Zochowski RJ, Pieniak M: Surface recording of electrical heart activity during the P-R segment in man by a computer averaging techniques. IRCS 11:73, 1973.
7. Flowers NC, Horan LG: His bundle and bundle branch recordings from the body surface (abstr). Circulation 48:IV-102, 1973.
8. Lazzara R, Campbell R, Berbari EJ, et al: Electrocardiogram of His-Purkinje system of man (abstr). Circulation 48:IV-22, 1973.
9. Berbari EJ, Lazzara R, Samet P, Scherlag BJ: Noninvasive technique for detection of electrical activity during the P-R segment. Circulation 48:-1005, 1973.
10. Flowers NC, Hand RC, Orander PC, et al: Surface recording of electrical activity from the region of the bundle of His. Am J Cardiol 33:384, 1974.
11. Flowers NC, Shvartsman V, Horan LG: A beat-by-beat recording of His-Purkinje waveform without digital averaging. Proceedings of 22nd Annual Meeting of the Association of University Cardiologists, Phoenix, Arizona, 1980.
12. Flowers NC, Shvartsman V, Kennelly BM, et al: Surface recording of

His-Purkinje activity on an every-beat basis without digital averaging. Circulation 63:948, 1981.

13. Shvartsman V, Barnes GR, Shvartsman L, Flowers NC: Multi-channel signal processing based on logic averaging. IEEE Trans Biomed Eng 29:531, 1982.

14. Schleher DC: Automatic Detection and Radar Data Processing. Dedham, MA; Artech, 1980, pp 3–297.

15. Harrington JV: An analysis of the detection of repeated signal in noise by binary integration. IEEE Trans Inform Theory IT-1:1, 1955.

16. Dillard GM: A moving-window detector for binary integration. IEEE Trans Inform Theory IT-13:2, 1967.

17. Worley R: Optimum threshold for binary integration. IEEE Trans Inform Theory IT-14:349, 1968.

18. Walker JF: Performance data for a double-threshold detector radar. IEEE Trans Aerosp Electron Syst AES-9:142, 1971.

19. Bogush AJ: Correlated clutter and resultant properties of binary signals. IEEE Trans Aerosp Electron Syst AES-9:208, 1973.

20. Santopietro RF: The origin and characterization of the principal signal, noise and interference sources in the high fidelity electrocardiogram. Proc IEEE 65:707, 1977.

21. Mehra R, Kelen G, El-Sherif N: Noninvasive beat to beat recording of diastolic and His-Purkinje potentials in man (abstr). Circulation 64:IV-239, 1981.

22. El-Sherif N, Mehra R, Gomes JAC, Kelen G: Appraisal of a low noise electrocardiogram. J Am Coll Cardiol 1:456, 1983.

23. Allor DR: A noninvasive method of recording a serial His-Purkinje study in man. CVP 8:16, 1980.

24. Kepski R, Plucinski Z, Walczak F: Noninvasive recording of His-Purkinje system (HPS) activity in man on beat-to-beat basis. PACE 5:506-511, 1982.

25. Erne SN, Fenici RR, Hahlbohm HD, et al: Beat to beat surface recording and averaging of His-Purkinje activity in man. J Electrocardiol 16:355, 1983.

26. Ishijima M, Kimata S, Kasanuki H, Sakurai Y: The feasibility of beat-to-beat detection of His-Purkinje activity by finite element method. PACE 10:1107, 1987.

27. Yang W, Wang K: Problems in noninvasive detection of His bundle electrograms on a beat-by-beat basis (abstr). Proceedings of the Chinese Association of Biomedical Electronics, Shanghai, China, 1985.

28. Flowers NC, Shvartsman V, Horan LG, et al: Analysis of PR subintervals in normal subjects and early studies in patients with abnormalities of the conduction system using surface His bundle recordings. J Am Coll Cardiol 2:939, 1983.

29. Flowers NC, Hand RC, Palakurthy PR, et al: Clinical aspects of single beat His recordings with examples. In Selvester RH, Geselowitz D (eds): Computerized Interpretation of the Electrocardiogram. Proceedings of the 1983 Engineering Foundation Conference. New York: Engineering Foundation, 1984, pp 193–207.

12

Detection of Ventricular Late Potentials on a Beat-to-Beat Basis: Methodological Aspects and Clinical Application

Marc Zimmermann, Richard Adamec, Jean Richez

Introduction

Time-domain signal averaging has been used for many years to detect ventricular late potentials from the body surface.[1-8] With this technique the signal-to-noise ratio is improved by repeated acquisition of the signal of interest; if the signal of interest has a constant time relationship to the event triggering the acquisition process, then the signal of interest will increase as n and the noise level as $\sqrt{n}$ (where n represents the number of averaged samples), thus improving the signal-to-noise ratio. However, time-domain signal averaging can only detect ventricular late potentials which are absolutely constant in duration, morphology, and timing relative to the QRS complex; therefore, this technique does not allow the detection of dynamic changes in ventricular late potentials which may occur either spontaneously[9] or during various diagnostic and therapeutic

From El-Sherif N, Turitto G (eds): *High-Resolution Electrocardiography*. Mount Kisco, NY, Futura Publishing Co., Inc., ©, 1992.

interventions. For these reasons, several investigators have attempted to detect these low amplitude high-frequency signals on a beat-to-beat basis using low-noise or high-resolution electrocardiographic systems. [10-20] The purpose of this chapter is to describe a new high-resolution electrocardiographic system developed at the University of Geneva, allowing a beat-to-beat online detection of ventricular late potentials without any averaging process. Acquisition is performed at the bedside, and a shielded room is not required. Emphasis will be put on various methodological aspects of the system, including its current limitations, clinical applications, and future perspectives.

Methodological Aspects

Description of the High–Resolution ECG Developed at Our Institution

The system was developed to record from the body surface low amplitude cardiac signals, at the microvolt level, without any averaging process. Three channels are recorded simultaneously and the analog input signal is fed through a preamplifier with a fixed gain of 1000. The filters are of the Sallen-Key type, allowing an easy selection of cut-off frequencies. The high-pass filter (-10 dB/octave in the first octave, -20 dB/octave in the second, and -35 dB in the third) is adjustable between 10 and 150 Hz in 10-Hz step increments. The low-pass filter (-20 dB/octave in the first octave and -50 dB in the second) is adjustable between 100 and 1000 Hz in 100-Hz step increments. A notch filter, specifically designed to eliminate 50-Hz noise, is inserted between the two bandpass filters, and used when necessary. A final amplifier with a gain of 100 to 1000 provides the gain required to obtain a 1 to 10 μV/cm trace on the ink-jet recorder (Mingograph Siemens 82). A high-resolution electrocardiogram with bandpass filters of 100 and 300 Hz is recorded on the first channel. A reference electrocardiogram (250 to 500 μV/cm on paper, bandpass filters of 1 and 1000 Hz with a 6 dB/octave slope) is recorded on the second channel. A high-resolution electrocardiogram with bandpass filters of 30 and 300 Hz is recorded on the third channel. An R wave detector is included in the system to synchronize signals for the time-domain averager. The averager is used during the same session at the same electrode position to compare beat-to-beat and signal-averaged recordings.

The following measurements are made on the recording to provide a quantitative approach:

A. the total duration of the filtered QRS complex;
B. the QRS voltage (peak-to-peak) 40 msec before the end of the QRS complex (V-40, expressed in microvolts);
C. the interval between the end of the QRS complex (including the ventricular late potentials eventually recorded) and the point (determined retrogradely) when the voltage of the terminal QRS falls below 40 μV (I-40, expressed in milliseconds).

Normal values for these quantitative parameters are derived from data obtained in normal subjects (mean $+2$ standard deviations) (see further in Table I).

Table I
Effect of High-Pass Filtering on the High-Resolution Electrocardiogram

High-Pass Filter	Parameter	Normal Subjects (n = 10)	CAD pts, no VLP (n = 11)	CAD pts, VLP + (n = 7)
40 Hz	QRS duration (msec)	115 ±15	116 ±8	146 ±28*#
	I-40 (msec)	25 ±10	19 ±5	35 ±12#
60 Hz	QRS duration (msec)	100 ±11	109 ±9*	142 ±29*#
	I-40 (msec)	22 ±8	18 ±7	38 ±18†#
80 Hz	QRS duration (msec)	91 ±9	99 ±8	136 ±21*#
	I-40 (msec)	21 ±8	18 ±6	46 ±19*#
100 Hz	QRS duration (msec)	88 ±6	91 ±5	132 ±21*#
	I-40 (msec)	21 ±5	19 ±6	49 ±22*#

CAD pts = coronary artery disease patients; VLP = ventricular late potentials; I-40 = interval between the end of the QRS and the voltage 40 μV; * = p <0.01 versus normal subjects; † = p <0.05 versus normal subjects; # = p < 0.01 versus CAD pts, no VLP.

Noise Reduction

In our experience important clues to noise reduction are the interface between patient skin and recording electrode, and the electrode itself; the skin is carefully prepared with an alcoholic solution and in selected cases lightly abraded with fine sandpaper. A pair of low-noise electrodes (ECEM recording electrodes with TECA electrode electrolyte) are applied to the skin in order to obtain a bipolar chest lead over the left precordium. The recording electrodes are then connected to the preamplifier and the connecting cables are arranged to minimize power-line interference. The patient is asked to relax and remain quiet during the recording, but no premedication is used. In optimal clinical conditions the noise level due to electromyographic activities and to power-line interference is 1 to 3 μV peak-to-peak. With our system the recording is made at the bedside and no shielded room is required.

The noise level is influenced by the bandpass filters (Table II): in ten normal subjects we observed a progressive decrease in the noise level when the high-pass filter was increased from 40 to 100 Hz; a similar tendency was observed in coronary artery disease patients with (n = 7) or without (n = 11) ventricular late potentials (Figure 1). These results are in agreement with data published by Gomes et al[21] with signal averaging and bidirectional four-pole Butterworth filters: the minimal noise level was observed with high-pass filters of

Table II
Effect of High-Pass Filtering on the Noise Level

	High-Pass Filter			
	40 Hz	60 Hz	80 Hz	100 Hz
Normal subjects (n = 10)	2.6 ±0.7 μV	2.4 ±0.52 μV	2.2 ±0.63 μV	1.6 ±0.52 μV
CAD pts, no VLP (n = 11)	3.5 ±0.69 μV	3.2 ±0.60 μV	2.3 ±0.47 μV	1.9 ±0.7 μV
CAD pts, VLP + (n = 7)	2.6 ±1.13 μV	2.6 ±0.79 μV	2.1 ±0.38 μV	1.9 ±0.69 μV

CAD pts = Coronary artery disease patients; VLP = ventricular late potentials; n = number of patients.

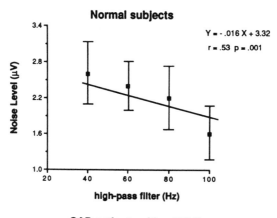

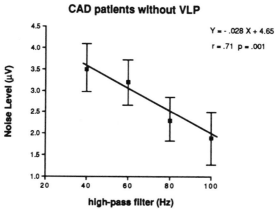

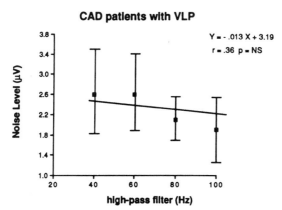

Figure 1. Influence of the high-pass filter on noise level of high-resolution recording. See text for details.

40, 80, and 100 Hz in normal subjects but with high-pass filters of 80 and 100 Hz in patients with organic heart disease with or without documented sustained ventricular arrhythmias. Although signal averaging and high-resolution electrocardiography are not comparable, the similar effect of high-pass filtering on noise level is interesting. Since noise reduction represents the main difficulty with the beat-to-beat technique, it seems reasonable to choose high-pass filters between 80 and 100 Hz in order to obtain a noise level of < 2 μV in clinical conditions.

Another way to improve the signal-to-noise ratio is to use spatial averaging[10–12,14,18]: the signals from multiple pairs of electrodes are averaged and if the electrodes are closely spaced, the signal recorded between any pair of electrode is assumed to be identical. With this approach the noise level could be reduced to 1–2 μV in clinical conditions.[11,12] Initial experiments in our laboratory with 4 and 16 pairs of closely spaced electrodes have been disappointing: the noise reduction was the same as with the aforementioned bipolar ECEM electrodes, and the spatial averaging approach was abandoned. Comparable results have been recently described by Lewis et al.[18]

Lead Selection

We, as others,[22,23] use bipolar chest leads placed over the left precordium because some data suggest that these leads are superior to the orthogonal system proposed by Simson for detection of ventricular late potentials.[24] In all cases, two bipolar chest leads are recorded, one between the conventional points V_2 and V_4, and one between the conventional V_4 and V_6; in selected cases additional bipolar chest leads are used for optimal detection of ventricular late potentials which have been shown to have a dipolar distribution by body surface potential mapping.[25] Berbari has suggested that the choice of the XYZ leads may provide insufficient information to assess the entire duration of the ventricular late potentials.[26,27] In fact, several lead positions on the precordium showed longer QRS (including the late potentials) durations than the XYZ leads.[26] Atwood et al[28] have observed more abnormal measurements and a longer interval between the end of the QRS complex and the voltage 40 μV (I-40) with bipolar chest leads than with the orthogonal lead system. In our system, great care has been taken to accurately position recording electrodes on the chest in order to minimize differences in QRS duration.[26]

Bandpass Filters

In high-gain electrocardiography, elimination of low-frequency components is mandatory to prevent extreme baseline drift. With time-domain signal averaging, high-pass filters have been chosen arbitrarily and no consensus exists regarding the optimal bandpass filtering for detection of ventricular late potentials.[26,29] With signal averaging and bidirectional four-pole Butterworth filters, it has been shown that a level of 25 Hz provides the best specificity, whereas a level of 80 Hz provides the best sensitivity.[21] No data exist concerning the optimal bandpass filtering for the beat-to-beat detection of ventricular late potentials. For this reason, we studied the effect of various high-pass filters on high-resolution recordings of 10 normal subjects, 11 coronary artery disease patients without ventricular late potentials, and 7 coronary artery disease patients with ventricular late potentials on time-domain signal-averaged recording (Table I). As the high-pass filter frequency increased from 40 to 100 Hz, the total filtered QRS duration decreased progressively in all three groups of subjects (Figures 2 and 3). The interval between the end of the QRS complex and the point where QRS voltage falls below 40 μV (I-40) showed a slight tendency to increase with increasing high-pass filtering in coronary artery disease patients with late potentials, but the results did not reach statistical significance (Figure 4). The optimal detection of ventricular late potentials occurred with high-pass filters of 80 and 100 Hz (Figure 5).

This observation, together with the results of high-pass filtering on noise level, prompted us to choose a high-pass filter of 100 Hz and a low-pass filter of 300 Hz for quantitative analysis of high-resolution recordings. However, in order to prevent loss of specificity a simultaneous recording with bandpass filters of 30 and 300 Hz was obtained in all cases. Similar findings have been reported by Gomes et al[21] with time-domain signal averaging. They found that a 80-Hz high-pass filter provides a larger percentage of abnormal quantitative variables compared with other filter settings, and that 80 Hz was the optimal high-pass filter to identify patients prone to ventricular tachycardia.[21]

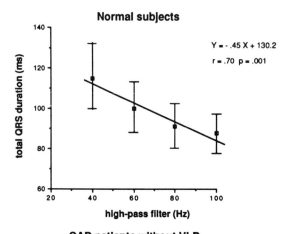

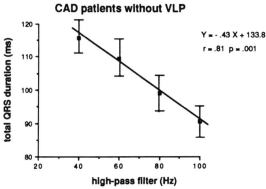

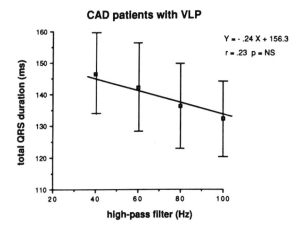

Figure 2. Influence of the high-pass filter on total QRS duration. As the high-pass filter is increased from 40 to 100 Hz a progressive decrease in total QRS duration is observed.

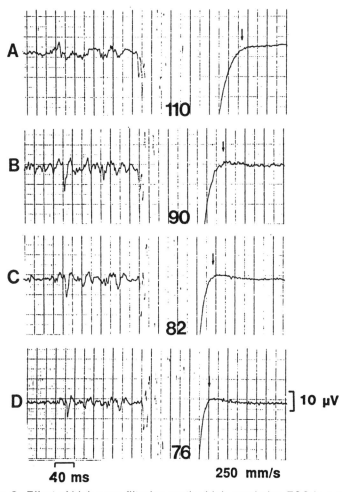

Figure 3. Effect of high-pass filtering on the high-resolution ECG in a normal subject. (A) High-pass filter of 40 Hz, QRS duration 110 msec. (B) High-pass filter of 60 Hz, QRS duration 90 msec. (C) High-pass filter of 80 Hz, QRS duration 82 msec. (D) High-pass filter of 100 Hz, QRS duration 76 msec. Paper speed 250 mm/sec, noise level <2 µV. Arrows indicate the end of the QRS complex.

Normal subjects

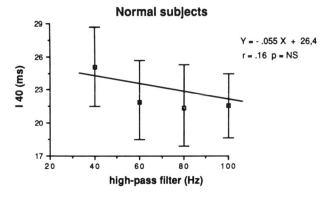

$Y = -.055 X + 26,4$
$r = .16 \ p = NS$

CAD patients without VLP

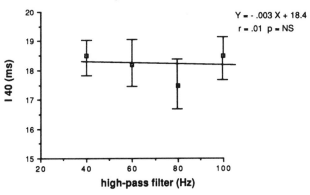

$Y = -.003 X + 18.4$
$r = .01 \ p = NS$

CAD with VLP

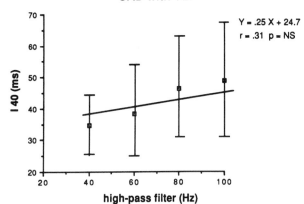

$Y = .25 X + 24.7$
$r = .31 \ p = NS$

Figure 4. Influence of the high-pass filters on the interval between the end of the QRS complex and the 40 µV voltage (I-40). See text for details.

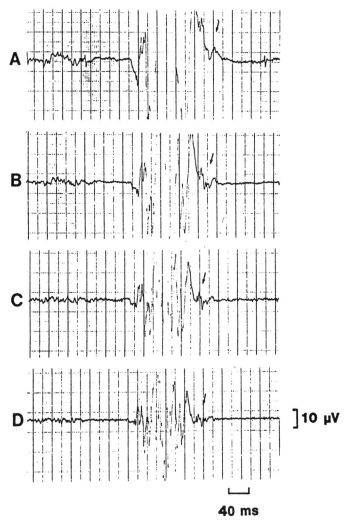

Figure 5. Effect of the high-pass filters on the high-resolution ECG in a patient with coronary artery disease and sustained monomorphic ventricular tachycardia. Ventricular late potentials are present (arrows) at each filter setting (A = 40 Hz, B = 60 Hz, C = 80 Hz, D = 100 Hz), but are best seen at 80 and 100 Hz. Paper speed 250 mm/sec.

Clinical Application

Validation

A close correlation has been observed between noninvasively recorded ventricular late potentials and delayed or fractionated potentials recorded during epicardial or endocardial mapping in patients with sustained monomorphic ventricular tachycardia.[30,31] These ventricular late potentials are thought to represent delayed conduction in localized areas of the myocardium and hence the sites for potential reentrant circuits.[32,33] Validation of repetitive abnormal signals is rather easy and is based on the reproducibility of abnormal signals in the time domain; thus, signal averaging itself provides a validation for constant signals. When one tries to detect dynamic changes of the signals, validation becomes a major problem and great caution should be used before drawing conclusions. Abnormal signals detected on the ST segment during sinus rhythm should be distinguished from artifacts. This distinction may not be easy when true abnormal signals occur just once or at some distance from the major QRS potential. Validation seems even more difficult for signals occurring during or after the T wave.[11] When a progressive increase in delay or duration of the ventricular late potential is observed (Wenckebach-like conduction delay), validation is possible only if the phenomenon is periodic and only if the same sequences are repeatedly recorded. Such dynamic patterns have been observed in animal experiments[9] but only rarely in humans[11,12] and the published recordings are not impressive. The same remarks apply to diastolic potentials observed only in the ST segment preceding a ventricular premature complex. Few recordings of this type have been obtained in humans[11,12]; in our experience, no significant change of ventricular late potentials was observed in the five cases exhibiting spontaneous premature ventricular complexes during the high-resolution recording. Failure to record any change before spontaneous premature ventricular complexes was also noted by El-Sherif et al on a beat-to-beat basis,[18] and by Lombardi et al by signal averaging of preextrasystolic beats.[34] They may be due to the fact that the observed ectopic beats were of focal origin and were not caused by reentry. Another explanation is that variations in ventricular late potentials are of too low amplitude to be detected by currently available techniques. Further studies are needed and solutions may be obtained by recording on a beat-to-beat basis during atrial or ventricular pacing, during programmed ventricular stimulation, or during spontaneous sustained monomorphic ventricular tachycardia.

Validation of beat-to-beat dynamic changes of ventricular late potentials detected on the body surface may be obtained by simultaneous recording with endocardial electrode catheter. However, agreement between intracavitary and body surface recordings is not perfect[35] and a complete endocardial mapping is necessary in order to localize the late potentials before any validation study.

Validation of high-resolution recordings by signal averaging is helpful but applicable only to repetitive signals (Figures 6A and 6B). In a preliminary study[19] performed in 31 normal subjects, 28 coronary artery disease patients without ventricular tachycardia, and 21 coronary artery disease patients with sustained monomorphic ventricular tachycardia, we observed concordant results between time-domain signal averaging and high-resolution recordings in 96% of the cases (77/80). Thirty-two patients were positive and 45 patients were negative for ventricular late potentials with both techniques. In three cases the high-resolution recording was considered abnormal whereas the signal-averaged recording was normal. These three patients had abnormal low amplitude high-frequency signals at the end of the QRS complex, but these late potentials were not constant in duration, morphology, and timing relative to the QRS complex and hence could not be recorded by time-domain signal averaging. In this study, the incidence of dynamic changes of ventricular late potentials was low (3/49 coronary artery disease patients), but only patients with chronic stable coronary artery disease have been included. The incidence may be much higher in unstable conditions such as ischemia, myocardial infarction, or during various therapeutic interventions. Thus, validation of abnormal signals detected on a beat-to-beat basis is difficult and caution is mandatory before interpreting the recordings.

Advantages of the High-Resolution Recordings

The main advantage of high-resolution recording systems is the possibility to obtain high-gain recording on a beat-to-beat basis, and hence to allow detection of dynamic variations of ventricular late potentials. The ability to record dynamic changes of these abnormal diastolic potentials may:

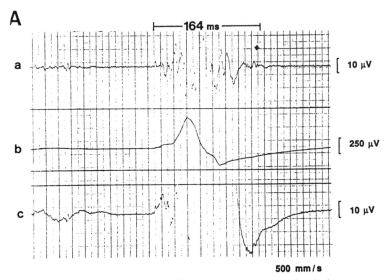

Figure 6A. High-resolution recording on a beat-to-beat basis in a coronary artery disease patient with recurrent episodes of sustained monomorphic ventricular tachycardia. Bipolar chest lead between V_3 and V_4. Paper speed 500 mm/sec. a = high-resolution recording (10 μV/cm) with a bandpass filtering of 100 and 300 Hz; b = reference ECG (250 μV/cm); c = high-resolution recording (10 μV/cm) with a bandpass filtering of 30 and 300 Hz. Ventricular late potentials are present (arrow) and prolong the total QRS duration to 164 msec.

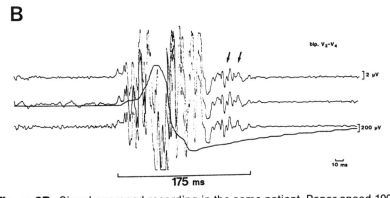

Figure 6B. Signal-averaged recording in the same patient. Paper speed 1000 mm/sec. Bandpass filtering of 100 and 300 Hz. Three successive high-gain (2 μV/cm) signal-averaged recordings (each one obtained by averaging 40 consecutive cardiac cycles) are displayed together with a reference ECG (200 μV/cm). Ventricular late potentials are present (arrows) and the total QRS duration is 175 msec. Concordance between high-resolution beat-to-beat recording and signal averaging is evident.

A. enhance the sensitivity for detection of ventricular late potentials since all variable late potentials are lost by the averaging process;
B. increase the specificity of late potentials for the identification of patients prone to malignant ventricular arrhythmias; indeed, variable late potentials may indicate electrical instability whereas stable late potentials may only indicate the presence of an organic substrate;
C. facilitate the study of the relationship between ventricular late potentials and the occurrence of spontaneous or induced reentrant ventricular arrhythmias;
D. allow to analyze the behavior of ventricular late potentials during ischemia, myocardial infarction, or reperfusion;
E. facilitate the evaluation of various therapeutic interventions. Specifically, our system has proven an effective means of noise reduction in clinical situations, allowing the noninvasive beat-to-beat detection of abnormal signals of more than 3 μV in amplitude; there is no need for a trigger and online recording is possible at the bedside, in a nonshielded room.

Limitations

The current limitations of the system are obvious and have been underlined above:

A. the noise level is reduced to 1 to 3 μV and this may be insufficient to detect low amplitude late potentials;
B. validation of abnormal signals remains difficult;
C. the optimal filter setting has not been sufficiently defined and further studies are needed;
D. an automatic determination of various quantitative parameters may be useful to avoid inter- and intraobserver variability.

Future Directions

Noninvasive recording of low amplitude abnormal signals on a beat-to-beat basis is feasible and large prospective trials should be started to evaluate the reliability and clinical usefulness of this new technique. Progress should be made to further increase the signal-to-noise ratio. Analysis of the behavior of ventricular late potentials under atrial or ventricular stimulation is under study in our laboratory and in others.[20] The results should clarify the exact role of late potentials in the genesis of reentrant ventricular arrhythmias. Finally, adaptation of high-resolution techniques to continuous electrocardiographic monitoring should help to understand the mechanism of spontaneous ventricular arrhythmias.

References

1. Fontaine G, Guiraudon G, Frank R, Vedel J, Grosgogeat Y, Cabrol C: Modern concepts of ventricular tachycardia. The value of electrocardiological investigations and delayed potentials in ventricular tachycardia of ischemic and nonischemic etiology (31 operated cases). Eur J Cardiol 8:565, 1978.
2. Simson MB, Untereker WJ, Spielman S: Relation between late potentials on the body surface and directly recorded fragmented electrograms in patients with ventricular tachycardia. Am J Cardiol 51:105, 1983.
3. Berbari EJ, Scherlag BJ, Hope RR, Lazzara R: Recording from the body surface of arrhythmogenic ventricular activity during the ST segment. Am J Cardiol 41:697, 1978.
4. Breithardt G, Becker R, Seipel L, Abendroth RR, Ostermeyer J: Noninvasive detection of late potentials in man—a new marker for ventricular tachycardia. Eur Heart J 2:1, 1981.
5. Simson MB: Use of signals in the terminal QRS complex to identify patients with ventricular tachycardia after myocardial infarction. Circulation 64:235, 1981.
6. Hombach V, Höpp HW, Braun V, Behrenbeck DW, Tauchert M, Hilger HH: Die Bedeutung von Nachpotentialen innerhalb des ST-Segmentes im Oberflächen-EKG bei Patienten mit koronarer Herzkrankheit. Dtsch Med Wschr 195:1457, 1980.
7. Rozanski JJ, Mortara D, Myerburg RJ, Castellanos A: Body surface detection of delayed depolarizations in patients with recurrent ventricular tachycardias and left ventricular aneurysm. Circulation 63:1172, 1981.
8. Zimmermann M, Adamec R, Simonin P, Richez J: Prognostic significance of ventricular late potentials in coronary artery disease. Am Heart J 109:725, 1985.
9. El-Sherif N, Scherlag BJ, Lazzara R, Hope RR: Reentrant ventricular arrhythmias in the late myocardial infarction period: 1. Conduction characteristics in the infarction zone. Circulation 55:686, 1977.
10. Flowers NC, Shvartsman V, Sohi GS, Horan LG: Signal averaged versus beat-to-beat recording of surface His-Purkinje potentials. In Hombach V, Hilger HH (eds): Signal-Averaging Technique in Clinical Cardiology. Stuttgart: FK Schattauer, 1981, pp. 329–349.
11. Hombach V, Kebbel U, Höpp HW, Winter U, Hirche H: Noninvasive

beat-by-beat registration of ventricular late potentials using high-resolution electrocardiography. Int J Cardiol 6:167, 1984.

12. El-Sherif N, Mehra R, Gomes JAC, Kelen G: Appraisal of a low noise electrocardiogram. J Am Coll Cardiol 1:456, 1983.

13. Chen WC, Zeng ZR, Chow C, Xine QZ, Kou LC: Application of a new spatial signal-averaging device for the beat-to-beat detection of cardiac late potentials. Clin Cardiol 9:263, 1986.

14. Edvardsson N, Hirsch I, Pettersson AS, Olsson SB: Noninvasive recording of continuous diastolic electrical activity during ventricular tachycardia (abstr). Circulation 70(Suppl II):II-252, 1984.

15. Adamec R, Zimmermann M, Richez J, Simonin P: A comparative study between non invasive registration of ventricular late potentials using beat-to-beat high-resolution electrocardiography and using signal-averaging technique. In Belhassen B, Feldmann S, Copperman Y (eds): Cardiac Pacing and Electrophysiology: Proceedings of the VIIIth World Symposium on Cardiac Pacing and Electrophysiology. Tel Aviv: R and L Creative Communications, 1987, pp 309–312.

16. Haberl R, Hengstenberg E, Steinbeck G: Single beat analysis of frequency content in the surface ECG for identification of patients with ventricular tachycardia (abstr). Circulation 72(Suppl III):III-433, 1985.

17. Oeff M, von Leitner ER, Erne SN, Hahlbohm HD, Lehmann HP, Schröder R: Einzelschlag-Registrierung Ventrikulärer Spätdepolarisationen von Der Körperoberfläche Koronarkranker Patienten (abstr). Z Kardiol 71:627, 1982.

18. Lewis SL, Lander PT, Taylor PA, Chamberlain DA, Vincent R: Identification of ventricular late potential activity in single cardiac cycles using spatial averaging and advanced filtering techniques (abstr). J Am Coll Cardiol 11:183A, 1988.

19. Zimmermann M, Adamec R, Simonin P, Richez J: Beat-to-beat detection of ventricular late potentials using high-resolution ECG and comparison with signal-averaging (abstr). Circulation 78(Suppl II):II-139, 1988.

20. Hombach V, Eggeling T, Höher M, Höpp HW, Kochs M, Giel I, Emsermann P, Hirche H, Hilger HH: Methoden zur Erfassung Ventrikulärer Spätpotentiale. Herz 13:147, 1988.

21. Gomes JA, Winters SL, Stewart D, Targonski A, Barreca P: Optimal bandpass filters for time-domain analysis of the signal-averaged electrocardiogram. Am J Cardiol 60:1290, 1987.

22. Olinic D, Olinic N, Nedevschi S, Vlaicu R: Signal averaging and beat by beat analysis of late potentials (abstr). Eur Heart J 9(Suppl 1):257, 1988.

23. Allor DR: A noninvasive method of recording a serial His-Purkinje study in man. CVP April/May: 16–19, 1980.

24. Oeff M, von Leitner ER, Sthapit R, Breithardt G, Borggrefe M, Karbenn U, Meinertz T, Zotz R, Clas W, Hombach V: Methods for noninvasive detection of ventricular late potentials—a comparative multicenter study. Eur Heart J 7:25, 1986.

25. Savard P, Faugere G, Nadeau RA, Derome D, Shenasa M, Page PL, Guardo R: The spatial distribution of late ventricular potentials. J Electrocardiol 20(Suppl):114, 1987.

26. Berbari EJ: Critical overview of late potential recordings. J Electrocardiol 20 (Suppl):125, 1987.
27. Berbari EJ, Friday KJ, Jackman WM, Hudgins P, Lazzara R: Precordial mapping of signal averaged late potentials compared to XYZ leads (abstr). J Am Coll Cardiol 7:127A, 1986.
28. Atwood JE, Myers J, Forbes S, Hall P, Friis R, Marcondes G, Mortara D, Froelicher VF: High-frequency electrocardiography: an evaluation of lead placement and measurements. Am Heart J 116:733, 1988.
29. Simson MB: Optimal identification of late potentials. In Santini M, Pistolese M, Alliegro A (eds): Progress in Clinical Pacing. Amsterdam: Excerpta Medica, 1988, pp 225–238.
30. Klein H, Karp RB, Kouchoukos NT, Zorn GL, James TN, Waldo AL: Intraoperative electrophysiologic mapping of the ventricles during sinus rhythm in patients with a previous myocardial infarction. Identification of the electrophysiologic substrate of ventricular arrhythmias. Circulation 66:847, 1982.
31. Josephson ME, Horowitz LN, Farshidi A, Spielman SR, Michelson EL, Greenspan AM: Sustained ventricular tachycardia: evidence for protected localized re-entry. Am J Cardiol 42:416, 1978.
32. Breithardt G, Borggrefe M: Pathophysiological mechanisms and clinical significance of ventricular late potentials. Eur Heart J 7:364, 1986.
33. Brugada P, Abdollah H, Wellens HJJ: Continuous electrical activity during sustained monomorphic ventricular tachycardia. Observations on its dynamic behaviour during the arrhythmia. Am J Cardiol 55:402, 1985.
34. Lombardi F, Finocchiaro ML, Dalla Vecchia L, Capiello E, Garimoldi M, Cerutti S, Malliani A: Signal-averaging of pre-extrasystolic beats in patients with ventricular arrhythmias (abstr). Circulation 78(Suppl II):II-237, 1988.
35. Zimmermann M, Friedli B, Adamec R, Oberhänsli I: Frequency of ventricular late potentials and fractionated right ventricular electrograms after operative repair of tetralogy of Fallot. Am J Cardiol 59:448, 1987.

Section III.

Late Potentials: Electrophysiologic Principles

13

Electrophysiologic Correlates of Ventricular Late Potentials

Nabil El-Sherif, William B. Gough, Mark Restivo

Introduction

The direct recording on the body surface of delayed depolarization potentials, usually referred to as late potentials, is a promising noninvasive technique which may be useful in identifying patients with the anatomic-electrophysiologic substrate for ventricular tachyarrhythmias based on a reentrant mechanism. The origin of late potentials is believed to be myocardial zones with slow and inhomogeneous activation patterns which may provide the substrate for reentrant excitation.[1] Delayed activation potentials were initially described from the ischemic regions of the canine post-infarction heart.[2-7] The relation between delayed ventricular activation in ischemic myocardial zones and ventricular arrhythmias based on a circus movement of excitation in the post-infarction heart has been extensively investigated.[8-15] Late potentials appear to correspond to delayed and fragmented activation, which has been observed in epicardial electrograms recorded from dogs with acute[16] or subacute myocardial infarction.[17] Several investigators have studied the relationship between late potentials in the body surface signal-averaged

From El-Sherif N, Turitto G (eds): *High-Resolution Electrocardiography*. Mount Kisco, NY, Futura Publishing Co., Inc., ©, 1992.

electrocardiogram (ECG) and the inducibility of ventricular tachyarrhythmias in a number of post-infarction canine models.[18–21] A thorough understanding of the electrophysiologic correlates of late potentials on the signal-averaged ECG is essential for defining the value and limitations of the technique as a marker of electrical instability.

The Relationship of Late Potentials to Activation Patterns of Sinus and Reentrant Rhythms

This relationship could be best studied in dogs 4-day post-ligation of the left anterior descending artery (LAD) which is a documented experimental model of reentrant rhythms. In this model the reentrant circuits are usually located in the surviving electrophysiologically abnormal epicardial layer overlying the infarction and are therefore accessible to detailed mapping of ventricular activation.[9,10] Reentrant rhythms could occur "spontaneously" during a regular cardiac rhythm[22] but are more commonly initiated by 1 or more premature stimulated beats. Figure 1 was obtained from a 4-day-old post-infarction canine heart and illustrates the epicardial activation pattern during sinus rhythm and reentrant excitation induced by a single premature stimulation (S_2) during regular ventricular pacing (S_1). Selected epicardial electrograms and a "simulated" high-resolution body surface ECG are also shown. During sinus rhythm, the majority of the epicardial surface of the right and

Figure 1 (opposite). Isochronal maps of epicardial activation from a dog with 4-day-old infarction. The map on the left represents epicardial activation of a sinus beat and the one on the right, the S_2 beat, that initiated a reentrant ventricular tachycardia. Selected epicardial electrograms as well as a simulated high-resolution body surface ECG recording are shown on the bottom. The epicardial electrograms enclosed between two dotted lines represent delayed activation of ischemic epicardial zones and are recorded during the early portion of the ST segment of the body surface ECG on the bottom. In this and subsequent maps, epicardial activation is displayed as if the heart is viewed from the apex located at the center of the circular map. The perimeter of the circle represents the atrio-ventricular junction. The epicardial outline of the ischemic zone is represented by the dotted line. Activation isochrones are drawn at 20-msec intervals. Arcs of functional conduction block are represented by heavy solid lines. See text for more details. (Modified with permission from El-Sherif et al, PACE 8:440, 1985.)

left ventricles was activated within 40 msec. This corresponded to the surface QRS duration of 42 msec. Most of the epicardial surface of the ischemic zone was also activated within 40 msec but a small paraseptal area showed late activation at 40 to 80 msec. Electrograms representing the 40 to 80 msec isochrones of delayed epicardial activation were recorded during the ST segment of the surface ECG. The epicardial activation pattern of the premature beat (S_2) that initiated the first reentrant cycle was markedly different from that during sinus rhythm. The premature beat resulted in a long arc of functional conduction block within the epicardial border of the ischemic zone (represented by the heavy solid line). The activation wave front circulated around both ends of the arc of block, coalesced, and advanced slowly from lateral to septal borders of the ischemic zone. The slow common reentrant wave front then reexcited normal myocardial zones on the septal side of the arc of block to initiate the first reentrant beat. Electrograms recorded from the reentrant pathway bridged the diastolic interval between the premature beat and the first reentrant beat as well as between successive reentrant beats as shown in the simulated high-resolution ECG.

The electrograms of delayed epicardial activation during sinus rhythm and those recorded from the reentrant pathway represented the bioelectric potentials generated by a relatively small mass of ischemic myocardial tissue. On the body surface, those ECG potentials would not be detected by routine measuring techniques because the signal is smaller than the electrical noise produced by various sources. Two different techniques could be utilized to improve signal-to-noise ratio: (1) ensemble averaging (routinely called signal averaging), which is applicable only to regular repetitive ECG signals and cannot detect moment-by-moment dynamic changes in the signal[23]; and (2) low-noise or high-resolution ECG, which utilizes spatial averaging techniques as well as other noise reducing measures to record the late potentials on the body surface on a beat-to-beat basis.[24,25] The simulated high-resolution ECG in Figure 1 illustrates the most optimal situation in which dynamic changes in the electrical signal can be faithfully recorded on the body surface on a beat-to-beat basis. In such a recording the classification of ventricular rhythms as due to focal discharge or reentrant activation could be easily accomplished by analysis of the diastolic interval preceding the ectopic beat. Diastolic depolarizations that reflect the activation wave front of the reentrant circuit will bridge the diastolic interval preceding the first reentrant beat as well as during successive reentrant beats.

At the present time, the techniques for reducing signal-to-noise level on a beat-to-beat basis are unable to provide a high degree of resolution as illustrated in the simulated ECG shown in Figure 1. Therefore, the signal-averaged technique has been utilized more often in the last few years for the detection of late potentials and the averaged signal has been analyzed in the time and frequency domain.[26,27] However, as mentioned earlier, signal averaging is only applicable to regular repetitive ECG signals. In the example shown in Figure 1, the signal-averaged technique could be utilized to detect the late potentials during sinus rhythm provided that all abnormal myocardial zones show a regular 1:1 conduction pattern. Also the technique could be applied to detect diastolic activity during a regular reentrant tachycardia with a stable reentrant pathway even though some technical problems may arise if atrial activity is asynchronous during the tachycardia.

Correlation of Late Potentials With Inducible Ventricular Tachyarrhythmia in the Post-Infarction Canine Model

Several studies have investigated the relationship of late potentials in the signal-averaged ECG during sinus rhythm and the results of programmed ventricular stimulation in different post-infarction canine models.[18–21] Yoh et al[20] studied a 7-day post-LAD ligation model. Dogs with inducible sustained ventricular tachycardia had a longer total QRS duration, lower terminal QRS amplitude, and a longer late potential duration compared to dogs with no inducible ventricular tachyarrhythmia. Epicardial activation of the ischemic zone was mapped with a patch electrode. Delayed epicardial activation was recorded after the end of the QRS at more sites in dogs with inducible tachycardia. The area of myocardial infarction was also more extensive in these dogs and the thickness of the surviving epicardial muscle in sites with delayed activation was usually ≤1 mm.

Kuchar et al[21] studied dogs following ligation of the LAD and all visible epicardial collateral vessels arising from the left circumflex and right coronary arteries. The signal-averaged ECG was recorded 1 hour after ligation and signal-averaged ECG and programmed stimulation were serially performed 3 to 21 days post-infarction. There was considerable day-to-day variability in the response to programmed stimulation and the results of the signal-averaged ECG. Late potentials during sinus rhythm were defined as a total QRS duration >58 msec, a terminal QRS amplitude in the last 20 msec <20 μV, and a late potentials duration >18 msec. Using this definition, late potentials were seen in two distinct phases; immediately after coronary ligation and then beyond the third post-infarction day. There was a close correlation between inducibility of ventricular tachycardia and the appearance of late potentials. The sensitivity of late potentials for the induction of monomorphic ventricular tachycardia was 100%, the specificity was 90%, and the positive predictive value was 86%. The authors concluded that the parallel time course of the inducibility of sustained ventricular tachycardia and the development of late potentials after myocardial infarction lend support to the concept that the signal-averaged ECG does identify an arrhythmogenic substrate.

In the study by Kuchar et al[21] dogs with inducible ventricular fibrillation had signal-averaged ECG characteristics that were intermediate between those of dogs with inducible monomorphic ventricular tachycardia and those of dogs with no inducible arrhythmias. These observations were different from those of Spear et al,[18] who studied a canine occlusion-reperfusion model 2 to 52 weeks after infarction and found that inducible ventricular fibrillation was a nonspecific end point. The characteristics of the signal-averaged ECG of these dogs were no different from dogs with no inducible tachyarrhythmias. On the other hand, all dogs with inducible sustained ventricular tachycardia had late potentials in the signal-averaged ECG during sinus rhythm defined as a QRS duration ≥64 msec, voltage in the last 20 msec of the QRS ≤13.5 μV, and duration of late activity below 30 μV ≥18.2 msec. All animals with infarction and late potentials had delayed and prolonged epicardial electrograms that extended into the time of late potentials recorded from 45 standard sites in the infarcted regions. The same group of investigators extended their observations on the correlation of signal-averaged ECG and inducibility of ventricular tachyarrhythmia to dogs 4 to 6 years after reperfused infarction and demonstrated that the substrate for reentrant tachycardia was present as shown by the inducibility of sustained ventricular tachycardia.[19] However, these dogs showed less abnormal electrophysiologic findings compared to dogs with 2- to 24-week-old infarction.

Correlation of Late Potentials in the Signal-Averaged ECG With Activation Patterns of Sinus and Induced Reentrant Rhythms

None of the studies mentioned above has correlated the presence of late potentials in the signal-averaged ECG with the ventricular activation patterns of sinus and induced reentrant rhythms. This was done in a study from our laboratory.[28] To assess the relative contribution of electrically active regions to their detection on the body surface in the canine post-infarction heart we constructed a synthesized root mean square (RMS) composite electrogram.[28] The composite was constructed by squaring the individual epicardial electrograms, adding them, then taking the square root of the sum. This eliminates the possibility of electrogram cancellation. Body surface X, Y, and Z leads were signal averaged, high-pass filtered, and vector summed to record a signal-averaged ECG. Late potentials in the signal-averaged ECG correlated in time with those in the epicardial electrograms and in the synthesized composite electrogram. Although the synthesized composite electrogram showed late potentials that bridged the diastolic interval, in the signal-averaged ECG, 20 to 80 msec of the middiastolic interval sometimes failed to show late potentials. The late potentials-free diastolic interval corresponded to slow conduction of the reentrant wave front and to electrograms <0.1 mV in amplitude.

The results from one of the experiments are shown in Figure 2. In this experiment a reentrant beat, V_1, was consistently induced by a single premature stimulus, S_2. On the left of the figure is shown the XYZ vector sum of the signal-averaged ECG. Diastolic activity is seen following the S_2 and preceding V_1. However, during a period of 70 msec in the middiastolic interval, activity was not present or was less than the noise level of the recording technique. The middiastolic interval corresponded in time to the slowly conducting common reentrant wave front as shown in the map to the right. On the other hand, continuous diastolic activity was evident in the epicardial electrograms and in the composite electrogram. The selected epicardial electrograms shown in the figure corresponded to the interval from 160 to 230 msec where surface activity was not detected. The electrograms in this interval were recorded from a thin (1–2 mm) surviving epicardial layer overlying the core of the infarct. Some

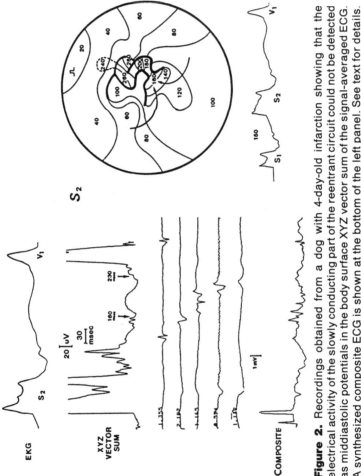

Figure 2. Recordings obtained from a dog with 4-day-old infarction showing that the electrical activity of the slowly conducting part of the reentrant circuit could not be detected as middiastolic potentials in the body surface XYZ vector sum of the signal-averaged ECG. A synthesized composite ECG is shown at the bottom of the left panel. See text for details.

electrograms in this area had relatively large amplitude (>1 mV), while some exhibited multiphasic electrotonic deflections, and others had low amplitude slow deflections (<0.1 mV). Those electrograms reflected slow conduction through a narrow pathway surrounded by functionally blocked tissue. The small mass of active tissue which comprised the slowest part of the reentrant circuit was not reflected in the body surface recording. The study shows that late potentials correlate with delayed epicardial activation in an area overlying the infarct. During reentrant activation, however, complete diastolic activity on the body surface may not be detected if the mass of electrically active cells is too small and/or if slow conduction in part of the circuit generates low amplitude extracellular potentials.

Activation Patterns of Sinus and "Spontaneous" Reentrant Rhythms

Activation of the ischemic zone during sinus rhythm in Figure 1 followed a regular 1:1 pattern. This is not the case, however, in all post-infarction canine hearts. Figure 3 was obtained from a dog 4 days post-infarction and illustrates that activation of the ischemic epicardial zone during sinus rhythm did not follow a regular 1:1 pattern. The activation pattern of the ischemic zone varied in successive sinus beats and was much more complex compared to the activation pattern shown in Figure 1. Zones of conduction block were seen during sinus rhythm, together with activation delays of up to 200 msec. Although most of the epicardial ischemic zone showed a 1:1 conduction pattern, there were areas that showed 2:1 conduction (electrograms #9 and #10) and others that showed a Wenckebach conduction pattern (electrograms #11 and #12). The signal averaging technique requires that the signal of interest be repeated in a regular fashion. This is obviously not the case during sinus rhythm in Figure 3. Although all electrograms showing a regular 1:1 pattern (#1-8) as well as those showing a 2:1 conduction pattern could be averaged, those showing the more dynamic Wenckebach pattern could not. The body surface signal-averaged ECG of the sinus rhythm in this case would still reveal late potentials. However, it will not faithfully reflect the degree nor the pattern of conduction delays of the entire ischemic zone.

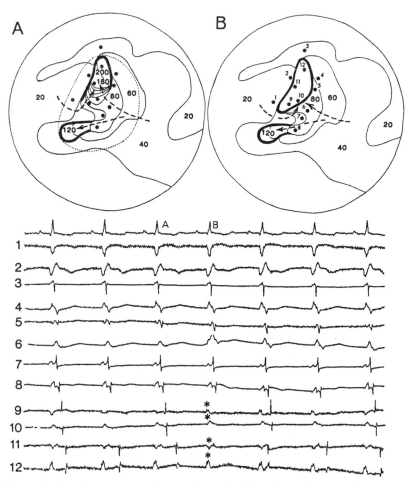

Figure 3. Isochronal maps of epicardial activation during 2 consecutive sinus beats (A and B) from a dog with a 4-day-old infarction. Selected epicardial electrograms are shown on the bottom. In contrast to Figure 1 where activation of the ischemic epicardial zone during sinus rhythm followed a regular 1:1 pattern, in Figure 3 the activation pattern of the ischemic zone varied in successive sinus beats. Some epicardial zones showed a 2:1 or a Wenckebach activation pattern. See text for more details. The asterisks refer to electrotonic potentials. (Reproduced with permission from El-Sherif et al, PACE 8:440, 1985.)

A Wenckebach conduction pattern in the ischemic myocardium may not be an uncommon occurrence. El-Sherif et al have shown that a Wenckebach conduction sequence is the initiating mechanism for "spontaneous" reentrant rhythms, that is, reentrant rhythms that occur during a regular cardiac rhythm (e.g., the sinus rhythm) as contrasted with reentrant rhythms induced by 1 or more premature beats that interrupt an otherwise regular cardiac rhythm. [6,7,22] For reentry to occur during regular cardiac rhythm, the heart rate should be within the relatively narrow critical range of rates during which conduction in a potentially reentrant pathway shows a Wenckebach-like pattern. [22] During a Wenckebach-like conduction cycle, a beat-to-beat increment in the length of the arcs of conduction block and/or the degree of conduction delay will occur until the activation wave front is sufficiently delayed for certain parts of the myocardium proximal to the arc of block to recover excitability and become reexcited by the delayed activation front. This is shown in Figure 4, which illustrates epicardial activation maps as well as selected electrograms from an experiment in which a reentrant trigeminal rhythm developed during sinus tachycardia. Once more, as is the case in Figure 3, the dynamic activation pattern in Figure 4 is not amenable to signal averaging techniques but theoretically can be represented on the body surface in a beat-to-beat fashion using a high-resolution ECG recording.

Are Regions of Delayed Activation During a Basic Rhythm the Responsible Arrhythmogenic Substrate for Reentry?

Restivo et al[29] conducted a study in the 4-day-old canine post-infarction model of reentry to determine if regions of delayed activation during a basic rhythm (sinus rhythm or regular ventricular pacing) are the responsible arrhythmogenic substrate for reentry. Reentrant rhythms were induced by programmed electrical stimulation. The signal-averaged ECG during basic rhythm at a cycle length of 400–500 msec detected late potentials which corresponded temporally with the region of latest epicardial activation. Subsequent signal averaging of reentrant circuits revealed that sites of late potentials during the basic rhythm were not always responsible for late potentials detected during reentrant activation. Examination of activation maps of these beats confirmed that the regions responsible for late potentials during a basic rhythm were not part of the final

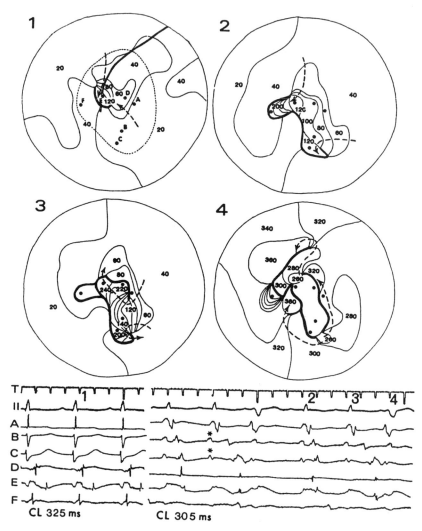

Figure 4. Isochronal maps of a reentrant trigeminal rhythm. The figure illustrates epicardial activation maps as well as selected electrographic recordings from a dog 4 days post-infarction in which a reentrant trigeminal rhythm developed during sinus tachycardia. The epicardial map of a sinus beat at a cycle length of 325 msec is labeled 1. Spontaneous shortening of the sinus cycle length to 305 msec resulted in the development of a single reentrant beat following every second sinus beat. The maps labeled 2, 3, and 4 represent the first and second sinus beats and the reentrant beat, respectively. Electrographic recordings from the reentrant pathway during the trigeminal rhythm (B, C, D, and E) illustrated a 3:2 Wenckebach conduction pattern while electrogram F showed 2:1 conduction. See text for more details. (Reproduced with permission from El-Sherif et al, J Am Coll Cardiol 6:124, 1985.)

common reentrant pathway during reentrant activation. Regions showing marked conduction delay in a 1:1 pattern or showing Wenckebach or 2:1 conduction patterns during the basic rhythm usually blocked during S_2 and did not participate in the reentrant process. This is illustrated in Figure 5 obtained from one of the experiments. Recordings on the left were obtained during basic right ventricular pacing at an $S_1 S_1$ cycle of 400 msec. Recordings on the right were obtained during premature stimulation (S_2) that initiated a reentrant beat (V_1). During S_1 stimulation the most delayed epicardial activation sites were in the center of the ischemic zone represented by epicardial electrograms C and D. These sites were reflected by late potentials in the signal-averaged ECG. However, during reentrant activation induced by S_2 stimulation, electrograms C and D showed conduction block and their sites did not participate in the reentrant circuit as shown in the activation map on the right. On the other hand, middiastolic activity during reentry is represented by electrograms A and B. These sites contributed to the diastolic potentials during reentry but not to the late potentials during the basic rhythm.

The results of the above study were corroborated by another recent study from our laboratory.[30] In this study, the correlation between myocardial sites critical for the prevention of initiation and/or termination of reentrant tachycardia by cryothermal techniques and sites of late activation during sinus rhythm was investigated in the canine post-infarction model. The sites correlated well in only 25% of the cases. The lack of correlation was explained by the fact that the critical sites during reentry were intimately related to the location and extent of the arcs of functional conduction block, which is one of two essential prerequisites for circus movement reentry besides slow conduction, while sites of delayed activation during sinus rhythm were not.

Electrophysiologic Mechanism of Fractionated Electrograms

Bioelectric signals are influenced by the recording method (i.e., electrode type, filter settings, and interelectrode spacing).[31] Depending on the recording technique employed, fractionated multicomponent and long duration electrograms can be recorded from diseased hearts and have been used as indirect evidence suggestive of reentry. Fractionated electrograms have been recorded from

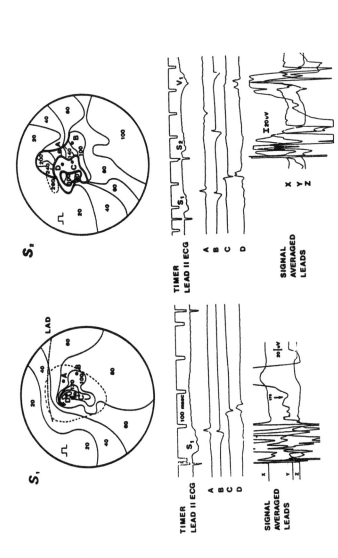

Figure 5. Recordings obtained from a dog 4 days post-infarction showing that regions responsible for late potentials during the basic rhythm (S_1, left panel) were not part of the slow common reentrant pathway during reentrant activation induced by a single premature stimulation (S_2, right panel). Shown from top to bottom are the epicardial activation map, surface ECG, selected epicardial electrograms and the X, Y and Z leads of the signal-averaged ECG. See text for details.

composite electrodes placed over a large area of the ventricular epicardial surface of 3- to 5-day-old canine infarcts,[5] ventricular endocardial surface in humans using wide bipolar (10 mm interpole) catheters,[32] the epicardial border zone of canine infarcts using 1-mm disk electrodes (2 mm interpole),[33] epicardial tissue from healed infarcts studied in in vitro,[34] subendocardial tissue from healed infarcts of human hearts,[35] and human atrial bundles infiltrated with collagenous septa.[36] In a study by Gardner et al[34] fractionated electrograms were recorded in epicardial preparations obtained from healed canine infarcts (2 weeks to 18-months old) utilizing bipolar electrodes with 0.5-mm interpolar distance (Figure 6). The fractionated electrograms were only rarely recorded in

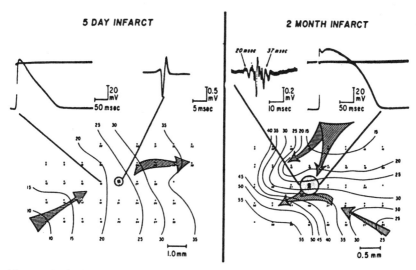

Figure 6. Activation maps of regions around bipolar electrodes in two different canine infarct preparations. The location and size of electrodes are indicated by the stippled circle and the electrograms recorded in each experiment are shown above. The points at which action potentials were recorded in each panel are indicated by the dots. Representative action potentials are also shown. The arrows and isochrones show the direction of activation. The stimulus sites are not included in the maps. The distance scale for each panel is shown below. The scale is two times larger for the 5-day-old infarct preparation than for the 2-month-old infarct preparation. In contrast to 5-day infarct, fractionated electrograms were recorded in the 2-month-old infarct and corresponded to slow and inhomogeneous conduction in the vicinity of the recording electrode. (Reproduced with permission from Gardner et al, Circulation 72:596, 1985.)

preparations from 5-day-old infarcts. Transmembrane action potentials from areas of fractionated electrograms were normal or nearly so. As originally proposed by Spach et al,[37] the authors suggested that the fractionated electrograms were the result of slowed and inhomogeneous conduction in the vicinity of the recording electrode resulting in superposition of temporally asynchronous depolarization potentials of normal muscle bundles that have been uncoupled by intervening fibrous tissue.

The fractionated electrograms recorded by the composite electrode or by a wide bipolar catheter electrode could also be explained by slowed and inhomogenous conduction in the vicinity of the electrode.[5] Since these electrodes register the activation of much larger myocardial areas the fractionated electrograms represent the superposition of temporally asynchronous activation potentials of relatively large myocardial zones. It is reasonable to assume that both slow and discontinuous propagation within small zones of scarred myocardium as well as temporally asynchronous activation over large electrophysiologically abnormal myocardial zones can potentially contribute to late potentials on the body surface. Fractionated electrograms from small isolated bundles in scarred myocardium usually have a low amplitude[34] and are less likely to be isolated from noise in the body surface signal-averaged ECG. More significant is the argument that areas of extensive fibrosis with disorganized, isolated, and uncoupled myocardial bundles may not provide the anatomic-electrophysiologic substrate for reentrant excitation.[30] This is not surprising since very slow and circuitous conduction is probably not tantamount to successful reentrant excitation compared to the presence of a critical zone of functional unidirectional conduction block. Areas of very slow conduction during a basic relatively slow cardiac rhythm do not usually participate in reentrant excitation induced by premature stimulation (see Figure 5).

Electrophysiologic Limitations of Late Potentials in the Signal-Averaged ECG

Most technical limitations of signal averaging could be improved by appropriate measures. However, it is important to understand the following electrophysiologic limitations of the signal-averaged ECG. (1) Since signal averaging can be applied only to regular repetitive signals, it is customarily applied to the QRS and ST-T segment of consecutive sinus beats. The recording will be able to average delayed activation signals that occur in a regular 1:1 or 2:1 pattern but not those with a dynamic Wenckebach sequence. Thus, the duration of late potentials may not reflect faithfully areas with marked but periodic conduction delays as shown in Figure 3. (2) The relationship between myocardial zones showing conduction delay during sinus rhythm on one hand and spontaneous or induced reentrant rhythms on the other hand is complex. Reentry requires a critical balance between the length of the zone of unidirectional block and the degree of conduction delay of the circulating wave front. The zones of unidirectional block are not represented in the signal-averaged ECG and the degree of conduction delay necessary for reentry may bear little relationship to the degree of conduction delay during sinus rhythm. There may be a significant difference between reentrant rhythms that occur spontaneously and those induced by premature stimulation in the same post-infarction heart.[22] Further, as discussed in the preceding section, fractionated electrograms from areas of scarred myocardium may contribute to late potentials in the signal-averaged ECG during sinus rhythm but these areas will probably not contribute to the anatomic-electrophysiologic substrate for reentrant excitation. Thus, late potentials in the signal-averaged ECG during sinus rhythm, at best, reflect myocardial zones with slow and inhomogeneous conduction and as such are only indirect markers for the propensity to develop reentrant tachyarrhythmias either spontaneously or following one or more premature stimulations. (3) Although reentrant arrhythmias commonly occur in the post-infarction heart and most probably are the underlying electrophysiologic mechanism for ventricular fibrillation and sudden cardiac death, some post-infarction arrhythmias may be caused by focal discharge of Purkinje fibers. The latter may be secondary to a mechanism of abnormal automaticity[38] or afterdepolarizations and triggered activity.[39] A ventricular tachycardia of nonreentrant origin may occur in hearts showing late potentials during sinus rhythm and bears no relationship to these potentials. (4) Late potentials during sinus rhythm have been shown to be a reliable indicator for the inducibility of sustained ventricular tachycardia.[18-21] However, their predictive accuracy for spontaneous tachyarrhythmias, particularly ventricular fibrillation, is rather low. This is undoubtedly related to the nature of the triggering mechanism(s) of spontaneous tachyarrhythmias which is not fully understood and may prove to be different and more complex compared to the technique of programmed stimulation. It is important to remember that late potentials reflect a fixed stable substrate of electrophysiologic abnormality. On the other hand, the eventual episode of ventricular fibrillation and sudden cardiac death may be a complex event that requires not only an established arrhythmogenic substrate, but also appropriate modulating and triggering factors, and/ or a de novo electrophysiologic perturbation.

Acknowledgment: This study was supported by NIH grants HL 31431 and HL 36680 and by Veterans Administration Medical Research Funds.

References

1. El-Sherif N, Gomes JAC, Restivo M, Mehra R: Late potentials and arrhythmogenesis. PACE 8:440, 1985.
2. Waldo AL, Kaiser GA: A study of ventricular arrhythmias associated with myocardial infarction in the canine heart. Circulation 47:1222, 1973.
3. Boineau JP, Cox JL: Slow ventricular activation in acute myocardial infarction. A source of reentrant premature ventricular contractions. Circulation 48:702, 1973.
4. El-Sherif N, Scherlag BJ, Lazzara R: Electrode catheter recordings during malignant ventricular arrhythmias following experimental acute myocardial ischemia. Circulation 51:1003, 1975.
5. El-Sherif N, Scherlag BJ, Lazzara R, Hope RR: Reentrant ventricular arrhythmias in the late myocardial infarction period. 1. Conduction characteristics in the infarction zone. Circulation 55:686, 1977.
6. El-Sherif N, Hope RR, Scherlag BJ, Lazzara R: Reentrant ventricular arrhythmias in the late myocardial infarction period. II. Patterns of initiation and termination of reentry. Circulation 55:702, 1977.
7. El-Sherif N, Lazzara R, Hope RR, Scherlag BJ: Reentrant ventricular arrhythmias in the late myocardial infarction period. III. Manifest and concealed extra-systolic grouping. Circulation 56:225, 1977.
8. Janse MJ, vanCapelle FJL, Morsink H, Kleber AG, Wilms-Schopman F, Cardinal R, D'Alnoncout CN, Durrer D: Flow of "injury" current and patterns of excitation during early ventricular arrhythmias in acute regional myocardial ischemia in isolated porcine and canine hearts. Circ Res 47:151, 1980.
9. El-Sherif N, Smith RA, Evans K: Ventricular arrhythmias in the late myocardial infarction period in the dog. 8 Epicardial mapping of reentrant circuits. Circ Res 49:255, 1981.
10. Wit AL, Allessie MA, Bonke FIM, Lammers W, Smeets J, Fenoglio JJ: Electrophysiologic mapping to determine the mechanism of experimental ventricular tachycardia initiated by premature impulses: experimental approach and initial results demonstrating reentrant excitation. Am J Cardiol 49:166, 1982.
11. El-Sherif N, Mehra R, Gough WB, Zeiler RH: Ventricular activation patterns of spontaneous and induced ventricular rhythms in canine one-day-old myocardial infarction. Evidence for focal and reentrant rhythms. Circ Res 51:152, 1982.
12. Mehra R, Zeiler RH, Gough WB, El-Sherif N: Reentrant ventricular arrhythmias in the late myocardial infarction period. 9. Electrophysi-

ologic-anatomical correlation of reentrant circuit. Circulation 67:11, 1983.

13. El-Sherif N, Mehra R, Gough WB, Zeiler RH: Reentrant ventricular arrhythmias in the late myocardial infarction period. Interruption of reentrant circuits by cryothermal techniques. Circulation 68:644, 1983.

14. Pogwizd SM, Corr BP: Reentrant and nonreentrant mechanisms contributing to arrhythmogenesis during early myocardial ischemia: results using three-dimensional mapping. Circ Res 61:352, 1987.

15. Restivo M, Gough WB, El-Sherif N: Ventricular arrhythmias in the subacute myocardial infarction period. High resolution activation and refractory patterns of reentrant rhythms. Circ Res 66:1310, 1990.

16. Simson MB, Euler D, Michelson EL, Falcone RA, Spear JF, Moore EN: Detection of delayed ventricular activation on the body surface in dogs. Am J Physiol 241:H363, 1981.

17. Berbari EJ, Scherlag BJ, Hope RR, Lazzara R: Recording from the body surface of arrhythmogenic ventricular activity during the S-T segment. Am J Cardiol 41:697, 1978.

18. Spear JF, Richards DA, Blake GJ, Simson MB, Moore EN: The effects of premature stimulation of the His bundle on epicardial activation and body surface late potentials in dogs susceptible to sustained ventricular tachyarrhythmias. Circulation 72:214, 1985.

19. Hanich RF, DeLangen CDJ, Kadish AH, Michelson EL, Levine JH, Spear JF, Moore EN: Inducible sustained ventricular tachycardia 4 years after experimental canine myocardial infarction: electrophysiologic and anatomic comparisons with early healed infarcts. Circulation 77:445, 1988.

20. Yoh S, Ogawa S, Satoh Y, Furuno I, Saeki K, Sadanaga T, Nakamura Y: Electrophysiological and anatomical substrates for late potential recorded by signal averaging in seven-day-old myocardial infarction in dogs. PACE 13:469, 1990.

21. Kuchar DL, Rosenbaum DS, Ruskin J, Garan H: Late potentials on the signal-averaged electrocardiogram after canine myocardial infarction: correlation with ventricular arrhythmias during the healing phase. J Am Coll Cardiol 15:1365, 1990.

22. El-Sherif N, Gough WB, Zeiler RH, Hariman R: Reentrant ventricular arrhythmias in the late myocardial infarction period. 12. Spontaneous versus induced reentry and intramural versus epicardial circuits. J Am Coll Cardiol 6:124, 1985.

23. Mehra R, El-Sherif N: Signal averaging of electrocardiographic potentials. A review. Acupuncture and Electrotherapeutics Res Int J 7:133, 1982.

24. El-Sherif N, Mehra R, Gomes JAC, Kelen G: Appraisal of a low noise electrocardiogram. J Am Coll Cardiol 1:456, 1983.

25. Hombach V, Kebbel U, Hopp H-W, Winter U, Hirche H: Noninvasive beat-by-beat registration of ventricular late potentials using high resolution electrocardiography. Int J Cardiol 6:167, 1984.

26. Cain ME, Ambos HD, Witkowski FX, Sobel BE: Fast-Fourier transform analysis of signal-averaged electrocardiograms for identification of patients prone to sustained ventricular tachycardia. Circulation 69:711, 1984.

27. Kelen GJ, Henkin R, Fontaine JM, El-Sherif N: Effects of analyzed

signal duration and phase on the results of Fast Fourier transform analysis of the surface electrocardiogram in subjects with and without late potentials. Am J Cardiol 60:1282, 1987.

28. Restivo M, El-Sherif N, Kelen GJ, Henkin R, Craelius W, Gough WB: Correlation of late potentials on the body surface and ventricular activation maps of reentrant circuits in the post-infarction dog heart (abstr). Circulation 72 (Suppl):III-11, 1985.

29. Restivo M, Henkin R, Craelius W, El-Sherif N: Are regions of delayed activation during a basic rhythm the responsible arrhythmogenic substrate for reentry? (abstr). J Am Coll Cardiol 7:85A, 1986.

30. Assadi M, Restivo M, Gough WB, El-Sherif N: Reentrant ventricular arrhythmias in the late myocardial infarction period. 17. Correlation of activation patterns of sinus and reentrant ventricular tachycardia. Am Heart J 119:1014, 1990.

31. Ideker RE, Mirvis DM, Smith WM: Late fractionated potentials. Am J Cardiol 55:1614, 1985.

32. Josephson ME, Horowitz LN, Farshidi A: Continuous local electrical activity: a mechanism of recurrent ventricular tachycardia. Circulation 57:659, 1978.

33. Dillon SM, Allessie MA, Ursell PC, Wit AL: Influences of anisotropic tissue structure in reentrant circuits in the epicardial border zone of subacute canine infarcts. Circ Res 63:182, 1988.

34. Gardner PI, Ursell PC, Fenoglio JJ, Jr, Wit AL: Electrophysiologic and anatomic basis for fractionated electrograms recorded from healed myocardial infarcts. Circulation 72:596, 1985.

35. DeBakker JMT, van Capelle FJL, Janse MJ, Wilde AAM, Coronel R, Becker AE, Dingemans KP, van Hemel NM, Haver RNW: Reentry as a cause of ventricular tachycardia in patients with chronic ischemic heart disease: electrophysiologic and anatomic correlation. Circulation 77:-589, 1988.

36. Spach MS, Dolber PC: Relating extracellular potentials and their derivatives to anisotropic propagation at a microscopic level in human cardiac muscle: evidence for electrical uncoupling of side to side fiber connections with increasing age. Circ Res 58:356, 1986.

37. Spach MS, Barr RC, Johnson EA, Kootsey JM: Cardiac extracellular potentials: analysis of complex wave forms about the Purkinje network in dogs. Circ Res 33:465, 1973.

38. Hoffman BF, Rosen MR: Cellular mechanisms for cardiac arrhythmias. Circ Res 49:1, 1981.

39. El-Sherif N, Gough WB, Zeiler RH, Mehra R: Triggered ventricular rhythms in 1-day-old myocardial infarction in the dog. Circ Res 52:566, 1983.

14

The Effect of Ischemia on the High-Frequency Potentials

Shimon Abboud

Introduction

Interpretation of conventional surface electrocardiogram (ECG) usually relies upon the recognition of grossly identifiable morphologic alterations in the QRS complexes and T waves. Since these changes typically involve frequencies below 100 Hz, the bandwidth employed in clinical electrocardiography is usually limited to 100 Hz. In the past several years, the terms "high frequency," "high fidelity," and "wide-band electrocardiography" have been used by several investigators[1-9] to refer to the process of recording ECGs with an extended bandwidth of up to 1000 Hz. Their analysis was based mainly on the temporal appearance of the notches and slurs in the conventional QRS complex and the term "high fidelity ECG" seems to be more accurate. The high fidelity ECG has been used to analyze the high-frequency details in the QRS complex with the hope that additional features seen in the QRS complex would provide information enhancing the diagnostic value of the ECG. Recent studies[10-14] from our laboratory analyzed the high-frequency components (150–250 Hz), which are beyond the visible notches and slurs, and showed that ischemia can be detected with more sensitivity by

From El-Sherif N, Turitto G (eds): *High-Resolution Electrocardiography.* Mount Kisco, NY, Futura Publishing Co., Inc., ©, 1992.

the high-frequency QRS complex than by visual inspection of the surface ECG alone. This high-frequency electrical activity present in the ECG signal is usually buried in random noise and high-gain amplification, signal filtering, and averaging is therefore necessary to improve the signal-to-noise ratio of the output signal.

We have previously reported[15-17] on the use of an advanced computerized method of signal averaging for recording His bundle activity[18,19] in patients with and without Wolff-Parkinson-White syndrome and for the recording of late potentials[20] in patients with a damaged mass of ventricular tissue. This method uses the fast Fourier transform algorithm and the cross correlation function[18] for accurate recording and filtering the averaged waveforms.[15-17] Based on our earlier experience with the signal averaging technique, several studies were designed to determine the extent to which the morphology of the high-frequency QRS potentials is affected by myocardial ischemia:

1. high-frequency electrocardiography in dogs during a coronary artery occlusion[10-12];
2. high-frequency electrocardiography in patients undergoing percutaneous transluminal coronary angioplasty[13];
3. high-frequency electrocardiography in patients with coronary artery disease and normal conventional ECG.[14]

The Signal Averaging Technique

The ECG waveforms are stored on an FM tape recorder for later playback and analysis. During playback of the recorded high fidelity ECGs, the analog data are passed through a low-pass six-pole Butterworth filter with a high-frequency cut-off at 360 Hz and then digitized by a 12-bit analog-to-digital converter with a sampling rate of 1024 Hz. The digitized waveforms are averaged together to reduce the relative contribution of the uncorrelated noise component. A detailed description of the averaging procedure is given in Chapter 6. In brief, the alignment of the waveforms to be averaged is accomplished via a normalized cross correlation technique.[15,17] Prior to averaging, the candidate waveforms are first passed through a nonrecursive digital bandpass filter[16] with low-frequency cut-off at 30 Hz and high-frequency cut-off at 250 Hz and subsequently cross correlated with a reference template[17] (a user chosen waveform). The point of maximum correlation for each waveform is taken as its fiducial point for averaging. Artifacts and abnormal complexes which cannot be correlated with the reference wave (cross correlation coefficients below a threshold value) are eliminated. The fiducial points are used to align the original (unfiltered) waveforms for averaging.

The averaged waveform is then bandpass filtered with low-frequency cut-off at 150 Hz and high-frequency cut-off at 250 Hz and is used to compute the envelope of the filtered QRS complex.

High–Frequency QRS Complex Envelope Determination

Averaged and filtered high-frequency QRS complexes obtained by the methods described are analyzed to determine the boundaries or envelopes of the waveforms. The upper and lower boundaries of the envelopes are defined as the line segments connecting local maxima and minima, respectively. A local maximum, V_{max}, is determined to be located at sample point t_i if and only if the amplitude of the high-frequency ECG, $V(t_i)$, at this point is exceeded by the amplitude of the three sample points preceding and following t_i:

$$[V(t_{i-3}), V(t_{i-2}), V(t_{i-1})] < V(t_i) > [V(t_{i+1}), V(t_{i+2}), V(t_{i+3})].$$

Similarly, a local minimum, V_{min}, is determined to be located at sample point t_1, if and only if the amplitude of the high-frequency $V(t_1)$, at this point is lower than the amplitude of three points preceding and following t_1. A reduced amplitude zone within the envelope of the averaged high-frequency QRS complex is considered to be present if at least two local maxima of the upper envelope or two local minima of the lower envelope are found. In such cases a zone of reduced amplitude (RAZ) is defined to be the region lying between two neighboring maxima or minima.

Figure 1 is a representative example of the signal-averaged non-filtered QRS complex of lead V_5 (top trace) from a normal individual without coronary artery disease. The middle and bottom traces in this figure are, respectively, the signal-averaged high-frequency QRS and the computer generated delineation of the envelope of the averaged high-frequency QRS. As it can be seen, no zones of reduced amplitude are apparent within the envelope of this signal (bottom

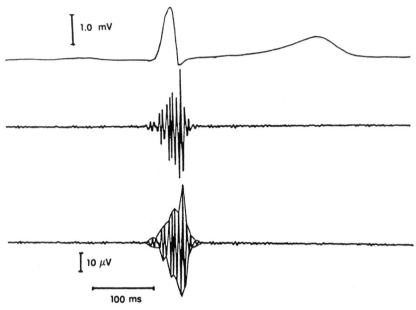

Figure 1. Signal-averaged nonfiltered ECG of surface lead V_5 (top), the signal-averaged high-frequency (150–250 Hz) QRS (middle), and the computer-generated delineation of the envelope of the high-frequency QRS (bottom) from a normal subject with no coronary artery disease. Note smooth contour of the envelope and absence of a zone of reduced amplitude.

trace, Figure 1). It is of interest to note that the high-frequency QRS complex (middle trace) is of low-amplitude (microvolts) compared to the standard QRS complex (millivolts).

Effects of Ischemia on the High-Frequency QRS Potentials

High-Frequency Electrocardiography in Dogs During Coronary Artery Occlusion

Ischemia is induced in dogs by a complete 5-minute occlusion of the left anterior descending coronary artery (LAD). The morphology of the high-frequency QRS complex components is examined before, during, and after occlusion of the coronary artery.

Experimental Procedure

Mongrel dogs weighing 15–25 kg were anesthetized with sodium pentobarbital (30 mg/kg body weight) and artificially ventilated through a cuffed endotracheal tube. The chest was opened via a lateral thoracotomy at the level of the fifth intercostal space and the pericardium was incised and reflected to expose the LAD. The artery was prepared for ligation by dissecting it free of the investing fascia and placing a balloon occluding cuff around it just distal to the first diagonal branch. The cuff was then tested to determine the level of inflation required to complete occlusion. The chest was closed and evacuated of air. The three orthogonal leads for the surface ECGs (X, Y, and Z) were monitored using an ECG laboratory station with the amplifiers set for 0.01- to 500-Hz bandpass filtering. The signals were recorded on an FM instrumentation recorder with bandwidth filters of 0–1250 Hz. Arterial blood pressure was monitored throughout the experiment.

Prior to inflation of the occluding cuff, a 5-minute recording of the three orthogonal electrocardiographic leads was made. The balloon cuff was then inflated to the predetermined level, resulting in a complete occlusion of the coronary artery. The cuff was maintained inflated for 5 minutes and then slowly deflated, allowing for reperfusion. The surface ECGs were recorded during the 5 minutes of ligation and during the subsequent 10 minutes of reperfusion. All recordings were made during normal sinus rhythm.

The recorded analog data were digitized and processed using a Masscomp MC-500 laboratory computer.

Data Analysis

The digitized data were divided into several segments lasting 10–15 seconds. The ECG waveforms from each segment, which contained about 20–30 waveforms (representing different stages of the ischemic state), were averaged together and then filtered between 150–250 Hz to obtain the high frequency QRS potentials.

Signal Averaging the High-Frequency ECG: Time-Domain Analysis

Examples of the waveforms obtained during various stages of the experiment are shown in Figure 2. The left traces are the re-

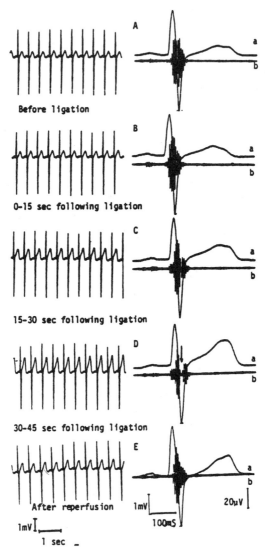

Figure 2. Tracing obtained from electrocardiographic recordings from lead Z during different stages of the ligation dog experiment. Traces on the left represent the ECG raw data. On the right traces are the averaged nonfiltered and filtered waveforms. A zone of reduced amplitude (arrow) can be seen in the averaged filtered waveform 30–45 seconds following ligation (trace d[b]). The millivolt scale relates to the averaged nonfiltered traces and the microvolt scale to the averaged and filtered traces.

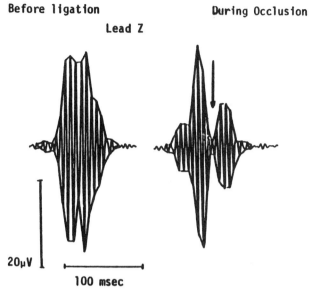

Before ligation   **During Occlusion**

Lead Z

20μV

100 msec

Figure 3. Envelopes of the high-frequency QRS complexes (shown in Figure 2) obtained before and during coronary ligation. The left trace is an example of a normal tracing without a reduced amplitude zone (RAZ). The trace on the right depicts a typical RAZ (arrow).

corded ECG waveforms. On the right, traces a and b show the unfiltered and the filtered (150–250 Hz) average waveforms, respectively. A zone of reduced amplitude, indicated by an arrow in panel D, is present in the filtered waveform obtained during the occlusion, 30–45 seconds following ligation. This reduced amplitude zone resolved following reperfusion (panel E). To delineate the reduced amplitude zone, the envelopes of the QRS complexes, obtained before ligation (Figure 2A) and during occlusion (Figure 2D) are displayed in Figure 3.

Beat-to-Beat Variability

Figure 4 represents beat-to-beat variability of nonaveraged high-frequency QRS complexes. Traces are the nonfiltered (left traces) and filtered (right traces) single waveforms (each tenth beat) obtained after occlusion. After 40 waveforms (about 20 seconds) the

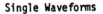

Single Waveforms

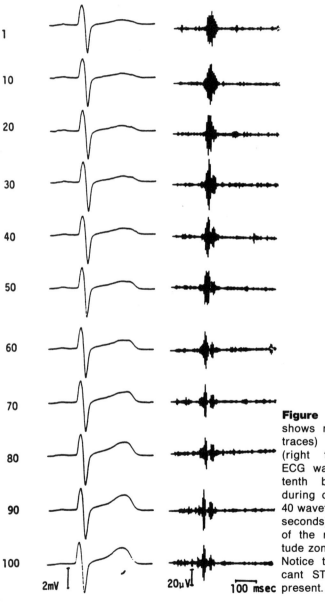

Figure 4. Traces shows nonfiltered (left traces) and filtered (right traces) single ECG waveforms (each tenth beat) obtained during occlusion. After 40 waveforms (about 20 seconds) the evolution of the reduced amplitude zone can be seen. Notice that no significant ST changes are present.

evolution of the reduced amplitude zone can be seen. It is of interest to note that these morphologic changes seen early in ischemia are not accompanied by significant changes in the QRS complex or ST segment of the conventional ECG. Figure 5A shows the beat-to-beat variability in the high-frequency QRS complex during the control stage (before the balloon was inflated) using normalized cross correlation scheme. The y axis represents the normalized cross correlation coefficient between a template filtered QRS complex and the following filtered QRS signals. No significant morphologic changes manifested by a decline in the cross correlation coefficient can be seen. Figure 5B shows the beat-to-beat variability during the occlusion of the coronary artery. Morphologic changes are present a few beats after balloon inflation.

Frequency-Domain Analysis

The high-frequency QRS complex can be represented as a multiplication of two sinusoidal waveforms: (A) the high-frequency component which simulated the rapid alterations (F_H = 160 Hz); and (B) the low-frequency component which represents the envelope of the high-frequency QRS complex (F_L = 16 Hz and 8 Hz for a QRS without and with reduced amplitude zone, respectively):

$$H(t) = A\sin(2\pi F_H t)\sin(2\pi F_L t).$$

The Fourier transform of a waveform separates the signal into a sum of sinusoids of two different frequencies, $F_H + F_L$ and $F_H - F_L$. The power spectrum diagram displays the amplitude square of each sinusoids:

$$P(F_1) = A^2(F_1) + B^2(F_1)$$

where $A(F_1)$ and $B(F_1)$ are the real and imaginary Fourier coefficients at frequency F_1 of the transformed signal.

Examples of the averaged waveforms and the power spectrum obtained from a dog before ligation are shown in Figure 6. As it can be seen, a broad spectral peak at approximately 160 Hz is present. Figure 7 shows the averaged waveforms (traces a and b) and the power spectrum (trace c) obtained following occlusion. Morphologic changes including a zone of reduced amplitude (arrow) can be seen in the high-frequency QRS complex and two separate peaks are present in the spectral curve at 145 Hz and 175 Hz. In the high-

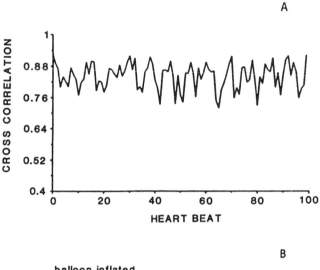

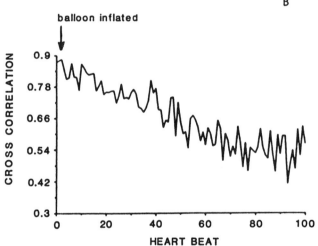

Figure 5. Beat-to-beat variability in the high-frequency (150–250 Hz) QRS complexes obtained before and during occlusion is present in traces A and B, respectively. The vertical axis represents the normalized cross correlation coefficient between the high-frequency QRS complex from a reference template and that of the following heart beats. No significant morphologic changes can be seen during the control stage before occlusion (trace a). Morphologic changes expressed as a reduction in the cross correlation coefficient can be seen a few beats after occlusion in trace b.

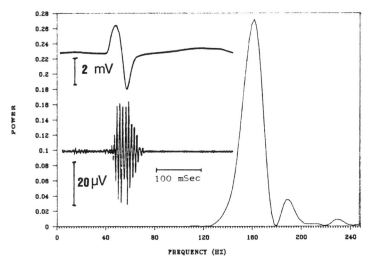

Figure 6. Averaged ECG waveforms and the power spectrum obtained from a dog before ligation. Traces a and b are the averaged nonfiltered and filtered (150–250 Hz) signals, respectively. Trace c is the power spectrum of the high-frequency QRS complex shown in trace b. A broad spectral peak at approximately 160 Hz can be seen.

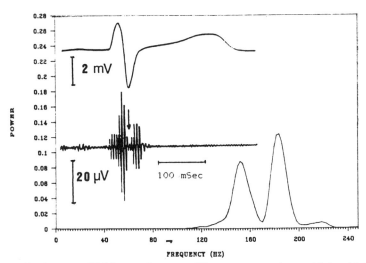

Figure 7. Averaged ECG waveforms and the power spectrum obtained following occlusion. A reduced amplitude zone (arrow) can be seen in the high frequency QRS complex (trace b). Two separate peaks are present in the spectral curve (trace c).

frequency QRS complex before occlusion, the low-frequency component (F_L), which represents the envelope, is approximately 8 Hz. The difference between the two sinusoidal components ($F_H - F_L$ and $F_H + F_L$) is too small and the power spectrum is displayed as one broad peak at a frequency equal to F_H (Figure 6 trace c). The high-frequency QRS with a reduce amplitude zone (Figure 7) consists of a higher low-frequency component ($F_L = 16$ Hz) and the power spectrum is displayed as two separated peaks at frequencies 145 Hz and 175 Hz.

Results

Results which were obtained using the above described method on ten dogs are presented in Table I. The Table summarizes the occurrence of the reduced amplitude zones on the envelope of the high-frequency QRS complex before ligation, during occlusion, and following reperfusion. In seven dog experiments, coronary artery

Table I

High-Frequency ECG and ST Changes During Coronary Ligation in Dogs

| Dog No. | The Presence of RAZ on the High-Frequency ECG | | | Presence of Significant ST Changes Following 2-minute Ligation |
	Before Ligation	During Ligation	Following Reperfusion	
1	—	lead Z	—	lead Z
2	—	lead X	—	leads X, Z
3	lead Z	lead Z	lead Z	lead Z
4	—	lead Z	—	lead Z
5	lead X	lead X	lead X	—
6	—	lead Z	—	lead Z
7	—	—	—	lead Z
8	—	lead Z	—	lead Y
9	—	lead X	—	leads X, Z
10	—	lead Z	—	lead Z

RAZ = reduced amplitude zone.

ligation resulted in a detectable zone of reduced amplitude during the time course of ligation, while no such zone was detected prior to ligation. In two experiments, ligation served to widen the zone of reduced amplitude. In one experiment, no reduced amplitude zone could be detected at any stage of the experiment. Figure 8 represents the high-frequency QRS complexes from a dog in which a zone of reduced amplitude is detected both before and after ligation. As it can be seen, ligation served to widen this zone. In six experiments, the zone was present in the Z lead, while in the remaining three it was found in the X lead. The presence of significant ST changes, defined as 0.2-mV J point elevation on the surface ECG leads during ligation is summarized in Table I. Five out of six experiments with reduced amplitude zones in lead Z also had ST changes after 2 minutes of ligation in lead Z. Two out of three experiments that showed reduced amplitude zones in lead X had ST changes in this lead.

High Frequency Electrocardiography in Patients Undergoing Percutaneous Transluminal Coronary Angioplasty

A study was designed to test the ability of computer-assisted analysis of standard as well as high-frequency ECGs to detect effects of transient ischemia in patients undergoing percutaneous transluminal coronary angioplasty (PTCA). Patients with disabling angina undergoing PTCA of a critical stenosis in the LAD were selected as subjects for the study after giving written informed consent. Patients underwent PTCA by a femoral approach according to previously described standard techniques.

Recording Protocol

In each patient surface electrocardiographic leads I, aVL, and V_5 were continuously monitored and recorded during PTCA by means of a photographic multichannel oscillographic recorder. Bandpass filters of the ECG amplifiers were set at 0.01 to 100 Hz for leads I and aVL. V_5 was recorded as a high fidelity signal with the use of bandpass filters between 0.01 to 500 Hz. In addition to three surface electrocardiographic leads, a local unipolar intracoronary ECG from myocardium distal to the LAD stenosis being dilated was

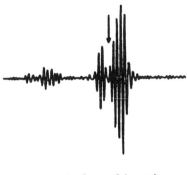

Before ligation

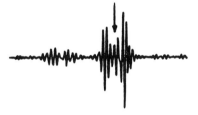

During Occlusion

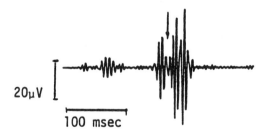

20μV

100 msec

After reperfusion

Figure 8. High-frequency ECG waveforms obtained from a dog that shows RAZ before ligation and during occlusion. Ligation served to widen the RAZ.

also continuously monitored and recorded.[21] The intracoronary unipolar ECG was obtained by positioning a standard PTCA guidewire and balloon catheter across the target stenosis and connecting the proximal end of the guidewire as it exited from the balloon catheter to a precordial lead of a standard surface electrocardiographic cable by means of a sterile double alligator connector. With the use of Wilson's Central Terminal for the indifferent electrode, the intracoronary ECG was filtered between 0.01 and 500 Hz and recorded simultaneously with the three surface electrocardiographic leads being monitored. In addition to real-time paper recordings, the surface and intracoronary ECGs were also stored on tape for later playback and analysis.

Before advancement of the guidewire and balloon catheter across the target LAD stenosis, the three surface electrocardiographic leads were recorded for a control period of 2 minutes. These leads and the intracoronary ECG were then recorded continuously immediately after the guidewire and balloon catheter had been positioned across the stenosis and during all subsequent balloon inflations and deflations. Throughout the procedure all patients were questioned repeatedly about the presence or absence of chest pain; these responses were recorded along with the surface and intracoronary ECGs. Ten minutes after completion of the dilatation and withdrawal of the guidewire and balloon catheter from the LAD, another recording of the surface electrocardiographic leads was obtained for 10 minutes.

Data Analysis

The digitized data from surface lead V_5 were divided into three time segments. The first segment consisted of records obtained during the initial control recording period before advancement of the guidewire or balloon catheter across the target stenosis. The second and third time segments were, respectively, records obtained during the last 30 seconds of initial balloon inflation and during the 10-minute recording period at the conclusion of the procedure. Electrocardiographic waveforms in each time segment were averaged together with the use of cross correlation scheme. Averaged original waveforms from each time segment were then bandpass filtered between 150 and 250 Hz and were used to compute the root mean square (RMS) voltage of the filtered QRS complex as well as the envelope of the filtered QRS complex.

Beat-to-Beat Variability of the ECG

A typical pattern of response of the surface and intracoronary ECGs to balloon inflation in the LAD, recorded during PTCA is illustrated in Figure 9. After advancement of the balloon catheter and guidewire across the stenosis but before balloon inflation only nonspecific ST segment and T wave abnormalities are apparent from visual inspection of the surface ECG (first two complexes, Figure

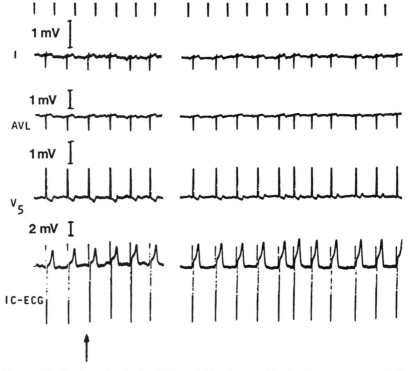

Figure 9. Surface leads I, aVL, and V₅ along with the intracoronary ECG (IC-ECG) during PTCA of an LAD. (A) Arrow denotes balloon inflation, which is followed by marked ST segment elevation in the IC-ECG with little change in the surface leads. (B) Records obtained after 30 seconds of balloon inflation.

analysis of the ST segment and T waves in lead V_5 of the individual depicted in Figure 9 in whom visual inspection of the surface ECG failed to reveal any ST segment or T wave abnormalities during balloon inflation, even though transient marked ST segment elevation developed on the intracoronary ECG. The morphology of each ST segment or T wave after balloon inflation is compared by cross correlation with the morphology of the ST segment and T wave of a single reference template waveform recorded before balloon inflation. As shown in Figure 10, 35 beats after balloon inflation the cross correlation coefficient fell from an initial value of 0.93 to a nadir of 0.83, indicating the appearance of a change in the ST segment and T wave morphology as compared with baseline. The cross correlation coefficient then returned to its control value within 20 beats after balloon deflation.

An example of computer-assisted cross correlation analysis of the ST segments and T waves of standard surface lead V_5 together with the high-frequency (150 to 250 Hz) nonaveraged QRS complex from surface lead V_5 during PTCA is illustrated in Figure 11. In the top panel of Figure 11, a change in morphology of the ST segment and T waves of standard surface lead V_5 becomes apparent 50 beats after balloon inflation, manifested by a precipitous decline in the cross correlation from its initial value of 0.99 to a nadir of 0.91. The cross correlation coefficient for the ST segments and T waves then returns to its control value within 20 beats after balloon deflation (Figure 11, top). Cross correlation analysis of the nonaveraged high-frequency QRS complex during PTCA in the same patient is shown in Figure 11, bottom. Nonaveraged high-frequency QRS complexes are characterized by low signal-to-noise ratios. Because of this problem, note that the initial cross correlation coefficient of complexes recorded before balloon inflation derived by comparison with a reference pre-PTCA complex is lower than the coefficient derived during analysis of ST segments and T waves of the standard surface ECG (0.74 before balloon inflation, Figure 10, bottom, vs. 0.99 before balloon inflation, Figure 11, top). Within several beats after balloon inflation cross correlation analysis of the high-frequency QRS complex reveals a prompt decline in the correlation coefficient to a nadir of 0.38, indicative of a morphologic change in this waveform in response to balloon inflation (Figure 11, bottom). After balloon deflation, the correlation coefficient returns to its control value within 20 beats (Figure 11, bottom). Thus, in spite of a lower initial cross correlation coefficient, beat-to-beat analysis of the high-frequency

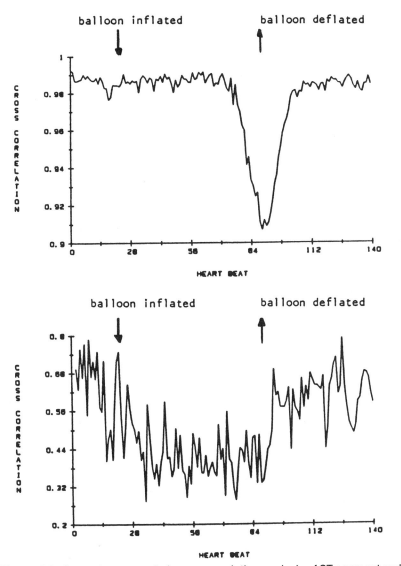

Figure 11. Computer-generated cross correlation analysis of ST segment and T wave morphology of the standard surface ECG (top) and of the nonaveraged high-frequency QRS complexes in lead V_5 (bottom) during PTCA. Balloon inflation was followed by a fall in the cross correlation coefficient for the ST segments and T waves after 50 beats (top). Cross correlation coefficient for the high-frequency nonaveraged QRS complexes fell more quickly after inflation (bottom). Note prompt return of cross correlation coefficients for both variables after balloon deflation.

QRS complex reveals a change in morphology more quickly than similar analysis of the ST segment and T waves of the standard surface ECG.

RMS Determination

The RMS value of the averaged high-frequency QRS complex is defined as:

$$\left[\frac{1}{n} \sum_{j=1}^{n} f^2(t_j) \right]^{1/2}$$

where $t_j = j^{th}$ sample point; $f(t_j)$ = electrocardiographic amplitude at the jth sample point. RMS values are computed from the averaged high-frequency QRS complex in each time segment, and a computer algorithm is used to define the time of onset and termination of the QRS complex. The computer accomplishes this by measuring RMS noise level in the TP segment and then searching between the PR interval and the ST segment for a signal with RMS amplitude greater than three times the RMS of the noise.

Signal-Averaged High-Frequency QRS Analysis

During the course of PTCA, striking changes are noted in the signal-averaged high-frequency QRS and in the calculated envelopes of these waveforms. A typical example of such changes is illustrated in Figure 12. During the control recording period in this patient, the calculated RMS value for signal-averaged high-frequency QRS was 3.97 μV and analysis of the envelope of the signal revealed the presence of a zone of reduced amplitude (Figure 12, left). The middle panel shows records obtained during the second time segment, after 30 seconds of balloon inflation in the LAD. Balloon inflation is associated with a reduction in the voltage of the high-frequency QRS (RMS = 2.26 μV, Figure 12, middle) and broadening of the zone of reduced amplitude in the envelope of the signal (Figure 12, middle). Records obtained during the third time segment, after balloon deflation and withdrawal of the balloon catheter from the LAD, are shown in Figure 12, right. At this stage of the procedure the RMS value of the high-frequency QRS had increased to 5.13

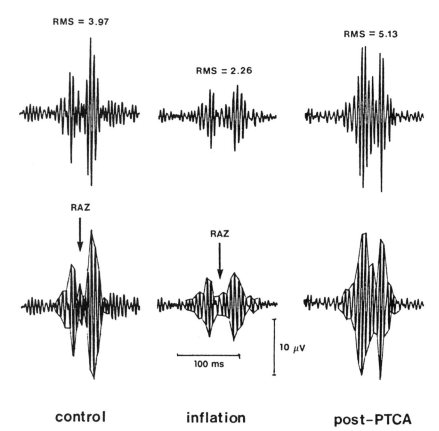

Figure 12. Signal-averaged high-frequency QRS (top) and envelope of the averaged high-frequency QRS (bottom) recorded during three different stages of angioplasty. RMS = root mean square voltage (μV) of the signal; RAZ = reduced amplitude zone. Balloon inflation is associated with a reduction in the voltage of the high-frequency QRS and broadening of the zone of reduced amplitude in the envelope of the signal which is also present during the control stage.

μV and the zone of the reduced amplitude in the envelope of the signal is less obvious (Figure 12, right). A slightly different sequence of events is observed during PTCA in another subject and is illustrated in Figure 13. Before PTCA, the envelope of the signal-averaged high-frequency QRS in this patient does not disclose a zone of reduced amplitude (Figure 13, left, lower panel). Balloon inflation is associated with a decline in the RMS value of the signal (3.54 μV to

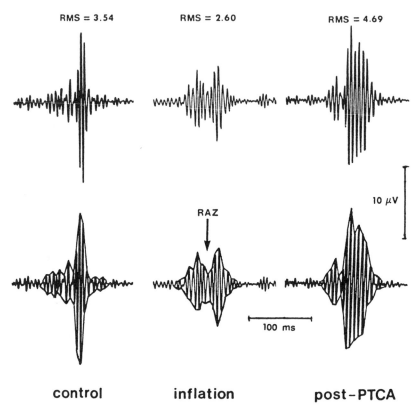

Figure 13. Signal-averaged high-frequency QRS (top) and envelope of the averaged high-frequency QRS (bottom) recorded during three different stages of angioplasty. RMS = root mean square voltage (µV) of the signal; RAZ = reduced amplitude zone. Balloon inflation is associated with a reduction in the voltage of the high-frequency QRS and broadening of the zone of reduced amplitude in the envelope of the signal which is not present during the control and the post-PTCA stages.

2.60 µV, Figure 13, left and middle, top traces) and the appearance of a new zone of reduced amplitude (Figure 13, middle, top trace). At the conclusion of PTCA, the zone of reduced amplitude disappears and the RMS returns to a value of 4.69 µV (Figure 13, right).

Results

Eleven patients with disabling angina undergoing PTCA of a critical stenosis in the LAD were selected as subjects for the study after giving written informed consent. All patients underwent PTCA by a femoral approach. The clinical characteristics of the patients studied are summarized in Table II. All patients were men with ages ranging between 42 and 71 years. The mean age for the group was 54 years. Seven patients had significant stenosis only of the LAD, whereas four patients had disease involving the circumflex or right coronary arteries as well as the LAD. In this latter group, the LAD stenosis was the most critical lesion and was the first lesion targeted for PTCA. Baseline 12-lead ECGs before PTCA were interpreted as within normal limits in four patients. Q waves suggestive of infarction were present in only one individual, although prior infarction had been documented by typical enzyme elevation in two patients. The remaining patients had nonspecific ST segment or T wave abnormalities on the resting ECG. Among the 11 patients studied, 10 individuals (90%) developed transient marked ST segment and T wave abnormalities that were obvious by visual inspection of the intracoronary ECG during balloon inflation (Table III). In contrast, visually apparent ST segment and T wave abnormalities in one or more of the surface leads during balloon inflation were found in only six patients (54%). When the intracoronary and surface ECG developed ST segment abnormalities during balloon inflation, the changes appeared earlier and were always of greater magnitude on the intracoronary ECG. Only a single patient was encountered in whom the intracoronary ECG remain unchanged during balloon inflation, even though ST segment elevation on the surface ECG appeared, accompanied by angina (Table III). In all 11 subjects visual analysis of QRS complexes in the surface leads failed to disclose any transient changes in response to balloon inflation or deflation.

The results of cross correlation analysis of the ST segment and T waves on the surface ECG for each of the 11 patients studied are listed in Table III. Nine of the 11 patients (82%) demonstrated ST segment and T wave abnormalities during PTCA by cross correlation analysis, whereas only six individuals (54%) developed transient ST segment and T wave abnormalities that were apparent by visual inspection of the surface ECG alone (Table III). No individuals were encountered in whom cross correlation analysis failed to detect transient abnormalities that were apparent by visual inspection.

The results of analysis of the signal-averaged high-frequency QRS in each of the 11 patients studied are listed in Table IV. In six individuals (patients 1, 2, 5, 7, 8, and 11, Table IV), zones of reduced

Table II
Clinical Profile of Patients Undergoing PTCA

Subject No.	Age (Yr)	Sex	Coronary Stenoses	Baseline ECG	Prior MI	Angina During PTCA
1	53	M	LAD	WNL	−	+
2	43	M	LAD	WNL	−	+
3	60	M	LAD	WNL	−	+
4	49	M	LAD	ST-TW-A	−	+
5	71	M	LAD,LCX	Q waves V_1-V_2	+	+
6	62	M	LAD,RCA	ST-TW-A	−	+
7	55	M	LAD,RCA	ST-TW-A	−	+
8	55	M	LAD	ST-TW-A	−	+
9	42	M	LAD,RCA	LVH,ST-TW-A	−	+
10	41	M	LAD	WNL	−	+
11	66	M	LAD	ST-TW-A	+	+

LCX = left circumflex artery; RCA = right coronary artery; WNL = within normal limits; ST-TW-A = nonspecific ST segment and T wave abnormalities; LVH = left ventricular hypertrophy; MI = myocardial infarction.

Table III
Intracoronary and Surface Electrocardiographic Changes During PTCA

Subject No.	ST-T Changes in IC-ECG	ST-T Changes in S-ECG by Visual Inspection	ST Changes in S-ECG by Cross Correlation
1	+	+	+
2	+		
3	+	+	+
4		+	+
5	+		+
6	+		
7	+		+
8	+	+	+
9	+		+
10	+	+	+
11	+	+	+

IC-ECG = intracoronary ECG; S-ECG = surface ECG; ST-T = ST segment and T wave.

Table IV
Signal-Averaged High-Frequency QRS Analysis During PTCA

Subject No.	Presence of RAZ			RMS (µV) QRS Complex		
	Before	During	After	Before	During	After
1	+	+	+	3.23	1.79	3.50
2	+	+	+	2.95	2.61	2.89
3	+	+		2.00	1.43	3.11
4				1.90	1.77	1.76
5	+	+	+	2.40	1.20	2.69
6		+		2.81	2.25	3.00
7	+	+	+	3.78	1.66	3.59
8	+	+	+	3.49	2.88	4.57
9	+	+		5.94	5.02	6.75
10		+		3.54	2.60	4.69
11	+	+	+	3.97	2.26	5.13

RAZ = reduced amplitude zone.

amplitude were present before PTCA, after 30 seconds of balloon inflation, and also at the conclusion of the procedure. In two individuals (patients 3 and 9, Table IV) zones of reduced amplitude that were present intially were no longer apparent after PTCA. Two subjects (patients 6 and 10, Table IV) developed a reduced amplitude zone only during balloon inflation and one patient (patient 4) had no evidence of such a zone at any time. In all 11 patients studied, balloon inflation was uniformly associated with a decrease in voltage of the high-frequency QRS, followed by a subsequent increase in voltage after conclusion of PTCA in all but one individual (Table IV). It is of interest to note that the single patient studied who had evidence of left ventricular hypertrophy on the standard surface ECG also had the largest calculated RMS value of the high-frequency QRS (patient 9, Tables II and IV). For the entire group, the mean value for RMS was $3.27 + 1.12$ µV before PTCA as compared with $2.31 + 1.04$ µV during balloon inflation ($p < 0.05$). The mean value for RMS after conclusion of PTCA was $3.79 + 1.30$ µV, a difference compared with the pre-PTCA value that was not significant, but that was significantly higher than the mean value during balloon inflation ($p < 0.01$).

High-Frequency Electrocardiography in Patients With Coronary Artery Disease and Normal Conventional Electrocardiogram

Conventional surface ECGs during angina-free intervals are often normal and do not accurately identify patients with coronary artery disease. Using high-frequency electrocardiography, we have attempted to determine whether it would be of value in the detection of coronary artery disease in patients with a normal, conventional ECG.

Recording Technique

Three unipolar precordial leads are positioned at the routine V_3, V_4, and V_5 locations. The ECG leads are recorded simultaneously by a common ECG recorder (bandpass of 0.3 to 500 Hz) and with a Hewlett Packard 3964A tape recorder (passband DC to 2500 Hz). The recorded analog data are digitized by a 10-bit analog-to-digital converter with a sampling rate of 1280 Hz onto a digital magnetic tape. The processing of the digitized data takes place off-line with a CDC 6600 computer.

Data Analysis

Four hundred ECG waveforms are averaged each time in order to reduce the random noise. Averaged waveforms, which are obtained in normal sinus rhythm from all patients at rest, are bandpass filtered between 150 and 250 Hz.

Three parameters are computed: (A) the RMS value over the high-frequency QRS complex; (B) the envelope of the filtered QRS complex; and (C) the RMS value over the envelope.

Signal-Averaged High-Frequency QRS Analysis

Examples of the averaged waveforms from a healthy subject and from a patient with coronary artery disease are illustrated in Figures 14 and 15, respectively. The upper traces of Figures 14A and 15A

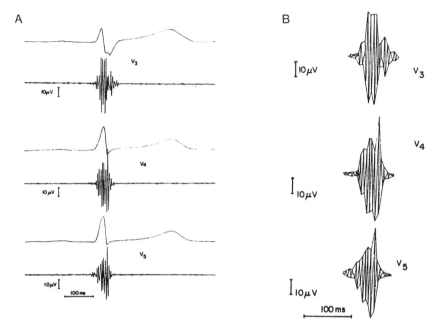

Figure 14. An example of the computer output tracing, which was obtained from ECG recording in leads V_3, V_4, and V_5 from a normal subject (group A). (A) The upper traces of the three leads are the averaged unfiltered ECG waveform. The lower traces are the same ECGs passed through a nonrecursive digital filter (150–250 Hz). (B) The envelopes over the high-frequency QRS complexes. No reduced amplitude zone is noted in the normal subject.

from leads V_3, V_4, and V_5 are the unfiltered, averaged waveforms, and the lower traces are the filtered waveforms (150–250 Hz). The high-frequency QRS complexes and their envelopes in ECG leads V_3, V_4, and V_5, obtained from the normal subject and from a patient with coronary artery disease are shown in Figures 14B and 15B, respectively. Zones of reduced amplitude, indicated by arrows, are present in leads V_4 and V_5 in the coronary artery disease patient (Figure 14B) but not in the healthy subject (Figure 15B).

Results

The study group included 45 subjects with normal resting 12-lead ECG who were divided into three groups. Group A (Table V)

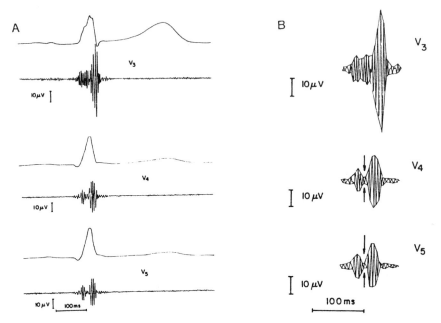

Figure 15. Similar recordings as in Figure 14 from a patient with coronary artery disease (group C). Reduced amplitude zones (panel B, arrows) are found in leads V_4 and V_5.

consisted of ten asymptomatic healthy subjects under the age of 30 (24 ±5 years; mean ±SD) with normal cardiovascular examination, who did not undergo coronary arteriography. Group B (Table VI) consisted of 15 consecutive patients (age: 52 ±9 years) with chest pain and angiographically normal coronary arteries. Group C (Table VII) consisted of 20 consecutive patients (age: 56 ±9 years) with chest pain and pathologic coronary arteries. No patients in this study had intraventricular conduction disturbances.

Table VIII summarizes the results obtained from the RMS values of the high-frequency QRS complex and over the envelope from subjects without (groups A and B) or with coronary artery disease (group C). There was no significant difference in the RMS values derived from subjects with and without coronary artery disease.

The frequency of reduced amplitude zones on the envelope of the high-frequency QRS complex of the subjects from groups A, B, and C are present in Tables V, VI, and VII, respectively. Table IX summarizes the number of patients who demonstrated a reduced amplitude

Table V
Results from High-Frequency Electrocardiograms

GROUP A

Patient No.	Sex/Age	RAZ ECG Lead		
		V_3	V_4	V_5
1	M/30	0	+	0
2	M/28	+	0	0
3	M/18	0	0	0
4	M/18	0	0	0
5	M/28	0	0	0
6	F/26	+	0	0
7	M/28	+	0	0
8	M/24	0	0	+
9	M/18	0	0	0
10	M/18	0	0	+

M = male; F = female; RAZ = reduced amplitude zone; ECG = electrocardiogram; + = presence of reduced amplitude zone; 0 = absence of reduced amplitude zone.

zone in one, two, and three ECG leads. When comparing the patients of group C with those of groups A and B, it appears that reduced amplitude of the QRS envelope in two ECG leads was the best criteria for coronary artery disease (Table IX). Reduced amplitude zones in two ECG leads were found in none of ten subjects of group A, in 3 of 15 patients (20%) of group B, and 15 of 20 patients (75%) of group C. The difference between the frequencies of reduced amplitude zones in subjects with and without coronary artery disease was highly significant (p <0.00003).

There was no significant difference between the mean left ventricular ejection fraction in the patients with and without reduced amplitude zone in the QRS envelope (66 ±11% vs 68 ±9%, respectively; Tables VI and VII). The presence of left ventricular wall abnormality was significantly greater in patients with than without reduced amplitude zone in the QRS envelope ($\frac{10}{18}$ = 55% vs $\frac{3}{7}$ = 18%, respectively; p <0.003; Tables VI and VII).

The mean QRS complex duration was not significantly different

Table VI
Results from High-Frequency Electrocardiograms

GROUP B

Patient No.	Sex/Age	LVEF (%)	LVW Abn	RAZ ECG Lead V₃	V₄	V₅
1	M/53	72	Normal	0	0	0
2	M/47	74	Normal	0	+	0
3	M/54	66	Normal	0	+	0
4	F/69	63	Normal	0	+	0
5	M/37	74	Normal	0	0	0
6	M/58	71	Normal	0	0	0
7	M/53	73	Normal	+	+	+
8	F/51	73	Normal	0	0	0
9	M/49	58	Normal	0	0	0
10	M/44	55	Normal	0	0	+
11	F/59	68	Normal	0	0	+
12	M/38	65	Ap Hypo	0	+	+
13	M/59	82	Normal	0	0	0
14	M/53	84	Normal	+	+	+
15	M/61	85	Normal	0	0	0

M = male; F = female; LVEF = left ventricular ejection fraction; LVW Abn = left ventricular wall abnormality; Ap Hypo = apical hypokinesia; RAZ = reduced amplitude zone.

in the three groups of subjects studied (86 ±3, 88 ±5 msec in group A + B and C, respectively).

Discussion

Early investigators[1-9] analyzed the notches and slurs in the QRS complex and investigated the possibility of utilizing these features in developing screening procedures for identifying the population with coronary artery disease. These investigators showed that the information contained in the notches and slurs was a valuable indication of different pathologic states of the heart, including transmural infarction, cardiomyopathies, and ventricular hypertro-

Table VII
Results from High-Frequency Electrocardiograms

Group C

Patient No.	Sex/Age	Percent Occlusion of Coronary Artery LAD	LCX	RCA	LVEF (%)	LVW Abn	RAZ ECG Lead V_3	V_4	V_5
1	M/63	75	25	100	59	Normal	0	+	+
2	M/58	90	100	100	41	Inf post Hypo	0	+	+
3	M/64	90	75	75	77	Mild Inf Hypo	+	+	+
4	M/48	90	50	–	60	Normal	0	0	0
5	M/58	100	100	75	67	Mild Inf Hypo	0	+	+
6	F/62	100	75	–	74	Ap Hypo	0	0	+
7	M/56	75	–	–	64	Normal	+	+	0
8	M/37	100	–	–	69	Ant Ap Hypo	+	+	+
9	M/47	75	75	–	65	Mild Ap Hypo	0	0	0
10	M/54	90	60	–	73	Normal	0	+	+
11	M/65	90	75	75	50	Inf bas Akin	0	+	0
12	M/41	75	75	–	71	Normal	+	+	+
13	M/63	25	100	100	46	Inf Hypo	+	+	+
14	M/56	–	–	100	55	Ap Hypo	+	+	+
15	M/60	100	50	100	63	Inf Hypo	+	+	+
16	F/64	100	–	50	78	Normal	0	+	+
17	M/68	50	–	–	71	Ap Hypo	+	+	+
18	M/63	25	90	50	68	Normal	0	0	0
19	M/46	100	90	100	68	Normal	+	+	0
20	M/56	–	90	100	58	Bas Akin	+	+	+

LAD = left anterior descending coronary artery; LCX = left circumflex artery; RCA = right coronary artery; Inf post = inferoposterior; Hypo = hypokinesia; Inf = inferior; Ap = apical; Ant ap = anteroapical; Inf bas = inferobasal; Akin = akinesia; Bas = basal; other abbreviations as in Figure 2.

Table VIII

Summarized Data of Root Mean Square Values

Group	Patients	RMS (μV) QRS Complex Mean ±SD ECG Lead			RMS (μV) Envelope Mean ±SD ECG Lead		
		V_3	V_4	V_5	V_3	V_4	V_5
A + B	25	6.95 ±3.22	6.04 ±3.74	4.78 ±2.72	8.92 ±4.15	7.85 ±4.81	6.35 ±3.69
C	20	6.65 ±2.76	6.23 ±2.25	4.98 ±2.21	8.47 ±3.37	8.14 ±2.86	6.57 ±2.92

RMS = root mean square value.

Table IX
Number of Subjects Showing Reduced Amplitude Zone in 1, 2, or 3
Electrocardiographic Leads

Group	RAZ in 1 Lead			RAZ in 2 Leads			RAZ in 3 Leads		
	n	%	P	n	%	P	n	%	P
A(10)	6	60	NS	0	0	<0.0002	0	0	<0.025
B(15)	8	53.3	<0.05	3	20	<0.0025	2	13.3	NS
A+B(25)	14	56	<0.04	3	12	<0.00003	2	8	<0.015
C(20)	17	85	–	15	75	–	8	40	–

n = number of subjects; P = compared with results in group C patients; RAZ = reduced amplitude zone.

phy. Goldberger et al[22,23] used signal averaging and filtering in the frequency range between 80 to 300 Hz to examine the effect of myocardial infarction on the high-frequency QRS potentials. They found that the high-frequency (80–300 Hz) RMS values were significantly greater in normal subjects than in patients with myocardial infarction.

Here we have focused on energies of higher frequency (150–250 Hz) contained with the ECG. Because these higher frequency ECGs are generally smaller in amplitude than the conventional ECG (microvolts vs millivolts), signal averaging techniques have been used to improve the signal-to-noise ratios. In this manner, the high-frequency ECG has been used to derive information on relatively localized events in the heart, such as myocardial ischemia, from the body surface. The signal averaging of the high-frequency (150–250 Hz) QRS, using a computerized cross correlation method,[17] was performed in dogs during occlusion of the LAD coronary artery; in patients undergoing PTCA, and in patients with coronary artery disease and normal conventional ECG. As described previously,[15–17] this method ensures accurate waveform alignments during the averaging process, and has been used successfully to record His bundle activity[18,19] and late potentials[20] within the ST segment from the body surface.

The effect of myocardial infarction on high-frequency QRS potentials has been studied previously.[22,23] Although prior infarction increases the number of notches and slurs in the QRS, presumably due to fragmentation of the depolarization wave front in scarred tissue, the overall voltage of the high-frequency components in the QRS is actually reduced by infarction.[22,23] This apparently paradoxical result might reflect on the fact that the notches and the slurs examined visually in earlier studies had most of their spectral contents below the high frequencies (150–250 Hz) and spectral analysis of ECG waveforms carried out by us[12–24] confirms this hypothesis. The attenuation of the high-frequency QRS voltage after infarction has been attributed to a decrease in overall electromotive force as well as slowing of conduction in and around the region of infarction.[22] Here we examine the effect of transient ischemia rather than infarction on high-frequency QRS. Using balloon inflation in the LAD in dogs experiments and in patients undergoing PTCA as models, we found that transient ischemia uniformly resulted in attenuation of the high-frequency component in the QRS, manifested by the appearance of reduced amplitude zone and by a decrease in the RMS value. An interesting finding is the presence of zones of reduced amplitude in the high-frequency QRS. Unlike late low-amplitude potentials in the terminal portion of the QRS or early part of the ST segment, which have been described in patients with prior infarction and which have been related to the occurrence of ventricular arrhythmias,[25,26] the reduced amplitude zones observed are generally located in the midportion of the high-frequency QRS. We observed areas of reduced amplitude in nine out of ten dogs with ischemia produced by experimental coronary occlusion. Additionally, these zones were usually found in the surface leads which eventually developed significant ischemic ST changes. These findings suggest an association between a reduced amplitude zone and ischemia. We also observed reduced amplitude zones in patients undergoing PTCA. Many of the patients who had reduced amplitude zones before PTCA developed widening of the zone during balloon inflation. These zones then became narrower after PTCA was completed and, in two individuals, actually disappeared altogether. In two other patients a zone of reduced amplitude was present only during balloon inflation. It is conceivable that reduced amplitude zones in some patients may reflect localized regions of ischemic-induced slow conduction. If this is the case, one would expect these zones to become more evident during interruption of coronary blood flow and to diminish or disappear after relief of obstruction to flow. On the other hand, it should be noted that many of the patients still had zones of reduced amplitude at the conclusion of an apparently successful PTCA procedure. Thus, in some patients, persistence of reduced amplitude zones after PTCA may reflect the presence of nonrevascularized viable myocardium in the distribution of other nondilated diseased vessels or, alternatively, regions of prior infarction rather than ischemia. We also recorded high-frequency (150–250 Hz) QRS complexes in patients with coronary artery disease (>50% coronary artery stenosis) and compared them to those recorded in patients with chest pain but without coronary disease, and in healthy normal subjects. We found that the shape of the high-frequency QRS envelope is a good indicator for the presence of coronary disease in patients with normal conventional ECG, since a reduced amplitude zone in at least two of the ECG leads, V_3, V_4, and V_5, was present in 15 of 20 (75%) patients with coronary artery disease but in only 3 of 25 (12%) subjects without coronary artery disease. The fact that the presence of left ventricular wall abnormality was significantly greater in patients with than without reduced amplitude zones in the QRS complex suggests that these zones may reflect small regions of prior infarction rather than ischemia. Spectral analysis of the high-frequency QRS complexes shows that the power spectrum can also be used to identify the morphologic changes present during transient ischemia.

During PTCA, we found that transient ischemia uniformly resulted in attenuation of the high-frequency component in the QRS, manifested by a decrease in calculated RMS values. When coronary blood flow was reestablished after balloon deflation, RMS values for high-frequency QRS complexes returned to their preischemic levels. Acute ischemia in myocardial cells leads to a decline in maximum diastolic potential and in the maximum upstroke velocity of phase 0 of the action potential, accompanied by slowing of conduction velocity.[27] Since reduction of conduction velocity in ventricular myocardium would be expected to shift high-frequency activity in the QRS to lower frequencies, slow conduction in the anterior wall may explain the transient decreases in RMS values that were observed during balloon inflation. On the other hand, in patients with coronary disease and with normal conventional ECG but without transient ischemia, the RMS values over the high-frequency QRS complex did not differ significantly from those recorded in subjects without coronary disease.

Beat-to-beat analysis of the ECG waveforms during balloon inflation in dog experiments and during PTCA confirms the clinical observation that the standard surface ECG is not always reliable in the diagnosis of myocardial ischemia. Visual inspection of the surface ECG revealed ST segment and T wave abnormalities suggestive of ischemia in only 54% of the patients undergoing PTCA of the LAD, even though every patient complained of angina during balloon inflation, and 90% of the patients had evidence of ischemia on the intracoronary ECG. As suggested in previous studies,[28,29] insensitivity of the surface ECG for detecting transient myocardial ischemia stems in part from the fact that the recorded magnitude of potentials generated by the heart falls precipitously with increasing distance between the recording electrode and the heart; leads on the body surface may simply be too distant to develop visually obvious changes due to ischemia in a localized area of myocardium. Computer-assisted cross correlation analysis of the surface ECG in dog experiments and in patients with transient ischemia during PTCA revealed beat-to-beat changes in the nonaveraged high-frequency QRS, and in the ST segment and T wave morphology in response to balloon inflation that were not apparent from visual inspection alone. Beat-to-beat analysis of the high-frequency QRS complex revealed a change in morphology more quickly than similar analysis of the ST segment and T wave. This morphologic change as reduced amplitude zones was seen early in ischemia and was not accompanied by significant changes in the QRS complex or ST segment of the conventional surface ECG. Cross correlation analysis of beat-to-beat ST segments, T waves, and high-frequency QRS complexes appears to be a noninvasive means of detecting transient abnormalities of the ECG with greater sensitivity than by simple visual inspection alone. Cross correlation analysis in patients with intermittent chest pain due to causes other than ischemia has not yet been done. However, noncardiac causes of chest pain may not cause the same changes in waveform morphology as they were encountered during myocardial ischemia. If such proves to be the case, computer-assisted electrocardiographic analysis may prove useful as a noninvasive diagnostic method in patients with chest pain of uncertain cause.

The origin and significance of the reduced amplitude zones is unknown at present. The conventional "low-frequency" ECG reflects primarily the global pattern of depolarization and repolarization in the heart. The high-frequency (150–250 Hz) signal may represent the degree of fragmentation of the depolarization wave front as it passes through tissue close to the recording electrode. This high-frequency activity is of smaller amplitude than the low-frequency ECG (microvolts vs millivolts) and may present a more local measurement. It also was found that this high-frequency signal left after filtering is the result of a subtle low amplitude constituent of the electrocardiographic signal, and a reduced amplitude zone is a result of changes in these components of the original signal.[10]

Further study is required to determined the true predictive value of the high-frequency ECG for the diagnosis of ischemia in humans. However, there is a potential clinical relevance in our findings: the high-frequency ECG may prove useful in diagnosing the effect of reperfusion therapy of acute myocardial infarction using thrombolytic agents or PTCA procedure, and it also may be used as a new noninvasive mean for detecting ischemic heart disease by studying the morphologic changes in the high-frequency QRS complex during exercise testing. These hypotheses require additional study.

References

1. Langner PH Jr, Geselowits DB, Mansure FT: High frequency components in the electrocardiograms of normal subjects and of patients with coronary heart disease. Am Heart J 62:746, 1961.
2. Langner PH Jr, Lauer JA: The relative significance of high-frequency and low-frequency notching in the electrocardiogram. Am Heart J 31:34, 1966.
3. Langner PH Jr, DeMott T, Hussey M: High-fidelity electrocardiography: effects of induced local myocardial injury in the dog. Am Heart J 71:790, 1966.
4. Reynolds EW, Muller BF, Anderson GJ, Muller BT: High-frequency components in the electrocardiogram: a comparative study of normals and patients with myocardial disease. Circulation 35:195, 1967.
5. Flowers NC, Horan LG, Thomas JR, Tolleson WJ: The anatomic basis for high frequency components in the electrocardiogram. Circulation 39:531, 1969.
6. Flowers NC, Horan LG, Tolleson WJ, Thomas JR: Localization of the site of myocardial scarring in man by high-frequency components. Circulation 40:927, 1969.
7. Flowers NC, Horan LG: Diagnostic import of QRS notching in high frequency electrocardiogram of living subjects with heart disease. Circulation 44:605, 1971.
8. Anderson GJ, Blieden MF: The high frequency electrocardiogram in coronary artery disease. Am Heart J 89:349, 1975.
9. Sapoznikov D. Tzivoni D, Weinman J, Penchas S, Gotsman MS: High frequency ECG in the diagnosis of occult coronary artery disease: a study

of patients with normal conventional ECG. J Electrocardiol 10:137, 1977.

10. Abboud S: Subtle alterations in the high frequency QRS potentials during myocardial ischemia in dogs. Comp Biomed Res 20:384, 1987.

11. Abboud S, Smith JM, Shargorodsky B, Laniado S, Sadeh D, Cohen RJ: High frequency electrocardiography of three orthogonal leads in dogs during a coronary artery occlusion. PACE 12:574, 1988.

12. Mor-Avi V, Shargorodsky B, Abboud S, Laniado S, Akselrod S: Effects of coronary occlusion on high frequency content of epicardial electrogram and body-surface ECG. Circulation 76:237, 1987.

13. Abboud S, Cohen RJ, Selwyn A, Ganz P, Sadeh D, Friedman PL: Detection of transient myocardial ischemia by computer analysis of standard and signal-averaged high-frequency electrocardiograms in patients undergoing percutaneous transluminal coronary angioplasty. Circulation 76:585, 1987.

14. Abboud S, Belhassen B, Miller HI, Sadeh D, Laniado S: High frequency electrocardiography using an advanced method of signal averaging for non invasive detection of coronary artery disease in patients with normal conventional electrocardiogram. J Electrocardiol 19:371, 1986.

15. Abboud S, Sadeh D: The waveform's alignment procedure in the external recording of the His bundle activity. Comp Biomed Res 15:212, 1982.

16. Abboud S, Sadeh D: The digital filtering process in the external recording of the His bundle activity. Comp Biomed Res 15:418, 1982.

17. Abboud S, Sadeh D: The use of cross-correlation function for the alignment of ECG waveforms and rejection of extrasystoles. Comp Biomed Res 17:258, 1984.

18. Abboud S, Belhassen B, Pelleg A, Laniado S, Sadeh D: An advanced noninvasive technique for the recording of His bundle potential in man. J Electrocardiol 16:397, 1983.

19. Abboud S, Belhassen B, Pelleg A, Laniado S, Sadeh D: Noninvasive recording of His bundle activity in patients with Wolff-Parkinson-White syndrome. PACE 7:40, 1984.

20. Abboud S, Belhassen B, Laniado S, Sadeh D: Non-invasive recording of late ventricular activity using an advanced method in patients with a damaged mass of ventricular tissue. J Electrocardiol 16:245, 1983.

21. Friedman PL, Shook TL, Kirshenbaum JM, Selwyn AP, Ganz P: Value of the intracoronary electrocardiogram to monitor myocardial ischemia during percutaneous transluminal coronary angioplasty. Circulation 74:330, 1986.

22. Goldberger AL, Bhargava V, Froelicher V, Covell J: Effect of myocardial infarction on high frequency ECG potentials. Circulation 64:34, 1981.

23. Goldberger AL, Bhargava V, Froelicher V, Covell J, Mortara D: Diminished peak to peak amplitude of the high frequency QRS in myocardial infarction. J Electrocardiol 31:367, 1980.

24. Mor-Avi V, Abboud S, Akselrod S: Frequency content of the QRS notching in high-fidelity canine ECG. Comput Biomed Res 22:18, 1989.

25. Berbari EJ, Scherlag BJ, Hope RR, Lazzara R: Recording from the body surface of arrhythmogenic ventricular activity during the ST segment. Am J Cardiol 41:697, 1978.

26. Simson MB, Untereker WJ, Spielman SR, Horowitz LN, Marcus NH, Falcone RA, Harken AH, Josephson ME: Relation between late potentials on the body surface and directly recorded fragmented electrograms in patients with ventricular tachycardia. Am J Cardiol 51:105, 1983.
27. Samson WE, Sher AM: Mechanism of ST segment alteration during acute myocardial injury. Circ Res 8:780, 1960.
28. Spach MS. Barr RC: Origin of epicardial ST-T wave potentials in the intact dog. Cir Res 39:475, 1976.
29. Spach MS, Barr RC, Lanning CF, Tucek PC: Origin of the body surface QRS and T wave potentials from epicardial potentials distributions in the intact chimpanzee. Circulation 55:268, 1976.

15

Late Potentials: Localization by Body Surface Potential Mapping

Pierre Savard, Gérard Faugère, René Cardinal, Dominique Lacroix, Pierre Pagé, Mohammad Shenasa

Introduction

From the early experimental studies[1] and clinical investigations,[2,3] late potentials have been mainly recorded with a few signal-averaged electrocardiographic leads. Obviously, a larger number of leads can provide more information than that provided by the standard three orthogonal leads, which are used essentially for detecting the presence or absence of late potentials.

Additional leads can first improve the sensitivity of the late potential detection, either by spatial averaging[4,5] or by selecting precordial leads having a better signal-to-noise ratio.[6] They can also provide new information about the spatial distribution of the late potentials over the entire torso surface.[7,8] Thus, indications about the location of the sources of late potentials can be obtained from the body surface potential maps (BSPM). This spatial information could be used, for example, to determine if activity terminates in an abnormal manner in patients with short filtered QRS duration. Past

From El-Sherif N, Turitto G (eds): *High-Resolution Electrocardiography*. Mount Kisco, NY, Futura Publishing Co., Inc., ©, 1992.

and current work on the localization of late potentials will be covered in this chapter using experimental and clinical results.

Methods

The basic data acquisition and processing techniques were similar to those currently used for the measurement of late potentials, with the exception that the body surface potentials were measured with 63 unipolar leads referenced to the Wilson central terminal. There were 43 electrodes distributed on the front and sides of the torso and 20 electrodes on the back. [7] The recordings were performed in the supine position during sinus rhythm. The electrocardiograms (ECGs) were amplified, filtered with a bandwidth of 0.05 to 200 Hz, sampled at 500 Hz, digitized with a resolution of 2.5 µV, and stored on a hard disk for periods of 52 seconds. The beats were automatically classified into different categories and averaged separately by using a cross correlation technique to align the beats. These averaged signals were corrected for baseline shift and digital filtering was then performed on each of the 63 ECGs to reject low-frequency components under 25 Hz (fourth-order Butterworth filter) and 60-Hz interference. Filtering was performed in the usual bidirectional manner [2] to reduce the effects of ringing on the measurement of the QRS duration.

To analyze the spatial distribution of the late potentials, isopotential maps (LP-BSPM) representing at one specific instant the value of the filtered signal on each of the 63 leads were drawn at each 2 msec between 80 and 170 msec after QRS onset. In these maps, the torso surface is represented in a rectangular format, the upper edge corresponds to the top electrode row, the lower edge to the lower row, and the side edges to the right midaxillary line. The zero line is identified by a heavier trace and the plus and minus signs indicate the maximum and minimum.

Animal Experiments

The experiments were carried out on 12 dogs, 3 to 15 days after occlusion of the left anterior descending coronary artery following methylprednisolone pretreatment. [9,10] On the day of the study, the dogs were anesthetized with sodium pentothal and chloralose. LP-

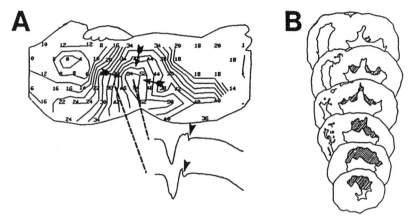

Figure 1. Epicardial isochronal map (A) and TTC-stained heart slices (B). The isochronal map depicts a typical activation sequence during sinus rhythm. The left part of the map represents the anterior portion of the ventricles, the right part represents the posterior portion, and the central part represents the left ventricle. Numbers indicate the local activation times in milliseconds relative to the epicardial breakthrough, isochronal lines join points having the same activation time at each 5 msec, and arrows indicate the progression of activation in the region overlying the infarct. Two unipolar electrograms from this area are shown. On the heart slices, the necrotic area which was identified by a TTC-staining technique is represented by the crosshatched region and it is located subendocardially in the anteroapical part of the left ventricle.

BSPM were recorded during sinus rhythm with 63 needle electrodes. A sternotomy was then performed and epicardial electrograms were recorded with a sock electrode array during sinus rhythm using 63 unipolar leads. Local activation times were automatically detected and manually edited on each electrogram in order to construct isochronal maps depicting the activation sequence (Figure 1A). After the study, a TTC-staining (triphenyl tetrazolium chloride) technique was used to identify necrotic tissue on heart slices spaced 1 cm apart (Figure 1B).

Clinical Studies

The studies were performed on 24 patients (20 men, 4 women) aged between 50 and 76 years who had documented sustained ventricular tachycardia (VT): 22 had an history of previous myocardial infarction, and 2 had a cardiomyopathy. None had conduction disturbances or antiarrhythmic treatment. For all these patients, BSPM was performed during sinus rhythm to record late potentials (LP-BSPM). At least two consecutive BSPM recordings were thus performed for each patient. For 17 patients, BSPM was also performed during different VT episodes induced in the electrophysiologic laboratory. These signals were corrected for baseline shift, but no filtering was performed. Isopotential maps (VT-BSPM) were plotted at each sampling instant after QRS onset. For 12 patients who underwent antiarrhythmia surgery, epicardial and endocardial activation mapping was performed with sock and balloon electrode arrays so as to localize the site of origin of VT (5 of these patients also had VT-BSPM).

Results

Animal Experiments

In the canine experiments, isochronal maps showed that terminal epicardial activity was located over the anterior and lateral parts of the left ventricle (Figure 1A), instead of near the base as in normal hearts. This terminal activation appeared to progress slowly in a well organized manner with isochronal lines forming concentric circles around the site of latest activity. The unipolar electrograms around this area showed that the terminal activation corresponded to a small RS notch appearing during the ST segment, after a large QS wave indicating the presence of a myocardial infarct. These RS deflections had amplitudes ranging between about 0.5 and 5 mV, and fragmentation was rarely observed.

The morphology of the late potentials seen on a given filtered ECG lead was similar to that of the neighboring leads. This was expressed on the maps by mostly dipolar distributions with single positive and negative regions. Dogs that showed terminal activity at similar epicardial sites showed similar isopotential maps at QRS offset. The BSPM extrema tended to be located over the inferior part of the torso for sites of terminal activity near the apex, superiorly for sites near the anterior base, over the right anterior part of the chest for sites near the right ventricle, to the back or the left of the torso for left lateral sites (Figure 2).

The TTC-stained heart slices showed that the infarct zone was

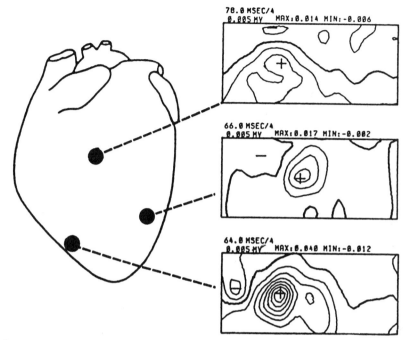

Figure 2. Body surface potential maps of the filtered late potentials (LP-BSPM) and the corresponding site of terminal epicardial activity in three dogs. The maps represent the potential distributions observed during two to four sampling instants before the filtered QRS offset in dogs where terminal activity was located at different sites in the anterior part of the left ventricle. Isopotential lines join points having the same potential value with an interval of 5 μV between the lines.

subendocardial (Figure 1B), extending transmurally in some dogs. The necrotic area was smaller (p <0.005) for the seven dogs investigated 3–5 days after coronary artery occlusion (11% ±5% of left ventricular mass) than for those investigated 10–15 days after (22 ±3% of LV), but the total epicardial activation durations were similar (42 ±9 and 48 ±10 msec).

Clinical Studies

The morphology of the different LP-BSPM from the same session was strictly reproducible. These maps were mostly dipolar, and patients showed either distant extrema (Figure 3A), or extrema close

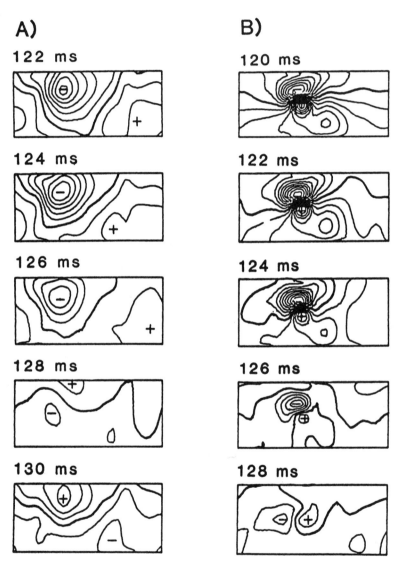

Figure 3. Typical LP-BSPM for two patients with coronary artery disease and VT during the last 10 msec of QRS (same format as Figure 2). (A) Morphology with two distant extrema. (B) Morphology with two close extrema. (Reprinted with permission from Faugère et al, Circulation 74:1323, 1986.)

together in the precordial or left midaxillary region (Figure 3B). For 13 patients with anterior myocardial infarction, the maps showed distant extrema for 7, and close extrema for 6. For eight VT patients with inferior myocardial infarction and one with anterior and inferior infarction, the maps always showed distant extrema. Maps with more than two extrema were found only once.

For the 17 patients who had BSPM performed during VT induced in the electrophysiologic laboratory (VT-BSPM), 6 patients showed a single morphology of sustained VT, 10 showed two distinct VT morphologies, and 1 patient showed three different morphologies. For 6 of these 17 patients, a map recorded during one of the different VT episodes (VT-BSPM) was similar to the map recorded during sinus rhythm (LP-BSPM). For example in Figure 4, the locations of the extrema and of the zero potential line in the VT1 map were similar to those of the LP-BSPM, whereas the VT2 map recorded during a different VT episode in the same patient did not correspond to the LP-BSPM. In contrast, for 11 of the 17 patients, none of the maps recorded during the different VT episodes was

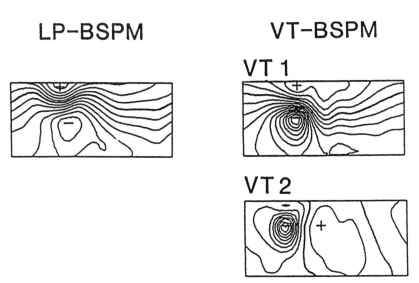

LP–BSPM   **VT–BSPM**

VT 1

VT 2

Figure 4. For the same patient with coronary artery disease and VT: at left, filtered isopotential map of the late potentials (LP-BSPM); and at right, unfiltered isopotential map at 20 msec after QRS onset (VT-BSPM) during two VT episodes with different morphology (VT1 and VT2). (Reprinted with permission from Savard et al, J Electrocardiol 20(Suppl):114, 1987

similar to the LP-BSPM. For the 12 patients who underwent antiarrhythmia surgery, 19 different sites of earliest VT activity were identified by epicardial and endocardial mapping. For the three patients who had LP-BSPM with close extrema, all had anterior or apical sites of VT origin, and one of them also had a posterior site. For the nine patients who showed distant extrema on the LP-BSPM, all had single or multiple posterior, lateral, or septal sites, with three additional anteroapical sites.

Discussion

So far, direct correlations between LP-BSPM and terminal intracardiac activity have been performed only in canine experiments. The observed patterns indicate that LP-BSPM does reflect the changes in the location of terminal activity that were observed in different animals. Thus, LP-BSPM has the potential to localize this activity noninvasively. However, criteria for the interpretation of LP-BSPM patterns must be developed specifically for man because of its particular torso geometry.

In man, LP-BSPM results have been shown for patients with different sites of myocardial infarction or different sites of origin of VT determined during surgery. The principal finding is that LP-BSPM patterns with close extrema in the precordial region are found mainly in patients with anterior or apical sites of myocardial infarction or VT origin. Since electrical sources that are close to the torso surface will produce thoracic potential distributions with sharp potential gradients and close precordial extrema, this suggests that terminal activity is located anteriorly, near the site of the infarct or the VT origin.

BSPM interpretation criteria that can provide a more precise localization of various cardiac sources have been proposed for the localization of ventricular pre-excitation in the Wolff-Parkinson-White syndrome,[11,12] the localization of myocardial infarction,[13,14] and the localization of initial activation during ventricular tachycardia.[8,15–17] BSPM can detect local abnormalities in ventricular activation sequence in patients with previous myocardial infarction[18] and in patients with coronary artery disease but normal electrocardiogram,[19] or abnormalities in ventricular repolarization such as idiopathic long QT syndrome.[20] Also, body surface potentials can be analyzed with computer models so as to estimate the potentials over the epicardium[21,22] or plot the trajectory of an equivalent moving dipole that can localize initial activation during ectopic beats,[23] ventricular pre-excitation,[24] or ventricular tachycardia.[16]

All these techniques constitute a framework for the detailed morphologic analysis of late potential distributions. However, physiologic and technical aspects are specific to late potential distributions. The physiologic particularity is caused by the nature of the late potential sources. In previous BSPM applications, the sources that generated the observed body surface potentials were mostly located in normal and homogeneous myocardium where extended activation wave front propagated in a uniform manner. For late potentials, the nature of the sources is different. Our results (Figure 1) indicate that late potentials are generated by a small epicardial wave front skirting over a subendocardial infarct. The concentric isochronal lines as well as the unipolar electrograms showing single RS notches suggest a fairly uniform wave front slowly propagating around a large obstacle. In canine preparations with 2-month-old infarct, isochronal maps show a nonuniform propagation accelerating and slowing along different directions, and the electrograms present multiple deflections.[25,26] These differences may be due to different infarct age, recording technique (unipolar vs bipolar) and mapping resolution (2 cm vs 5-mm electrode spacing). But whatever is the complexity of the sources of late potentials in man, as the recording electrode is moved from the surface of the heart to the surface of the torso, the electrocardiographic contribution of the higher order multipole components is drastically reduced and dipolar components dominate, as can be seen on Figures 2 to 4. The electrocardiographic particularity of late potentials is that changes in relative amplitude and orientation of the equivalent dipole can take place more rapidly than for other sources.

The technical aspect of the morphologic analysis of late potentials is relatively new and unsettled. The late potentials, which have amplitudes of about 0 to 25 μV, are superimposed over the ST segment (about 50 to 200 μV) and their onset is totally masked by the QRS. Isopotential maps of the signal-averaged ECG would mainly show the ST segment distribution instead of the late potential distribution. To extract the late potentials, signal processing must be performed either in the time domain or in the space domain.

In the time domain, the low-frequency component of the ST segment can be eliminated separately on each lead by high-pass filtering, which is the standard electrocardiographic practice. However, the morphology of the late potentials is altered by the high-pass filtering, whatever the type and cut-off frequency of the filter. For example, a late potential signal composed of a series of positive peaks with no repolarization component will appear after filtering as a series of positive and negative peaks. This can explain the polarity reversals that can be seen on some series of maps (Figure 3). Numerous types of high-pass filters are available and filter design is essentially a question of compromises.[27] Bidirectional infinite impulse response (IIR) filters such as the one used in this study will prevent ringing outside the QRS but not within the QRS, and will also produce phase shifts. Symmetrical finite impulse response (FIR) filters can prevent ringing and phase shifts but their response will be affected by the proximity of the QRS. Different filters may thus be selected for different applications such as QRS duration measurement (IIR) or morphologic analysis (FIR).

In the space domain, two BSPM analysis techniques are relevant to the morphologic analysis of late potentials. The first was proposed by Horan et al[28] for the extraction of the low level His potentials from the larger atrial repolarization potentials. A spatial filter is first adapted to the morphology of atrial depolarization distribution, and is then used to detect and cancel the atrial repolarization. The second technique was recently proposed by Horacek et al.[29] It consists in detecting local extrema on the unfiltered BSPM and plotting their trajectory over the torso during the entire heart beat. These techniques merit further investigation. High-pass filtering in the time domain was employed in this study because a high-frequency content is specific to late potentials and also because filtering is the usual technique in clinical studies.

The morphologic analysis of late potential distributions provides new information with respect to the usual measurements such as duration, amplitude, and frequency content of late potentials recorded with three leads.[30] This new information can be applied in different contexts. For example, LP-BSPM can distinguish between some normal and abnormal patterns of terminal activity[7] and may be applied for the identification of patients with borderline filtered QRS duration. BSPM can also indicate that the region of initial activation during VT corresponds approximately to that of terminal activity (Figure 4), which can be useful information during arrhythmia surgery. The effects of various interventions can be described more precisely with LP-BSPM than with the standard three lead

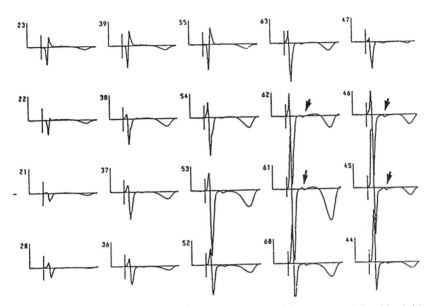

Figure 5. Signal-averaged ECG from a young girl (8-years old) with right ventricular dysplasia. The ECGs were recorded on the upper part of the anterior torso: the middle electrode of the upper row is located over the suprasternal notch and the other electrodes are spaced 5 cm apart. Arrow heads indicate delayed activation in the leads from the left parasternal region.

technique. For example, Faugère et al[7] reported that arrhythmia surgery shortens the filtered QRS duration and alters the late potential maps, whereas amiodarone prolongs the QRS but does not alter the maps, which indicates respectively the presence or absence of alterations in the terminal activation sequence.

In conclusion, late potentials are a new feature in the history of electrocardiography. Recording techniques, measurements, nomenclature, and significance are not as widely accepted as for the other characteristics of the ECG. In this context, BSPM is an appropriate technique for the detailed study of terminal activity in a wide range of conditions in addition to coronary artery disease with VT,[31] such as nonischemic congestive cardiomyopathy,[32] myotonic dystrophy,[33] heart transplant,[34] and ventricular dysplasia (Figure 5).

Acknowledgments: The authors gratefully acknowledge the contributions of Dr. Reginald Nadeau for the clinical studies, and of Denis Derome and Lise Legendre for technical assistance. This work was supported in part by the Medical Research

Council of Canada, the Canadian Heart Foundations, and the Fonds de la recherche en santé du Québec.

References

1. Berbari EJ, Scherlag BJ, Hope RR, Lazzara R: Recording from the body surface of arrhythmogenic ventricular activity during the ST segment. Am J Cardiol 41:697, 1978.
2. Simson MB: Use of signals in the terminal QRS complex to identify patients with ventricular tachycardia after myocardial infarction. Circulation 64:235, 1981.
3. Rozanski JJ, Mortara D, Myerburg RJ, Castellanos A: Body surface detection of delayed depolarizations in patients with recurrent ventricular tachycardia and left ventricular aneurysm. Circulation 63:1172, 1981.
4. Flowers NC, Shvartsman V, Kenelly BM, Sohi GS, Horan LG: Surface recording of His-Purkinje activity on an every-beat basis without digital filtering. Circulation 63:948, 1981.
5. Mehra R, Restivo M, El-Sherif N: Electromyographic noise reduction for high-resolution electrocardiography. Proceedings Fifth IEEE EMBS, 248–253, 1983.
6. Berbari EJ: Critical overview of late potential recordings. J Electrocardiol 20 (Suppl):125, 1987.
7. Faugère G, Savard P, Nadeau RA, Derome D, Shenasa M, Pagé P, Guardo R: Characterization of the spatial distribution of late ventricular potentials by body surface potential mapping in patients with ventricular tachycardia. Circulation 74:1323, 1986.
8. Savard P, Faugère G, Nadeau RA, Derome D, Shenasa M, Pagé P, Guardo R: The spatial distribution of late ventricular potentials. J Electrocardiol 20 (Suppl):114, 1987.
9. Cardinal R, Savard P, Carson L, Perry JB, Pagé P: Mapping of ventricular tachycardia induced by programmed stimulation in canine preparations of myocardial infarction. Circulation 70:136, 1984.
10. Pagé P, Cardinal R, Savard P, Shenasa M: Sinus rhythm mapping in a canine model of ventricular tachycardia. PACE 11:632, 1988.
11. De Ambroggi L, Taccardi B, Macchi E: Body surface maps of heart potentials: tentative localization of pre-excited area in forty-two Wolff-Parkinson-White patients. Circulation 54:251, 1976.
12. Benson DW, Sterba R, Gallagher JJ, Walston A, Spach MS: Localization of the site of ventricular pre-excitation with body surface maps in patients with the Wolff-Parkinson-White syndrome. Circulation 65:1259, 1982.
13. Montague TJ, Smith ER, Spencer CA, Johnstone DE, Lalonde LD, Bessoudo RM, Gardner MJ, Anderson RN, Horacek BM: Body surface electrocardiographic mapping in inferior myocardial infarction. Manifestation of left and right ventricular involvement. Circulation 67:665, 1983.
14. Ackaoui A, Nadeau R, Sestier F, Savard P, Primeau R, Lemieux R, Descary MC: Myocardial infarction diagnosis with body surface poten-

tial mapping, electrocardiography, vectorcardiography and Thallium-201 scintigraphy: a correlative study with left ventriculography. Clin Invest Med 8:68, 1985.

15. Savard P, Boucher S, Cardinal R, Giasson R: Localization of cardiac electrical activity by a single moving dipole during ventricular tachycardia in dog: validation by epicardial activation mapping. In van Dam RT, van Oosterom A (eds): Electrocardiographic Body Surface Mapping. Boston: Martinus Nijhoff, 1986, pp. 109-112.

16. Savard P, Shenasa M, Pagé P, Cardinal P, Derome D, Nadeau R: Body surface potential mapping of induced ventricular tachycardia in man: electrocardiographic and surgical correlations (abstr). Circulation 76(Suppl IV):438, 1987.

17. Sippens Groenewegen A, Spekhorst H, Hauer RNW, van Hemel NM, Kingma JH, de Bakker JMT, Janse MJ: Body surface mapping of ventricular tachycardia: localization of the site of origin compared with intraoperative mapping (abstr). Circulation 76(Suppl IV):437, 1987.

18. Ikeda K, Kubota I, Igarashi A, Yamaki M, Tsuiki K, Yasui S: Detection of local abnormalities in ventricular activation sequence by body surface isochrone mapping in patients with previous myocardial infarction. Circulation 72:801, 1985.

19. Green LS, Lux RL, Haws CW: Detection and localization of coronary artery disease with body surface potential mapping in patients with normal electrocardiograms. Circulation 76:1290, 1987.

20. De Ambroggi L, Bertoni T, Locati E, Stramba-Badiale M, Schwartz P: Mapping of body surface potentials in patients with the idiopatic long QT syndrome. Circulation 74:1334, 1986.

21. Barr R, Spach MS: Inverse calculation of QRS-T epicardial potentials from body surface potential distributions from normal and ectopic beats in the intact dog. Circ Res 42:661, 1978.

22. Rudy Y: The relationship between body surface and epicardial potentials: a theoretical model study. In van Dam RT, van Oosterom A (eds): Electrocardiographic Body Surface Mapping. Boston: Martinus Nijhoff, 1986, pp 247-258.

23. Savard P, Ackaoui A, Gulrajani RM, Nadeau RA, Roberge FA, Guardo R, Dubé B: Localization of cardiac ectopic activity in man by a single moving dipole, comparison of different computation techniques. J Electrocardiol, 18:211, 1985.

24. Nadeau RA, Savard P, Faugère G, Shenasa M, Pagé P, Gulrajani RM, Guardo RA, Cardinal R: Localization of pre-excitation sites in the Wolff-Parkinson-White syndrome by body surface potential mapping and a single moving dipole representation. In van Dam RT, van Oosterom A (eds): Electrocardiographic Body Surface Mapping. Boston: Martinus Nijhoff, 1986, pp 95-98.

25. Gardner PJ, Ursell PC, Pham TD, Fenoglio JJ, Wit AL: Experimental chronic ventricular tachycardia: anatomic and electrophysiologic substrates. In Josephson ME, Wellens HJJ (eds): Tachycardias: Mechanisms, Diagnosis, Treatment. Philadelphia: Lea and Febiger, 1984.

26. Wit AL, Josephson ME: Fractionated electrograms and continuous ac-

tivity: fact or artifact. In Zipes DP, Jalife J (eds): Cardiac Electrophysiology and Arrhythmias. Philadelphia, Grune and Stratton, 1985.

27. Oppenheim AV, Schafer RW: Digital Signal Processing. Englewood Cliffs, Prentice Hall Publ, 1975.

28. Horan LG, Flowers NC, Sohi GS: A dynamic electrical record of the pathway of human His bundle activation from surface mapping. Circ Res 50:47, 1982.

29. Horacek BM, Montague TJ, Gardner MJ, Smith ER: Arrhythmogenic conditions. In Mirvis D (ed): Electrocardiographic Body Surface Mapping. Boston: Martinus Nijhoff, 1988.

30. Breithardt G, Borggrefe M: Recent advances in the identification of patients at risk of ventricular tachyarrhythmias: role of ventricular late potentials. Circulation 75:1091, 1987.

31. Cardinal R, Vermeulen M, Shenasa M, Roberge F, Pagé P, Hélie F, Savard P: Anisotropic conduction and functional dissociation of ischemic tissue during reentrant ventricular tachycardia in canine myocardial infarction. Circulation 77:1162, 1988.

32. Poll DS, Marchlinski FE, Falcone RA, Josephson ME, Simson MB: Abnormal signal-averaged electrocardiograms in patients with nonischemic congestive cardiomyopathy: relationship to sustained ventricular tachyarrhythmias. Circulation 72:1308, 1985.

33. Baciarello G, Villani M, Di Maio F, Sciacca A: Late surface potentials in myotonic dystrophy with ventricular tachycardia. Am Heart J 111:-413, 1986.

34. Keren A, Gillis AM, Freedman RA, Baldwin JC, Billingham ME, Stinson EB, Simson MB, Mason JW: Heart transplant rejection monitored by signal averaged electrocardiography in patients receiving cyclosporine. Circulation 70(Suppl I):124, 1984.

Section IV.

Late Potentials in the Post-Infarction Period

16

Late Potentials in the Post-Infarction Period: Natural History

Dennis L. Kuchar

Introduction

Late potentials, detected by signal averaging of the surface electrocardiogram (ECG), are associated with the spontaneous occurrence of sustained ventricular tachycardia (VT) in patients with
chronic healed myocardial infarction and have been shown to identify patients with coronary artery disease who have inducible VT at
electrophysiology study.[1-4] These signals, which are thought to
arise from small areas of myocardium at the periphery of myocardial
infarction, have also been shown to correspond in timing with signals recorded from the endocardium at the site of origin of VT and
to disappear with successful endocardial resection.[5,6] This provides
compelling evidence that these signals originate from the anatomic
substrate for reentrant ventricular arrhythmias complicating
healed myocardial infarction. As discussed elsewhere in this volume, late potentials have been shown to differentiate patients with
and without VT, with a high sensitivity and specificity.

Several questions remained unanswered from these studies: (1)

From El-Sherif N, Turitto G (eds): *High-Resolution Electrocardiography*. Mount
Kisco, NY, Futura Publishing Co., Inc., ©, 1992.

do late potentials detected soon after infarction predict which patients will develop subsequent spontaneous ventricular arrhythmias? and (2) what is the time course of late potentials after myocardial infarction?—as clearly they had been reported to occur in around 30%–40% of patients with an acute infarction but seemed to be uncommon in patients with remote infarction, being fairly specific for those who had sustained VT. A number of recent experimental observations has shed light on these questions.

Changes in Terminal QRS Activation in Acute Myocardial Infarction

Animal Studies

Much attention has been focused on the recording of fractionated electrograms in the perinfarction zone in dogs after occlusion of the left anterior descending coronary artery and their association with ventricular arrhythmias. Harris[7] described two distinct time periods after creation of infarction during which ventricular arrhythmias were noted. Subsequent studies[8-11] demonstrated that the early phase (within minutes of occlusion and lasting up to 30 minutes) was associated with the recording of low amplitude fragmented electrograms within the "ischemic zone" in the subepicardium which were closely correlated with the subsequent occurrence of ventricular ectopy and often ventricular fibrillation (VF). Furthermore, these electrograms were shown to bridge the diastolic interval with electrical activity preceding the ectopic beats, giving rise to the hypothesis that such arrhythmias are reentrant in nature. Kaplinsky et al[12] showed that peak epicardial delay occurred within the first 5–10 minutes after occlusion and that the degree of delay (after the inscription of the surface QRS complex) correlated with the type of spontaneous arrhythmia that occurred: VT and VF were associated with longer epicardial signals with delays of up to 320 msec. These were often seen to occur with a Wenckebach-type periodicity before the onset of ventricular arrhythmia. Subsequent conduction delay was then noted to diminish after a further 10 minutes, presumably because of electrical silence (absence of electrical activity) in this severely ischemic tissue.

Simson et al[13] performed a similar experiment but analyzed this epicardial delay from the body surface using the signal-averaged ECG. After injecting latex into the left anterior descending coronary artery, prolongation of epicardial and surface electrograms was noted and persisted for up to 80 minutes in 9 of 11 dogs. Beyond this time period, electrograms were no longer recorded in the ischemic zone although some fractionated activity was recorded at the border of cyanotic and normal myocardium with a total area of 1.7 cm^2 (Figure 1).

Murdock et al[14] subsequently demonstrated reemergence of fractionated epicardial potentials following reperfusion of the ischemic zones, suggesting a possible mechanism for the arrhythmias frequently seen in the setting of successful thrombolytic therapy.

Ventricular arrhythmias observed in the dog after this initial period are thought to be due to increased automaticity of Purkinje fibers and myocardial cells associated with such factors as hypoxia,

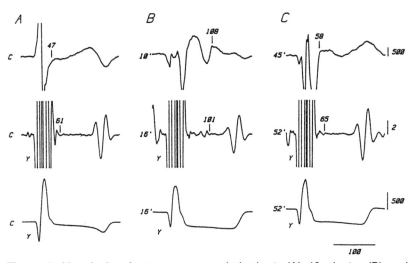

Figure 1. Ventricular electrograms recorded prior to (A), 10 minutes (B), and 45 minutes (C) following acute occlusion of the left anterior descending coronary artery of the dog. The top tracing is a direct epicardial recording, the middle tracing is signal-averaged surface lead Y, and the bottom tracing is the unprocessed Y lead.

acidic pH, anaerobic metabolism, potassium concentration, and catecholamines.[15,16] These arrhythmias do not appear to be associated with significant epicardial delay suggesting that conduction disorders are not operative during this period.

Beyond the first 24 hours, a third stage of electrical instability is then noted. El-Sherif et al[17] have extensively studied this period and have demonstrated the presence of localized conduction disorders in the infarction zone with characteristics similar to those noted during the acute phase; they showed that fractionated electrical activity could be shown to span diastole after introduction of an early atrial depolarization in turn giving rise to brief periods of VT which displayed continuous activity consistent with a reentrant mechanism. Such arrhythmias are thought to be analogous to the sustained ventricular arrhythmias typically seen in humans with chronic myocardial infarction. Histologic and microelectrode techniques have suggested that these delayed depolarizations result from slowed asynchronous conduction in areas containing surviving myocardial cells which have normal resting potentials, but are uncoupled by interstitial fibrosis and connected to the larger mass of myocardium at the edges of the infarction.[18]

Berbari et al[19] studied dogs 3–6 days after infarction. In 7 out of 9 dogs, epicardial and signal-averaged surface electrograms were recorded during atrial pacing. This correlated with the induction of ventricular arrhythmia using an electrical stimulation protocol. In one animal, a Wenckebach periodicity was seen in the electrogram recorded from the epicardium during successive beats, but not from the body surface; this highlights one drawback of the signal averaging technique which relies on consistent beat-to-beat occurrence of a signal for its full registration.

Preliminary data from our laboratory in dogs with apical infarction using a bidirectional filter similar to that used in prior clinical studies showed that low amplitude signals < 20 µV in the last 20 msec of the filtered (40–250 Hz) QRS complex identified those animals with inducible VT using stimulation protocols similar to those used in clinical studies in humans. Late potentials were not seen prior to or 1 hour following ligation of the left anterior descending coronary artery but did appear 3–14 days later in those dogs in whom sustained monomorphic VT was induced (Figure 2). In contrast to the study of Berbari et al,[19] we could not demonstrate changes in conduction delay with incremental atrial pacing.

preMI

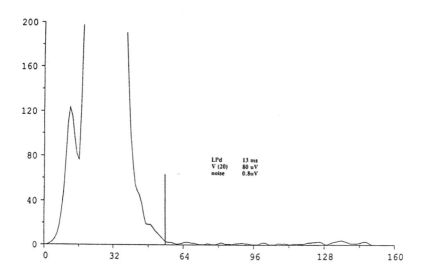

post-MI

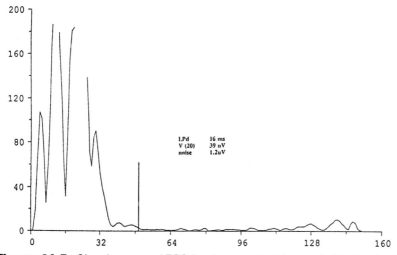

Figures 2A,B. Signal-averaged ECG (vector magnitude) recorded before (top) and over several days (bottom) after occlusion of the left anterior descending coronary artery in the dog.

day 4

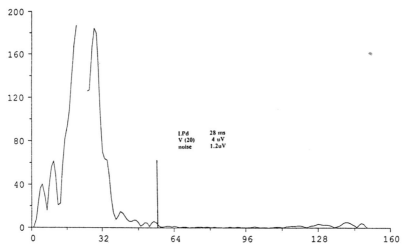

Figure 2C. Programmed ventricular stimulation led to induction of sustained monomorphic VT on day 4 with two extrastimuli.

day 19

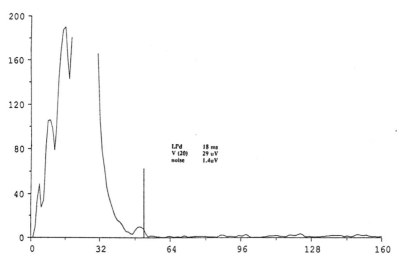

Figure 2D. On day 19 no monomorphic VT could be induced, but VF was induced with three extrastimuli. LPd = duration of signals < 40 μV from the end of the QRS; V (20) = root mean square voltage in the terminal 20 msec of the QRS.

Human Studies

Although the electrophysiologic characteristics of VT in chronic myocardial infarction are similar in the dog model and in man, little is known of the precise mechanism of VT and VF and its relationship to conduction delay occurring in the early phase of infarction.

Kertes et al[20] recorded signal-averaged ECGs in patients within hours of onset of myocardial infarction soon after admission to the coronary care unit. They frequently observed late potentials in the terminal QRS complex but found that the presence of these signals did not correlate with subsequent occurrence of VF and noted that they were transient in nature. When recordings were obtained during the next few days, Gomes et al[21] found a clear association between late potentials and the occurrence of sustained and nonsustained VT during the hospital stay. One could speculate that the electrophysiologic milieu of the infarct zone is constantly changing with progression of ischemia and development of myocardial necrosis, and that late potentials measured at one instant in the first few hours after coronary artery occlusion may well be a transient phenomena. Late potentials detected several days after infarction, on the other hand, may represent the early development of a chronic substrate for arrhythmia—although fibrosis may not be evident at this early stage, myocardial cell uncoupling probably occurs due to interstitial edema and inflammatory infiltrate which may well lead to asynchronous electrical activation providing a substrate for arrhythmia, a precursor to the chronic substrate described above.[22,23]

We recorded signal-averaged ECGs in a group of 35 patients on each day after presentation of acute myocardial infarction.[24] Of these, 11 had a late potential (mean voltage < 20 μV in the last 40 msec of the filtered [40–250 Hz] QRS complex) at the time of hospital discharge, 8–10 days after infarction. During the initial recording (within 36 hours of onset of chest pain), six of these patients had voltage criteria for a late potential; in one of these, a late potential was recorded 3 hours after onset of chest pain in a patient without previous history of an infarction. On the third day, 7 patients had a late potential, and by the sixth day, 9 of the 11 had a late potential. In addition, two patients with late potentials during the first 3 days after myocardial infarction "normalized" their QRS complexes by the time of discharge. One patient with a late potential on day 1 developed refractory VT and died on the third day after presentation with infarction. In the group of patients overall, there was a gradual increase in the total filtered QRS duration, a reduction in terminal QRS voltage, and a gradual increase in the duration of low amplitude signal in the terminal portion of the QRS from the first recording to the final recording just prior to discharge. Hence, there are dynamic changes in the terminal activation of the QRS during the first 10 days after myocardial infarction with appearance and disappearance of late potentials. However, the majority of patients who will leave hospital alive with a late potential already have this ECG characteristic within the first 3 days of their infarction.

Late Changes in Ventricular Activation After Myocardial Infarction

In order to document the changes in late potentials during the first year after recovery from myocardial infarction, we studied 165 consecutive patients who were managed in the coronary care unit who survived the hospital phase of recovery.[25] The signal-averaged ECG was performed at an average of 10.5 ±6.1 (SD) days after initial presentation. Subsequent studies were performed 6 weeks after hospital discharge and then at 3, 6, and 12 months. The signal-averaged ECG was obtained using a high-resolution ECG (ART 101, Arrhythmia Research Technology, Bellevue, WA) based on methods described by Simson and Denes and coworkers. The ECG was recorded in sinus rhythm with standard bipolar, orthogonal leads X, Y, and Z in an unshielded room. Signals from 200–300 beats were amplified, digitized, averaged, and then filtered with a fourth-order bidirectional Butterworth filter with a high bandpass frequency of 40 Hz. This filter does not produce ringing artifacts, commonly seen with conventional high order digital filters, which may obscure late potentials and produce an artifactual signal that may mimic a late potential.[3] The filtered leads were then combined into a vector magnitude tracing derived as the square root of the sum of squares of the amplitude of individual leads, and from which QRS duration and terminal voltages were automatically derived by computer algorithm. In accordance with previous studies,[3,26] we defined a late potential as a low amplitude signal (< 20 µV) in the last 40 msec of the QRS complex. A filtered QRS > 120 msec was defined as abnormally prolonged. Hence, an abnormal signal-averaged ECG included the presence of a late potential or a prolonged filtered QRS complex. Patients with bundle branch block on the standard ECG were not included in these analyses, so that a prolonged filtered QRS implies that there is abnormal delayed activity that is undetectable from the standard surface ECG.

Two important points about the technique need to be emphasized before serial changes in signal-averaged ECG parameters can be interpreted correctly. The noise level in the ST segment, which was automatically determined by the computer, was always ≤ 0.5 μV. In fact for each individual patient, we attempted to closely match the noise levels for each tracing. This can be achieved by averaging a similar number of beats if the patient is well relaxed or by progressively increasing the number of beats sampled until the desired noise level is attained. An estimated noise level is continuously supplied by the computer to the technician during data aquisition. Once the noise level is kept constant and well below the amplitude of the desired signals (generally < 1 μV), it is important to realize the degree of variability of the parameters derived from the recording system. We found that in a group of patients without recent infarction, who underwent repeat signal-averaged ECG recordings separated by 1 hour to 3 months, the mean coefficient of variability for the voltage in the last 40 msec of the QRS was 6.6% with 95% confidence intervals of ± 3.8 μV, and for the filtered QRS duration were 1.0% and ± 2 msec, respectively.[27] Day-to-day changes outside these limits can therefore be interpreted as true biological changes.

Of the 165 patients entered into the study at the time of discharge from hospital, 65 had an abnormal signal-averaged ECG (group I), 92 had a normal tracing (group II), and 8 had bundle branch block. In group I patients, the mean duration of the filtered QRS complex did not change significantly during the 12-month period (Figure 3). However, the mean voltage in the terminal QRS increased significantly from the initial study to the second study performed 6 weeks after hospital discharge (from 12.8 ± 7.5 μV to 20.0 ± 12.6 μV, p < 0.001) (Figures 3 and 4); this increase was well outside the 95% confidence limits of reproducibility. No further significant change in voltage occurred in the group overall over the remaining follow-up period. In group II, the mean filtered QRS duration was 100 ± 9 msec at the discharge study and did not change significantly during the year after infarction. Similarly, no change in the terminal QRS voltage was noted in those patients whose

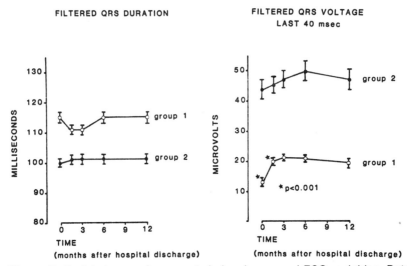

Figure 3. Serial changes in computed signal-averaged ECG variables. Data are presented as mean ± SEM. (Reproduced with permission from Kuchar et al. Circulation 74:1280, 1986.)

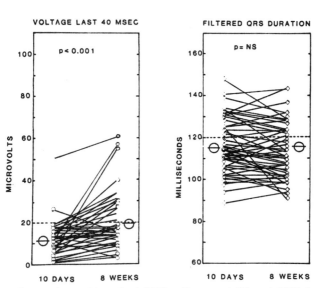

Figure 4. Comparison of terminal QRS voltage and filtered QRS duration 10 days and 8 weeks after myocardial infarction. The horizontal dashed line indicates the criteria used to define abnormal values. (Reproduced with permission from Kuchar et al. Circulation 74:1280, 1986.)

signal-averaged ECG was normal at the time of discharge from hospital.

In contrast to previous studies in patients with remote infarctions, where patients with late potentials appeared to constitute a small minority group who were distinguishable by a history of serious ventricular arrhythmia, we found that 41% of patients with a recent infarction (i.e., within 10 days) had a late potential. A similar prevalence of late potentials in this type of population has been reported by others.[28] By the time of the 6-week study, however, 11 patients (18%) had undergone spontaneous "normalization" of the QRS complex (loss of late potential). Examples of this phenomenon are shown in Figure 5. Over the next 12 months, there was a gradual decrease in the prevalence of late potentials; 1 year after the infarction, only 70% of group I patients still had a late potential (Figure 6). In those patients whose tracing was normal at the time of hospital

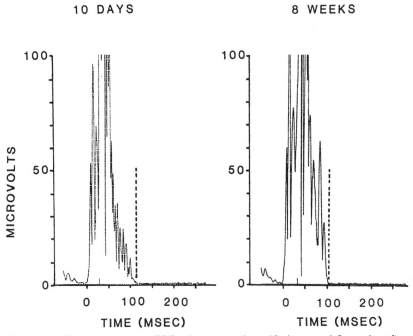

Figure 5. Signal-averaged ECGs from a patient 10 days and 8 weeks after myocardial infarction. Note the increase in the terminal QRS voltage, with "loss" of the late potential. (Reproduced with permission from Kuchar et al. Circulation 74:1280, 1986.)

discharge, between 2% and 4% of patients were found to develop a late potential over the following year. In two patients these abnormalities coincided with a recurrent myocardial infarction (Figure 7); however, in the remainder, there was no obvious precipitant or change in treatment to explain the changes in terminal QRS voltage.

It should be noted that, although many patients had an obvious decrease in QRS duration and "normalized" their terminal QRS voltage, some patients had signal-averaged ECG parameters which were close to the cut-off values that defined normal and abnormal. These defined values however were shown to accurately predict those patients who subsequently developed symptomatic VT and those who died suddenly (arrhythmic events): 11 patients with an abnormal signal-averaged ECG at hospital discharge had an arrhythmic event (17% of group I) compared with only one patient (1% of group II) with a normal tracing. None of the patients who initially had a late potential which subsequently normalized had an arrhythmic event.

These results have been recently confirmed in a preliminary study by Grigg et al,[29] who reported findings in 60 patients with reduced left ventricular function (LVEF < 40%). The initial signal-averaged ECG performed within 5 days of myocardial infarction identified late potentials in 30% of cases, and after 3 weeks in 33%. A decline in incidence of late potentials to 23% was noted after 12 months. No patients in their study developed a late potential de novo after the 3-week recording.

The temporal changes noted in the signal-averaged ECG may share a common cause to the temporal changes noted in the inducibility of VT after myocardial infarction. Whereas induction of VT in patients with chronic infarction and clinical VT is a highly specific finding, in patients with recent infarction induction of VT has been reported in about 20%–30% of cases. Denniss et al have shown that in fact a close correlation exists between the finding of late potentials and the inducibility of sustained VT early after infarction.[30] In addition, Roy et al[31] showed that an induced sustained ventricular arrhythmia during programmed stimulation 8 days after infarction, could only be reproduced in 70% of cases after 6 months. Similar findings were also noted by Bhandari et al.[32] A recent study by Duff et al[33] in canine infarction noted that of 19 dogs with anteroapical infarction, which had inducible VT 4 days after coronary artery occlusion, 8 dogs did not continue to have sustained ventricular arrhythmias with repeat testing over the next 26 days. Differential

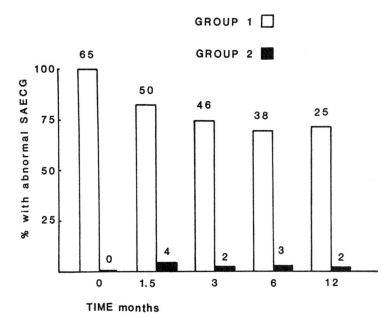

Figure 6. Prevalence of late potentials at each follow-up assessment in patients without change in antiarrhythmic therapy or surgical intervention. (Reproduced with permission from Kuchar et al. Circulation 74:1280, 1986.)

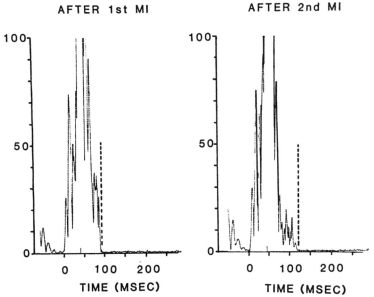

Figure 7. Signal-averaged ECG after initial and then after a second myocardial infarction. Note the new appearance of a late potential. (Reproduced with permission from Kuchar et al. Circulation 74:1280, 1986.)

changes in local refractoriness and repolarization time in the infarct region were noted between the dogs with and without persistently inducible VT. Persistence of abnormal electrophysiologic findings appeared to be related to the degree of LV dysfunction, with mono-morphic VT being more reproducible in dogs with larger infarcts and depressed LV systolic function. [33,34] These studies suggest that a significant change occurs in the electrophysiologic properties of the anatomic substrate for reentrant VT during the months after infarc-tion. This change probably reflects the long-term healing phase of infarction possibly due to amelioration of ischemia from develop-ment of collateral circulation or recovery of stunned myocardium in the peri-infarct border zone. Alterations of the cellular constituents or metabolism of cells within the infarct zone could also account for these changes. The disappearance of late potentials may also be due to electrical isolation of the areas responsible for fractionated elec-trical activity by progression of fibrosis.

These data suggest that for the prognostic evaluation of pa-tients after myocardial infarction, maximal information is obtained by performance of the signal-averaged ECG at about 8–10 days after the infarction. Whether the subsequent disappearance of late poten-tials is associated with a good prognosis cannot be satisfactorily answered with the data currently available. In patients susceptible to lethal arrhythmias, the disappearance of late potentials might serve as a marker for cessation of antiarrhythmic therapy.

References

1. Fontaine G, Frank R, Gallais Hamono F, Allali I, Phan-Tuc H, Gros-gogeat Y: Electrocardiographie des potentiels tardifs du syndrome de postexcitation. Arch Mal Coeur 71:854, 1978.
2. Breithardt G, Becker R, Seipel L, Abendroth RR, Ostermeyer J: Noninva-sive detection of late potentials in man—a new marker for ventricular tachycardia. Eur Heart J 2:1, 1981.
3. Simson MB: Use of signals in the terminal QRS complex to identify patients with ventricular tachycardia after myocardial infarction. Circu-lation 64:235, 1981.
4. Rozanski JJ, Mortara D, Myerburg RJ, Castellanos A: Body surface de-tection of delayed depolarizations in patients with recurrent ventricular tachycardia and left ventricular aneurysm. Circulation 63:1172, 1981.
5. Breithardt G, Seipel L, Ostermeyer J, Karbenn V, Abendroth R-R, Borg-grefe M, Yeh HL, Birks W: Effects of antiarrhythmic surgery on late ventricular potentials recorded by precordial signal averaging in pa-tients with ventricular tachycardia. Am Heart J 104:996, 1982.

6. Simson MB, Untereker WJ, Spielman SR, Horowitz LN, Marcus NH, Falcone RA, Harken AH, Josephson ME: Relation between late potentials on the body surface and directly recorded fragmented electrograms in patients with ventricular tachycardia. Am J Cardiol 57:105, 1983.
7. Harris AS: Delayed development of ventricular ectopic rhythms following experimental coronary occlusion. Circulation 1:1318, 1950.
8. Boineau JP, Cox JL: Slow ventricular activation in acute myocardial infarction: a source of reentrant premature ventricular contraction. Circulation 48:702, 1973.
9. Waldo AL, Kaiser GA: A study of ventricular arrhythmias associated with acute myocardial infarction in the canine heart. Circulation 47:1222, 1973.
10. Scherlag BJ, El-Sherif N, Hope RR, Lazzara R: Characterization and localization of ventricular arrhythmias resulting from myocardial ischaemia and infarction. Circ Res 35:372, 1974.
11. El-Sherif N, Scherlag BJ, Lazzara R: Electrode catheter recording during malignant ventricular arrhythmias following experimental acute myocardial ischemia: evidence for reentry due to conduction block in ischemic myocardium. Circulation 51:1003, 1975.
12. Kaplinsky E, Ogawa S, Balke CW, Dreifus LS: Two periods of early ventricular arrhythmia in the canine acute myocardial infarction model. Circulation 60:397, 1979.
13. Simson MB, Euler D, Michelson EL, Falcone RA, Spear JF, Moore EN: Detection of delayed ventricular activation on the body surface in dogs. Am J Physiol 241:H363, 1981.
14. Murdock DK, Lamb JM, Euler DE, Randall WC: Electrophysiology of coronary artery reperfusion: a mechanism for reperfusion arrhythmias. Circulation 61:175, 1980.
15. Wit AL: Electrophysiological mechanisms of ventricular tachycardia caused by myocardial ischemia and infarction in animals. In Josephson ME (ed): Ventricular Tachycardia: Mechanism and Management. Mt Kisco, NY: Futura Publishing Co, 1982, p. 33.
16. Janse MJ, Kleber AG: Electrophysiological changes and ventricular arrhythmias in the early phase of regional myocardial ischemia. Circ Res 49:1069, 1981.
17. El-Sherif N, Scherlag BJ, Lazzara R, Hope RR: Reentrant ventricular arrhythmias in the late myocardial infarction period. I. Conduction characteristics in the infarction zone. Circulation 55:686, 1977.
18. Fenoglio JJ, Pham TD, Harken AH, Horowitz LN, Josephson ME, Wit AL: Recurrent sustained ventricular tachycardia. Structure and ultrastructure of subendocardial regions in which tachycardia originates. Circulation 68:518, 1983.
19. Berbari EJ, Scherlag BJ, Hope RR, Lazzara R: Recording from the body surface of arrhythmogenic ventricular activity in the ST segment. Am J Cardiol 41:697, 1978.
20. Kertes PJ, Glabus M, Murray A, Julian DG, Campbell RWF: Delayed ventricular depolarization—correlation with ventricular activation and relevance to ventricular fibrillation in acute myocardial infarction. Eur Heart J 5:974, 1984.
21. Gomes JA, Mehra R, Barreca P, El-Sherif N, Hariman R, Holtzmann R:

Quantitative analysis of the high frequency components of the signal-averaged QRS complex in patients with acute myocardial infarction: a prospective study. Circulation 72:105, 1985.

22. Fishbein MC, Maclean D, Maroko PR: The histopathological evolution of acute myocardial infarction. Chest 73:843, 1978.

23. Ursell PC, Gardner PI, Albala A, Fenoglio JJ, Wit AL: Structural and electrophysiological changes in the epicardial border zone of canine myocardial infarcts during infarct healing. Circ Res 56:436, 1985.

24. Kuchar D, McGuire M, Ganis J, Thorburn C, Sammel N: Evolution of late potentials during the first 10 days after acute myocardial infarction. J Am Coll Cardiol 9:224A, 1987.

25. Kuchar DL, Thorburn CW, Sammel NL: Late potentials detected after myocardial infarction: natural history and prognostic significance. Circulation 74:1280, 1986.

26. Denes P, Santarelli P, Hauser RG, Uretz EF: Quantitative analysis of the high frequency components of the terminal portion of the body surface QRS in normal subjects and in patients with ventricular tachycardia. Circulation 67:1129, 1983.

27. Kuchar DL: Comprehensive noninvasive risk stratification after myocardial infarction. MD Thesis, University of Sydney, 1986.

28. Breithardt G, Schwarzmaier J, Borgrefe M, Haerten K, Seipel L: Prognostic significance of ventricular late potentials after acute myocardial infarction. Eur Heart J 4:487, 1983.

29. Grigg L, Chan W, Summers P, Murphy A, Hunt D: Changes in the signal averaged ECG in the first year post myocardial infarction: a prospective study (abstr). Aust NZ J Med 17:576, 1987.

30. Denniss AR, Richards DAB, Farrow RH, Davison A, Uther JB: The use of signal-averaged vectorcardiography to predict patients with electrical instability after myocardial infarction (abstr). Aust NZ J Med 12:307, 1982.

31. Roy D, Marchand E, Theroux P, Waters DD, Pelletier GB, Bourassa MG: Reproducibility and significance of ventricular arrhythmias induced after an acute myocardial infarction (abstr). Circulation 70(Suppl II):II-18, 1984.

32. Bhandari AK, Au PK, Rose JS, Rahimtoola SH: Decline in inducibility of sustained ventricular tachycardia from 2 to 20 weeks after acute myocardial infarction. Am J Cardiol 59:284, 1987.

33. Duff HJ, Martin JME, Rahmberg M: Time-dependent changes in electrophysiologic milieu after myocardial infarction in conscious dogs. Circulation 77:209, 1988.

34. Garan H, Ruskin JN, McGovern B, Grant G: Serial analysis of electrically induced ventricular arrhythmias in a canine model of myocardial infarction. J Am Coll Cardiol 5:1095, 1985.

17

Late Potentials in the Post-Infarction Period: Correlation with the Ejection Fraction, Holter Monitoring, and Inducibility of Ventricular Tachycardia

J. Anthony Gomes, Stephen L. Winters

Introduction

Sustained ventricular tachycardia and ventricular fibrillation are the major cardiac rhythm disturbances that auger sudden death following an acute myocardial infarction. Although the ultimate factors that initiate a malignant ventricular arrhythmia are incompletely understood, the occurrence of acute ischemia, reinfarction, and the presence of an arrhythmic substrate characterized by inhomogenous and slow propagation of conduction in scarred myocardium, play a major role. Approximately 6%–10% of patients have sudden cardiac death in the first year following a myocardial infarction; however, the risk of developing a malignant arrhythmia is likely much higher in certain high-risk subsets of patients. Thus, identification of the patients at low- and high-risk is of clinical

From El-Sherif N, Turitto G (eds): *High-Resolution Electrocardiography*. Mount Kisco, NY, Futura Publishing Co., Inc., ©, 1992.

relevance, since appropriate therapeutic modalities may be applied to the high-risk group of patients. Thus, several investigators have attempted to risk stratify patients post-myocardial infarction by using clinical and a variety of noninvasive and invasive tests.[1-8] The noninvasive tests that have been used include 24-hour Holter monitoring, exercise testing, and radionuclide angiography. The invasive tests include programmed electrical stimulation and coronary angiography. Recently, the technique of signal averaging with high-gain amplification and filtering has been used to detect late potentials in the terminal QRS complex and the ST segment.[9-41] Late potentials detected by signal averaging of the surface QRS complex is an attractive noninvasive test for risk stratifying patients post-myocardial infarction because it is considered a noninvasive marker of the "arrhythmic substrate." Evidence for this concept is based on the following observations: (1) experimental and clinical studies have documented that the electrophysiologic basis of late potentials is slow and inhomogenous propagation of conduction in scarred myocardium; (2) late potentials seen in animal infarction models and in patients with ventricular tachycardia have been correlated with fragmented electrograms recorded from the epicardial and endocardial surface; (3) removal of the substrate by endocardial resection abolishes late potentials and this has been shown to correlate with noninducibility of ventricular tachycardia; (4) a good correlation has been observed between late potentials recorded by signal averaging of endocardial and epicardial electrograms and signal averaging of the surface QRS complex; and (5) late potentials have been recorded in a high proportion of patients with spontaneous as well as induced ventricular tachycardia.

The purpose of this chapter is to review the incidence and significance of late potentials relative to 24-hour ambulatory Holter monitoring, ejection fraction, site of myocardial infarction, and inducibility of ventricular tachycardia.

The Incidence of Late Potentials Following an Acute Myocardial Infarction

The incidence of late potentials or an abnormal signal-averaged electrocardiogram (ECG) has varied from study to study. This is related to several factors which include time of recording following an acute myocardial infarction, technique of recording, and variable definitions of what constitutes late potentials, or an abnormal signal-averaged ECG. McGuire and coworkers[34] assessed the natural history of late potentials in the first 10 days after acute myocardial infarction in 50 patients. The signal-averaged ECG was filtered at 40 Hz and late potentials were defined if the total filtered QRS complex was >120 msec in duration or the root mean square voltage of the terminal 40 msec (RMS40) was <20 μV. Late potentials were present in 32% of patients on day 1 post-acute infarction and increased progressively throughout the hospital stay. Late potentials were present in 52% of patients 7–10 days post-myocardial infarction. Recent prospective studies[40,41] on the natural history of late potentials suggest the following: (1) an initial normal signal-averaged ECG rarely becomes abnormal; and (2) 18% to 67% of abnormal signal-averaged ECGs become normal at 6 weeks to 3 months. At 6 months and 1 year, there is concordance between 3 months; however, Kuchar et al reported that 30% of abnormal recordings prior to discharge can become normal at 1 year.[40]

It is important to note that the incidence of an abnormal signal-averaged ECG is dependent on the high-pass filtering as well as on the quantitative variable. In a study of 115 patients (10 ±6 days post-myocardial infarction) reported from our laboratory,[35] the duration of the signal-averaged QRS was abnormal (>114 msec) in 26 of 115 patients (23%), whereas the RMS40 was abnormal (<20 μ v) in 40 of 115 patients (35%), and the duration of low amplitude signals (>38 msec) was abnormal in 34 of 115 patients (30%) at 40-Hz high-pass filtering. If an abnormal signal-averaged ECG was defined as ≥1 abnormal parameter, then 48 of 115 (42%) had an abnormal signal-averaged ECG; ≥2 abnormal parameters, then 31 of 115 patients (27%) had an abnormal signal averaged ECG. Whereas, if an abnormal duration of the signal-averaged QRS complex as well as an abnormal RMS40 were used to define an abnormal signal-averaged ECG, only 16 of 115 patients (14%) were classified as abnormal. These observations are of considerable importance since the predictive value of late potentials or an abnormal signal-averaged ECG will depend on the variables used to define the abnormality.

The incidence of an abnormal signal-averaged ECG (≥1 quantitative variable) is greater in patients with inferior or inferoposterior infarcts when compared to patients with anteroseptal or anterior infarcts (56% vs 27%) (Table I). This observation is likely related to two factors. (1) Differences in depolarization of the inferoposterior segments of the left ventricle relative to the anteroseptal and ante-

Table I

Clinical and Other Noninvasive Variables in Patients With Abnormal Signal-Averaged ECG and a Normal Signal-Averaged ECG

	Abnormal SA-ECG	Normal SA-ECG	P Value
No	48	68	
Age (yrs)	64 ± 10	62 ± 13	n.s.
Sex (m/f)	38/10	42/24	
Site of MI			
Anterior	15	48	0.002
Inferior	28	22	0.006
Non-Q wave	5	5	n.s.
Peak CK (u/L)	1417 ± 1215	1219 ± 1373	n.s.
EF (%)	35 ± 13	39 ± 12	n.s.
VPCs			
0 or < 10/hr	17/40	24/54	n.s.
≥ 10/hr	2/40	4/54	n.s.
Couplets	11/40	18/54	n.s.
Triplets	10/40	8/54	n.s.

CK = creatine kinase; EF = ejection fraction; MI = myocardial infarction; SA = signal averaged; n.s. = not significant; VPCs = ventricular premature complexes. (Modified from Gomes et al, J Am Coll Cardiol 13:377, 1988.)

rior segments of the left ventricle. Because activation of the infero-posterior segments of the left ventricle is later than that of the anterior segments, patients with inferior wall myocardial infarction are more likely to demonstrate abnormalities in the terminal QRS complex, whereas patients with anterior wall myocardial infarction may reveal abnormalities in the initial part of the QRS complex. For patients with anterior wall infarctions to demonstrate significant abnormalities in the terminal QRS complex, they will need conduction delays to outlast depolarization of the inferoposterior walls. (2) In anteroseptal or anterior wall infarction, a higher voltage generated by normal inferoposterior wall activation during slow regional depolarization of the anterior wall may mask low amplitude signals in the terminal QRS complex due to superimposition effect. These are important considerations that have clinical significance, since the predictive value of the signal-averaged ECG will also depend on the site of myocardial infarction.[35]

The Relationship Between the Signal-Averaged ECG and Left Ventricular Ejection Fraction Post-Myocardial Infarction

In patients post-myocardial infarction, we have found no relationship between the signal-averaged ECG and left ventricular ejection fraction (EF) determined by radionuclide ventriculography. In a study[35] of 110 patients post-myocardial infarction in whom the signal-averaged ECG and radionuclide ventriculography were performed within 10 ±6 days of the index infarction, patients with an abnormal signal-averaged ECG had similar EFs when compared to patients with a normal signal-averaged ECG (Table II). No significant correlation was noted between the RMS40 and EF (r = 0.198), between the duration of the low amplitude signals and EF (r = 0.063), and between the duration of the signal-averaged QRS complex and the EF (r = 0.326). These observations concur with our findings that patients with an abnormal signal-averaged ECG did not reveal significant differences in the peak CPK when compared to patients with a normal signal-averaged ECG.

Some previous studies have noted a good correlation between the presence of late potentials and wall motion abnormalities in patients with coronary artery disease. Breithardt et al[42] found late potentials in 34% of their patients without ventricular tachycardia, of whom 42% had dyskinesis, 22% had hypokinesis, and 40% had akinesis. Zimmerman et al[32] and Abboud et al[43] reported a higher

Table II
Left Ventricular Wall Motion Abnormalities in Patients With and Without Late Potentials

	EF (%)	Dyskinesis	Akinesis	N/H
Late potentials (+)	38 ±14	57%	29%	14%
Late potentials (−)	36 ±12	62%	10%	28%
P value	n.s.	n.s.	n.s.	n.s.

EF = ejection fraction; N/H = normal or hypokinetic; n.s. = not significant. (Modified with permission from Gomes et al, Am J Cardiol 59:1071, 1987.)

incidence of late potentials in patients with left ventricular aneurysm in the absence of ventricular tachycardia. We performed a prospective study[20] in 50 patients with acute myocardial infarction to determine the relationship between late potentials and wall motion abnormalities. Signal averaging of the surface QRS complex and radionuclide ventriculography were performed within 8 ± 5 days of the acute myocardial infarction. A wall motion score was constructed according to the method of Hecht and Hopkins[44] and Currie et al.[45] The left and right ventricles were separated into a total of 21 segments (Figure 1) in the anterior, left anterior oblique, and lateral views. Wall motion was scored in the following manner: normal segment = 4; hypokinesis = 3; akinesis = 2; and dyskinesis = 1. Thus, a normal segment had the best score and a dyskinetic segment the worst score. A patient with a normal right and left ventricle would have a total score of 84. The prevalence of dyskinesis, akinesis, hypokinesis, and normal wall motion was also assessed. There was no significant difference in the distribution of wall motion abnormalities in patients with and without late potentials (Table II). The total wall motion score for the left ventricle (47 ± 13 vs 49 ± 10) and right ventricle (13 ± 3 vs 14 ± 3) and the combined wall motion scores were not significantly different in patients with and without late potentials. Thus, our observations suggest that the type and degree of wall motion abnormalities is not the source of late potentials in patients post-myocardial infarction. It is possible that the source of late potentials in these patients is the amount of viable myocardium in the infarcted zone or the regional slow ventricular activation in the border zone of the infarct.

RADIONUCLIDE VENTRICULOGRAM

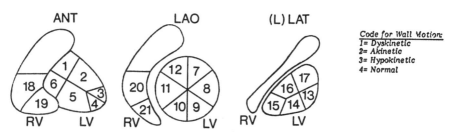

Figure 1. Code for wall motion scores on radionuclide ventriculography. The left and right ventricles are separated into 21 segments. ANT = anterior; LAO = left anterior oblique; (L) LAT = left lateral; RV = right ventricle; LV = left ventricle. (Modified with permission from Gomes et al, Am J Cardiol 59:1071, 1987.)

Of considerable interest is our observation that the ejection fraction and signal-averaged ECG reveal opposing information in relation to the site of myocardial infarction. Whereas a higher proportion of patients with an anterior wall myocardial infarction have an abnormal EF of <40% when compared to patients with an inferior wall myocardial infarction (66% vs 32%), a higher number of patients with an inferior wall myocardial infarction have an abnormal signal-averaged ECG when compared to patients with an anterior wall myocardial infarction (56% vs 27%).[35] Thus, the predictive value of the two tests will depend on the site of myocardial infarction.[35]

The Relationship Between the Signal-Averaged ECG and Results of 24-Hour Holter Monitoring

In a prospective study[35] of 94 patients post-infarction in whom a signal-averaged ECG and 24-hour Holter was obtained within 10 ±6 days of the index infarction, we found no relationship between the presence or absence of an abnormal signal-averaged ECG and the frequency and characteristics of ventricular premature complexes (Table I).

Thus, our studies suggest that the signal-averaged ECG, ejection fraction, and the frequency and characteristics of ventricular premature complexes on a Holter are independent of each other.

The Prognostic Significance of the Signal-Averaged ECG

Prospective follow-up studies[21,22,30,33,35,40] in a large number of patients post-myocardial infarction have shown that patients with an abnormal signal-averaged ECG (assessed qualitatively or quantitatively) have a significantly greater arrhythmic event rate of 17% to 27%, when compared to patients with a normal signal-averaged ECG in whom the event rates were 1% to 4% for a follow-up period of 14 ±5 months. However, the predictive value of the signal-averaged ECG is dependent on the quantitative variable, high-pass filtering, site of myocardial infarction, and time of recording in the post-infarction period. To assess these aspects prospectively, we studied[35] 115 patients in whom a signal-averaged ECG was obtained within 10 ±6 days of the index infarction and the patients were followed for 14 ± 8 months. Sixteen patients or 14%, had an arrhythmic event defined as sustained ventricular tachycardia or sudden death, or both, within 8 to 150 days of the infarction. Both at 25- and 40-Hz high-pass filtering, patients with abnormal quantitative parameters had higher event rates (Table III). The sensitivity of an abnormal signal-averaged ECG (≥1 variable) was 81% and the specificity was 65% at 40-Hz high-pass filtering. Sensitivity and specificity values were slightly better at 40 Hz when compared to 25-Hz high-pass filtering. Kuchar et al[40] reported a higher sensitivity of 92% than that noted in our study; however, the specificity was quite comparable in the two studies. The sensitivity and specificity of the signal-averaged ECG was dependent on the quantitative variable (Table III). A marked improvement in specificity (95%) occurred if an abnormal signal-averaged ECG was defined as a combination of abnormal signal-averaged QRS duration and RMS40. This combination also provided the highest positive predictive value of 58%.

Table III

Relation Between Quantitative Signal-Averaged Variables and Arrhythmic Event Rates

	Event Rate		Sn	Sp
SA-Variables (25 Hz)	Abnormal	Normal	%	%
SA-QRS duration	10/26	6/89	63	84
RMS40	9/31	7/84	56	78
LAS	12/33	4/82	75	78
≥1 variable	12/51	4/64	75	61
≥2 variables	10/26	6/89	62	84
SA-QRS + RSMS40	8/16	8/99	50	92
SA-Variables (40 Hz)				
SA-QRS duration	10/26	6/89	63	84
RMS40	13/40	3/75	81	73
LAS	11/34	5/81	69	77
≥1 variable	13/48	3/67	81	65
≥2 variables	11/31	5/84	69	80
SA-QRS + RMS40	9/16	7/99	56	95

LAS = low amplitude signals of <40 μV; RMS40 = root mean square voltage of last 40 msec of QRS; Sn = sensitivity; Sp = specificity. (Modified with permission from Gomes et al, J Am Coll Cardiol 13:377, 1988.)

Of considerable importance was our observation[35] that the signal-averaged ECG had a sensitivity of 100% in patients with inferior wall myocardial infarction and a lower sensitivity of 75% in patients with anterior infarction. In contrast, the specificity was better in patients with anterior wall infarction than inferior wall infarction (80% vs 50%) in predicting arrhythmic events post-myocardial infarction. The predictive value of the EF in relation to the site of myocardial infarction markedly contrasts with that of the signal-averaged ECG. Whereas the EF had a higher sensitivity than the signal-averaged ECG (87% vs 75%) in predicting arrhythmic events in anterior wall myocardial infarction, the signal-averaged ECG had a better specificity than the EF (80% vs 38%). Similarly, whereas the signal-averaged ECG had a better sensitivity than the EF (100% vs 50%) in predicting arrhythmic events in inferior wall myocardial infarction, the specificity of the EF was better than that of the signal-averaged ECG (71% vs 50%). Clearly, these observations are of considerable clinical importance, since they raise important issues regarding the usefulness of these two tests in predicting arrhythmic events in different types of myocardial infarction. Further studies in a large number of patients are needed to confirm our observations.

The prognostic significance of the signal-averaged ECG relative to its time of recording in the post-infarction period has been recently assessed by El-Sherif et al.[46] Serial recordings of the SA-ECG and 24-hour ambulatory ECG were obtained in 156 patients with myocardial infarction in 3 phases: phase 1 (0–5 days); phase 2 (6–30 days); and phase 3 (31–60 days). Left ventricular EF was determined in phase 2. Eight patients developed VT/VF in the first 48 hours of myocardial infarction, only one of these patients had an abnormal signal-averaged ECG. Twelve patients developed late arrhythmic events during the first year of follow-up. Stepwise logistic regression analysis showed that an abnormal signal-averaged ECG in phase 2 had the most significant relationship to late arrhythmic events.

Independent Prognostic Value of the Signal-Averaged ECG

The independent prognostic value of the signal-averaged ECG in predicting arrhythmic events post-myocardial infarction has been confirmed in three large prospective studies.[33,35,40,46] In one of these,[40] the radionuclide EF and an abnormal signal-averaged ECG, defined as the presence of an RMS40 <20 μV or a filtered QRS of >120 msec at 40-Hz high-pass filtering, were independently significant by logistic regression analysis. In contrast, the frequency and characteristics of ventricular premature complexes on a 24-hour Holter were not independently significant. Our initial study[33] in 102 patients showed that the EF, the signal-averaged ECG and the presence of nonsustained ventricular tachycardia (≥3 ventricular premature complexes in a row) were independently significant when assessed in the Cox survivorship analysis. Subsequently, we assessed the independent prognostic value of 27 clinical and noninvasive variables, including quantitative signal averaging at 25-Hz and 40-Hz high-pass filtering in the Cox model in 115 patients.[35] This analysis showed that the total duration of the signal-averaged QRS complex at 40-Hz high-pass filtering (improvement X^2 = 16.5, p = 0.0001), couplets on 24-hour Holter recording (improvement X^2 = 5.39, p = 0.04), and EF (improvement X^2 = 4.1, p = 0.04) had the most significant relationship to an arrhythmic event. This suggests that the duration of the signal-averaged QRS complex is the most important single variable relative to other signal-averaged variables and the results of 24-hour Holter monitoring and EF determined by radionuclide ventriculography. It is possible that an abnormal duration of the signal-averaged QRS complex in the absence of bundle branch block reflects a greater mass of ventricular myocardium with abnormally slow and inhomogenous propagation of conduction, thereby facilitating the occurrence of reentrant ventricular tachycardia or fibrillation.

The Combined Noninvasive Index in Predicting Ventricular Arrhythmias

Because of the independent nature of the signal-averaged ECG, EF, and results of 24-hour Holter monitoring in relation to each other and to future arrhythmic events, we assessed the combination of these three tests to risk stratify patients. The signal-averaged ECG was considered as abnormal if ≥1 variable was abnormal; an abnormal EF was dichotomized at <40% and an abnormal 24-hour

Holter was taken as the presence of high grade ventricular ectopy (i.e., the presence of ≥10 ventricular premature complexes/hour and/or couplets and/or triplets). Although the presence of any abnormal test was associated with a higher arrhythmic event rate than when a test was normal, the combination of two abnormal tests provided with an arrhythmic event rate of 35% to 37% (Table IV). The combination of an abnormal EF and an abnormal signal-averaged ECG was associated with the highest odds ratio of 30.1.[35] When these two tests were normal, no arrhythmic events were noted. Likewise, Kuchar et al[30] found a 34% event rate when these two tests were abnormal. When all three tests were abnormal (Figure 2) the arrhythmic event rate was 50%, as compared to no events when these three tests were normal.[34] These original observations have been confirmed in a recent study by El-Sherif et al.[46] These investigators have noted a 54% event rate in patients with an abnormal SA-ECG, EF of <40%, and complex ectopy. In contrast, the event rate was only 2% in patients in whom these tests were normal. We believe that the combined noninvasive index may be useful in clinical practice in selecting high-risk patients for extended coronary care unit monitoring. Furthermore, these high-risk patients are optimally suited to assess the role of antiarrhythmic therapy and antitachycardia devices.

Table IV

Relationship Between the Signal-Averaged ECG, Ejection Fraction, Holter Monitoring, and Arrhythmic Events

	Normal (%)	Abnormal (%)	P Value	Odds Ratio
SA-ECG	1/57(3.5%)	13/45(29%)	0.003	11
EF	3/47(6%)	12/50(24%)	0.01	4.6
Holter	3/32(91%)	12/52(23%)	0.09	2.9
SA-ECG + EF	0/26(0%)	10/28(36%)	0.0007	30.1
SA-ECG + Holter	0/14(0%)	9/26(35%)	0.01	15.7
EF + Holter	1/16(6%)	11/30(37%)	0.025	8.7
SA-ECG + EF + Holter	0/9(0%)	8/16(50%)	0.01	19

EF = ejection fraction; SA-ECG = signal-averaged ECG. (Reprinted with permission from Gomes et al, J Am Coll Cardiol 13:377, 1988.)

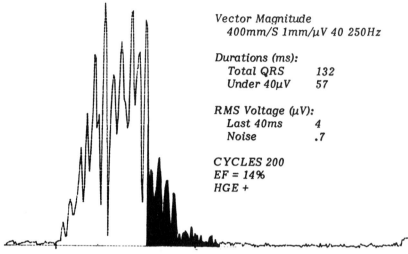

Vector Magnitude
400mm/S 1mm/μV 40 250Hz

Durations (ms):
  Total QRS   132
  Under 40μV   57

RMS Voltage (μV):
  Last 40ms   4
  Noise   .7

CYCLES 200
EF = 14%
HGE +

Figure 2. Vector magnitude showing late potentials in a patient post-myocardial infarction. The patient had a markedly abnormal signal-averaged ECG (SA-QRS = 132 msec; duration of low amplitude signals = 57 msec and RMS voltage = 4 μV). Additionally, the patient had an EF of 14% and high grade ectopy on the Holter. This patient subsequently developed recurrent sustained ventricular tachycardia 3 weeks post-myocardial infarction. (Modified with permission from Gomes et al, J Am Coll Cardiol 10:349, 1987.)

Relationship Between Late Potentials and Inducibility of Ventricular Tachycardia in Patients With High-Grade Ventricular Ectopy Post-Myocardial Infarction

Several studies [47–52] have shown that the results of programmed ventricular stimulation in patients with complex forms of ventricular ectopy, including nonsustained ventricular tachycardia, have prognostic long-term significance. In a few of these studies which discussed subgroups of patients who were status post-remote myocardial infarction, the lack of inducible ventricular tachycardia was associated with spontaneous episodes of ventricular tachyarrhythmias or sudden death in only 2% to 12% over long-term follow-up. While most of the patients who had no inducible ventricular tachyarrhythmias did not receive antiarrhythmic therapy, most of those with inducible arrhythmias received electrophysiologic guided therapy. In this latter group, there was an event rate of 12% to 32% for follow-up periods of up to 3 years, despite therapy (antiarrhythmic agents only in most cases). In view of the aforementioned findings, we sought to extend our observations to individuals referred for evaluation of complex ventricular ectopy post-remote myocardial infarction. This group was comprised of 46 individuals without documented sustained ventricular arrhythmias or sudden death who had no bundle branch block and were on no antiarrhythmic therapy. All individuals had complex ventricular ectopy defined as the presence of nonsustained ventricular tachycardia, 10 or more ventricular premature complexes/hour, or paired ventricular premature beats. With the exception of three patients who were 3 to 4-weeks status post-myocardial infarction, all were months to years post-myocardial infarction.

All individuals underwent signal-averaged electrocardiography prior to programmed ventricular stimulation. Thirty patients had an abnormal (≥ 1 abnormal parameter), and 16 had a normal signal-averaged ECG. The mean ages, sites of myocardial infarction, presence of prior syncopal episodes, and left ventricular ejection fraction were similar in the two groups of individuals (Table V). Regardless of the results of the signal-averaged ECGs, all individuals underwent programmed ventricular stimulation in the fasting, antiarrhythmic drug-free state. Standard quadripolar electrode catheters were positioned at multiple sites of the right heart. Programmed stimulation was performed at basic drive cycle lengths of 600 msec and 400 msec, or 450 msec with single and double premature stimuli, as previously described. If no ventricular tachyarrhythmia was initiated, burst ventricular pacing was done to cycle lengths where ventricular pacing exit block occurred or to 220 msec. When no ventricular tachycardia was initiated from the right ventricular apex, stimulation was carried out from the right ventricular outflow tract. The impact of aggressive (i.e., S_4, left ventricular, or post-isoproterenol infusion) stimulation was not evaluated in this study.

None of the individuals with normal signal-averaged ECGs had inducible ventricular tachycardia, whereas 16 (53%) of those with abnormal signal-averaged ECGs had inducible ventricular tachycardia. Twelve of the inducible patients had sustained monomorphic ventricular tachycardia and four patients had reproducible nonsustained monomorphic ventricular tachycardia (i.e., five or more repetitive ventricular responses). Ventricular fibrillation or polymorphous ventricular tachycardia was not induced in any of the

Table V

Characteristics of Individuals With Complex Ventricular Ectopy Remotely Post-Myocardial Infarction

	Abnormal SA-ECG (n = 30)	Normal SA-ECG (n = 16)
Age	64 + 12 yrs	58 + 8 yrs
AWMI	10(33%)	5(31%)
IWMI	18(60%)	8(50%)
Other MI	2(7%)	3(18%)
Syncope	6(20%)	5(31%)
LVEF	34 ± 15%	41 ± 15%
Ak./Dysk.	18(60%)	9(56%)
Dysk.	11(37%)	5(32%)

Ak./Dysk. = one or more akinetic or dyskinetic left ventricular segments; Dysk. = one or more dyskinetic left ventricular segments; AWMI = anterior wall myocardial infarction; IWMI = inferior wall myocardial infarction; MI = myocardial infarction; LVEF = left ventricular ejection fraction; SA-ECG = signal-averaged electrocardiogram.

patients. Patients who had no inducible ventricular tachycardia were recommended no antiarrhythmic therapy. Patients who had ventricular tachycardia induced underwent antiarrhythmic drug therapy by serial electrophysiologic studies.

Stepwise multivariate regression analysis was performed to determine the most significant independent parameter for predicting inducibility. The parameters evaluated included: age; site of myocardial infarction; presence of prior syncope; left ventricular EF; and the presence of akinetic or dyskinetic left ventricular wall segments. The significant variables in order of greatest confidence levels were: the presence of an abnormal signal-averaged ECG ($p = 0.0001$); the presence of a prior syncopal episode ($p = 0.019$); and age ($p = 0.035$). Among the 30 patients with abnormal signal-averaged ECGs, 12 (75%) who had inducible ventricular tachycardia had two or more abnormal variables, whereas 6 of the 14 (45%) noninducible patients had two or more abnormal variables. The optimal sensitivity (75%) and specificity (80%) were found when two or more of the three signal-averaged electrocardiographic parameters were evaluated. A predictive accuracy of 78% was associated with the presence of two or more abnormal signal-averaged parameters. Of note, 6 of the 16 (38%) inducible patients had had prior syncopal episodes, whereas none of the patients with abnormal signal-averaged electrocardiograms who were noninducible had syncope (p <0.05).

Follow-up of the group of individuals with abnormal signal-averaged ECG was completed over 20 ±12 months and 16 ±12 months for those with normal signal-averaged ECGs. During this time period, 3 of the 16 (19%) inducible patients in this group had a sustained ventricular tachyarrhythmia or sudden death. Of the other 14 individuals, 11 (79%) received no antiarrhythmic agents, and 1 of these died secondary to a malignant neoplasm. The other three were treated with antiarrhythmic agents for control of supraventricular tachyarrhythmias, or at the referring physician's discretion, and had no significant arrhythmic events. Of the 16 patients with normal signal-averaged ECGs and no inducible ventricular tachycardia, 1 patient (on no therapy) was lost to follow-up. Of the other ten individuals not treated with antiarrhythmic agents, no sustained ventricular tachyarrhythmic events occurred. Three patients received antiarrhythmic therapy, either for control of a supraventricular arrhythmia or at the referring physician's preference. One of these latter patients developed sustained ventricular tachycardia for the first time while on treatment with procainamide.

Previous work reported by several independent investigators has demonstrated a role for risk stratification using programmed electrical stimulation in patients with high grade ventricular ectopy and various cardiac disorders.[47-52] However, breakdown of the patient groups demonstrated that individuals with prior myocardial infarction were at greatest risk for inducible ventricular tachycardia. Thus, this study focused specifically on individuals with prior myocardial infarction. Due to the possible fluctuations in the underlying myocardial substrate in the first few weeks post-myocardial infarction, this time period was excluded. Furthermore, the results of programmed stimulation have also been considered to be controversial in this early post-infarction period. Thus, with the exception of three patients, all individuals had been months or years post-myocardial infarction. Mean intervals from the time of myocardial infarction could not be estimated, since the date of myocardial infarction could not be documented in one-third of the patients.

Of marked significance and clinical utility, none of the individuals with a normal signal-averaged ECG had inducible ventricular tachycardia or a significant clinical arrhythmic event on follow-up. Thus, support is provided for consideration of withholding antiarrhythmic treatment from such patients without the need for invasive programmed ventricular stimulation. In agreement with previous studies, the presence of syncope in patients with normal signal-averaged ECGs and high grades of ventricular ectopy portends a low likelihood of inducible ventricular tachycardia or spontaneous sustained ventricular tachycardia, despite prior myocardial infarction. With respect to the presence of an abnormal signal-averaged ECG in patients with a prior myocardial infarction and complex ventricular ectopy, the only clinical variable which differed significantly between the groups with and without inducible ventricular tachycardia was syncope. Yet, the majority of patients with inducible ventricular tachycardia (10 out of 16 or 63%) did not have a history of syncope. The lack of inducible ventricular tachycardia in these patients with an abnormal signal-averaged ECG was still associated with a good prognosis. In this study, one of the patients who underwent nonrecommended antiarrhythmic therapy not guided by electrophysiologic testing developed a significant arrhythmic event. Although this may or may not have been a cause and effect relationship, the occurrence of a higher incidence of sustained arrhythmic events was found in a group of patients with nonsustained ventricular tachycardia who underwent nonelectrophysiologic guided antiarrhythmic therapy reported by Buxton et al.[50] The incidence of clinically significant ventricular arrhythmias in our patients with abnormal signal-averaged ECGs and inducible ventricular tachycardia who underwent antiarrhythmic therapy guided by electrophysiologic study was approximately 20%. Similar findings to ours have been reported in patients with high grades of ventricular ectopy and inducible ventricular tachycardia.

The absence of inducible ventricular tachycardia or spontaneous arrhythmic events in 14 of the 30 (47%) patients with an abnormal signal-averaged ECG makes the management of patients with a prior myocardial infarction and complex ventricular ectopy difficult. One approach might be to perform programmed ventricular stimulation in individuals with abnormal signal-averaged ECGs and high grades of ventricular ectopy, and base further therapy on the results of stimulation studies. While an abnormal signal-averaged ECG may well reflect the underlying substrate capable of sustaining ventricular tachyarrhythmias, attention needs to be given to identification of possible triggers in this group, such as specific patterns of ectopic beats, beat-to-beat cycle length variability, and fluctuations in autonomic tone.

References

1. Fioretti P, Brower RW, Simonson ML, et al: Relative value of clinical variables, bicycle ergometry, rest radionuclide ventriculography, 24-hour ambulatory electrocardiographic monitoring at discharge to predict 1 year survival after myocardial infarction. J Am Coll Cardiol 8:40, 1986.
2. Schultze RA, Strauss HW, Pitt B: Sudden death in the year following myocardial infarction. Am J Med 62:192, 1977.
3. Bigger JT, Fleiss JL, Kleiger R, Miller JP, Rolnitzky LM, the Multicenter Post-Infarction Research Group: The relationship among ventricular arrhythmias, left ventricular dysfunction and mortality in the 2 years after myocardial infarction. Circulation 69:250, 1984.
4. Mukarji J, Rude RE, Poole WK, Gustafsen N, Thomas LJ, Jr, Strauss HW, Jaffe AS, Muller JE, Roberts R, Raabe DS, Jr, Crofe CH, Passamani E, Braunwald E, the MILIS Study Group: Risk factors for sudden death after acute myocardial infarction: two year follow-up. Am J Cardiol 54:31, 1984.
5. Hamer A, Vohra J, Hunt D, Sloman G: Prediction of sudden death by electrophysiologic studies in high-risk patients surviving acute myocardial infarction. Am J Cardiol 50:223, 1982.
6. Richards DA, Cody DV, Denniss AR, Russell PA, Young AA, Uther JB: Ventricular electrical instability: a predictor of death after myocardial infarction. Am J Cardiol 51:75, 1983.
7. Gomes JAC, Hariman RI, Kang PS, El-Sherif N, Chowdhry I, Lyons J: Programmed electrical stimulation in patients with high-grade ventricular ectopy: electrophysiologic findings and prognosis for survival. Circulation 70:43, 1984.
8. Waspe LE, Seinfeld D, Feerick A, Kim SG, Matos JA, Fisher JD: Prediction of sudden death and spontaneous ventricular tachycardia in survivors of complicated myocardial infarction: value of the response to programmed stimulation using a maximum of three ventricular extrastimuli. J Am Coll Cardiol 5:1292, 1985.
9. Berbari BJ, Scherlag RJ, Hope RR, Lazzara R: Recording from the body surface of arrhythmogenic ventricular activity during the ST segment. Am J Cardiol 41:697, 1978.
10. Fontaine G, Frank R, Gallais Hammono F, Allali I, Phan-Thuc H, Grosgogeat Y: Electrocardiographie des potentiels tardifs du syndrome de post-excitation. Arch Mal Coeur 78:854, 1978.
11. Rozanski JJ, Mortara D, Myerburg RJ, Castellanos A: Body surface detection of delayed depolarizations in patients with recurrent ventricular tachycardia and left ventricular aneurysm. Circulation 63:1172, 1981.

12. Simson MB: Use of signals in the terminal QRS complex to identify patients with ventricular tachycardia after myocardial infarction. Circulation 64:235, 1981.
13. Breithardt G, Becker R, Seipel L, Abendroth RR, Ostermeyer J: Noninvasive detection of late potentials in man: a new marker for ventricular tachycardia. Eur Heart J 2:1, 1981.
14. Denes P, Santarelli P, Hauser RG, Uretz EF: Quantitative analysis of the high-frequency components of the terminal portion of the body surface QRS in normal subjects and in patients with ventricular tachycardia. Circulation 67:1129, 1983.
15. Gomes JAC, Mehra R, Barreca P, El-Sherif N, Hariman R, Holtzman R: Quantitative analysis of the high frequency components of the signal-averaged QRS complex in acute myocardial infarction. Circulation 72: 102, 1985.
16. El-Sherif N, Gomes JAC, Restivo M, Mehra R: Late potentials and arrhythmogenesis. PACE 8:440, 1985.
17. Simson MB, Untereker WJ, Spielman SR, Horowitz LN, Marcus NH, Falcone RA, Harken AH, Josephson ME: Relation between late potentials on the body surface and directly recorded fragmented electrograms in patients with ventricular tachycardia. Am J Cardiol 57:105, 1983.
18. Kanovsky MS, Falcone RA, Dresden CA, Josephson ME, Simson MB: Identification of patients with ventricular tachycardia after myocardial infarction: signal-averaged electrocardiogram, Holter monitoring and cardiac catheterization. Circulation 79:264, 1984.
19. Gomes JAC, Mehra R, Barreca P, Winters SL, Ergin A, Estioko M, Minditch BP: A comparative analysis of signal averaging of the surface QRS complex and intracardiac electrode recordings in patients with ventricular tachycardia. PACE 11:271, 1988.
20. Gomes JAC, Horowitz S, Milner, M, Machac J, Winters SL, Barreca P: Signal averaging of the QRS complex in myocardial infarction: relationship between ejection fraction and wall motion abnormalities. Am J Cardiol 59:1071, 1987.
21. Breithardt G, Borggrefe M, Haarten K: Role of programmed ventricular stimulation and non-invasive recording of ventricular late potentials for the identification of patients at risk of ventricular arrhythmias after acute myocardial infarction. In Zipes DP, Jalife J (eds); Cardiac Electrophysiology and Arrhythmias. Orlando, FL: Grune & Stratton, 1984, pp 553–561.
22. Denniss AR, Richard DA, Cody DV, Russell PA, Young AA, Cooper MJ, Ross DL, Uther JB: Prognostic significance of ventricular tachycardia and fibrillation induced at programmed stimulation and delayed potentials detected on the signal-averaged electrocardiograms of survivors of acute myocardial infarction. Circulation 74:731, 1986.
23. Gomes JA, Winters SL, Stewart D, Targonski A, Barreca P: Optimal band pass filters for time domain analysis of the signal-averaged electrocardiogram. Am J Cardiol 60:1290, 1987.
24. Nalos PC, Gang ES, Mandel WJ, Ladenheim ML, Lass Y, Peter T: The signal-averaged electrocardiogram as a screening test for inducibility of sustained ventricular tachycardia in high-risk patients: a prospective study. J Am Coll Cardiol 9:539, 1987.
25. Lindsay BD, Ambos HP, Schectman KB, Cain ME: Improved selection

of patients for programmed ventricular stimulation by requiring analysis of signal-averaged electrocardiograms. Circulation 73:675, 1986.

26. Gomes JAC, Winters SL: Clinical uses of the signal-averaged electrocardiogram. CVR&R 25:8, 1988.

27. Winters SL, Stewart D, Gomes JAC: Signal averaging of the surface QRS complex predicts inducibility of ventricular tachycardia in patients with syncope of unknown origin: a prospective study. J Am Coll Cardiol 10:775, 1987.

28. Gang ES, Peter T, Rosenthal ME, Mandel WJ, Lass Y: Detection of late potentials on the surface electrocardiogram in unexplained syncope. Am J Cardiol 58:1014, 1986.

29. Kuchar DL, Thorburn CW, Sammel NL: Signal-averaged electrocardiogram for evaluation of recurrent syncope. Am J Cardiol 58:949, 1986.

30. Kuchar DL, Thorburn CW, Sammel NL: Prediction of serious arrhythmic events after myocardial infarction: signal-averaged electrocardiogram, Holter monitoring and radionuclide ventriculography. J Am Coll Cardiol 9:531, 1987.

31. Itoh S, Kobayaski K, Fukuzak H: Clinical study of late potentials: serial changes of late potentials in relation to ventricular arrhythmias and hemodynamic findings in acute myocardial infarction. Jpn Circ J 51:15, 1987.

32. Zimmerman M, Adamec R, Simonin P, Richez J: Prognostic significance of ventricular late potentials in coronary artery disease. Am Heart J 109:725, 1985.

33. Gomes JA, Winters SL, Stewart D, Horowitz S, Milner M, Barreca P: A new noninvasive index to predict sustained ventricular tachycardia and sudden death in the first year after myocardial infarction: based on signal-averaged electrocardiogram, radionuclide ejection fraction and Holter monitoring. J Am Coll Cardiol 10:349, 1987.

34. McGuire M, Kuchar D, Ganes J, Sammel N, Thorburn C: Natural history of late potentials in the first ten days after acute myocardial infarction and relation to early ventricular arrhythmias. Am J Cardiol 61:1187, 1988.

35. Gomes JA, Winters SL, Martinson M, Machac J, Stewart D, Targonsky A: The prognostic significance of quantitative signal-averaged variables relative to clinical variables, site of myocardial infarction, ejection fraction and ventricular premature beats: a prospective study. J Am Coll Cardiol 13:377, 1988.

36. Grimm M, Billhardt RA, Mayerhofer KE, Denes P: Prognostic significance of signal-averaged ECG's during acute myocardial infarction: a preliminary report. J Electrocardiol 21:283, 1988.

37. Gomes JA, Winters SL, Ergin A, Targonski A, Stewart D, Cohen M, Estioko M, Sherman W: The clinical electrophysiologic determinants and survival of patients with sustained ventricular tachycardia early post myocardial infarction (abstr). J Am Coll Cardiol 11:182A, 1988.

38. Vatterott PJ, Hammill SC, Bailey KA, Berbari EJ, Matheson SJ: Signal-averaged electrocardiography: a new non-invasive test to identify patients at risk for ventricular arrhythmias. Mayo Clin Proc 63:931, 1988.

39. Hall PAX, Atwood E, Myers J, Froelicher VF: The signal-averaged surface electrocardiogram and the identification of late potentials. Progr Cardiovasc Dis 31:295, 1989.

40. Kuchar DL, Thorburn CW, Sammel NL: Late potentials detected after myocardial infarction: natural history and prognostic significance. Circulation 74:1280, 1986.

41. Hong MA, Gang ES, Wang FZ, et al: Reproducibility of the signal-averaged ECG in the acute phase of myocardial infarction and at long-term follow-up (abstr). J Am Coll Cardiol 13:190A, 1988.

42. Breithardt G, Borggrefe M, Karbenn U, Abendroth RR, Yeh HL, Seipel L: Prevalence of late potentials in patients with and without ventricular tachycardia: correlation with angiographic findings. Am J Cardiol 49:-1932, 1982.

43. Abboud S, Belhassen B, Laniado S, Sadeh D: Non-invasive recording of late ventricular activity using an advanced method in patients with a damaged mass of ventricular tissue. J Electrocardiol 16:245, 1983.

44. Hecht HS, Hopkins JM: Exercise induced regional wall motion abnormalities on radionuclide angiography: index of reliability for detection of coronary artery disease in the presence of ventricular heart disease. Am J Cardiol 47:861, 1981.

45. Currie PJ, Kelly MU, Harper RW, et al: Incremental value of clinical assessment, supine exercise electrocardiography, and biplane exercise radionuclide ventriculography in the prediction of coronary artery disease in men with chest pain. Am J Cardiol 52:927, 1983.

46. El-Sherif N, Ursell SN, Bekheit S, Fontaine J, Turitto G, Henkin R, Caref EB: Prognostic significance of the signal-averaged electrocardiogram depends on the time of recording in the post-infarction period. Am Heart J 118:256, 1989.

47. Gomes JAC, Hariman RI, Kang PS, El-Sherif N, Chowdhry I, Lyons J: Programmed electrical stimulation in patients with high grade ventricular ectopy: electrophysiologic findings and prognosis for survival. Circulation 70:43, 1984.

48. Buxton AE, Marchlinski FE, Waxman HL, Flores BT, Cassidy DM, Josephson ME: Prognostic factors in non-sustained ventricular tachycardia. Am J Cardiol 53:1275, 1984.

49. Zheutlin TA, Roth H, Chua W, Steinman R, Summers C, Lesch M, Kehoe RF: Programmed electrical stimulation to determine the need for antiarrhythmic therapy in patients with complex ventricular ectopic activity. Am Heart J 111:860, 1986.

50. Buxton AE, Marchlinski FE, Flores BT, Miller JM, Doherty JU, Josephson ME: Nonsustained ventricular tachycardia in patients with coronary artery disease: role of electrophysiologic study. Circulation 75:-1178, 1987.

51. Winters SL, Stewart D, Targonski A, Gomes JA: Role of signal averaging of the surface QRS complex in selecting patients with nonsustained ventricular tachycardia and high-grade ventricular arrhythmias for programmed ventricular stimulation. J Am Coll Cardiol 12:1481, 1988.

52. Turitto G, Fontaine JM, Ursell SN, Carf EB, Henkin R, El-Sherif N: Value of the signal-averaged electrocardiogram as a predictor of the results of programmed stimulation in nonsustained ventricular tachycardia. Am J Cardiol 61:1272, 1988.

18

Late Potentials in the Post-Infarction Period: Correlation with Programmed Electrical Stimulation

A. Robert Denniss

Introduction

There has been considerable interest in recent years in the prognostic implications of inducible ventricular tachyarrhythmias[1-7] and late potentials[6,8-11] in survivors of recent myocardial infarction.

Most studies of programmed electrical stimulation in the post-infarction period, especially those with large patient numbers and a large number of study end points, have shown that inducible ventricular tachyarrhythmias sustained for at least 10 to 30 seconds can predict subsequent occurrence of death or spontaneous ventricular tachyarrhythmias.[7] Inducible monomorphic ventricular tachycardia (VT), but not inducible ventricular fibrillation (VF) is associated with adverse prognostic implications in survivors of recent myocar-

From El-Sherif N, Turitto G (eds): *High-Resolution Electrocardiography*. Mount Kisco, NY, Futura Publishing Co., Inc., ©, 1992.

dial infarction, at least in patients who have not exhibited spontaneous arrhythmias at the time of study.[6,8]

Although late potentials detected by the signal-averaged electrocardiogram (ECG) in the post-infarction period appear to have similar prognostic implications to inducible VT,[6] there have been few studies examining specifically the correlation between the presence of inducible VT and the presence of late potentials in the post-infarction period.

Most studies which have sought to relate the findings on signal-averaged ECG with the results of programmed stimulation have concentrated on patients with spontaneous ventricular tachyarrhythmias, many of whom did not have coronary artery disease, let alone myocardial infarction.[12-15] In some of these studies, it appears that patients were selected for signal averaging of the ECG only if they were found to have inducible as well as spontaneous arrhythmias. Moreover, programmed stimulation was sometimes terminated prematurely when as few as 4 nonstimulated ventricular beats were induced.[12] This is a common response even in normal patients studied at twice diastolic threshold stimulation.[16] As pointed out previously,[15] the usefulness of many of these correlative studies has clearly been limited by small sample sizes and bias in patient selection, as well as differences in protocols and techniques for programmed stimulation and signal processing.

This chapter will concentrate on experience from Westmead Hospital correlating the signal-averaged ECG with programmed stimulation in 389 survivors of myocardial infarction with (n = 65) and without (n = 324) spontaneous ventricular tachyarrhythmias. The Westmead patients to be presented were a relatively homogeneous group of patients who fulfilled the following criteria: previous transmural (Q wave) myocardial infarction; age < 76 years; no bundle branch block on 12-lead ECG; no angina requiring treatment with beta blockers or revascularization; no cardiac failure, or else cardiac failure controlled by diuretics; no significant comorbidity; and no antiarrhythmic medications or beta blockers for at least 1 week prior to study.

The Westmead protocols for signal averaging and programmed stimulation have been described in detail previously.[16-19] The protocols were applied without variation to all 389 patients in this study, with signal averaging and programmed stimulation being performed on the same day in all patients.

Patients With Spontaneous Ventricular Tachyarrhythmias

Programmed electrical stimulation and signal averaging of the Frank ECG were performed in 65 patients with spontaneous sustained VT or VF (lasting at least 10 seconds).[19] These arrhythmias had occurred more than 1 week after transmural myocardial infarction in the absence of chest pain or electrocardiographic evidence of fresh ischemia. Mean age of this group was 58 years and anterior infarction was present in 36 patients (55%). An example of the signal-averaged ECG in a patient with ventricular tachycardia after myocardial infarction is provided in Figure 1.

As shown in Table I, 58 patients (89%) had late potentials and 51 (78%) had inducible VT. There was a significant correlation between the presence of late potentials and the ability to induce VT. As a predictor of inducible VT, late potentials had high sensitivity (94%) but low specificity (29%) in this group of patients. Seven

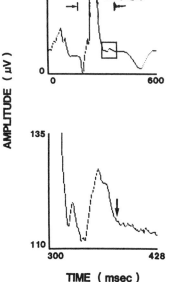

Figure 1. Signal-averaged Y trace from a patient who developed ventricular tachycardia late after myocardial infarction. *Top.* Averaged Y trace at low amplification. Ventricular activation time in this lead was 198 msec, the determinations of QRS onset and offset being made at high amplification. *Bottom.* QRS offset shown at high amplification. QRS offset (arrow) occurs at the end of low amplitude signals that extend into the ST segment. These signals were well above the noise level of 0.5 μV (not shown).

Table I

Correlation Between Late Potentials and Inducible Ventricular Tachycardia (VT) in 65 Survivors of Myocardial Infarction With Spontaneous Ventricular Tachyarrhythmias

	VT Inducible	No VT Inducible*	Total
Late potentials	48	10	58
No late potentials	3	4	7
Total	51	14	65
	p = 0.03		

*This category includes patients with inducible ventricular fibrillation as well as patients with no inducible arrhythmias.

patients (11%) had inducible VF, including four patients with late potentials.

Two major differences were found between patients with inducible VT and patients with inducible VF.

Ventricular activation time (measured from QRS onset to the end of the late potentials) was longer for patients with inducible VT than for patients with inducible VF (Figure 2). In addition, patients with inducible VT had lower mean left ventricular ejection fraction than did patients with inducible VF (Figure 3).

Not only was left ventricular ejection fraction related to the morphology of the inducible arrhythmia, but in patients with inducible VT there was also a correlation between ejection fraction and cycle length of inducible VT.[20] However, ejection fraction was not correlated with ventricular activation time (Figure 4), and there was also no correlation found between ventricular activation time and cycle length of inducible VT (Figure 5).

Ventricular activation time in sinus rhythm and left ventricular ejection fraction were not only important factors influencing the morphology of inducible arrhythmias, but they also influenced the morphology of the spontaneous arrhythmias.[20] Thus, patients with spontaneous and inducible VT had more marked prolongation of ventricular activation time and more marked derangement of left ventricular function than did patients with a combination of spontaneous VF and inducible VF.

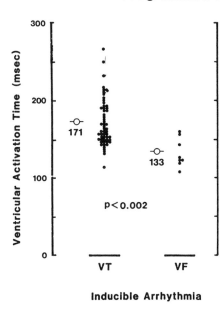

Figure 2. Ventricular activation time determined from the signal-averaged electrocardiogram in patients with spontaneous arrhythmias and inducible ventricular tachycardia (VT) or inducible ventricular fibrillation (VF).

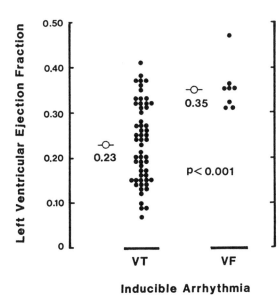

Figure 3. Left ventricular ejection fraction in patients with spontaneous arrhythmias and inducible ventricular tachycardia (VT) or inducible ventricular fibrillation (VF).

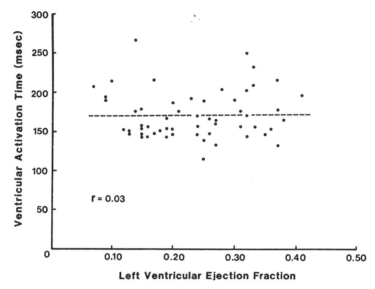

Figure 4. Lack of correlation between ventricular activation time and left ventricular ejection fraction in patients with spontaneous arrhythmias.

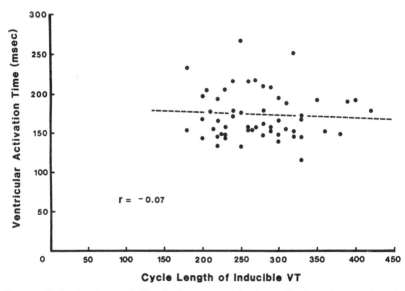

Figure 5. Lack of correlation between ventricular activation time and cycle length of inducible ventricular tachycardia (VT) in patients with spontaneous arrhythmias.

Patients Without Spontaneous Ventricular Tachyarrhythmias

The results of signal averaging and programmed electrical stimulation were also correlated in 324 patients who had had an acute myocardial infarction within the previous year and who had not had spontaneous ventricular tachyarrhythmias. Mean age of this group was 52 years and anterior infarction was present in 129 patients (40%).

As shown in Table II, 84 patients (26%) had late potentials and 67 (21%) had inducible VT. There was a highly significant correlation between the presence of late potentials and the ability to induce VT. As a predictor of inducible VT, late potentials had a sensitivity of 54% and a specificity of 81%. The incidence of late potentials and the incidence of inducible VT were each significantly lower (at p < 0.001) in this group of patients without spontaneous arrhythmias than in the group with spontaneous arrhythmias. Forty-seven patients (15%) had inducible VF, including 15 patients with late potentials.

Mean ventricular activation time was highest (152 ± 4 msec) in the 67 patients with inducible VT and lower at 137 ± 4 msec (p < 0.001) and 127 ± 2 msec (p < 0.001), respectively, in the groups with inducible VF (n = 47) and no inducible arrhythmias (n = 210).

As in the patients with spontaneous arrhythmias (Figures 2 and 3), patients with inducible VT not only had longer mean ventricular activation time than did patients with inducible VF, but patients with inducible VT also had lower left ventricular ejection fraction

Table II
Correlation Between Late Potentials and Inducible Ventricular Tachycardia (VT) in 324 Survivors of Myocardial Infarction Without Spontaneous Ventricular Tachyarrhythmias

	VT Inducible	No VT Inducible	Total
Late potentials	36	48	84
No late potentials	31	209	240
Total	67	257	324
	p < 0.001		

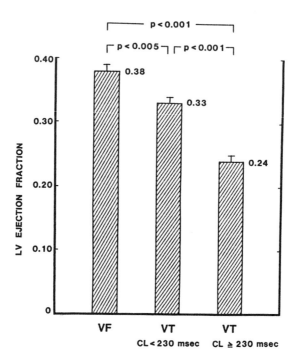

Figure 6. Left ventricular (LV) ejection fraction in patients whose inducible arrhythmias were ventricular fibrillation (VF) or ventricular tachycardia (VT). The patients with inducible ventricular tachycardia were divided into those with VT of cycle length (CL) <230 msec ("ventricular flutter") and cycle length of at least 230 msec.

than did patients with inducible VF (Figure 6). Of the patients with inducible VT, those with inducible slow VT (cycle length of at least 230 msec) had lower mean ejection fraction than did patients with inducible fast VT ("ventricular flutter").

Late Potentials as Noninvasive Predictors of Inducible Ventricular Tachycardia

From the Westmead results presented above it was evident that in patient groups with and without spontaneous ventricular tachyarrhythmias after myocardial infarction, there was a significant correlation between the presence of late potentials and the ability to induce VT, although overlap was not complete. Sensitivity of late potentials for prediction of VT was particularly high at the expense of specificity in the patients with spontaneous arrhythmias, while the reverse was true in the patients without spontaneous arrhythmias.

In view of the significant correlation between late potentials and inducible VT, it was not surprising that the prognostic implications of late potentials and inducible VT were found to be similar in patients without spontaneous arrhythmias.[6]

Late potentials and inducible VT appeared, however, to identify slightly different patient groups,[19] and the observation that VT could be induced in the absence of late potentials and vice versa may reflect imperfections in the techniques of signal averaging and programmed stimulation. The signal-averaged ECG might miss late potentials if they varied from beat-to-beat[21] or if the late potentials arose from areas of the heart not covered adequately by the ECG leads used.[22] Alternatively, the protocol of programmed stimulation might not be sufficiently aggressive for induction of VT in susceptible patients.[23]

Computer modeling of ventricular tachyarrhythmia induction[24] has suggested that the degree of conduction delay in sinus rhythm is the single most important variable influencing arrhythmia induction. The other important variables (in decreasing order of importance) were found to be infarct size, prematurity of extrastimuli, and proximity of the pacing site to the edge of the infarct.

Incomplete correspondence between the presence of late potentials and the ability to induce VT may therefore be due partly to a variation from patient to patient in the relative contribution of these variables to arrhythmia induction.

Recent evidence from an ongoing Westmead Hospital study[25] suggests that multilead signal averaging (of 28 body surface leads) is superior for identification of patients with inducible slow VT than either signal averaging using a bidirectional digital filter[26] or signal averaging of the Frank ECG without filtering.[18] Use of a multilead ECG system increases the information content available for averaging,[22] and promises to give better coverage of the body surface than conventional ECG lead systems.

The Westmead studies did not address the question of whether the signal-averaged ECG was useful in predicting inducibility of VT in patients with conduction disease on ECG. However, there is preliminary evidence to suggest that the signal-averaged ECG is useful in the setting of intraventricular conduction delay, but parameters in addition to ventricular activation time have to be considered during analysis of the averaged ECG in patients with conduction disease.[15]

Do Changes in Late Potentials and Inducibility of VT Occur in Parallel With Each Other?

The changing incidence of late potentials in the 12 months after myocardial infarction[11,27] has been found to parallel the changing incidence of inducible VT during the same time period.[6] However, it cannot always be assumed that perturbations in late potentials observed over a period of time after myocardial infarction will be accompanied by a change in inducibility of VT. More studies will be required to investigate whether serial signal averaging or programmed stimulation studies will be useful in assessing a patient's ongoing risk of spontaneous ventricular tachyarrhythmias.

Even allowing for deficiencies in the techniques for detection of late potentials and inducible VT, it is clear that late potentials are not necessarily reliable predictors of inducible VT in the presence of antiarrhythmic therapies (especially medical).

Several studies have shown that antiarrhythmic drug therapies had no consistent effects on either late potentials or ventricular activation time, even when ability to induce VT was suppressed after treatment.[28–30] This would suggest a limited role for the signal-averaged ECG in assessing efficacy of the currently available antiarrhythmic drugs.

Following surgical excision of electrically abnormal ventricular myocardium for VT, changes in inducibility of VT were not necessarily accompanied by abolition of late potentials. Loss of ability to induce VT post-operatively was associated with a reduction in ventricular activation time, but not necessarily complete abolition of late potentials.[31,32] In one surgical series,[32] one-third of patients had abolition of late potentials and inducible VT post-operatively, while another one-third of patients had the ability to induce VT abolished without late potentials being abolished as well.

Clinical Implications

There is clearly a significant correlation between the presence of late potentials on signal-averaged ECG and inducible VT at programmed electrical stimulation in survivors of myocardial infarction not taking antiarrhythmic medications or beta blockers. This correlation applies to patients with or without spontaneous ventricular tachyarrhythmias. The data from the signal-averaged ECG provides significant additional information regarding inducibility of VT over and above the information provided by clinical variables and left ventricular ejection fraction.[15]

There is not, however, complete correspondence between the presence of late potentials and inducible VT, and the degree of noncorrespondence increases following institution of antiarrhythmic therapies, especially drug therapies.

Detection of late potentials using the signal-averaged ECG appears likely to be most useful as a noninvasive predictor of inducibility of VT in patients with previous myocardial infarction who are not on antiarrhythmic medications at the time of study. Patients who are identified as having late potentials and who are under consideration for antiarrhythmic drug therapies would, however, still need to undergo programmed stimulation to enable optimization of antiarrhythmic therapy.[33]

Acknowledgement: The typographical assistance of Mrs. Heather Marshall is gratefully acknowledged.

References

1. Richards DA, Cody DV, Denniss AR, Russell PA, Young AA, Uther JB: Ventricular electrical instability: a predictor of death after myocardial infarction. Am J Cardiol 51:75, 1983.
2. Hamer A, Vohra J, Hunt D, Sloman G: Prediction of sudden death by electrophysiologic studies in high risk patients surviving acute myocardial infarction. Am J Cardiol 50:223, 1982.
3. Marchlinski FE, Buxton AE, Waxman HL, Josephson ME: Identifying patients at risk of sudden death after myocardial infarction: value of the response to programmed stimulation, degree of ventricular ectopic activity, and severity of left ventricular dysfunction. Am J Cardiol 52:1190, 1983.

4. Roy D, Marchand E, Theroux P, Waters DD, Pelletier GB, Bourassa MG: Programmed ventricular stimulation in survivors of an acute myocardial infarction. Circulation 72:487, 1985.

5. Waspe LE, Seinfeld D, Ferrick A, Kim SG, Matos JA, Fisher JD: Prediction of sudden death and spontaneous ventricular tachycardia in survivors of complicated myocardial infarction: value of the response to programmed stimulation using a maximum of three ventricular stimuli. J Am Coll Cardiol 5:1292, 1985.

6. Denniss AR, Richards DA, Cody DV, Russell PA, Young AA, Cooper MJ, Ross DL, Uther JB: Prognostic significance of ventricular tachycardia and fibrillation induced at programmed stimulation and delayed potentials detected on the signal-averaged electrocardiograms of survivors of acute myocardial infarction. Circulation 74:731, 1986.

7. Uther JB, Richards DA, Denniss AR, Ross DL: The prognostic significance of programmed ventricular stimulation after myocardial infarction. Circulation 75(Suppl III):161, 1987.

8. Breithardt G, Borggrefe M, Haerten K: Role of programmed ventricular stimulation and non-invasive recording of ventricular late potentials for the identification of patients at risk of ventricular tachyarrhythmias after acute myocardial infarction. In Zipes DP, Jalife J (eds): Cardiac Electrophysiology and Arrhythmias. New York: Grune and Stratton, 1985, pp 53–61.

9. Gomes JA, Mehra R, Barreca P, El-Sherif N, Hariman R, Holtzman R: Quantitative analysis of the high frequency components of the signal-averaged QRS complex in patients with acute myocardial infarction: a prospective study. Circulation 72:105, 1985.

10. Kuchar DL, Thorburn CW, Sammel NL: Late potentials detected after myocardial infarction: natural history and prognostic significance. Circulation 74:1280, 1986.

11. Gomes JA, Winters SL, Stewart D, Horowitz S, Milner M, Barreca P: A new noninvasive index to predict sustained ventricular tachycardia and sudden death in the first year after myocardial infarction: based on signal-averaged electrocardiogram, radionuclide ejection fraction and Holter monitoring. J Am Coll Cardiol 10:349, 1987.

12. Breithardt G, Borggrefe M, Quantius B, Karbenn U, Seipel L: Ventricular vulnerability assessed by programmed ventricular stimulation in patients with and without late potentials. Circulation 68:275, 1983.

13. Denes P, Santarelli P, Hauser RG, Uretz EF: Quantitative analysis of the high frequency components of the terminal portion of the body surface QRS in normal subjects and in patients with ventricular tachycardia. Circulation 67:1129, 1983.

14. Freedman RA, Gillis AM, Keren A, Soderholm-Difatte V, Mason JW: Signal-averaged electrocardiographic late potentials in patients with ventricular fibrillation or ventricular tachycardia: correlation with clinical arrhythmia and electrophysiologic study. Am J Cardiol 55:1350, 1985.

15. Nalos PC, Gang E, Mandel WJ, Ladenheim ML, Lass Y, Peter T: The signal-averaged electrocardiogram as a screening test for inducibility of

sustained ventricular tachycardia in high risk patients: a prospective study. J Am Coll Cardiol 9:539, 1987.

16. Richards DA, Cody DV, Denniss AR, Russell PA, Young AA, Uther JB: A new protocol of programmed stimulation for assessment of predisposition to spontaneous ventricular arrhythmias. Eur Heart J 4:376, 1983.

17. Denniss AR, Ross DL, Uther JB: Reproducibility of measurements of ventricular activation time using the signal-averaged Frank vectorcardiogram. Am J Cardiol 57:156, 1986.

18. Denniss AR, Richards DA, Farrow RH, Davison A, Ross DL, Uther JB: Technique for maximising the frequency response of the signal averaged Frank vectorcardiogram. J Biomed Eng 8:207, 1986.

19. Denniss AR, Richards DA, Cody DV, Russell PA, Young AA, Ross DL, Uther JB: Correlation between signal-averaged electrocardiogram and programmed stimulation in patients with and without spontaneous ventricular tachyarrhythmias. Am J Cardiol 59:586, 1987.

20. Denniss AR, Ross DL, Richards DA, Holley LK, Cooper MJ, Johnson DC, Uther JB: Differences between patients with ventricular tachycardia and ventricular fibrillation as assessed by signal-averaged electrocardiogram, radionuclide ventriculography and cardiac mapping. J Am Coll Cardiol 11:276, 1988.

21. El-Sherif N, Mehra R, Gomes JAC, Kelen G: Appraisal of a low noise electrocardiogram. J Am Coll Cardiol 1:456, 1983.

22. Lux RL, Smith CR, Wyatt RF, Abildskov JA: Limited lead selection for estimation of body surface potential maps in electrocardiography. IEEE Trans Biomed Eng 25:2707, 1978.

23. Richards DA, Taylor A, Fahey P, Irwig L, Koo CC, Ross DL, Cooper MJ, Kiat H, Skinner M, Uther JB: Identification of patients at risk of sudden death after myocardial infarction: the continued Australian experience. In Brugada P, Wellens HJJ (eds): Cardiac Arrhythmias. Where to Go From Here? Mount Kisco, NY: Futura, 1987, pp 329–341.

24. Holley LK, Uther JB: A computer model of ventricular electrical activity and its application to ventricular arrhythmias. Australasian Physical Eng Sci Med 8:88, 1985.

25. Richards DA, Haeusler P, Wallace E, Denniss AR, Ross DL, Uther JB: Which method of signal averaging best identifies patients with inducible ventricular tachycardia? Aust N Z J Med 18: 1988.

26. Simson MB: Use of signals in the terminal QRS complex to identify patients with ventricular tachycardia after myocardial infarction. Circulation 64:235, 1981.

27. Denniss AR, Ross DL, Richards DA, Uther JB: Changes in ventricular activation time on signal-averaged electrocardiogram in the first year after acute myocardial infarction. Am J Cardiol 60:580, 1987.

28. Simson MB, Waxman HL, Falcone R, Marcus NH, Josephson ME: Effects of antiarrhythmic drugs on non-invasively recorded late potentials. In Breithardt G, Loogen F (eds): New Aspects in the Medical Treatment of Tachyarrhythmias. Role of Amiodarone. Munich: Urban and Schwarzenberg, 1983, pp 80–86.

29. Denniss AR, Ross DL, Richards DA, Cody DV, Russell PA, Young AA, Uther JB: Effect of antiarrhythmic therapy on delayed potentials de-

tected by the signal-averaged electrocardiogram in patients with ventricular tachycardia after acute myocardial infarction. Am J Cardiol 58:261, 1986.

30. Breithardt G, Borggrefe M, Karbenn U, Schwarzmaier J: Effects of pharmacological and non-pharmacological interventions on ventricular late potentials. Eur Heart J 8(Suppl A):97, 1987.

31. Marcus NH, Falcone RA, Harken AH, Josephson ME, Simson MB: Body surface late potentials: effects of endocardial resection in patients with ventricular tachycardia. Circulation 70:632, 1984.

32. Denniss AR, Johnson DC, Richards DA, Ross DL, Uther JB: Effect of excision of ventricular myocardium on delayed potentials detected by the signal-averaged electrocardiogram in patients with ventricular tachycardia. Am J Cardiol 59:591, 1987.

33. Mason JW, Winkle RA: Accuracy of ventricular tachycardia—induction study for predicting long-term efficacy and inefficacy of antiarrhythmic drugs. N Engl J Med 303:1073, 1980.

19

Late Potentials in the Post-Infarction Period: Prognostic Significance

Gunter Breithardt, Martin Borggrefe,
Antoni Martinez-Rubio

Introduction

For many years, high-gain amplification and subsequent signal averaging for reduction of randomly occurring noise have been used for the detection of low amplitude signals from the body surface. It has attracted a great deal of interest since the initial reports by Fontaine et al[1,2] and Berbari et al.[3] Subsequently, Simson et al,[4,5] Rozanski et al,[6] Breithardt et al,[7-10] Uther et al,[11] and Hombach et al[12] presented their initial experience in patients with ventricular tachyarrhythmias. Since then, experimental and clinical studies have improved our understanding of the pathophysiologic mechanisms as well as of the clinical significance of ventricular late potentials.[13]

Pathophysiologic Background

The anatomic substrate for the occurrence of ventricular late potentials in patients after myocardial infarction, obviously, is the

From El-Sherif N, Turitto G (eds): *High-Resolution Electrocardiography*. Mount Kisco, NY, Futura Publishing Co., Inc., ©, 1992.

appearance of interstitial fibrosis forming insulating boundaries between muscle bundles in the border zone of myocardial infarction.[14,15] The individual components of fragmented electrograms most probably represent asynchronous electrical activity in each of the separate bundles of surviving muscle under the electrode. The intrinsic asymmetry of cardiac activation due to fiber orientation may be accentuated by infarction and may predispose to reentry.[14,15] The slow activation might result from conduction over circuitous pathways caused by the separation and distortion of the myocardial fiber bundles. The low amplitude of the electrograms from the border zone of myocardial infarction probably results from the paucity of surviving muscle fibers under the electrode because of the large amount of connective tissue, and not from depression of the action potentials.[14] The anatomic substrate for reentry seems to be present in regions where fragmented electrograms can be recorded which, thus, indicate slow inhomogenous conduction. However, fragmented electrograms are probably found wherever myocardial fibers are separated by connective tissue, even if reentry does not occur in the region. This has been recently shown by Kienzle et al[16] who concluded that these electrograms may be associated with, but are not specific for sites of origin of ventricular tachycardia.

The time course with which late potentials appear during acute myocardial infarction has only been studied in a small groups of patients. Kertes et al[17] found late potentials in 16% of patients with myocardial infarction without ventricular fibrillation. In five of six patients in whom late potentials were present on the admission averaged electrocardiogram (ECG), they had either disappeared or they were prominently reduced in duration on the second averaged ECG. This may be due to ongoing fibrosis in the infarct area which may lead to devitalization of surviving muscle fibers.

Late Potentials in Patients Without a History of Ventricular Tachyarrhythmias

Ventricular late potentials cannot only be detected in patients with previously documented ventricular tachycardia but also in asymptomatic patients[9] (i.e., patients without a history of ventricular tachycardia or fibrillation outside acute myocardial infarction). In this setting, late potentials were detected in 49 of 146 patients

(37.6%). These data indicate that in many of these patients, most of them having coronary artery disease with previous myocardial infarction, there is a substrate for reentrant arrhythmias which, however, has not yet manifested itself. Obviously, some trigger factor is needed to initiate ventricular tachycardia or fibrillation. These results have subsequently been confirmed by others.[10,17–21] Figures 1 and 2 are examples of the signal-averaged electrocardiogram in a patient with ventricular tachycardia and in a healthy volunteer.

Since late potentials were not only found in patients with but also without previously documented ventricular tachycardia, their presence did not prove to be highly specific for patients with clinically evident ventricular tachyarrhythmias. Additionally, there was a large overlap in the duration of late potentials among patients with ventricular tachycardia or fibrillation and patients without a

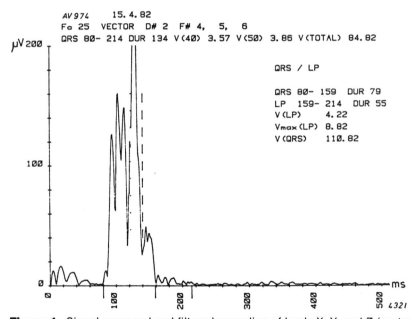

Figure 1. Signal-averaged and filtered recording of leads X, Y, and Z (vector magnitude) using the software developed by M. Simson in a patient with ventricular tachycardia. QRS duration (DUR) in the highly amplified and filtered recording was 134 msec. The program automatically identified the end of the total QRS complex at 214 msec on the X axis. The amplitude in the terminal 40 msec was low (V[40] = 3.57 μV). The onset of low amplitude activity was automatically identified at 159 msec by the automatic recognition program.[52]

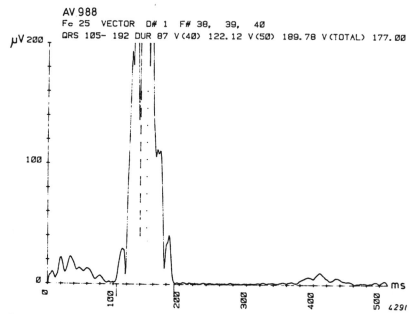

Figure 2. Signal-averaged and filtered recording of leads X, Y, and Z (vector magnitude) using the software developed by M. Simson in a patient without a history of ventricular tachycardia and without structural heart disease. There is no low amplitude activity at the end of the high amplitude portion of the QRS complex. The voltage in the last 40 msec of QRS was 122.12 μV. The QRS duration was 87 msec.

history of these arrhythmias.[9] The longer duration of late potentials in patients with ventricular tachycardia may indicate that in these cases, regional abnormal activation was more fragmented and possibly slower than in those without previously documented ventricular tachycardia.

Prognostic Significance of Late Potentials

The major impact for the use of signal averaging is not so much in the field of retrospective analysis of patients with documented sustained ventricular tachycardia,[4-9,11,12,17,19-24] but in its application for predicting prognosis in patients after recent myocardial infarction who have been hitherto free of ventricular tachyarrhythmias. During recent years, several studies have addressed this issue.[25–32] The results of these studies are summarized in Table I.

Our own experience is based on two prospective studies. First, a prospective trial was initiated at Düsseldorf University in 1980 that used the methodology for recording of signal-averaged ECGs that had been developed in our department between 1978 and 1979. This system was primarily based on a hard-wired signal averager[8–10,25,29] which, subsequently, has also been used by other groups.[33–35] The second study was started in January 1983. This study included only male patients after recent Q wave myocardial infarction. Signal averaging was performed using the software program developed by M. Simson[5] which includes bidirectional filtering and automated analysis of signal-averaged ECGs. This multicenter noninterventional study has been called the PILP-Study (Post-Infarction Late Potential-study). It has recently been completed after inclusion of almost 800 patients. Data analysis has not yet been completed.

The long-term results of our first study group have recently been reported in a preliminary fashion.[36–38] Six hundred and twenty-eight patients without a history of sustained ventricular tachycardia or fibrillation outside the acute phase of myocardial infarction, without a history of syncope, and without complete bundle branch block were included. The patients were selected if they either had survived recent myocardial infarction or if they were referred to our department because of a clinical indication for coronary angiography to establish or exclude the presence of coronary artery disease. In the first subgroup, only patients with acute myocardial infarction that were admitted to the hospital were included on a primary referral basis. Thus, patients referred from other hospitals because of major complications of myocardial infarction were not included. Signal averaging was done as described previously.[8,10] Mean age of these patients was 54 ± 7.6 years. Four hundred and sixty-nine patients had a history of previous myocardial infarction; 258 patients were included within the first 4 weeks after myocardial infarction, another 52 patients within the second month, whereas the remaining 259 patients were studied after more than 2 months after their myocardial infarction. Three hundred and seventy-nine patients (60%) had no late potentials whereas 191 patients (30%) had late potentials of < 40 msec in duration and 58 patients (9%) had late potentials of 40 msec duration or more.

Mean follow-up duration was 39 ± 15.0 months. At the end of follow-up, 21 patients (3.3%) had died suddenly within 1 hour, mostly

Table I

Prognostic Value of Ventricular Late Potentials for Predicting Cardiac Mortality, Sudden Death, and/or Occurrence of Sustained Ventricular Tachycardia

Authors	n	Interval after MI	Follow-up Duration		Prognostic Value of Late Potentials		
					Cardiac mortality	Sudden death	Sust. VT
Breithardt et al[36-38]	628	<1 mo n = 258 2 mo n = 52 3–12 mo n = 60 >12 mo n = 99 no MI n = 159	39 ±15 months (mean ±SD)	No LP <40 msec >40 msec	4.5% 7.3% 12.1%	1.6% 5.2% 8.6%	0.8% 1.6% 13.8%
Von Leitner et al[28]	518	6 to 8 weeks	10 months (mean)	LP absent LP present	1.5% 7.3%	0.9% 3.6%	No event
Denniss et al[26]	110	7 to 28 days (mean 11)	2–12 months (mean 5)	LP absent LP present	No inf.		1.1% 17.4%
Kacet et al[27]	104	No inf.	8.5 ±4 months (6–15)	LP absent LP present	No inf.	0% 13%	4.5% 28.9%
Kuchar et al[32]	123	10 days	3–12 months	LP absent LP present	Sudden death or symptomatic VT 1.4% 20.5%		
Höpp et al[31]	50	<4 weeks	24 ±5 months	LP absent LP present		Sudden death 0% 40%	

Table I (Continued)

Authors	n	Interval after MI	Follow-up Duration		Prognostic Value of Late Potentials
Höpp et al [31]	200	Chronic CAD	20 ±5 months	LP absent LP present	Sudden death 4.3% 13.9%
Denniss et al [39]	403	11–12 days	2 years	LP absent LP present	Sudden death or VT/VF At 1 year At 2 years 2% 4% 15% 21%
Eldar et al [40]	121	till 48 h	2–10 days	QRS <110 msec QRS >110 msec RMS 40 msec >8.3 μV RMS 40 msec <8.3 μV	sudden death 4.1% 29.2% 6.9% 19%
Hong et al [41]	240	3 ± 2 days	1–10 days	LP absent LP present	VT/VF 23% 65%
Denniss et al [43]	250	<2 months	3 years	LP absent LP present	Sudden death or VT/VF 1.5 7.4 (odds ratio)

CAD = coronary artery disease; LP = late potentials; VF = ventricular fibrillation; VT = ventricular tachycardia.

occurring either instantaneously or during sleep whereas another 3 patients (0.5%) died within 1 to 24 hours. There were another 14 cardiac deaths mostly due to reinfarction and myocardial failure. In addition, there were 14 patients (2.2%) who had survived an episode of symptomatic spontaneous sustained ventricular tachycardia that required some type of emergency intervention. Thus, in a total of 35 patients, a major arrhythmic event occurred during follow-up. The risk of major arrhythmic complications was 2.8 times greater in patients with late potentials of <40 msec-duration compared to those without, and 9.3 times greater in those with a duration of 40 msec or more. The chance of sudden cardiac death within 1 hour was 3.3 and 5.4 times greater, respectively, whereas the chance for symptomatic sustained ventricular tachycardia was 2.0 and 17.4 times greater, respectively, depending on the duration of late potentials (<40 msec or greater). The chance of major arrhythmic complications such as sudden cardiac death or sustained symptomatic ventricular tachycardia was greatest in those patients who were studied within the first 4 to 8 weeks after their qualifying myocardial infarction. The results of follow-up were significantly correlated with the presence and duration of late potentials, the site of (anterior wall) and the interval after myocardial infarction (1–2 months), and the degree of left ventricular dysfunction. The 4-year arrhythmic event free rate in patients with late potentials was 72% (ejection fraction below 40%) and 93% (ejection fraction >40%) versus 98% in patients without late potentials. Thus, the presence of late potentials predicted the subsequent occurrence of arrhythmic events during long-term follow-up in post-myocardial infarction patients with impaired left ventricular function.

Denniss et al,[26,30] using a recording system developed by their group, studied 110 patients 7 to 28 days after acute myocardial infarction. The median day of study was 11. Follow-up of these patients ranged between 2 to 12 months (mean: 5 months). There was a significant difference in the subsequent occurrence of symptomatic sustained ventricular tachycardia during follow-up in patients without late potentials (1.1%) compared to those with late potentials (17.4%). The incidence of sudden cardiac death was not reported in the study. In a more recent report, the same group presented the results of long-term observation in 403 clinically well survivors of transmural infarction who were 65-years old or younger.[39] In these patients, signal averaging and programmed ventricular stimulation were compared. Twenty-six percent of the patients had late potentials. Mean ventricular activation time was longer in patients with inferior infarcts (137 ±2 msec) than in those with anterior infarcts (127 ±3 msec; p <0.005). The mean time after infarction at which signal averaging was performed was similar in patients with and without late potentials (12 and 11 days, respectively). There was a significant (p <0.001) correlation between the presence of late potentials and the ability to induce ventricular tachycardia. At 2 years, the probability of remaining free from cardiac death or nonfatal ventricular tachycardia or fibrillation was 0.73 for patients with late potentials and 0.95 for patients without. For patients with late potentials, the probability of remaining free from instantaneous death or nonfatal ventricular tachycardia or fibrillation was 0.85 at 1 year and 0.79 at 2 years, much lower than the corresponding figures of 0.98 (p <0.001) and 0.96 (p <0.001) for patients without late potentials.[39] Among those with late potentials, patients who either died instantaneously or had nonfatal ventricular tachycardia or fibrillation had a longer mean ventricular activation time, a lower mean left ventricular ejection fraction, and a higher incidence of left ventricular aneurysms than patients who were event free. The incidence of antiarrhythmic therapy was similar in the group with primarily tachyarrhythmic events (33%) and the group without such events (26%).[39] However, a policy of obtaining a signal-averaged ECG only in patients with a poor left ventricular ejection fraction (0.30 or less) would have missed 43% of the patients with late potentials who either died instantaneously or had nonfatal ventricular tachycardia/fibrillation during follow-up. A cut-off point for left ventricular ejection fraction of 0.40 or less would have been more appropriate for a screening test since only 7% of patients with late potentials who developed a ventricular tachyarrhythmia had an ejection fraction >0.40.[39]

Kacet et al[27] studied a population of 104 patients by use of the algorithm developed by M. Simson.[5] These patients were followed for 8.5 ±4 months. The incidence of subsequent symptomatic sustained ventricular tachycardia in patients without late potentials was 4.5% compared to 28.9% in patients with late potentials. None of the patients without late potentials died suddenly compared to 13% of patients with late potentials.

In another study, Kuchar et al[32] reported the results of follow-up (3 to 12 months) of 123 patients that were studied 10 days (mean) after acute myocardial infarction. The incidence of major arrhythmic complications such as sudden death or symptomatic sustained ventricular tachycardia was only 1.4% in patients without late potentials compared to 20.5% in patients with late potentials.

In a study by Höpp et al,[31] 50 patients were studied in the early post-infarction period. These patients were followed for 24 ±5 months. Twelve of 30 patients who had late potentials (37%) died suddenly. On the contrary, none of the 20 patients without late potentials died suddenly. The same authors studied another group of 200 patients with chronic, stable coronary artery disease.[31] Mean follow-up was 20 ±5 months. One hundred and eight of 200 patients had ventricular late potentials. Fifteen of these patients (13.9%) died suddenly compared to 4 of 92 patients (4.3%) without late potentials (p <0.001).

Von Leitner et al[28] followed 518 patients who took part in a rehabilitation program after myocardial infarction. These patients were studied between 6–8 weeks after onset of infarction. During a mean follow-up period of 10 months, cardiac mortality was 1.5% in patients without late potentials compared to 7.3% in patients with ventricular late potentials. Sudden cardiac death occurred in 0.9% of patients without late potentials compared to 3.6% of patients with late potentials. In none of these patients was symptomatic sustained ventricular tachycardia reported.

To identify patients at risk of dying in the early post-myocardial infarction period, Eldar et al[40] performed signal averaging of the 12-lead ECG in 121 patients within 48 hours of their first myocardial infarction. Eleven patients died within the first 2 to 10 days of myocardial infarction (5 patients of ventricular fibrillation, 3 of electromechanical dissociation, 1 of atrio-ventricular block, and 2 patients of cardiogenic shock) and 110 patients survived. Patients in whom the duration of the filtered QRS complex was longer than the average duration +1 standard deviation (109.8 msec) in the precordial leads had an almost seven-fold probability of dying within 2 to 10 days of myocardial infarction (7 of 24 patients, 29.2%) compared with patients having a duration of the filtered QRS complex <110 msec (4 of 97 patients, 4.1%). Similarly, a voltage of the terminal 40 msec lower than the average −1 standard deviation (<8.3 µV) identified a subgroup of patients with an almost three times greater probability of dying during this period (4 of 19 patients vs 7 of 102 patients, 19% vs 6.9%, respectively).

Hong et al[41] examined the relationship between the presence of ventricular late potentials and the occurrence of spontaneous ventricular tachycardia or fibrillation in the prehospital and in-hospital

(<10 days) phases of acute myocardial infarction. Two hundred and forty consecutive patients were included in the study. The signal-averaged ECG was performed in all patients at 3 ±2 days after admission using 25 to 250-Hz bandpass filtering and 200-beat signal averaging. Sustained ventricular tachycardia or fibrillation occurred in 17 of 240 patients (7%). Late potentials were recorded in 63 patients (26%). The incidence of late potentials was significantly higher among patients with ventricular tachycardia or ventricular fibrillation than among those without (11 of 17 patients, 65% vs 52 of 223 patients, 23%, p <0.01). The subgroup of patients with prehospital ventricular tachycardia or ventricular fibrillation also showed a higher incidence of late potentials (7 of 11 patients, 64% vs 56 of 229 patients, 24 %, p <0.01). The authors were able to show that the presence of late potentials in this setting was independent of infarct size.

Role of Thrombolytic Therapy

With an increasing use of thrombolytic therapy in the acute phase of myocardial infarction, there might be a change in the anatomic and functional substrate of infarction. This might have implications for the evaluation of these patients and may also be the reason for the improved prognosis in many patients after acute thrombolysis in myocardial infarction. To address this question, Lew et al[42] studied the relation between the presence or absence of ventricular late potentials and the patency of the infarct-related artery in 203 consecutive patients with acute myocardial infarction in whom coronary angiography had been performed after their admission. A patent infarct-related artery was found in 76 of 140 patients (54.3%) with no intervention aimed at reperfusion and was achieved in 50 of 63 patients (79.4%) treated by acute thrombolysis or angioplasty. Late potentials were recorded in 10 of the 128 patients (8%) with a patent infarct-related artery compared to 23 of the 77 patients (30%) with an occluded infarct-related artery (p <0.001). In addition, there was a low incidence of late potentials in those patients with a patent infarct-related artery whether or not the patency of this vessel was spontaneous or by intervention. The reduced incidence of late potentials in patients with a patent infarct-related artery was independent of CK-MB-estimated myocardial infarction size and Q or non-Q wave myocardial infarction. Thus, the incidence of late potentials was reduced in patients with patent infarct-related coronary arteries even when patency was spontaneous. This may explain the recently reported reduced mortality following late reperfusion which may be in part due to enhanced electrical stability.

Comparison With Other Parameters

Denniss et al[43] recently assessed the relative values of signal averaging and exercise testing in predicting death and arrhythmias after myocardial infarction in 250 clinically well patients aged <66 years. Signal averaging and exercise testing had been done within 2 months of myocardial infarction. An abnormal finding was defined as late potentials on the signal-averaged ECG being present, ST segment changes of 2 mm or more, or impaired hemodynamics or angina on exercise testing. Patients were followed for 3 years. They reported that the signal-averaged ECG was superior to exercise testing. The odds ratio for death or sustained ventricular tachycardia or fibrillation was 7.4 in patients with compared to those without late potentials; in contrast, it was only 1.5 in patients with compared to those without ST segment depression or in those in whom any of these parameters (ST segment depression or impaired hemodynamics or angina) were present.

Similar results were recently reported by Cripps et al.[44] These authors prospectively investigated the relative value of exercise testing, late potentials recorded using the algorithm by M. Simson[5] and simple clinical assessment in predicting ischemic and arrhythmic events during follow-up after acute myocardial infarction. One hundred and seventy-six consecutive patients surviving at least 7 days after acute myocardial infarction were studied. The presence of late potentials was defined as the presence of one or more of the following criteria: (1) filtered QRS duration of 120 msec or more; (2) duration of the filtered QRS complex after the voltage had decreased below 40 μV, of 40 msec or more; and (3) a root mean square voltage during the last 40 msec of the filtered QRS complex of 20 μV or less. A prolonged filtered QRS alone was not considered a positive result if QRS duration in the standard ECG was more than 120 msec in duration. Patients with bundle branch block were excluded. No investigations or therapy were instituted on the basis of the results of signal averaging, and no patient received prophylactic antiarr-

hythmic therapy before the occurrence of arrhythmic events. Treadmill exercise testing was carried out within 6 weeks of infarction. In
108 of 172 patients (63%), this was a symptom-limited test using the
Bruce protocol and the test was carried out after discharge at about
1 month after infarction. In the remaining patients, exercise testing
was carried out before discharge using a 9-minute 3-stage protocol.
The latter protocol was introduced after the death of a number of
patients after discharge but before the time of the planned post-
discharge exercise test. The age of the patients was 56 ±9 years
(range 28 to 70), 20% of the patients were female. The site of infarction was anterior in 90 (52%), inferior or posterior or both in 76
(44%), and indeterminate in 8 patients (4%). Signal averaging was
performed 12 ±19 days after infarction in all 176 patients. Late
potentials were present in 41 patients (24%). All but two of the
patients with arrhythmic events (sudden death defined as witnessed
instantaneous sudden death not preceded by chest pain or sustained
ventricular tachycardia associated with symptomatic hypotension
or requiring emergency intervention or both) had late potentials
whereas 32 of 165 patients without arrhythmic events had late potentials. However, only 5 of 23 patients with ischemic events (including
coronary artery bypass grafting) had late potentials. Exercise testing was performed 21 ±14 days after infarction. There were two
patients who where unable to perform the test due to cardiovascular
instability at the time of the test. Test results were positive in 18 of
23 patients with ischemic events, but only in 6 of 11 patients with
arrhythmic events. There were four positive exercise test results in
63 of 153 patients. The duration of follow-up was 15 ±7 months
(range 3 to 24 months). Using multivariate analysis, the only independent variable predicting ischemic events was the exercise test
result. Arrhythmic events were independent of the exercise test result but the Killip class on admission, presence of late potentials,
previous infarction, occurrence of in-hospital complications, and
non-Q wave infarction were independently associated with arrhythmic events. The independent variables predicting any event (reinfarction, coronary artery bypass grafting, symptomatic ventricular
tachycardia, and sudden death) included, in the order of importance,
Killip class, exercise test result, presence of late potentials, and
non-Q wave infarction.

Based on these results, the authors[44] concluded that exercise
testing is sensitive although of low positive predictive accuracy in
predicting *ischemic* events and that, similarly, the presence of late

potentials is sensitive yet inaccurate in predicting *arrhythmic* events. Only about one out of five patients with late potentials will suffer an arrhythmic event. Therefore, they suggested that more specific tests are required in the group identified by noninvasive screening. They suggested that the addition of clinical observations and the occurrence of a positive result in the exercise test also enhanced the predictive accuracy of this test. In contrast, patients at low risk were those free of complications during the acute phase of myocardial infarction, with a negative result in the exercise test, and no late potentials. In the presence of this combination of parameters, a course free of subsequent arrhythmic or ischemic events could be predicted with a certainty of 99%.[44]

In our prospective study, several parameters were evaluated in 552 patients with coronary artery disease but without a history of ventricular tachycardia or ventricular fibrillation outside the acute phase of myocardial infarction. Using a combination of signal averaging and programmed ventricular stimulation, we were able to show that the predictive value for subsequent arrhythmic events could be markedly increased.[29,45] During a mean follow-up period of 30 ± 19 months, 53 patients (10%) died. There were 21 sudden deaths and 16 patients had documented symptomatic sustained ventricular tachycardia (total arrhythmic event rate 7%). The prevalence of a subsequent arrhythmic event was 2.8% in patients without late potentials and without inducible ventricular tachycardia whereas in patients with late potentials and inducible ventricular tachycardia the prevalence was 25%. Compared to patients without late potentials the relative risk (odds ratio) of patients with late potentials was 2.6, of those with late potentials and inducible sustained ventricular tachycardia 4.5. The predictive value of these tests as well as the odds ratios were markedly higher if only the subgroup of patients with subsequent symptomatic sustained ventricular tachycardia was evaluated. In this subgroup, the relative risk of late potentials and inducible ventricular tachycardia was 19.4 compared to those without late potentials. This means that these patients had a 19.4 times greater chance of developing sustained symptomatic ventricular tachycardia than those without a positive finding. Thus, this combined approach helped to identify subgroups at high risk of subsequent arrhythmic events. Using ejection fraction as an additional parameter, the predictive value of these parameters could even be increased (unpublished data).

Significance of Late Potentials to Predict Rejection After Heart Transplantation

Recently, Haberl et al[46,47] reported the use of frequency-domain analysis of low-noise electrocardiographic recordings as a new noninvasive approach to detect early rejection after cardiac transplantation. Thirty-six acute rejection crises requiring treatment in heart transplanted patients were diagnosed by cytoimmunologic monitoring and endomyocardial biopsy. In 33 of 36 cases, a significant increase in the frequency content of the QRS complex between 70 and 110 Hz was observed on the days of rejection. The frequency content of the ST segment in a 300-msec window was found to be decreased between 10 and 30 Hz. These changes in the frequency content were reversible within 1–2 weeks in most patients after successful treatment. They found only two false-positive results (two patients with acute mediastinitis). The mechanism of these changes and the potential use of this method for the evaluation of acute and chronic rejection after orthotopic heart transplantation seems a promising new approach that still needs further evaluation.

Conclusions and Clinical Implications

Based on these presently available prospective studies, the presence of ventricular late potentials obviously heralds an increased risk for subsequent occurrence of sudden cardiac death or symptomatic sustained ventricular tachycardia. This mainly applies to patients who have been studied after recent myocardial infarction[25–27,31,32] whereas patients who are included later and/or who are considered eligible for a cardiac rehabilitation program,[28] obviously have a much lower incidence of arrhythmic events. Thus, the predictive value of the presence of ventricular late potentials largely depends on the clinical circumstances under which they can be detected. Patients who have survived for a long period after their myocardial infarction have a much lower risk of subsequent development of sudden cardiac death or symptomatic sustained ventricular tachycardia. This is obviously based on a selection process as patients at greater risk might have died in the meanwhile. In addition, our own results show that the duration of late potentials might be of prognostic significance. The chance for development of an arrhythmic event, mainly symptomatic sustained ventricular tachycardia, has been proportional to the duration of the late potentials (unpublished data).

Sudden cardiac death is a multifactorial problem. It may be due to chronic electrophysiologic abnormalities as a consequence of regional slow conduction in the border zone of a previous myocardial infarction which is conventionally considered to be the electrophysiologic substrate for ventricular late potentials. The presence of regional slow conduction is mostly not sufficient for the spontaneous occurrence of ventricular tachyarrhythmias. Instead, some trigger factor such as spontaneous ventricular ectopic beats are necessary to alter the electrophysiologic milieu in a way that it originates tachycardia. However, most spontaneous ventricular arrhythmias detected during long-term ECG recording are not harmful to the patient as they obviously do not induce ventricular tachycardia. Instead, some change in, for instance, the coupling interval or the sequence of ectopic beats, including the occurrence of short runs, may alter the electrophysiologic milieu in a way that the prerequisites for reentry are met. Such transient occurrence of complex ventricular arrhythmias acting as trigger factor might also be induced by short, regional episodes of ischemia induced by embolization of platelet aggregates into the peripheral coronary system.[48]

Another mechanism that may lead to sudden cardiac death is the occurrence of extensive ischemia due to reinfarction. This may cause a transient electrophysiologic abnormality that is able to sustain ventricular tachyarrhythmias. Thus, this mechanism may also lead to sudden cardiac death. Such a type of event, of course, cannot be predicted on the presence of pre-existing indicators of regional slow conduction such as late potentials. However, it has been shown that pre-existing myocardial damage increases the chance of ventricular fibrillation if regional ischemia occurs at a site remote from that of pre-existing cardiac damage.[49]

Thus, it seems unjustified to expect any single method to be able to identify the individual patient at risk of sustained ventricular tachycardia and/or sudden death. Instead, a combination of various parameters including late potentials, spontaneous ventricular arrhythmias during long-term ECG recording, extent of myocardial contractile disturbance (ejection fraction), exercise test, electrophysiologic study, and estimates of central nervous activity[50,51] might serve for further risk stratification in patients after recent myocardial infarction.

Acknowledgment: This work was supported by the Johann A. Wülfing-Stiftung, the Berta and Ernst Grimmke-Stiftung, the Sonderforschungsbereich 30 (Kardiologie) and the Sonderforschungsbereich 242 (Koronare Herzkrankheit—Prophylaxe und Therapie akuter Komplikationen) of the Deutsche Forschungsgemeinschaft, Bonn-Bad Godesberg (Germany, F.R.).

References

1. Fontaine G, Guiraudon G, Frank R: Intramyocardial conduction defects in patients prone to ventricular tachycardia. In Sandoe E, Julian DG, Bell JW (eds.): Management of Ventricular Tachycardia—Role of Mexiletine. Amsterdam: Excerpta Medica, 1978, pp 67–69.
2. Fontaine G, Frank R, Gallais-Hamonno F, Allali I, Phan-Thuc H, Grosgogeat Y: Electrocardiographie des potentiels tardifs du syndrome de post-excitation. Arch Mal Coeur 71:854, 1978.
3. Berbari EJ, Scherlag BJ, Hope RR, Lazzara R: Recording from the body surface of arrhythmogenic ventricular activity during the ST-segment. Am J Cardiol 41:697, 1978.
4. Simson M, Horowitz L, Josephson M, Moore EN, Kastor J: A marker for ventricular tachycardia after myocardial infarction (abstr). Circulation 62:III-262, 1980.
5. Simson MB: Use of signals in the terminal QRS-complex to identify patients with ventricular tachycardia after myocardial infarction. Circulation 64:235, 1981.
6. Rozanski JJ, Mortara D, Myerburg RJ, Castellanos A: Body surface detection of delayed depolarizations in patients with recurrent ventricular tachycardia and left ventricular aneurysm. Circulation 63:1172, 1981.
7. Breithardt G, Becker R, Seipel L: Non-invasive recording of late ventricular activation in man (abstr). Circulation 62:III-320, 1980.
8. Breithardt G, Becker R, Seipel L, Abendroth RR, Ostermeyer J: Non-invasive detection of late potentials in man—a new marker for ventricular tachycardia. Eur Heart J 2:1, 1981.
9. Breithardt G, Borggrefe M, Karbenn U, Abendroth RR, Yeah HL, Seipel L: Prevalence of late potentials in patients with and without ventricular tachycardia: correlation to angiographic findings. Am J Cardiol 49:1932, 1982.
10. Breithardt G, Borggrefe M, Quantius B, Karbenn U, Seipel L: Ventricular vulnerability assessed by programmed ventricular stimulation in patients with and without late potentials. Circulation 68:275, 1983.
11. Uther JB, Dennett CJ, Tan A: The detection of delayed activation signals of low amplitude in the vectorcardiogram of patients with recurrent ventricular tachycardia by signal averaging. In Sandoe E, Julian D, Bell JW (eds): Management of Ventricular Tachycardia—Role of Mexiletine. Amsterdam, Oxford: Excerpta Medica, 1978, pp 80–82.
12. Hombach V, Höpp HW, Braun V, Behrenbeck DW, Tauchert M, Hilger HH: Die Bedeutung von Nachpotentialen innerhalb des ST-Segmentes

im Oberflächen-EKG bei Patienten mit koronarer Herzkrankheit. Dtsch med Wschr 105: 1457, 1980.

13. Breithardt G, Borggrefe M: Pathophysiological mechanisms and clinical significance of ventricular late potentials. Eur Heart J 7: 364, 1986.

14. Gardner PHJ, Ursell PHC, Pham TD, Fenoglio JJ, Wit AL: Experimental chronic ventricular tachycardia: anatomic and electrophysiologic substrates. In: Tachycardias: Mechanisms, Diagnosis, Treatment. Philadelphia: Lea and Febiger, 1984, pp 29–60.

15. Richards DA, Blake GJ, Spear JF, Moore EN: Electrophysiologic substrate for ventricular tachycardia: correlation of properties in vivo and in vitro. Circulation 69: 369, 1984.

16. Kienzle MG, Miller J, Falcone R, Harken A, Josephson ME: Intraoperative endocardial mapping during sinus rhythm: relationship to site of origin of ventricular tachycardia. Circulation 70:957, 1984.

17. Kertes PJ, Glaubus M, Murray A, Julian DG, Campbell RWF: Delayed ventricular depolarization-correlation with ventricular activation and relevance to ventricular fibrillation in acute myocardial infarction. Eur Heart J 5:974, 1984.

18. Abboud S, Belhassen B, Laniado S, Sadeh D: Non-invasive recording of late ventricular activity using an advanced method in patients with a damaged mass of ventricular tissue. J Electrocardiol 16:245, 1983.

19. Höpp HW, Hombach V, Deutsch HJ, Osterspey A, Winter U, Hilger HH: Assessment of ventricular vulnerability by Holter ECG, programmed ventricular stimulation and recording of ventricular late potentials. In Steinbach K, Glogar D, Laszkovics A, Scheibelhofer W, Weber W (eds): Cardiac Pacing. Darmstadt: Steinkopff Verlag, 1983, pp 625–632.

20. Freedman RA, Gillis AM, Keren A, Soderholm-Difatte V, Mason JW: Signal-averaged ECG late potentials correlate with clinical arrhythmia and electrophysiological study in patients with ventricular tachycardia or fibrillation (abstr). Circulation 70: II-252, 1984.

21. Kanovsky MS, Falcone RA, Dresden CA, Josephson ME, Simson ME: Identification of patients with ventricular tachycardia after myocardial infarction: signal-averaged electrocardiogram, Holter monitoring, and cardiac catheterization. Circulation 70: 264, 1984.

22. Cain ME, Ambos D, Witkowski FX, Sobel BE: Fast-Fourier transform analysis of signal-averaged electrocardiograms for identification of patients prone to sustained ventricular tachycardia. Circulation 69: 711, 1984.

23. Poll DS, Marchlinski FE, Falcone RA, Simson MB: Abnormal signal averaged ECG in nonischemic congestive cardiomyopathy: relationship to sustained ventricular tachyarrhythmias (abstr). Circulation 70: II-253, 1984.

24. Cain ME, Ambos HD, Markham J, Fischer AE, Sobel BE: Quantification of differences in frequency content of signal-averaged electrocardiograms in patients with compared to those without sustained ventricular tachycardia. Am J Cardiol 55: 1500, 1985.

25. Breithardt G, Schwarzmaier J, Borggrefe M, Haerten K, Seipel L: Prognostic significance of ventricular late potentials after acute myocardial infarction. Eur Heart J 4: 487, 1983.

26. Denniss AR, Cody DV, Fenton SM, Richards DA, Ross DL, Russell PA, Young AA, Uther JB: Significance of delayed activation potentials in survivors of myocardial infarction (abstr). J Am Coll Cardiol 1: 582, 1983.

27. Kacet S, Libersa C, Caron J, Bondoux d'Haute-Fenille B, Marchand X, Dagano J, Lekieffre J: The prognostic value of averaged late potentials in patients suffering from coronary artery disease (personal communication).

28. Von Leitner ER, Oeff M, Loock D, Jahns B, Schröder R: Value of non invasively detected delayed ventricular depolarizations to predict prognosis in post myocardial infarction patients (abstr). Circulation 68: III-83, 1983.

29. Breithardt G, Borggrefe M, Haerten K: Role of programmed ventricular stimulation and noninvasive recording of ventricular late potentials for the identification of patients at risk of ventricular tachyarrhythmias after acute myocardial infarction. In Zipes DP, Jalife J (eds): Cardiac Electrophysiology and Arrhythmias. Orlando: Grune and Stratton, 1985, pp 553–61.

30. Denniss AR, Cody DV, Russell PA, Young AA, Ross DL, Uther JB: Prognostic significance of inducible ventricular tachycardia after myocardial infarction. J Am Coll Cardiol 3: 610, 1984.

31. Höpp HW, Hombach V, Osterspey A, Deutsch H, Winter U, Behrenbeck DW, Tauchert M, Hilger HH: Clinical and prognostic significance of ventricular arrhythmias and ventricular late potentials in patients with coronary heart disease. In Hombach, Hilger HH (eds): Holter Monitoring Technique. Technical Aspects and Clinical Applications. Stuttgart-New York: Schattauer, Stuttgart-New York: 1985, pp 297–307.

32. Kuchar D, Thorburn C, Sammel N: Natural history and clinical significance of late potentials after myocardial infarction (abstr). Circulation 72: III-477, 1985.

33. Oeff M, Von Leitner ER, Brüggemann T, Andresen D, Sthapit R, Schröder R: Methodische Probleme bei der Registrierung ventrikulärer Spätpotentiale (abstr.). Z Kardiol 71: 204, 1982.

34. Jauernig RA, Senges J, Langfelder W, Rizos J, Hoffmann E, Brachmann J, Kübler W: Effect of antiarrhythmic drugs on ventricular late potentials at sinus rhythm and at constant heart rate. In Steinbach K, Glogar D, Laszkovics A, Scheibelhofer W, Weber W (eds): Cardiac Pacing. Darmstadt: Steinkopff Verlag, 1983, pp 767–772.

35. Oeff M, Von Leitner ER, Sthapit R, Breithardt G, Borggrefe M, Karbenn U, Meinertz T, Zotz R, Clas W: Methods for non-invasive detection of ventricular late potentials—A comparative multicenter study. In Steinbach K, Glogar D, Laszkovics A, Scheibelhofer W, Weber W (eds): Cardiac Pacing. Darmstadt: Steinkopff Verlag, 1983, pp 641–647.

36. Breithardt G, Borggrefe M, Haerten K, Seipel L: Value of electrophysiologic testing, recording of late potentials by averaging techniques and Holter monitoring for the identification of high risk patients after acute myocardial infarction. In Kulbertus HE (ed): Medical Management of Cardiac Arrhythmias. Edingburgh, London, Melbourne, and New York: Churchill Livingstone, 1986, pp 228–246.

37. Breithardt G, Borggrefe M: Recent advances in the identification of patients at risk of ventricular tachyarrhythmias: role of ventricular late potentials. Circulation 75: 1091, 1987.

38. Breithardt G, Borggrefe M, Podczeck A, Schwarzmaier J, Karbenn U: Prognostic significance of late potentials in patients with coronary heart disease (abstr). Circulation, 76:IV-344, 1987.

39. Denniss AR, Richards DA, Cody DV, Russell PA, Young AA, Cooper MJ, Ross DL, Uther JB: Prognostic significance of ventricular tachycardia and fibrillation induced at programmed ventricular stimulation and delayed potentials detected on the signal-averaged electrocardiogram of survivors of acute myocardial infarction. Circulation 74:731, 1986.

40. Eldar M, Leor J, Rotstein Z, Hod H, Truman S, Abboud S: Signal averaging identifies increased mortality risk at early post-infarction period. Circulation 78(Suppl):II-51, 1988.

41. Hong M, Gang ES, Wang FZ, Siebert C, Xu YX, Simonson J, Peter T: Ventricular late potentials are associated with ventricular tachyarrhythmias in the early phase of myocardial infarction. Circulation 78(Suppl):II-302, 1988.

42. Lew AS, Hong M, Xu YX, Peter T, Gang E: The relation of ventricular late potentials to patency of the infarct artery: possible implications for late reperfusion (abstr). Circulation 78(Suppl):II-578, 1988.

43. Denniss AR, Cody DV, Richards DA, Ross DL, Russell PA, Young AA, Uther JB: Signal-averaged electrocardiogram is superior to exercise testing in predicting death and arrhythmias after myocardial infarction (abstr). Circulation 78(Suppl):II-301, 1988.

44. Cripps T, Bennett D, Camm J, Ward D: Prospective evaluation of clinical assessment, exercise testing and signal-averaged electrocardiogram in predicting outcome after acute myocardial infarction. Am J Cardiol 62:995, 1988.

45. Breithardt G, Borggrefe M, Haerten K, Martínez-Rubio A: Value of late potentials and programmed ventricular stimulation in predicting long-term arrhythmic complications in patients with coronary artery disease (abstr). Circulation 78(Suppl):II-301, 1988.

46. Haberl R, Weber M, Kemkes B, Steinbeck G: Frequency analysis of the QRS-complex and ST-segment for noninvasive detection of acute rejection after orthotopic heart transplantation (abstr). Circulation 76(Suppl IV):204, 1987.

47. Haberl R, Weber M, Reichenspurner H, Kemkes BM, Osterholzer G: Aufhuber M, Steinbeck G: Frequency analysis of the surface electrocardiogram for recognition of acute rejection after orthotopic cardiac transplantation. Circulation 76:101, 1987.

48. Davies MJ, Path FRC, Thomas AC, Path MRC, Knapman PA, Hangartner JR: Intramyocardial platelet aggregation in patients with unstable angina pectoris suffering sudden ischemic cardiac death. Circulation 73:418, 1986.

49. Patterson E, Holland K, Eller BT, Lucchesi BR: Ventricular fibrillation resulting from ischemia at a site remote from previous myocardial infarction. A conscious canine model of sudden coronary death. Am J Cardiol 50:1414, 1982.

50. Malliani A, Schwartz PJ, Zanchetti A: Neural mechanisms in life-threatening arrhythmias. Am Heart J 100: 705, 1980.
51. Tavazzi L, Zotti AM, Rondanelli R: The role of psychologic stress in the genesis of lethal arrhythmias in patients with coronary artery disease. Eur Heart J 7(Suppl A):99, 1986.
52. Karbenn U, Breithardt G, Borggrefe M, Simson MB: Automatic identification of late potentials. J Electrocardiol 18:123, 1985.

20

Late Potentials in the Post-Infarction Period: Role in Risk Stratification Strategies

Nabil El-Sherif, Soad Bekheit,
Gioia Turitto, John M. Fontaine,
Shantha N. Ursell, Bassiema Ibrahim,
Edward B. Caref

Introduction

Serious arrhythmic events (AE) defined as sudden cardiac death, documented ventricular fibrillation (VF) and symptomatic ventricular tachycardia (VT) remain a significant risk in patients who survive an episode of acute myocardial infarction (AMI). The risk is highest for several weeks after AMI but continues to remain high during the first year post-MI. The current incidence of serious AE in the first year post-MI is probably lower than what has been quoted often,[1] which could be attributed to the changing strategies in the management of AMI during the past few years. Nevertheless, accurate stratification of post-MI patients into low- and high-risk groups for future AE is of marked significance because specific management strategies could be applied to high-risk patients.

From El-Sherif N, Turitto G (eds): *High-Resolution Electrocardiography*. Mount Kisco, NY, Futura Publishing Co., Inc., ©, 1992.

The occurrence of serious AE in post-MI patients, can be hypothesized as being due to the interaction of at least four major factors: (1) A fixed anatomic-electrophysiologic substrate for reentrant arrhythmias. This factor could be evaluated by time-domain analysis of late potentials (LPs) in the signal-averaged electrocardiogram (SAECG), and probably more accurately, by recent spectral analysis techniques[2]; (2) The initiating or triggering factor for reentrant tachyarrhythmias in the form of spontaneous premature beats. This could be evaluated from ambulatory ECG recordings; (3) Left ventricular function, which could be evaluated noninvasively by radionuclide or echocardiographic measurement of left ventricular ejection fraction. A ventricular tachyarrhythmia in the presence of a low ejection fraction is more likely to result in hemodynamic compromise and sudden cardiac death; (4) Factors that modulate the degree of electrical instability. In this regard the role of the autonomic nervous system may be paramount.

In recent years a number of invasive and noninvasive tests have been utilized singly or in combination for risk stratification of post-MI patients for serious AE. In this chapter the value of the SAECG in this risk stratification strategy will be specifically examined and correlated with the role of ambulatory ECG, left ventricular function, electrophysiologic study, and the autonomic nervous system.

The Signal-Averaged Electrocardiogram

The concept of late potentials (LPs) in the SAECG as a marker of ventricular electrical instability was developed as a consequence of studies of reentrant rhythms in the canine post-infarction model using composite electrode recordings.[3] Late potentials are low amplitude fragmented signals occurring at the terminal part of the QRS complex/early ST segment. These signals represent electrical activation of abnormal myocardial regions showing slow and inhomogeneous conduction.[4] These regions are thought to provide the anatomic-electrophysiologic substrate for reentrant tachyarrhythmias. Therefore, the detection of LPs in the SAECG could be utilized as a noninvasive marker to identify patients at risk of future spontaneous ventricular tachyarrhythmias and sudden cardiac electrical death.[5]

Prognostic Significance of the SAECG in the Early Post-Infarction Period

The value of the SAECG in predicting ventricular tachyarrhythmias during the first 48 hours of myocardial infarction is controversial. In a study by El-Sherif et al,[6] the SAECG was abnormal in only one of eight patients who had VT/VF during the first 48 hours of AMI. Similar observations have been reported by other investigators.[7-10] For example, Kertes et al[7] recorded an SAECG within hours of onset of AMI and observed that the presence of LPs did not correlate with subsequent occurrence of VF. On the other hand, McGuire et al,[11] in a small series of patients, suggested that the SAECG may be useful in identifying patients at high risk of developing early ventricular tachyarrhythmias. The prevalence of an abnormal SAECG in this series was 52%, which is much higher than the incidence of abnormal recording during the acute phase reported by other studies. In another report[12] the SAECG was recorded in 75 patients within 24 hours from the onset of AMI and LPs were found in 20 patients (26.7%). Out of this group, eight (40%) developed VF compared to one incidence of VF among patients without LPs (1.8%).

One of the difficulties in interpreting the relationship between the SAECG and ventricular tachyarrhythmias in the early post-MI period is that the recording was sometimes obtained after the arrhythmic event.[11] The possible effects of interventions such as electrical cardioversion or antiarrhythmic medication will be difficult to assess. The electrophysiologic substrate of ventricular tachyarrhythmias in the early post-MI period is probably different from the substrate that underlies late AE. Furthermore, the use of the SAECG to predict early post-MI ventricular tachyarrhythmias may be of limited clinical relevance. The majority of these arrhythmias will occur while patients are under continuous ECG monitoring and in an environment where successful resuscitative measures should be available.

Prognostic Significance of the SAECG in the Subacute Post-Infarction Period

In contrast to the controversial value of the SAECG in the early post-MI period, several prospective studies have documented the prognostic significance of the SAECG recorded during the subacute post-MI period for predicting late AE.[6,13,18] Patients with an abnormal SAECG have a significantly higher AE rate of 17% to 29% compared to patients with a normal SAECG of 1%–4% during approximately 1 year of follow-up. Table I summarizes the results of four studies reported between 1987–1989 that utilized a similar signal averaging equipment.[6,15–17] Although there were few differences in the type of high-pass filter applied to the averaged signal and in the scoring criteria for an abnormal recording, all the studies have shown an approximately similar sensitivity, specificity, and predictive accuracy of the SAECG.

Table I

Studies of the Prognostic Significance of the Signal-Averaged (SA) ECG in the Post-Infarction Period

	Kuchar et al 1987[15]	Gomes et al 1987[16]	Cripps et al 1988[17]	El-Sherif et al 1989[6]
No. of patients	200	102	159	156
Time post-MI (days)	7–40 (11)	10 ±6	3 ±2	6–30
Follow-up (months)	6–24 (14)	12 ±6	12 ±6	12
Bandpass filters (Hz)	40–250	40–250	25–250	25–250
Definition of LPs:				
QRSD (msec)	> 120	> 114	≥ 120	≥ 120
RMS40 (µV)	and/or < 20	and/or ≤ 20	and/or ≤ 25	and/or ≤ 25
LAS40 (msec)	—	and/or > 38	and/or ≤ 40	—
SAECG:				
Sensitivity	93	87	91	75
Specificity	65	63	81	79
PPA	17	29	26	23

LAS = low amplitude signals <40 µV; LP = late potential; QRSD = total filtered QRS duration; PPA = positive predictive accuracy; RMS40 = root mean square voltage of the signals in the last 40 msec of the filtered QRS.

The Prognostic Significance of the SAECG Depends on the Time of Recording in the Post-Infarction Period

El-Sherif et al conducted a study to determine whether the prognostic significance of the SAECG depends on the time of recording in the post-MI period.[6] Serial recordings of the SAECG and a 24-hour ambulatory ECG were obtained in 156 patients with AMI up to 5 days (phase 1), 6 to 30 days (phase 2), and 31 to 60 days (phase 3) post-MI. The study showed the dynamic nature of the SAECG in the first 2 months post-MI. Of 51 patients with an abnormal SAECG during the first 2 months post-MI, 35 patients (69%) changed categories between normal and abnormal recordings. The changes were mainly in the direction of either a delayed appearance of an abnormal recording after the first 5 days post-MI (26 of 51 patients; 50%) (Figure 1) or reversal of the abnormality after the first 30 days post-MI (13 of 51 patients; 25%). The dynamic changes in the SAECG were similar to those reported by other investigators.[10,14,19] A significant finding of the study was that a transient abnormality of the SAECG during the first 5 days post-MI and the late appearance of an abnormal recording during the second month after infarction were not associated with AE. The highest incidence of an abnormal SAECG occurred 6 to 30 days post-MI during which an abnormal recording had the most significant relation to AE. Ninety-three percent of abnormal recordings during this phase including all recordings in patients who had an AE were obtained 6 to 14 days after infarction. The study suggested that the optimal window for obtaining the SAECG is between 6 and 14 days post-MI which corresponds approximately to the time of hospital discharge. The importance of this timing was emphasized by the fact that 58% of AE in this study occurred between 7 and 28 days post-MI.

Limitations of Studies of the Prognostic Significance of Time-Domain SAECG in the Post-Infarction Period

There are several technical and electrophysiologic limitations of time-domain SAECG in post-MI patients. There is a lack of agreement in the literature as to the optimal filter characteristics as well

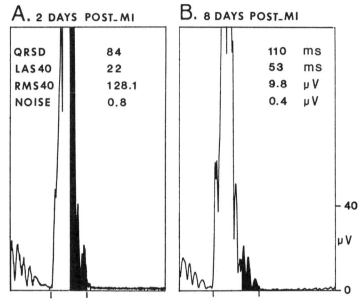

A. 2 DAYS POST-MI   **B.** 8 DAYS POST-MI

	A		B	
QRSD	84		110	ms
LAS 40	22		53	ms
RMS 40	128.1		9.8	µV
NOISE	0.8		0.4	µV

Figure 1. Time course of the SAECG in a patient with acute myocardial infarction and late arrhythmic event. SAECG was normal 2 days after infarction (A) but was abnormal 8 days after infarction (B). Note decrease in amplitude of root mean square voltage of signals in last 40 msec (RMS40) from 128.1 to 9.8 µV and increase in filtered QRS duration (QRSD) from 84 to 110 msec. Duration of low amplitude signal <40 µV (LAS) also increased from 22 to 53 msec. The patient died with documented ventricular tachycardia/ventricular fibrillation 23 days after infarction. (Reproduced with permission from El-Sherif et al, Am Heart J 119:1014, 1989.)

as the best numeric criteria of abnormality. In a study from our laboratory[20] we established normal values for SAECG parameters over a wide range of high-pass filters in a large group of normal subjects. The effects of different high-pass filters on the SAECG were identified. The normal values were then applied in a systematic approach to optimize the accuracy of the SAECG to predict the results of programmed stimulation. A combination of SAECG parameters analyzed at more than one high-pass filter was found to enhance the total predictive accuracy of the technique to up to 89%. However, a major limitation of this study, and of the time-domain analysis technique in general, was that patients with bundle branch block (BBB) and/or QRS duration >120 msec were excluded. In the presence of BBB, which many patients at high risk have, interpretation of time-domain LP analysis is difficult and most published studies have specifically excluded such patients. In another study from our laboratory, we have demonstrated that the numeric measurements for time-domain analysis of SAECG are sensitive to the specific algorithm used for determining QRS termination.[21] This was a major factor to explain differences in numeric criteria provided by various commercial SAECG devices when the same set of SAECG data was analyzed. Other limitations of current methods of time-domain analysis of SAECG are the occasional loss of information when a composite vector complex is analyzed instead of individual X, Y, and Z leads[22] and a lack of information on the ideal number and configuration of ECG leads to record body surface signals.[23]

An important electrophysiologic limitation in studies of the prognostic significance of the SAECG in the post-MI period is that the recording is used to predict AE including sustained monomorphic VT and VF. The relationship of LPs to spontaneous sustained VT[24,25] as well as to sustained VT induced by programmed stimulation[26] is consistent with known electrophysiologic mechanisms. However, the relationship between the fixed electrophysiologic substrate of LPs and the future occurrence of VF is less clear. Because of this and other electrophysiologic limitations optimizing the SAECG technique is not expected to increase significantly its positive predictive accuracy. We probably will still be faced with the fact that a majority of patients with an abnormal SAECG will not develop late AE in the post-MI period. This argument provides the rationale for the utilization of a battery of tests for risk stratification in the post-MI period.

The Prognostic Significance of SAECG and Complex Ventricular Arrhythmias (CVA)

Several studies have shown that there is no correlation between CVA in the ambulatory ECG and abnormal SAECG in the post-MI period.[6,8,18] In a study by El-Sherif et al,[6] the time course of CVA and abnormal SAECG in the post-MI period was quite different (Figure 2). The highest incidence of abnormal SAECG occurred 6 to 30 days post-MI but was associated with the lowest incidence of CVA. The lack of correlation between CVA and an abnormal SAECG may be explained by the difference in the electrophysiologic basis of the two phenomena. An abnormal SAECG represents ischemic myocardial zones with delayed activation that can provide the electrophysiologic substrate for reentrant tachyarrhythmias.[27] On the other

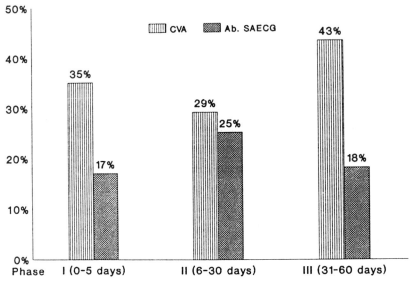

Figure 2. Frequency of complex ventricular arrhythmias (CVA) and abnormal signal-averaged ECG (Ab. SAECG) during phases 1 to 3 after infarction. (Reproduced with permission from El-Sherif et al, Am Heart J 119:1014, 1989.)

hand, the underlying electrophysiologic mechanism(s) for CVA in the ambulatory ECG may include reentry and abnormal or triggered automaticity. Complex ventricular arrhythmias caused by focal pacemaker discharge rather than reentry are not expected to be associated with an abnormal SAECG. Moreover, VT of nonreentrant origin may occur in the presence of an abnormal SAECG and does not have a cause-and-effect relationship with the abnormal recording.

In three large multicenter studies,[28–30] CVAs were found to be an independent predictor of sudden cardiac death in the post-MI period, although in one study,[30] the risk was only limited to patients with non-Q wave infarction. Some studies that investigated the prognostic significance of abnormal SAECG and CVA in the post-MI period found that both are independently significant.[25,26] However, in the study by El-Sherif et al, the presence of CVA or nonsustained VT 6 to 30 days post-MI was not an independent predictor of late AE.[27] On the other hand, all studies showed that the positive predictive value of the combination of abnormal SAECG and CVA is significantly higher compared to either factors alone (Table II)[6,15–17]

Table II

Studies of the Combined Prognostic Significance of the Signal-Averaged (SA) ECG, Complex Ventricular Arrhythmias (CVA), and Left Ventricular Ejection Fraction (LVEF) in the Post-Infarction Period

	Kuchar et al 1987[15]	Gomes et al 1987[16]	Cripps et al 1988[17]	El-Sherif et al 1989[6]
SAECG + CVA				
Sensitivity	65	100	73	88
Specificity	89	45	97	88
PPA	31	35	62	27
SAECG + LVEF				
Sensitivity	80	100	—	86
Specificity	89	59	—	87
PPA	34	36	—	37
SAECG + CVA + LVEF				
Sensitivity	—	100	—	80
Specificity	—	53	—	94
PPA	—	50	—	50

PPA = positive predictive accuracy.

The Prognostic Significance of SAECG and Left Ventricular Ejection Fraction (LVEF)

Several studies have shown that an abnormal SAECG and LVEF <40% independently predict the probability of late AE in the post-MI period.[6,15,16] In the study by El-Sherif et al,[6] the rate of AE in patients with an abnormal LVEF and a normal SAECG was as low as the event rate in patients with normal LVEF (7% vs 5%, respectively). Similar findings were reported by Kuchar et al[15] and Gomes et al[16] and suggest that left ventricular dysfunction alone does not carry a high risk of future AE. In a study by Gomes et al,[18] the predictive value of LVEF in relation to the site of AMI contrasted markedly with that of the SAECG. Whereas LVEF had a higher sensitivity than the SAECG (87% vs 75%) in predicting AE in anterior wall MI, the SAECG had a better specificity than LVEF (80% vs 38%). On the other hand, whereas the SAECG had a better sensitivity than LVEF (100% vs 50%) in predicting AE in inferior wall MI, the specificity of LVEF was better than that of the SAECG (71% vs 50%).

The combination of an abnormal SAECG and an abnormal LVEF was associated with a higher event rate than either abnormality[6,15–17] (Table II). This makes sense since the occurrence of a ventricular tachyarrhythmia in the presence of a low LVEF is more likely to result in hemodynamic compromise and may thus strongly correlate with sudden cardiac death. On the other hand, a possible correlation between the combined abnormality and a higher incidence of sustained VT is more difficult to explain.

The Prognostic Significance of SAECG + CVA + LVEF

Both Gomes at al[16] and El-Sherif et al[6] have shown that the combination of an abnormal SAECG, CVA in the ambulatory ECG and an abnormal LVEF has the highest positive predictive accuracy for AE of 50% to 57%. An important limitation of this combined index, however, is illustrated in the study of El-Sherif et al.[6] In this study 210 consecutive patients admitted to the coronary care unit with documented AMI were screened and 54 patients were excluded for a variety of reasons that included age > 79 years, BBB, cardiogenic shock, advanced cancer or renal disease, and refusal or inability to participate in the protocol. Of the remaining 156 patients who were prospectively followed for up to 1 year only 9 patients (4.5%) had a combination of an abnormal SAECG, CVA, and low LVEF. Of these nine patients, five (57%) suffered an AE. Thus in a fairly representative sample of post-MI patients the percentage of patients with all three abnormal indices was relatively low and hence the positive predictive value of the combined index is limited. On the other hand, a much larger cohort of patients (47 of 156 patients, 30%) had a normal SAECG, LVEF > 40% and no CVA. This group had a low incidence of AE of 2%.

Role of Electrophysiologic Study (EPS)

This technique is based on the assumption that the induction of ventricular tachyarrhythmia by programmed ventricular stimulation in post-MI patients can serve as a surrogate marker for the future occurrence of spontaneous ventricular tachyarrhythmias. However, the nature of the triggering mechanism(s) for spontaneous ventricular tachyarrhythmias is not fully understood and may prove to be different and more complex than the technique of programmed ventricular stimulation. Therefore, it is not surprising that the sensitivity, specificity, and positive predictive accuracy of the technique could be less than optimal.

Several studies have been published in the last decade on the value of programmed ventricular stimulation in risk stratification of post-MI patients for future AE.[14,31–37] The results of these studies have been highly controversial (see Table III). The report by Hamer et al,[31] Waspe et al,[32] Breithardt et al,[33] Denniss et al,[14] and Cripps et al[34] suggest that the technique has a relatively high sensitivity although the positive predictive accuracy was usually rather low. On the other hand, the studies by Marchlinski et al,[35] Roy et al,[36] and Bhandari et al[37] found that the response to programmed ventricular stimulation is not helpful in identifying patients at risk for future AE in the post-MI period. All of the reports, however, suffered from a number of limitations concerning study design and rationale:

1. Size of study groups: With the exception of Denniss et al[14] who studied 403 patients, most other investigators reported the results of relatively small study groups. This frequently resulted in few AE available for analysis. For example, in the report by Roy et al,[36] only two AE occurred in a group of 35 patients who had inducible nonsustained and sustained VT while two additional AE occurred in 115 post-MI with no inducible tachyarrhythmia. This limits the validity of the conclusions that could be drawn from such studies.

2. Clinical characteristics of study population: Different studies included post-MI patients with varying clinical characteristics. Some studies had an overall representative sample of post-MI patients[14] while others included either predominantly low[37] or high-risk groups[32] based on a battery of clinical evidence of uncomplicated or complicated post-MI course, respectively. The incidence of AE is expected to be higher in patients with clinical evidence of major infarction.[34] In fact, some studies suggest that simple clinical indicators of major MI could be a sensitive index of AE even though these usually have a low positive predictive accuracy.[34] Another confusing factor in some studies is the inclusion of patients on various pharmacologic regimens or who have undergone interventional procedures that could conceivably affect the incidence of AE in the post-MI period. These include the use of beta adrenergic blocking

Table III

Studies of the Prognostic Significance of Electrophysiologic Studies (EPS) in the Post-Infarction Period

Author	Pt No	Time Post-MI (days)	Follow-Up (months)	EPS Protocol	EPS Endpoint	Sensitivity (%)	Specificity (%)	PPA (%)
Hamer et al 1982[31]	37	7–20(11)	12	2 ES	≥5 RVR	80	75	33
Marchlinski et al 1983[35]	46	8–60(22)	(18)	2 ES	≥4 RVR	17	78	10
Roy et al 1985[36]	150	8–20 (14)	10 (5)	2 ES	≥6 RVR	29	77	6*
Waspe et al 1985[32]	50	7–36 (16)	(22.8)	3 ES	≥7 RVR	100	57	41
Breithardt et al 1986[33]	132	<6 weeks	(15)	2 ES	≥4 RVR	77	57	16
Denniss et al 1986[14]	403	7–28	24(12)	2 ES, 20 mA	VT >10 sec, VF	52	82	18
Cripps et al 1989[34]	75	(21)	(16)	3 ES	VT/VF	100	97	75
Bhandari et al 1989[37]	75	9–21 (14)	(18)	3 ES	VT/VF	71	60	15

ES = extrastimuli; RVR = repetitive ventricular responses; PPA = positive predictive accuracy; VT = ventricular tachycardia; VF = ventricular fibrillation; * = small number of events. Numbers in parentheses are mean values.

drugs, calcium channel blocking drugs, antiarrhythmic drugs, digoxin, diuretics, angioplasty, and coronary artery bypass surgery. The use of antiarrhythmic drugs in those studies can be particularly disturbing not only because of their potential protective effect but more significantly in view of the recent evidence of proarrhythmic effects of some of the drugs in post-MI patients.[38]

3. Time of EPS in the post-MI period: This ranged from as early as 7 days[31,32,34] up to 60 days post-MI.[35] There is some evidence that the inducibility of VT/VF is higher in the first few weeks post-MI and may significantly decrease several months later.[39] This may be related to the evolution of the electrophysiologic substrate. On the other hand, the failure to induce a tachyarrhythmia 2 weeks after MI was found to have a long-term reproducibility.[39] Another unsettling issue is the day-to-day reproducibility of inducible tachyarrhythmias. In one study, inducible sustained VT with cycle length ≥ 240 msec was highly reproducible while the inducibility of rapid VT or VF showed a significant day-to-day variability.[40]

4. The protocol for programmed ventricular stimulation: The site of stimulation, current strength, number of extrastimuli, and use of burst pacing can significantly affect the incidence and type of induced arrhythmias. A stimulation protocol with optimal sensitivity and specificity in post-MI patients is not established. However, there seems to be an agreement that a stimulation protocol with up to three extrastimuli can increase the sensitivity of the test without necessarily decreasing its specificity.[34,37]

5. End point of programmed ventricular stimulation and the relationship to future AE: In patients with a history of spontaneous VT, the induction of sustained monomorphic VT is highly specific, whereas repetitive ventricular responses, nonsustained VT, polymorphic VT or VF are relatively nonspecific.[41] In the post-MI patient, the specific end point for programmed stimulation seems to depend on the expected outcome. Several studies have shown that the induction of sustained monomorphic VT with relatively long cycle length ≥ 240–270 msec can predict the future occurrence of spontaneous sustained monomorphic VT in post-MI patients.[33,34] Another clear conclusion is that the induction of VF seems to represent a nonspecific response in these patients.[14,34,37] The most significant question, however, is whether a specific end point of programmed stimulation can predict future sudden arrhythmic death. It is quite likely that sudden arrhythmic death in the post-MI period is a complex event that requires not only an established arrhythmo-

genic substrate, but also appropriate modulating and triggering factors and/or a de novo electrophysiologic derangement. The prognostic significance in the post-MI period of the spontaneous occurrence of hypotensive VT/VF that would result in sudden arrhythmic death unless appropriately interrupted, should be clearly distinguished from that of hemodynamically stable VT.

The unresolved question regarding the value of EPS in predicting sudden arrhythmic death, in addition to the invasive nature of the test could limit the utility and the scope of its application for risk stratification in the post-MI period. Besides, some studies suggest that a similar degree of predictive accuracy could be obtained from a number of clinical variables and noninvasive tests like the signal-averaged ECG.[14,34] In the study by Denniss et al[14] a significant correlation was found between the presence of LPs and inducible sustained monomorphic VT in post-MI patients not receiving antiarrhythmic medications or beta blockers. This correlation applied to patients with or without spontaneous ventricular tachyarrhythmias. There was not, however, complete correspondence between the presence of LPs and inducible VT, and the degree of noncorrespondence increased following institution of antiarrhythmic drug therapies. To provide a more definitive answer regarding the role of EPS in the risk stratification strategy of post-MI patients would require a multicenter study with a large study group that follows a standardized protocol and utilizes powerful statistical techniques.

Role of the Autonomic Nervous System

It has been proposed that myocardial infarction and/or ischemia can result in abnormal sympathovagal imbalance and predispose the heart to serious AE.[42,43] Direct measurements of vagal or sympathetic activity in humans are not readily available. However, instantaneous heart rate depends on the interaction between sympathetic and parasympathetic efferent activities and the cardiac pacemaker properties. Analysis of beat-to-beat oscillations which characterize heart rate and arterial blood pressure could lead to a noninvasive assessment of the autonomic nervous system.[44] Various approaches have been proposed to evaluate the contributions of parasympathetic and sympathetic discharges to heart rate variability (HRV).

Respiratory sinus arrhythmias[45] and time-domain analysis of HRV[46,47] have been utilized to noninvasively assess parasympathetic activity. Recent studies suggest that analysis of HRV may contribute to identification of patients at increased risk of sudden death. Kleiger et al analyzed HRV, defined as the standard deviation of all normal RR intervals in a 24-hour ECG recording in a large population of post-MI patients.[48] Patients with decreased HRV had a significantly higher mortality. This was explained by suggesting that decreased HRV correlated with increased sympathetic or decreased vagal tone which may predispose the heart to VF.

Nonpower spectral methods of HRV analysis appear to lump together several components which may result in the loss of valuable information.[49] Spectral techniques have been suggested to assess the frequency components of the HRV signal.[44,50,51] A major advantage of spectral analysis is the finding that, in addition to assessing parasympathetic activity, changes in sympathetic activity to the heart can be recognized and quantified and some index of the balance between sympathetic and vagal activity can be obtained. High-frequency component of the HRV power spectrum (>0.15 Hz) is synchronous with the respiration and has been considered as a quantitative evaluation of respiratory arrhythmia.[44,52] The high-frequency component markedly diminishes on standing or tilt position and disappears after atropine and represents a clinically useful index of vagal activity.[50] On the other hand, low-frequency components of the HRV power spectrum (<0.15 Hz) seem to reflect parasympathetic and sympathetic activity.[50] However, the increase in low-frequency peak during standing or passive tilting to upright position seems to reflect primarily sympathetic activity.[53,54] We and others have shown that this component of the HRV power spectrum could be markedly reduced by beta adrenergic blocking agents.[50,53,54] In a recent study from our laboratory we have shown that the calcium channel blocker, diltiazem, but not nifedipine, could also depress the low-frequency component of the HRV power spectrum during tilt.[54]

In a preliminary study, Lombardi et al[55] using spectral analysis of HRV showed that sympathetic activity is increased while parasympathetic activity is decreased 2 weeks after AMI and that normalization of the sympathovagal imbalance occurred after 6 to 12 months. However, the prognostic significance of this sympathovagal imbalance has not been investigated. A future study to test the hypothesis that post-MI patients, who have a fixed electrophysiologic substrate of reentrant arrhythmias as identified by the SAECG, will be more likely to develop serious AE if they also have abnormal sympathovagal tone could provide significant information.

Conclusions

The role of EPS for risk stratification of post-MI patients for future AE is still controversial. On the other hand, several prospective studies have documented the prognostic significance of the SAECG recorded during the subacute post-MI phase for predicting future AE. The technique has a high negative predictive accuracy but the positive predictive accuracy is rather low. An abnormal SAECG, combined with CVA in the ambulatory ECG and low LVEF had a high positive predictive accuracy for future AE but the combined index is of limited value because it only identifies a small number of post-MI patients. The development of accurate measurements of sympathovagal tone may enhance the predictive accuracy of other risk factors.

Acknowledgment: This study was supported by National Institute of Health Grants HL36680 and HL31341 and the Veterans Administration Medical Research Funds.

References

1. Kannel WB, Sorlie P, McNamara PM: Prognosis after initial myocardial infarction: The Framingham study. Am J Cardiol 44:53, 1979.
2. Kelen G, Henkin R, Caref E, Starr A-M, Bloomfield D, El-Sherif N: Spectral turbulence analysis of the signal-averaged electrocardiogram and its predictive accuracy for inducible sustained monomorphic ventricular tachycardia. Am J Cardiol 67:965, 1991.
3. El-Sherif N, Scherlag BJ, Lazzara R, Hope RR: Reentrant ventricular arrhythmias in the late myocardial infarction period. 1. Conduction characteristics in the infarction zone. Circulation 55: 686, 1977.
4. El-Sherif N, Gough WB, Restivo M, Craelius W, Henkin R: Electrophysiological basis of ventricular late potentials. In Santini M, Pistolese M, Alliegro A (eds): Progress in Clinical Pacing. New York: Excerpta Medica, 1988, pp 209–223.
5. El-Sherif N, Restivo M, Craelius W, Mehra R, Henkin R, Caref EB, Kelen G: The high resolution electrocardiogram. Technical and basic aspects.

In El-Sherif N, Samet P (eds): Cardiac Pacing and Electrophysiology. Philadelphia: WB Saunders, 1990, pp 349–371.

6. El-Sherif N, Ursell SN, Bekheit S, Fontaine J, Turitto G, Henkin R, Caref EB: Prognostic significance of the signal-averaged ECG depends on the time of recording in the post-infarction period. Am Heart J 118:-256, 1989.

7. Kertes P, Glabus M, Murray A, Julian D, Campbell R: Delayed ventricular depolarization—correlation with ventricular activation and relevance to ventricular fibrillation in acute myocardial infarction. Eur Heart J 5:974, 1984.

8. Turitto G, Caref EB, Macina G, Fontaine JM, Ursell SN, El-Sherif N: Time course of ventricular arrhythmias and the signal-averaged electrocardiogram in the post infarction period: a prospective study of correlation. Br Heart J 60:17, 1988.

9. Grimm M, Billhart RA, Mayerhofer KE, Denes P: Prognostic significance of signal-averaged ECGs during acute myocardial infarction: a preliminary report. J Electrophysiol 21:283, 1988.

10. Lewis SL, Lander PT, Taylor PA, Chamberlin DA, Vincent R: Evolution of late potential activity in the first six weeks after acute myocardial infarction. Am J Cardiol 63:647, 1989.

11. McGuire M, Kuchar D, Ganis J, Sammel N, Thorburn C: Natural history of late potentials in the first ten days after acute myocardial infarction and relation to early ventricular arrhythmias. Am J Cardiol 61:1187, 1988.

12. Dluzniewski M, Kulchowski P, Senatorski M, Ceremuzynski L: Late potentials in the acute phase of myocardial infarction indicate the risk of early ventricular fibrillation. Eur Heart J 9:1175, 1988.

13. Breithardt G, Schwarzmayer J, Borggrefe M, Haerten K, Seipel L: Prognostic significance of late ventricular potentials after acute myocardial infarction. Eur Heart J 4:487, 1983.

14. Denniss AR, Richards DA, Cody DV, Russell PA, Young AA, Cooper MJ, Ross DL, Uther JB: Prognostic significance of ventricular tachycardia and fibrillation induced at programmed stimulation and delayed potentials detected on the signal-averaged electrocardiograms of survivors of acute myocardial infarction. Circulation 74:731, 1986.

15. Kuchar D, Thorburn C, Sammel N: Prediction of serious arrhythmic events after myocardial infarction: signal-averaged electrocardiogram, Holter monitoring, and radionuclide ventriculography. J Am Coll Cardiol 9:531, 1987.

16. Gomes JA, Winters SL, Stewart D, Horowitz S, Milner M, Barreca P: A new noninvasive index to predict sustained ventricular tachycardia and sudden death in the first year after myocardial infarction: based on signal-averaged electrocardiogram, radionuclide ejection fraction and Holter monitoring. J Am Coll Cardiol 10:349, 1987.

17. Cripps T, Bennett ED, Camm AJ, Ward DE: High-gain signal-averaged electrocardiogram combined with 24 hour monitoring in patients early after myocardial infarction for bedside prediction of arrhythmic events. Br Heart J 60:181, 1988.

18. Gomes JA, Winters SL, Marinson M, Machac J, Stewart D, Targonsky

A: The prognostic significance of quantitative signal-averaged variables relative to clinical variables, site of myocardial infarction, ejection fraction and ventricular premature beats: a prospective study. J Am Coll Cardiol 13:377, 1989.

19. Kuchar D, Thorburn C, Sammel N: Late potentials detected after myocardial infarction: natural history and prognostic significance. Circulation 6:1280, 1986.

20. Caref EB, Turitto G, Ibrahim BB, Henkin R, El-Sherif N: Role of band-pass filters in optimizing the value of the signal-averaged electrocardiogram as a predictor of the results of programmed stimulation. Am J Cardiol 64:16, 1989.

21. Henkin R, Caref EB, Kelen GJ, El-Sherif N: The signal-averaged electrocardiogram and late potentials. A comparative analysis of commercial devices. J Electrocardiol 22(Suppl 1):19, 1990.

22. Lander P, Deal RB, Berbari EJ: The analysis of late potentials using orthogonal recordings. IEEE Biomed Eng 35:629, 1988.

23. Atwood AE, Myers JJ, Forbes S, Hall F, Marcondes G, Mortara D, Froelicher VF: High frequency electrocardiography. An evaluation of lead placement and measurements. Am Heart J 116:733, 1988.

24. Simson MB: Use of signals in the terminal QRS complex to identify patients with ventricular tachycardia after myocardial infarction. Circulation 64:235, 1981.

25. Denes P, Santarelli P, Hauser RG, Uretz EF: Quantitative analysis of the high-frequency components of the terminal portion of the body surface QRS in normal subjects and in patients with ventricular tachycardia. Circulation 67:1, 1983.

26. Turitto G, Fontaine JM, Ursell SN, Caref EB, Henkin R, El-Sherif N: Value of the signal-averaged electrocardiogram as a predictor of the results of programmed stimulation in nonsustained ventricular tachycardia. Am J Cardiol 61:1272, 1988.

27. El-Sherif N, Gomes JAC, Restivo M, Mehra R: Late potentials and arrhythmogenesis. PACE 8:440, 1985.

28. Bigger JT, Kleiger R, Miller JP, Rolnitzky LM, Multicenter Post-Infarction Research Group: The relationship among ventricular arrhythmias, left ventricular dysfunction and mortality in the 2 years after myocardial infarction. Circulation 69:250, 1984.

29. Mukarji J, Rude RE, Pool WK, Gustafson N, Thomas LJ, Jr, Strauss HW, Jaffe AS, Muller JE, Roberts R, Raabe DS, Jr, Croft CH, Passamani E, Braunwald E, Willerson JT, the MILIS Study Group: Risk factors for sudden death after acute myocardial infarction: two-year follow-up. Am J Cardiol 54:31, 1984.

30. Maisel AS, Scott N, Gilpin E, Ahnve S, Winter ML, Henning H, Collins D, Ross J Jr: Complex ventricular arrhythmias in patients with Q wave versus non-Q wave myocardial infarction. Circulation 72:983, 1985.

31. Hamer A, Vohra J, Hunt D, Sloman G: Prediction of sudden death by electrophysiologic studies in high risk patients surviving acute myocardial infarction. Am J Cardiol 50:223, 1982.

32. Waspe LE, Seinfeld D, Ferrick A, Kim SG, Matos JA, Fisher JD: Prediction of sudden death and spontaneous ventricular tachycardia in survi-

vors of complicated myocardial infarction: value of the response to programmed stimulation using a maximum of three ventricular extrastimuli. J Am Coll Cardiol 5:1292, 1985.

33. Breithardt G, Borggrefe M, Haerten K: Ventricular late potentials and inducible ventricular tachyarrhythmias as a marker for ventricular tachycardia after myocardial infarction. Eur Heart J 7(Suppl A):127, 1986.

34. Cripps T, Bennett ED, Camm AJ, Ward DE: Inducibility of sustained, monomorphic ventricular tachycardia as a prognostic indicator in survivors of myocardial infarction: a prospective evaluation in relation to other prognostic variables. J Am Coll Cardiol 14:289, 1989.

35. Marchlinski FE, Buxton AE, Waxman HL, Josephson ME: Identifying patients at risk of sudden death after myocardial infarction: value of the response to programmed stimulation, degree of ventricular ectopic activity and severity of left ventricular dysfunction. Am J Cardiol 52:1190, 1983.

36. Roy D, Marchand E, Theroux P, Waters D, Pelletier G, Bourassa M: Programmed ventricular stimulation in survivors of an acute myocardial infarction. Circulation 72:487, 1985.

37. Bhandari AK, Hong R, Kotlewski A, McIntosh N, Av PK, Sankoorikal A, Rahimtoola S: Prognostic significance of programmed ventricular stimulation in survivors of acute myocardial infarction. Br Heart J 61:410, 1989.

38. The Cardiac Arrhythmia Suppression Trial (CAST) Investigators: Preliminary report: effect of encainide and flecainide on mortality in randomized trial of arrhythmia suppression after myocardial infarction. N Engl J Med 321:406, 1989.

39. Bhandari AK, Au PK, Rose JS, Kotlewski A, Blue S, Rahimtoola S: Decline in inducibility of sustained ventricular tachycardia from two to twenty weeks after acute myocardial infarction. Am J Cardiol 59:284, 1987.

40. Bhandari AK, Hong R, Kulick D, Peterson R, Rubin JN, Leon C, McIntosh N, Rahimtoola SH: Day to day reproducibility of electrically inducible ventricular arrhythmias in survivors of acute myocardial infarction. J Am Coll Cardiol 15:1075, 1990.

41. Wellens HJJ, Brugada P, Stevenson WG: Programmed electrical stimulation of the heart in patients with life-threatening arrhythmias: what is the significance of induced arrhythmias and what is the correct stimulation protocol? Circulation 72:1, 1985.

42. Ryan C, Hollenberg M, Harvey DB, Gwynn R: Impaired parasympathetic responses in patients after myocardial infarction. Am J Cardiol 37:1013, 1976.

43. LaRovere MT, Specchia G, Mortara A, Schwarz PJ: Baroreflex sensitivity, clinical correlates and cardiovascular mortality among patients with a first myocardial infarction: a prospective study. Circulation 78:816, 1988.

44. Akselrod S, Gardner D, Ubel FA, Shannan DI, Bayer AC, Cohen RJ: Power spectrum analysis of heart rate fluctuation: a quantitative probe of beat-to-beat cardiovascular control. Science 213:220, 1981.

45. Katona P, Jih F: Respiratory sinus arrhythmia: noninvasive measure of parasympathetic cardiac control. J App Physiol 39:801, 1976.
46. Fouad FM, Tarazi RC, Ferrario CM, Fighaly S, Alicandri C: Assessment of parasympathetic control of heart rate by non-invasive method. Am J Physiol 246:H838, 1984.
47. Ewing DJ, Nellson JMM, Travis P: New method for assessing cardiac parasympathetic activity using 24-hour electrocardiograms. Br Heart J 52:396, 1984.
48. Kleiger RE, Miller JP, Bigger JT Jr, Moss AJ, Multicenter Post-Infarction Research Group: Decreased heart rate variability and its association with increased mortality after acute myocardial infarction. Am J Cardiol 59:256, 1987.
49. Myers GA, Martin GJ, Magid NM, Barnett PS, Schadd JW, Weiss JS, Leach M, Singer DH: Power spectral and heart rate variability in sudden cardiac death: comparison to other methods. IEEE Trans Biomed Eng 33:1149, 1986.
50. Pomeranz N, Macaulay RJB, Caudill A, Kutz I, Adam D, Gordon Killborn KM, Barger AG, Shannon DC, Cohen RJ, Benson H: Assessment of autonomic functions in humans by heart rate spectral analysis. Am J Physiol 248:H151, 1985.
51. Craelius W, Chen VK-H, Restivo M, El-Sherif N: Rhythm analysis of arterial blood pressure. IEEE Trans Biomed 33:1166, 1986.
52. Bigger JT Jr, Albrecht P, Steinmann RC, Rolnitzky LM, Fleiss JL, Cohen RJ: Comparison of time and frequency domain-based measures of cardiac parasympathetic activity in Holter recordings after myocardial infarction. Am J Cardiol 64:536, 1989.
53. Pagani M, Lombardi F, Guzzetti S, Rimoldi O, Furian R, Pizzinelli P, Sandrone G, Malfatto G, Dell'Orto S, Piccaluga E, Turiel M, Bassell G, Cerutti S, Malliani A: Power spectral analysis of heart rate and arterial pressure variabilities as a marker of sympathovagal interaction in man and conscious dog. Circ Res 59:178, 1986.
54. Bekheit S, Tangella M, El-Sakr A, Rasheed Q, Craelius W, El-Sherif N: Use of heart rate spectral analysis to study the effects of calcium channel blockers on sympathetic activity after myocardial infarction. Am Heart J 119:79, 1990.
55. Lombardi F, Sandrone G, Pernpruner S, Sale R, Garimoldi M, Cerutti S, Basellini G, Pagani M, Malliani A: Heart rate variability as an index of sympathovagal interaction after acute myocardial infarction. Am J Cardiol 60:1239, 1987.

21

Late Potentials in Acute Ischemic Syndromes

Gioia Turitto, Edward B. Caref, Nabil El-Sherif

Introduction

Delayed and fractionated activation potentials were initially observed in ischemic regions of the canine heart, where they provided the electrophysiologic basis for reentrant ventricular rhythms.[1,2] These late potentials were found to correspond to low amplitude, high-frequency signals detected at the end of the QRS complex on the signal-averaged electrocardiogram (ECG).[2,3] Late potentials on the signal-averaged ECG correlated with the occurrence of spontaneous and electrically induced ventricular tachyarrhythmias in patients with coronary artery disease and prior myocardial infarction.[4,5] On the other hand, the role of myocardial ischemia and reperfusion in the genesis of late potentials on the signal-averaged ECG is poorly understood. This subject has significance, since studies on the relationship between acute ischemic syndromes and late potentials may provide an insight into the pathogenesis of ischemia related ventricular tachyarrhythmias. Finally, the influence of reperfusion mediated by thrombolysis on late potentials as well as

From El-Sherif N, Turitto G (eds): *High-Resolution Electrocardiography.* Mount Kisco, NY, Futura Publishing Co., Inc., ©, 1992.

on ventricular arrhythmias in survivors of myocardial infarction is still under investigation.

Ventricular Arrhythmias and Myocardial Ischemia

There is extensive literature describing the incidence, time course, and malignancy of complex ventricular arrhythmias during episodes of transient myocardial ischemia with ST elevation[6,7] or ST depression.[8] On the other hand, the electrophysiologic mechanisms of these arrhythmias have not been clarified. Furthermore, myocardial ischemia seems to play an important role in the occurrence of sudden cardiac death. It has been estimated that approximately one-third of sudden cardiac deaths is due to ventricular tachycardia/fibrillation precipitated by myocardial ischemia.[9] Ischemia-induced ventricular tachyarrhythmias may show different characteristics with respect to chronic recurrent sustained ventricular tachycardias. While the latter are inducible by programmed stimulation of the heart in the vast majority of cases, ischemic arrhythmias may not be electrically reproducible. In fact, up to one-third of survivors of sudden cardiac death has a negative electrophysiologic evaluation.[10] Arrhythmias induced by programmed stimulation, specifically sustained monomorphic ventricular tachycardias, are thought to indicate the presence of a reentrant substrate.[11] Thus, noninducible patients may lack a chronic reentrant substrate. However, they may still develop a transient arrhythmogenic substrate during myocardial ischemia.

The hypothesis that myocardial ischemia may facilitate induction of reentrant ventricular tachyarrhythmias by programmed ventricular stimulation was tested in a limited number of studies that showed conflicting results. One retrospective analysis concerning 32 patients with stable coronary artery disease concluded that pacing-induced angina did not result into the induction of ventricular tachyarrhythmias.[12] Significant shortcomings of this study were that none of the included patients had a history of spontaneous sustained ventricular tachycardia/fibrillation and that the diagnosis of ischemia was based solely on the occurrence of chest pain during pacing. Another study of 19 survivors of cardiac arrest suggested that transient myocardial ischemia was a requirement for the induction of ventricular tachyarrhythmias in some patients.[13] The onset of myocardial ischemia during ventricular stimulation was assessed by measuring arterial-coronary sinus lactate difference and was reflected by the presence of net lactate production. Programmed stimulation induced sustained monomorphic ventricular tachycardia in six cases, sustained polymorphic ventricular tachycardia in seven, and nonsustained polymorphic ventricular tachycardia in two patients. Myocardial ischemia was documented before initiation of ventricular tachycardia in 8 of the 15 patients with inducible tachyarrhythmias. Ventricular stimulation was repeated in the absence of ischemia in five patients with net lactate production during the first induction of ventricular tachycardia, and the arrhythmia was no longer inducible. Caution must be used to interpret these results, since the reproducibility of ventricular tachyarrhythmias induced during electrophysiologic testing is by no means absolute.[14]

Late Potentials and Myocardial Ischemia

Noninvasive evaluation for the presence of a reentrant substrate may be performed through signal-averaged electrocardiography. Late potentials on signal-averaged ECG recordings appeared to be strictly associated with the presence of such a substrate.[1,2] The search for a link between transient myocardial ischemia and late potentials on the signal-averaged ECG was the objective of a small number of investigations. They focused on ischemia induced during percutaneous transluminal coronary angioplasty,[15] dipyridamole infusion,[16] and exercise test.[17]

The Signal-Averaged ECG During Coronary Angioplasty

In a study from Abboud et al,[15] a single surface ECG lead (V_5) was recorded, averaged, filtered between 150 and 250 Hz, and used to compute the "envelope," i.e., the root mean square (RMS) voltage of QRS complex. Ischemia was induced by inflation of an angioplasty balloon positioned into the left anterior descending coronary artery; signal-averaged ECG recordings were obtained at baseline, prior to advancement of the balloon catheter across the target lesion, during the last 30 seconds of the initial balloon inflation, and at the end of the procedure. Ischemia secondary to balloon inflation was reported to lead to a statistically significant reduction ($p < 0.05$) in the calculated RMS voltage of QRS, as well as to the appearance of zones of reduced amplitude located in the midportion of QRS. This was attributed to the development of slow conduction during transient myocardial ischemia. No QRS prolongation or onset of late potentials was reported in this study. The significance of these findings is uncertain, since they were based on equipment for signal averaging, filter setting, and calculated parameters which were substantially different from those utilized in most studies involving averaging of ECG signals.

The Signal-Averaged ECG During Dipyridamole Test

In the report from Turitto et al,[16] the correlation between transient myocardial ischemia and late potentials was prospectively studied in a series of patients with coronary artery disease, by analyzing serial recordings of the signal-averaged ECG obtained before, during, and after provocation of ischemia by means of dipyridamole test. The study population included 100 patients with myocardial infarction and/or angina pectoris and ECG documentation of transient myocardial ischemia, no bundle branch block, QRS duration < 120 msec, and absence of electrolyte imbalance, antiarrhythmic or beta blocker treatment, and acute or chronic heart failure. The dipyridamole test was performed after withdrawal of all therapy for ≥ 24 hours and consisted of the intravenous administration of a "low dose" of dipyridamole (0.56 mg/kg body weight over 4 minutes), followed by a 4-minute observation period; an additional "high dose" of dipyridamole (0.28 mg/kg over 2 minutes) was used when the low dose failed to induce ischemic ST changes. After an observation period of 4 minutes, intravenous aminophylline (240 mg over 2 minutes) was administered to prevent any further effects from dipyridamole. Aminophylline was also utilized to relieve induced myocardial ischemia in case of a positive test. Endpoints of the dipyridamole test were completion of the protocol, or induction of transient ischemic ST changes (ST elevation or rectilinear or downsloping ST depression ≥ 1 mm in ≥ 1 conventional ECG lead, lasting ≥ 1 minute). The signal-averaged ECG was performed at baseline ("pretest" recording), after the low dose, after the high dose when appropriate ("test" recordings), and after aminophylline ("post-test" recording). Standard bipolar X, Y, and Z leads were recorded, filtered at 25–250 Hz, and combined into a vector magnitude. An abnormal signal-averaged ECG was defined as a recording showing a QRS duration

> 115 msec, a RMS voltage of last 40 msec of QRS (RMS40) < 25 μV, or both.[18] Late potentials were defined as signals with abnormal RMS40. In each patient, tracings were accepted for analysis if the noise level was ≤0.8 μV and showed a ≤0.2 μV difference between all of them. During dipyridamole test, 47 patients developed transient myocardial ischemia, while 53 patients did not. Transient ischemic ST elevation was noted in 14 cases and ST depression in the remaining 33. Ischemia appeared after the low dipyridamole dose in 17 patients and after the high dose in 30. Baseline signal-averaged ECG was abnormal in 20 of 100 study patients (20%), with no significant differences between those with or without transient myocardial ischemia (respectively: 12 of 47 [26%] vs 8 of 53 [15%]). A prolonged QRS duration was seen in six cases, a late potential in nine, and both abnormalities in five patients. Values of the signal-averaged ECG parameters obtained before, during, and after dipyridamole test were compared in both groups of patients by means of analysis of variance and Student's t-test for paired data (Tables I and II). None of these comparisons revealed any significant differences regarding QRS duration, RMS40, or the noise level. Absence of significant differences was also observed when cases with transient ischemic ST elevation or depression were analyzed separately. All 20 patients (100%) with or without induced ischemia who had abnormal QRS duration and/or RMS40 at baseline maintained abnormal values on all subsequent recordings; similarly, 78 of 80 patients (98%) with a normal baseline recording retained normal parameters during dipyridamole test and afterwards. In only two cases with induced ischemia, a borderline RMS40 value at baseline (25.7 and 29.9 μV) became abnormal during the test (respectively, 21.6 and 24.1 μV) and returned to normal value on the post-test recordings (28.4 and 28.2 μv, respectively). Figures 1 and 2 present serial signal-averaged ECGs obtained during the dipyridamole test in two patients from group 1. There were no significant changes between the baseline recordings and those performed during induced transient myocardial ischemia: both were normal in Figure 1 and abnormal in Figure 2. This study showed that the short-term reproducibility of signal-averaged ECG parameters is high. Using dipyridamole test and achieving an optimal noise level (≤0.8 μV for all recordings), there were no significant differences in QRS duration and RMS40 on serial signal-averaged ECGs obtained before, during, and after the test in the group without induced ischemia. These results were not influenced by the presence or absence of abnormal parameters at

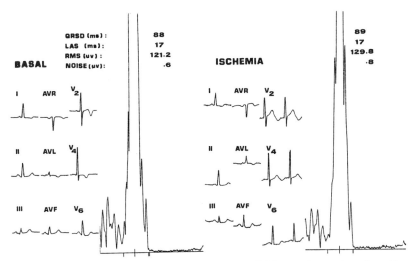

Figure 1. Conventional and signal-averaged ECGs performed at baseline (left) and during dipyridamole-induced transient ischemic ST elevation (right). The signal-averaged ECG is normal at baseline and does not show any significant changes during ischemia. LAS = duration of low amplitude signals <40 μV; QRSD = high-frequency QRS duration; RMS = root mean square voltage of last 40 msec of QRS. (Reproduced with permission from Turitto et al, Am J Cardiol 65:290, 1990.)

(corresponding to the test recording) and its resolution (corresponding to the post-test recording), as well as for the two types of ischemia, expressed by ST elevation (transmural ischemia) or ST depression (subendocardial ischemia).

The Signal-Averaged ECG During Stress Test

Caref et al[17] reported the effects of exercise-induced ischemia on the signal-averaged ECG in a series of 52 patients with coronary artery disease, documented by evidence of previous myocardial infarction and/or coronary angiography, and stable angina. These patients underwent conventional 12-lead and signal-averaged ECGs at baseline and within 1 minute of completion of a treadmill stress test. The latter was considered to be positive for transient myocardial ischemia when downsloping or horizontal ST depression ≥1 mm at 60–80 msec after the J point was recorded. Techniques for signal

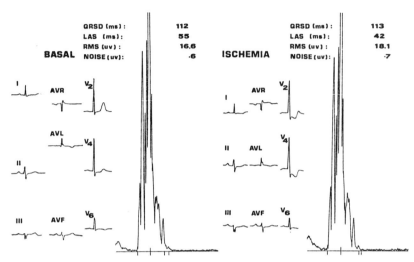

Figure 2. Conventional and signal-averaged ECGs performed at baseline (left) and during dipyridamole-induced transient ischemic ST depression (right). The signal-averaged ECG is abnormal at baseline, due to the presence of late potentials, and does not show any significant changes during ischemia. Abbreviations as in Figure 1. (Reproduced with permission from Turitto et al, Am J Cardiol 65:290, 1990.)

averaging were similar to those described by Turitto et al,[16] with the exception that data were analyzed with two different filter settings, namely between 25–250 Hz and 40–250 Hz. Late potentials were defined as signals with RMS40 < 25 μV at 25 Hz or < 16 μV at 40 Hz.[18] Signal-averaged ECGs were included in the study if the noise level was ≤0.8 μV at 25 Hz and ≤0.6 μV at 40 Hz, and the difference in the noise level between baseline and post-exercise recordings was ≤0.3 μV at 25 Hz and ≤0.2 μV at 40 Hz. Patients were divided into different subgroups, based on the outcome of exercise test (positive or negative), the presence or absence of prior myocardial infarction, the location of infarction (anterior vs inferior), and the presence or absence of exercise-induced ventricular arrhythmias. The latter were defined as a greater than or equal to four-fold increase in ventricular premature complexes compared to baseline and/or development of couplets or ventricular tachycardia (≥3 ventricular premature complexes at a rate ≥100/min). Among the 52 patients, 28 had a positive stress test, while 24 had not; 36 had a prior myocardial infarction (inferior in 20, anterior in 15, non-Q in 1 case). During exercise, ten patients developed a significant arrhythmic response. Table III summarizes the effects of stress testing on signal-averaged ECG parameters in all the study subgroups. There were no significant differences in any of the signal-averaged ECG parameters recorded pre- and post-exercise and analyzed at 40–250 Hz in any of the study subgroups. In particular, no significant variations between the baseline and the post-exercise signal-averaged ECGs were observed in the 28 patients with a positive exercise test. In 26 of 28 patients with a positive test, significant ST depression was maintained during the period of recording the post-exercise signal-averaged ECG (Figure 3). When the signal-averaged ECG was analyzed at 25–250 Hz, there was a tendency for the QRS duration and duration of low amplitude signals < 40 µV to shorten slightly and for the RMS40 amplitude to increase following exercise. These changes were statistically significant in 8 of 24 determinations (Table III). However, the changes were not related to the presence or absence of a positive exercise test, prior myocardial infarction, site of myocardial infarction, or exercise-induced ventricular arrhythmias. Seven patients (13%) had late potentials at baseline; four patients lost them on the post-exercise recording, due to an increase of RMS40 at 25–250 Hz. On the other hand, two patients developed late potentials after exercise, due to a slight decrease of RMS40 at 25–250 Hz. In all these cases, visual inspection of baseline and post-exercise signal-averaged ECGs revealed only minor changes in the terminal QRS morphology.

These studies from Turitto et al[16] and Caref et al[17] were concordant in showing that transient myocardial ischemia did not significantly affect the signal-averaged ECG. This phenomenon was independent of the presence or absence of abnormal signal-averaged ECG parameters at baseline, the mechanisms of induced ischemia (dipyridamole vs exercise test), the type of ischemia (transmural vs nontransmural), the presence and location of previous myocardial infarction, and the presence or absence of complex ventricular arrhythmias during ischemia. On the other hand, the results of these reports must be interpreted bearing in mind several methodological and technical issues. First, the sensitivity and specificity of dipyridamole and exercise tests for transient myocardial ischemia are not optimal. Selection of both study populations among patients with documented coronary artery disease was aimed to lower the risk for false-positive tests. The occurrence of false-negative tests could not be ruled out, but it would not have changed the results. In fact, they

Table III (Continued)

	Subgroup 1			Subgroup 2			Subgroup 3			Subgroup 4		
	Pos EX n = 28	Neg EX n = 24	p Value	MI n = 36	No MI n = 16	p Value	Ant MI n = 15	Inf MI n = 20	p Value	VA n = 10	No VA n = 34	p Value
40–250Hz												
QRS-BL (msec)	101	95	NS	100	96	NS	99	100	NS	101	99	NS
QRS-EX (msec)	101	95	NS	100	95	NS	99	101	NS	102	99	NS
Δ (msec)	0	0	NS	0	−1	NS	0	1	NS	1	0	NS
p value			NS			NS			NS			NS
LAS-BL (msec)	32	29	NS	31	30	NS	31	31	NS	31	31	NS
LAS-EX (msec)	31	28	NS	31	25	NS	31	32	NS	30	30	NS
Δ (msec)	−1	−1	NS	0	−5	NS	0	1	NS	−1	−1	NS
p value			NS			NS			NS			NS
RMS-BL (μV)	43	41	NS	40	48	NS	45	34	NS	49	39	NS
RMS-EX (μV)	44	42	NS	40	50	NS	46	36	NS	47	39	NS
Δ (μV)	1	1	NS	0	2	NS	1	2	NS	−2	0	NS
p value			NS			NS			NS			NS

Ant = anterior; BL = baseline; EX = post-exercise; Inf = inferior; LAS = low amplitude signal < 40 μV of the terminal filtered QRS; MI = myocardial infarction; neg = negative; NS = not statistically significant; pos = positive; QRS = filtered QRS duration; RMS = root mean square voltage of the last 40 msec of the filtered QRS; VA = exercise-induced ventricular arrhythmias.

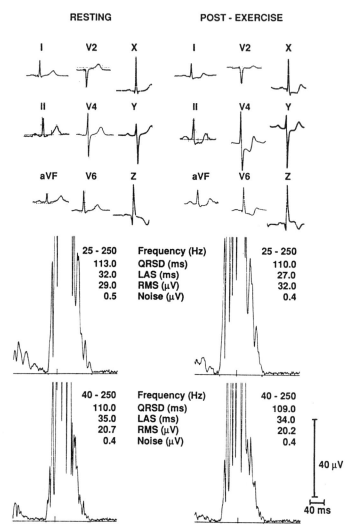

Figure 3. Conventional and signal-averaged ECGs performed at baseline (top left) and during exercise-induced transient ischemic ST depression (top right). The signal-averaged ECG was analyzed at 25 to 250 Hz (middle) and 40 to 250 Hz (bottom). Exercise-induced ischemic ST changes were not associated with significant changes in the signal-averaged ECG. Abbreviations as in Figure 1. (Reproduced with permission from Caref et al, Am J Cardiol 66:54, 1990.)

were comparable in all groups with or without induced ischemia in showing no significant differences between serial recordings obtained before and during the provocative tests (dipyridamole infusion or exercise). The signal averaging technique has some important electrophysiologic limitations. A conduction delay in the ischemic myocardium with a Wenckebach pattern may not be amenable to a technique which requires that the signal of interest be repeated at regular intervals. Finally, it may be argued that induced ischemia was not severe enough to induce significant myocardial conduction changes that could be detected as late potentials on the signal-averaged ECG. On the other hand, brief periods of ischemia may well precipitate complex ventricular arrhythmias. Arrhythmias were seen during exercise-induced ischemia in a proportion of patients studied by Caref et al (ten cases)[17]; however, they were not associated with the onset of late potentials on the signal-averaged ECG. Furthermore, in the study by Turitto et al, ischemia elicited by dipyridamole infusion was similar, in type and duration, to episodes of spontaneous ischemia which were documented to provoke arrhythmias;[6-8] however, late potentials failed to appear on the signal-averaged ECG during positive dipyridamole test. Extensive studies on the signal-averaged ECG during episodes of spontaneous ischemia with ST elevation or depression are not available; however, most recent data suggest that late potentials are not evoked, thus duplicating findings relative to dipyridamole and exercise-induced ischemia.[19] In the report from Turitto et al,[19] the effects of spontaneous transient myocardial ischemia on the signal-averaged ECG were investigated in 13 patients with coronary artery disease and spontaneous angina who had transient ischemic attacks (ST elevation or depression ≥ 1 mm for ≥ 1 minute) during three-channel ambulatory ECG. A total of 61 ischemic attacks was recorded: 17 had ST elevation and 44 ST depression. The mean duration and magnitude of ischemic ST changes were, respectively, 14.5 ± 9.7 minutes and 2.3 ± 1.6 mm. They lasted > 10 minutes during 31 ischemic attacks and were > 2 mm during 20 of them. The location of ischemia was anterior in five patients, inferior in four, and undetermined in four, based on electrocardiographic and angiographic findings. Signal-averaged ECGs with noise levels ≤ 1 µV were obtained from Holter tapes at baseline and during 54 of 61 ischemic attacks (88%). Baseline signal-averaged ECGs were normal in eight patients (62%), showed a long QRS duration (> 115 msec) in two (15%), and both a long QRS duration and a late potential (RMS40 < 25 µV) in the remaining three

(23%). Comparison of recordings obtained at baseline and during ischemic attacks revealed no significant changes in QRS duration and RMS40. Absence of significant differences was also noted when analysis was performed separately according to the type of ischemic attacks (with ST elevation or ST depression), their location (anterior or inferior), their duration ($\leq$10 minutes or longer), and their magnitude ($\leq$2 mm or greater). It was concluded that spontaneous transient myocardial ischemia, independent of its type, location, duration, and magnitude, does not generate a substrate for late potentials.

Late potentials may not provide an electrophysiologic basis for ischemia related arrhythmias, in patients with coronary artery disease. Possible mechanisms for these arrhythmias include focal pacemaker discharge due to abnormal automaticity or triggered activity; furthermore, reentrant activation may play a role, even though the pathways for reentry may differ in the acutely ischemic heart, with respect to the heart with chronic infarction. The relevance of each of these mechanisms to the clinical setting still awaits confirmation. However, it may be suggested that electrophysiologic changes associated with transient myocardial ischemia do not bear any relationship with the anatomic-electrophysiologic substrate that underlies late potentials on the signal-averaged ECG.

Late Potentials and Myocardial Reperfusion

During acute myocardial infarction, reperfusion induced by thrombolytic agents has been shown to decrease the infarct size and to improve survival. On the other hand, little is known about the effect of thrombolysis mediated reperfusion on markers for electrical instability, namely late potentials on the signal-averaged ECG [20,21] and complex ventricular arrhythmias on the ambulatory ECG. [22,23]

Turitto et al [20] conducted a prospective study to determine if thrombolysis reduces the prevalence of late potentials or ventricular arrhythmias. They compared recordings of the signal-averaged and ambulatory ECGs in patients treated with or without thrombolytic therapy in the setting of acute myocardial infarction. The study population included 118 patients who presented with acute myocardial infarction, absence of prior myocardial infarction, QRS duration <120 msec and no bundle branch block on 12-lead ECG, and survived until completion of the protocol. Among them, 46 patients admitted within 6 hours of the onset of chest pain received intravenous thrombolytic therapy with urokinase (35 cases), recombinant tissue plasminogen activator (7 cases), or streptokinase (4 cases); the remaining 72 patients did not receive thrombolysis, due to their late hospital arrival or to the presence of contraindications. All patients had signal-averaged and ambulatory ECGs within 24 hours of each other. The tests were performed before hospital discharge, 13 ± 2 days after the index infarction and ≥ 24 hours after withdrawal of all therapy. For signal averaging, standard bipolar X, Y, and Z leads were recorded, filtered at 25–250 Hz and combined into a vector magnitude. An abnormal signal-averaged ECG was defined as a recording showing one or more of the following: QRS duration >115 msec; duration of low amplitude signals (<40 μV) >32 msec; and RMS voltage of last 40 msec of QRS (RMS40) <25 μV.[18] Late potentials were defined as signals with abnormal RMS40. Complex ventricular arrhythmias were defined as frequent ventricular premature complexes (≥ 10/hour), ventricular tachycardia (≥ 3 ventricular premature complexes at a rate >100/min), or both.[24] A cardiac catheterization was performed before discharge in all 46 patients subjected to thrombolysis and in 39 patients not subjected to this intervention. When patients who received thrombolysis (group 1) were compared to patients who did not receive it (group 2), they were not significantly different with regard to their age and sex distribution, type and location of myocardial infarction, maximum increase in serum cardiac enzymes, and prevalence of ventricular fibrillation during hospitalization (Table IV). An abnormal signal-averaged ECG was recorded in 22 of the 118 study patients (19%), with no significant difference between groups 1 and 2 (respectively: 7 of 46 [15%] vs 15 of 72 [21%]). No significant differences were found regarding the prevalence of abnormal signal-averaged ECG parameters, or their mean values in the two groups. An abnormal signal-averaged ECG was slightly more common in patients with inferior than in those with anterior infarctions (respectively: 19% vs 10% in group 1 and 24% vs 18% in group 2); however, comparison of the signal-averaged ECG data according to the site of infarction did not reveal any significant differences between groups. Complex ventricular arrhythmias on the ambulatory ECG were observed in 25 of the 118 study patients (21%), with no significant difference between groups 1 and 2 (respectively: 9 of 46 [20%] vs 16 of 72 [22%]). On the other hand, the mean hourly number of ventricular premature complexes

Table IV *(Continued)*

	Thrombolysis *(n = 46)*	No Thrombolysis *(n = 72)*	*p Value*
1 abnormal parameter (%)	7 (15)	15 (21)	NS
2 abnormal parameters (%)	7 (15)	13 (18)	NS
3 abnormal parameters (%)	4 (19)	9 (13)	NS

Continuous variables are expressed as mean ±standard deviation; CK = creatine kinase; ECG = electrocardiogram; LAS40 = duration of low amplitude signals <40 µV; MB-CK = creatine kinase-MB isoenzyme; MI = myocardial infarction; NS = not significant; RMSQRS = root mean square voltage of total QRS; RMS40 = root mean square voltage of last 40 msec of QRS; VF = ventricular fibrillation; VPCs = ventricular premature complexes; VT = ventricular tachycardia.

was lower in group 1 than in group 2 (p <0.05). Complex ventricular arrhythmias were equally common in patients with or without an abnormal signal-averaged ECG in both groups. Complex ventricular arrhythmias were present in 29% of cases in group 1 and 27% of cases in group 2 who had an abnormal signal-averaged ECG, as well as in 18% of cases in group 1 and 21% of cases in group 2 who had a normal signal-averaged ECG. These differences were not statistically significant.

Thrombolysis was successful in restoring patency of the infarct related coronary artery in 26 cases (group 1A), while it failed to do so in 20 cases (group 1B). Table V summarizes angiographic and electrocardiographic variables in groups 1A and 1B. Left ventricular ejection fraction was higher (p <0.05), while a/dyskinesia in the infarcted area and collateral circulation to the infarct related vessel were less common (p <0.001) in the presence than in the absence of successful thrombolysis. Abnormalities of the signal-averaged ECG tended to be less frequent in group 1A than in group 1B, but none of the observed differences reached statistical significance. On the other hand, both the mean root mean square voltage of total QRS and RMS40 were significantly higher in group 1A than in group 1B. No significant differences were found between groups 1A and 1B regarding the prevalence of complex ventricular arrhythmias (respectively: 19% vs 20%). On the other hand, the mean hourly number

Table V
Characteristics of Patients With or Without Successful Thrombolysis
During Acute Myocardial Infarction

	Successful Thrombolysis (n = 26)	No Successful Thrombolysis (n = 20)	p Value
Angiographic Data			
Ejection fraction	0.62 ±0.13	0.54 ±0.12	<0.05
A/dyskinesia in infarcted segment(s) (%)	8 (31)	17 (85)	<0.001
Collateral circulation to infarct related artery (%)	4 (15)	16 (80)	<0.001
Ambulatory ECG Data			
VPCs/hour (n)	1.11 ±0.88	4.49 ±2.61	<0.01
Frequent VPCs (%)	1 (4)	3 (15)	NS
Nonsustained VT (%)	4 (15)	2 (10)	NS
Complex ventricular arrhythmias (%)	5 (19)	4 (20)	NS
Signal-averaged ECG Data			
QRS duration (msec)	99 ±13	106 ±13	NS
LAS40 (msec)	23 ±11	29 ±12	NS
RMSQRS (µV)	136 ±51	94 ±32	<0.01
RMS40 (µV)	73 ±50	45 ±25	<0.05
Prolonged QRS duration (%)	1 (4)	3 (15)	NS
Prolonged LAS40 (%)	2 (8)	5 (25)	NS
Late potentials (%)	2 (8)	5 (25)	NS
Abnormal signal-averaged ECG (%)	2 (8)	5 (25)	NS
1 abnormal parameter (%)	2 (8)	5 (25)	NS
2 abnormal parameters (%)	2 (8)	5 (25)	NS
3 abnormal parameters (%)	1 (4)	3 (15)	NS

Abbreviations as in Table IV.

of ventricular premature complexes was lower in group 1A than in group 1B (p <0.01). In group 1A, complex ventricular arrhythmias were seen in no cases with an abnormal signal-averaged ECG and in 21% of cases with a normal signal-averaged ECG; in group 1B, they were noted in 40% of cases with an abnormal signal-averaged ECG and in 13% of cases with a normal signal-averaged ECG (differences not significant).

In order to assess if patency of the infarct related artery, whether or not mediated by thrombolysis, influenced the signal-averaged ECG and complex ventricular arrhythmias, the characteristics of 42 patients with patency of the infarct related artery (26 from group 1A and 16 from group 2) were compared with those of 33 patients with occlusion of the infarct related artery (20 from group 1B and 13 from group 2) (Table VI). This analysis showed no significant differences in the prevalence of abnormal signal-averaged ECG parameters, although the mean root mean square voltage of total QRS and RMS40 were significantly higher in the presence than in the absence of a patent artery. Similarly, no significant differences were found in the prevalence of complex ventricular arrhythmias between patients with or without patency of the infarct related artery, although the mean hourly number of ventricular premature complexes was lower (p <0.05) in the former than in the latter group. These results led to several conclusions: (1) Thrombolysis favorably influences some signal-averaged ECG parameters, namely root mean square voltage of total QRS and root mean square voltage of last 40 msec of QRS. In fact, these indices are significantly higher in the presence than in the absence of successful thrombolysis, possibly a reflection of reduced loss of myocardial mass due to necrosis. Thus, they may be helpful in estimating myocardial salvage after thrombolysis. (2) No significant differences in the prevalence of an abnormal signal-averaged ECG may be observed between patients with or without thrombolysis, although there is a tendency toward a lesser number of abnormal signal-averaged ECG parameters in the group with than in the group without successful thrombolysis. These findings are at variance with those from Gang et al,[21] who performed a signal-averaged ECG within 48 hours of admission in 44 patients with and 62 patients without thrombolytic treatment and found abnormal parameters, respectively, in 2 and 14 patients (5% vs 23%, p = 0.01). An abnormal signal-averaged ECG was associated with future arrhythmic events when observed in the late hospital period (6–30 days after infarction) rather than in the early phase (0–5 days

Table VI

Characteristics of Patients With or Without Patency of the Infarct Related Coronary Artery After Acute Myocardial Infarction

	Patency of the Infarct Related Coronary Artery (n = 42)	Occlusion of the Infarct Related Coronary Artery (n = 33)	p Value
Ambulatory ECG Data			
VPCs/hour (n)	3.16 ±6.15	6.39 ±7.00	<0.05
Frequent VPCs (%)	3 (7)	5 (15)	NS
Nonsustained VT (%)	5 (12)	3 (9)	NS
Sustained VT (%)	0	1 (3)	NS
Complex ventricular arrhythmias (%)	7 (17)	6 (18)	NS
Signal-averaged ECG Data			
QRS duration (msec)	99 ±14	106 ±18	NS
LAS40 (msec)	24 ±10	29 ±14	NS
RMSQRS (μV)	140 ±50	104 ±38	<0.01
RMS40 (μV)	72 ±54	47 ±27	<0.05
Prolonged QRS duration (%)	4 (10)	7 (21)	NS
Prolonged LAS40 (%)	5 (12)	9 (27)	NS
Late potentials (%)	5 (12)	8 (24)	NS
Abnormal signal-averaged ECG (%)	6 (14)	9 (27)	NS
1 abnormal parameter (%)	6 (14)	9 (27)	NS
2 abnormal parameters (%)	5 (12)	8 (24)	NS
3 abnormal parameters (%)	3 (7)	5 (15)	NS

Abbreviations as in Table IV.

after infarction)[25]; thus, data from Gang et al may not be relevant to long-term prognosis of post-infarction patients. Furthermore, in their investigation the signal-averaged ECG repeated before discharge remained abnormal in 2 cases with and in only 11 cases without thrombolysis (5% vs 18%, difference not significant). (3) The prevalence of late potentials is independent of the patency of the infarct related coronary artery. This is different from a study by Lange et al,[26] who performed a signal-averaged ECG in 109 subjects, 1 to 48 months after their first myocardial infarction (mean: 19 ±14). They found late potentials in 4 of 49 cases with antegrade flow in the infarct artery and in 24 of 60 cases with no or minimal flow (8% vs 40.5%, p <0.001). However, this study is affected by a significant limitation, namely the long time interval between the infarction and the recording of the signal-averaged ECG. (4) The effects of thrombolysis on the signal-averaged ECG are not related to those on left ventricular function, since the prevalence of an abnormal signal-averaged ECG is similar in patients with or without a/dyskinesia in the infarcted area. This duplicates observations from Gomes et al, who documented no correlation between the signal-averaged ECG and left ventricular ejection fraction or wall motion abnormalities in a group of 50 post-infarction patients.[27] It may be speculated that late potentials arise from viable myocardium interspersed in the infarct zone, showing delayed conduction, or from slow activation in the infarct border zone; thus, any intervention aimed to reduce the extent of myocardial infarction and wall motion abnormalities may not be expected to modify the substrate for late potentials. (5) Thrombolysis may not represent an antiarrhythmic intervention. Complex ventricular arrhythmias may be equally common in the presence or in the absence of successful thrombolysis. The lack of a net antiarrhythmic efficacy of thrombolysis is not surprising, because the consequences of pharmacologic reperfusion may not be uniform. In some cases, ventricular arrhythmias may be improved due to reversal of ischemic damage, while in other cases they may be exacerbated as a result of enhanced heterogeneity in the infarct zone. The fact that arrhythmias are as frequent in patients with as in those without an abnormal signal-averaged ECG confirms the absence of correlation between late potentials and complex ventricular arrhythmias previously documented in studies not focused on thrombolysis.[24] It also supports the concept that late potentials on the signal-averaged ECG and complex ventricular arrhythmias may reflect two different electrophysiologic substrates.

References

1. El-Sherif N, Gomes JAC, Restivo M, Mehra R: Late potentials and arrhythmogenesis. PACE 8:440, 1985.
2. El-Sherif N, Gough WB, Restivo M, Craelius W, Henkin R: Electrophysiological basis of ventricular late potentials. In Santini M, Pistolese M, Alliegro A (eds): Progress in Clinical Pacing. Amsterdam: Excerpta Medica, 1988, pp 209–223.
3. Simson MB, Untereker WJ, Spielman SR, Horowitz LN, Marcus NH, Falcone RA, Harken AH, Josephson ME: Relation between late potentials on the body surface and directly recorded fragmented electrograms in patients with ventricular tachycardia. Am J Cardiol 51:105, 1983.
4. Simson MB: Use of signals in the terminal QRS complex to identify patients with ventricular tachycardia after myocardial infarction. Circulation 64:235, 1981.
5. Turitto G, Fontaine JM, Ursell SN, Caref EB, Henkin R, El-Sherif N: Value of the signal-averaged electrocardiogram as a predictor of the results of programmed stimulation in nonsustained ventricular tachycardia. Am J Cardiol 61:1272, 1988.
6. Turitto G, El-Sherif N: Alternans of the ST segment in variant angina: incidence, time course and relation to ventricular arrhythmias during ambulatory electrocardiographic recording. Chest 93:587, 1988.
7. Turitto G, Dini P, Prati PL: The R on T phenomenon during transient myocardial ischemia. Am J Cardiol 63:1520, 1989.
8. Turitto G, Zanchi E, Maddaluna A, Pellegrini A, Risa AL, Prati PL: Prevalence, time course and malignancy of ventricular arrhythmias during spontaneous ischemic ST-segment depression. Am J Cardiol 64: 900, 1989.
9. Goldstein S, Vanderbrug Medendorp S, Landis JR, Wolfe RA, Leighton R, Ritter G, Vasu CM, Acheson A: Analysis of cardiac symptoms preceding cardiac arrest. Am J Cardiol 58:1195, 1986.
10. Gottlieb C, Josephson ME: The preference of programmed stimulation-guided therapy for sustained ventricular arrhythmias. In Brugada P, Wellens HJJ (eds): Cardiac Arrhythmias: Where To Go From Here? New York: Futura Publishing, 1987, pp 421–434.
11. Wellens HJJ, Brugada P, Stevenson WG: Programmed electrical stimulation of the heart in patients with life-threatening ventricular arrhythmias: what is the significance of induced arrhythmias and what is the correct stimulation protocol? Circulation 72:1, 1985.
12. Kowey PR, Friehling TD, Kline RA, Engel TR: Pacing-induced angina pectoris and induction of ventricular arrhythmias in coronary artery disease. Am J Cardiol 58:90, 1986.
13. Morady F, DiCarlo LA, Jr, Krol RB, Annesley TM, O'Neill WW, de Buitleir M, Baerman JM, Kou WH: Role of myocardial ischemia during programmed stimulation in survivors of cardiac arrest with coronary artery disease. J Am Coll Cardiol 9:1004, 1987.
14. de Buitleir M, Morady F, DiCarlo LA, Jr, Baerman JW, Krol RB: Immediate reproducibility of clinical and nonclinical forms of induced ventricular tachycardia. Am J Cardiol 58:279, 1986.

15. Abboud S, Cohen RJ, Selwyn A, Ganz P, Sadeh D, Friedman PL: Detection of transient myocardial ischemia by computer analysis of standard and signal-averaged high-frequency electrocardiograms in patients undergoing percutaneous transluminal coronary angioplasty. Circulation 76:585, 1987.
16. Turitto G, Zanchi E, Risa AL, Maddaluna A, Saltarocchi ML, Vajola SF, Prati PL: Lack of correlation between transient myocardial ischemia and late potentials on the signal-averaged electrocardiogram. Am J Cardiol 65:290, 1990.
17. Caref EB, Goldberg N, Mendelson L, Hanley G, Okereke R, Stein RA, El-Sherif N: Effects of exercise on the signal-averaged electrocardiogram in coronary artery disease. Am J Cardiol 66:54, 1990.
18. Caref EB, Turitto G, Ibrahim BB, Henkin R, El-Sherif N: Role of bandpass filters in optimizing the value of the signal-averaged electrocardiogram as a predictor of the results of programmed stimulation. Am J Cardiol 64:16, 1989.
19. Turitto G, Caref EB, Zanchi E, Menghini F, Kelen G, El-Sherif N: Spontaneous myocardial ischemia and the signal-averaged electrocardiogram. Am J Cardiol 67:676, 1991.
20. Turitto G, Risa AL, Zanchi E, Prati PL: The signal-averaged electrocardiogram and ventricular arrhythmias after thrombolysis for acute myocardial infarction. J Am Coll Cardiol 15:1270, 1990.
21. Gang ES, Lew AS, Hong M, Wang FZ, Siebert CA, Peter T: Decreased incidence of ventricular late potentials after successful thrombolytic therapy for acute myocardial infarction. N Engl J Med 321:712, 1989.
22. Cercek B, Lew AS, Laramee P, Shah PK, Peter TC, Ganz W: Time course and characteristics of ventricular arrhythmias after reperfusion in acute myocardial infarction. Am J Cardiol 60:214, 1987.
23. Theroux P, Morrissette D, Juneau M, de Guise P, Pelletier G, Waters DD: Influence of fibrinolysis and percutaneous transluminal angioplasty on the frequency of ventricular premature complexes. Am J Cardiol 63:797, 1989.
24. Turitto G, Caref EB, Macina G, Fontaine JM, Ursell SN, El-Sherif N: Time course of ventricular arrhythmias and the signal-averaged electrocardiogram in the post-infarction period: a prospective study of correlation. Br Heart J 60:17, 1988.
25. El-Sherif N, Ursell SN, Bekheit S, Fontaine J, Turitto G, Henkin R, Caref EB: Prognostic significance of the signal-averaged ECG depends on the time of recording in the postinfarction period. Am Heart J 118:-256, 1989.
26. Lange RA, Cigarroa RG, Wells PJ, Kremers MS, Hillis LD: Influence of antegrade flow in the infarct artery on the incidence of late potentials after acute myocardial infarction. Am J Cardiol 65:554, 1990.
27. Gomes JA, Horowitz SF, Millner M, Machac J, Winters SL, Barreca P: Relation of late potentials to ejection fraction and wall motion abnormalities in acute myocardial infarction. Am J Cardiol 59:1071, 1987.

Section V.

Late Potentials and Ventricular Arrhythmias

22

Late Potentials in Patients with Nonsustained Ventricular Tachycardia

Gioia Turitto, John Fontaine,
Shantha Ursell, Soad Bekheit,
Nabil El-Sherif

Prevalence of Late Potentials in Nonsustained Ventricular Tachycardia

The prevalence of late potentials in patients with complex ventricular ectopy and/or nonsustained ventricular tachycardia (VT) is 0% to 45% (mean: 29%) (Table I).[1-11] This is much lower than the prevalence of late potentials in patients with spontaneous sustained VT or ventricular fibrillation (see Chapter 23). The prevalence of late potentials also varies according to the presence and type of heart disease (Table I).[1-11] An abnormal signal-averaged electrocardiogram (ECG) is least frequent when nonsustained VT occurs in the setting of an apparently normal heart, and is most common when this arrhythmia is observed in post-infarction patients. Limited data are available on the prevalence of late potentials in patients with dilated cardiomyopathy and nonsustained VT. In one report,[1] the

From El-Sherif N, Turitto G (eds): *High-Resolution Electrocardiography*. Mount Kisco, NY, Futura Publishing Co., Inc., ©, 1992.

Table I

Prevalence of Late Potentials in Subjects With Complex Ventricular Arrhythmias and/or Nonsustained VT

Author	Organic Heart Disease	Population (n) With Late Potentials/Total	Prevalence of Late Potentials
Turitto, 1988[1]	miscellaneous	23/105	23%
	—with CAD	15/60	25%
	—with dilated CMP	6/26	23%
	—none	2/19	11%
Turitto, 1988[2]	CAD, post-MI	8/33	24%
Gomes, 1987[3]	CAD, post-MI	23/52	44%
Buxton, 1987[4]	CAD, post-MI	23/43	53%
Denes, 1987[5]	miscellaneous	15/84	18%
Nalos, 1987[6]	miscellaneous	9/24	38%
Poll, 1985[7]	dilated CMP	2/11	18%
Coto, 1985[8]	miscellaneous	5/11	45%
Zimmermann, 1985[9]	CAD	0/6	0
Kertes, 1985[10]	miscellaneous	6/22	27%
Denes, 1984[11]	CAD	3/10	30%
Total		117/401	29%

CAD = coronary artery disease; CMP = cardiomyopathy; MI = myocardial infarction.

prevalence did not differ from that described in subjects with coronary artery disease (Table I).

Late Potentials and Left Ventricular Function

A close relationship between late potentials and the degree of left ventricular dysfunction was described in several studies of patients with or without documented VT.[12–15] Early reports suggested the possibility that the presence of late potentials was mainly related to left ventricular ejection fraction and wall motion abnormalities, rather than to VT. Breithardt et al[16] studied 209 patients with organic heart disease (mostly coronary artery disease), of whom 63 had a history of sustained ventricular tachyarrhythmias, while 146 did not. They found that the main factor associated with the occurrence of late potentials was the presence of left ventricular wall motion abnormalities. In fact, the prevalence of late potentials in the group without arrhythmias was as low as 9% in those with a normal contraction pattern of the left ventricle, approached 22% in patients with hypokinesia, and reached 54% and 42%, respectively, in those with akinesia or left ventricular aneurysm. A similar trend was noted in patients with spontaneous sustained ventricular tachyarrhythmias: late potentials were present in 33% of patients with wall motion abnormalities; 67% of those with akinesia; and 83% of those with aneurysm. However, more recent studies utilizing multivariate statistical analysis techniques have shown that late potentials are able to identify patients with spontaneous sustained VT independent of left ventricular ejection fraction and wall motion abnormalities. [13–15]

Late Potentials and Programmed Ventricular Stimulation

In earlier studies, the signal-averaged ECG showed a strong correlation with the outcome of programmed ventricular stimulation in patients with spontaneous sustained VT or ventricular fibrillation. [11,17,18] In these subjects, an abnormal signal-averaged ECG had a predictive value for the induction of sustained ventricular tachyarrhythmias of 71% to 75%. [11,17] The high predictive accuracy of late potentials for the induction of sustained VT was confirmed by Nalos et al[6] in 100 "high-risk" patients, presenting with syncope (38 cases), nonsustained VT (24 cases), sustained VT (25 cases), or sudden cardiac arrest (13 cases). In the experience of these authors, stepwise logistic regression analysis identified the signal-averaged ECG as the best predictor of the induction of sustained monomorphic VT, independent of left ventricular ejection fraction, presence of left ventricular aneurysm, myocardial infarction, and other clinical variables. The sensitivity and specificity of the signal-averaged ECG for predicting induced sustained monomorphic VT were, respectively, 93% and 94%.

Buxton et al[4] studied 43 patients with spontaneous nonsustained VT after healing of myocardial infarction. Prior infarction was inferior in 29 cases and anterior in 14. Programmed stimulation was performed in all patients and VT was induced in 22. Patients with inferior infarctions and induced sustained VT had significantly longer filtered QRS durations and significantly lower voltage in the last 40 msec of the filtered QRS complex, compared to patients without induced sustained VT. In contrast, the signal-averaged ECG in patients with anterior infarctions and induced sustained VT did not differ significantly from those without induced sustained VT. It was concluded that the signal-averaged ECG may be useful in identifying patients with nonsustained VT after inferior infarction who had induced sustained VT; however, it may not distinguish patients with or without induced sustained VT, among those with nonsustained VT after anterior infarction. These results from Buxton et al[4] may be partly related to the small size of the group with anterior infarction (eight cases with and six without induced sustained VT).

Winters et al[19] performed signal averaging of the QRS complex prior to programmed ventricular stimulation in 53 individuals with high grade ventricular arrhythmias (frequent ventricular premature complexes or couplets) and/or nonsustained VT. An abnormal signal-averaged ECG was recorded in 22 patients and was associated with induced VT in 12 (55%). In contrast, a normal signal-averaged ECG was seen in 31 cases and was associated with induced VT in only 1 patient (3%). This difference was statistically significant (55% vs 3%, $p < 0.005$). These authors concluded that signal averaging of the surface QRS complex is useful in identifying patients with high grade ventricular ectopy or nonsustained VT who will have induced VT on programmed stimulation.[19]

A series of 274 patients subjected to programmed stimulation and signal-averaged ECG was reported by Vatterott et al.[20] The patients underwent electrophysiologic testing because of syncope (146 cases), complex ventricular ectopy (83 cases), VT (21 cases), wide complex tachycardia (15 cases), or out-of-hospital cardiac arrest (9 cases). Sustained monomorphic VT was induced in 70 patients. A stepwise logistic regression analysis was utilized to rank eight clinical and nine signal-averaged electrocardiographic variables. The best predictors for the induction of sustained VT were ejection fraction, history of infarction, ventricular ectopic pairs or nonsustained VT on Holter monitoring, QRS duration after 25–Hz filtering, and root mean square voltage of last 40 msec of the QRS complex after 40- and 80–Hz filtering. Cross validation (a statistical technique that can be used to accurately evaluate how a predictive model will perform on a prospective patient population) was used to validate the model. After cross validation, the sensitivity of the model was 95% and its specificity was 59% for VT during electrophysiologic testing. This model was compared with established 25–Hz late potential criteria (QRS duration >110 msec and root mean square voltage of last 40 msec of QRS <25 µV; sensitivity, 64%; specificity, 85%) and with established 40–Hz late potential criteria (QRS duration >114 msec or root mean square voltage of last 40 msec of QRS <20 µV or duration of the low amplitude (<40 µV) signal >38 msec; sensitivity, 84%; specificity, 54%).

We prospectively studied a consecutive series of 105 patients with nonsustained VT.[1] Patients included in this study fulfilled the following criteria: (1) one or more episodes of spontaneous nonsustained VT, defined as three or more ventricular premature complexes, <30 seconds, at a rate >100/min, during a 24-hour ambulatory ECG; (2) QRS duration <120 msec with absence of bundle branch block pattern and QT prolongation on the 12-lead ECG; and (3) absence of recent (<3 weeks) myocardial infarction, electrolyte imbalance, antiarrhythmic drug treatment at the time of the ambulatory ECG, and documented sustained VT/ventricular fibrillation/sudden death. Using stepwise discriminant function analysis, we examined several clinical variables (age, sex, etiology of underlying heart disease, history of syncope/presyncope), electrocardiographic characteristics of the spontaneous arrhythmia, left ventricular function indices (ejection fraction, segmental a/dyskinesia), and the signal-averaged ECG to assess their predictive accuracy for the induction of sustained ventricular tachyarrhythmias by programmed stimulation.

The study group consisted of 60 patients with coronary artery disease, 26 with nonischemic dilated cardiomyopathy, and 19 with no identifiable heart disease. All patients had radionuclide ventriculography, signal-averaged ECG, and programmed electrical stimulation. The signal-averaged ECG (vector magnitude of X, Y, and Z bipolar leads, filtered between 25 and 250 Hz) was considered to be abnormal if the filtered QRS duration was ≥120 msec, the duration of low amplitude signals of <40 µV (LAS40) was ≥38 msec, or the root mean square voltage of signals in the last 40 msec of the filtered QRS (RMS40) was ≤25 µV. Late potentials were defined as signals with abnormal LAS40 and RMS40. Patients were divided into three groups according to the results of programmed stimulation (three extrastimuli delivered to two right ventricular sites during basic rhythm and ventricular pacing at cycle lengths of 600, 500, and 400 msec). Group 1 included 22 patients with induced sustained monomorphic VT ($\geq$ 30 seconds), group 2 comprised 14 patients with induced ventricular fibrillation, and group 3 consisted of 69 patients without induced sustained ventricular tachyarrhythmias. Table II shows the characteristics of patients in the three groups. When compared to patients without induced sustained VT/ventricular fibrillation (group 3), patients with induced sustained monomorphic VT (group 1) showed a significantly higher frequency of syncope/ presyncope, left ventricular ejection fraction < 40%, and late potentials on the signal-averaged ECG. The etiology of underlying heart disease, the electrocardiographic characteristics of the spontaneous arrhythmia (number, duration, morphology, and cycle length of nonsustained VT runs), and the prevalence of left ventricular wall motion abnormalities were not significantly different in groups 1 and 3. On the other hand, when patients with induced ventricular fibrillation (group 2) were compared to patients without induced sustained VT/ventricular fibrillation (group 3), none of the variables showed significant differences. Further analysis of group 3 patients revealed no significant differences in clinical and electrocardiographic variables, left ventricular function indices, and the signal-averaged ECG between patients in whom monomorphic nonsustained VT, polymorphic nonsustained VT, or no VT (< 6 repetitive ventricular responses) were induced.

The signal-averaged ECG parameters were analyzed singly or in combination to obtain the best predictive accuracy for inducible sustained monomorphic VT (Table III). Abnormal filtered QRS duration showed the least specificity and predictive accuracy. Abnormal RMS40 alone, LAS40 alone, or a combination of both (defined as late potentials) had a similar sensitivity (64%), specificity (87% to 89%), and predictive accuracy (82% to 84%). The combination of abnormal QRS, RMS40, or both, did not increase the predictive accuracy. Late potentials were recorded in 23 patients (22%): 14 in group 1; 3 in group 2; and 6 in group 3. Among the 23 patients with late potentials, 14 patients (61%) had induced sustained monomorphic VT, 3 (13%) had induced ventricular fibrillation, while 6 (26%) showed no induced sustained ventricular tachyarrhythmias (Figure 1). Among the 82 patients without late potentials, 8 patients (10%) had induced sustained monomorphic VT, 11 (13%) had induced ventricular fibrillation, and 63 (77%) showed no induced sustained ventricular tachyarrhythmias (Figure 2). When only the episodes of sustained

Table II

Characteristics of Patients With or Without Induced Sustained
Ventricular Tachyarrhythmias

	Group 1* (n = 22)	Group 2† (n = 14)	Group 3‡ (n = 69)	p Value	
				1 vs 3	2 vs 3
Clinical Data					
Age (yrs)	59 ±12	66 ±9	62 ±11	NS (AVa)	
Male/Female	21/1	10/4	53/16	NS	NS
Coronary artery disease (%)	16 (73)	7 (50)	37 (54)	NS	NS
Previous MI (%)	12 (55)	5 (36)	26 (38)	NS	NS
Idiopathic dilated cardiomyopathy (%)	5 (23)	3 (21)	18 (26)	NS	NS
No identifiable heart disease (%)	1 (5)	4 (29)	14 (20)	NS	NS
History of syncope or presyncope (%)	11 (50)	7 (50)	15 (22)	<0.05	NS
Holter Data					
VPCs/hour (n)	232 ±376	192 ±274	249 ±345	NS (AVa)	
Repetition index	0.06 ±0.12	0.07 ±0.08	0.07 ±0.15	NS (AVa)	
Runs of NS-VT/24 hours (n)	11 ±21	63 ±208	12 ±30	NS (AVa)	
1 run (%)	10 (45)	8 (57)	32 (46)	NS	NS
2–10 runs (%)	7 (32)	3 (21)	25 (36)	NS	NS
>10 runs (%)	5 (23)	3 (21)	12 (17)	NS	NS
Duration of NS-VT runs (complexes)	10 ±7	11 ±14	10 ±11	NS (AVa)	
3–9 complexes (%)	11 (50)	11 (79)	41 (59)	NS	NS
≥10 complexes (%)	11 (50)	3 (21)	28 (41)	NS	NS
Uniformity of NS-VT (%)	18 (82)	11 (79)	52 (73)	NS	NS
Cycle length of NS-VT (msec)	455 ±74	417 ±68	439 ±91	NS (AVa)	
LV Function Studies					
Ejection fraction	0.30 ±0.11	0.48 ±0.16	0.44 ±0.18	<0.0005 (AVa)	
Ejection fraction <0.40 (%)	19 (86)	5 (36)	25 (36)	<0.0001	NS
Segmental a/dyskinesia (%)	11 (50)	3 (21)	16 (23)	NS	NS
Signal-Averaged ECG Data					
QRS duration ≥ 120 msec (%)	16 (73)	5 (36)	17 (25)	<0.0001	NS
LAS40 ≥38 msec (%)	14 (64)	3 (21)	6 (9)	<0.0000	NS
RMS40 ≤25 µV (%)	14 (64)	4 (29)	7 (10)	<0.0000	NS

Table II (Continued)

	Group 1* (n = 22)	Group 2† (n = 14)	Group 3‡ (n = 69)	p Value 1 vs 3	2 vs 3
Late potentials (%)	14 (64)	3 (21)	6 (9)	<0.0000	NS
QRS duration (msec)	128 ±28	107 ±16	105 ±16	<0.001 (AVa)	
LAS40 (msec)	38.9 ±17.4	27.5 ±13.2	23.6 ±11.0	<0.0000 (AVa)	
RMS40 (µV)	24.5 ±24.3	68.5 ±49.9	72.1 ±50.4	<0.0000 (AVa)	

Continuous variables are expressed as mean ± standard deviation.
AVa = analysis of variance; LAS40 = duration of low amplitude signals of <40 µV; LV = left ventricular; MI = myocardial infarction; NS = not significant; NS-VT = nonsustained ventricular tachycardia; RMS40 = root mean square voltage in the last 40 msec of the QRS; VPCs = ventricular premature complexes; *group 1 = induced sustained monomorphic ventricular tachycardia; †group 2 = induced ventricular fibrillation; ‡group 3 = no induced sustained ventricular tachyarrhythmias.

VT with a cycle length ≥200 msec were taken into consideration, the positive predictive accuracy of late potentials did not change (61%), while the negative predictive accuracy increased from 90% to 94%.

The frequency of late potentials was similar in patients with coronary artery disease (15 of 60 cases, or 25%) and in those with dilated cardiomyopathy (6 of 26, or 23%). Their predictive accuracy was also comparable in the two groups: 85% in coronary artery disease and 81% in cardiomyopathy patients. Among the 43 patients with prior myocardial infarction, late potentials showed high predictive accuracy when the site of infarction was inferior (14 of 16, or 88%), as well as when the site was anterior (11 of 15, or 73%). The predictive accuracy of late potentials was also comparable when runs of nonsustained VT were short (3–9 complexes) or long (≥10 complexes): 84% versus 83%, respectively.

Using stepwise discriminant function analysis, late potentials proved to be the variable most strongly correlated (p <0.00001) with the induction of sustained monomorphic VT. The other significant variables were ejection fraction and history of syncope/presyncope. When late potentials, ejection fraction and syncope/presyncope were entered into the equation, 84% of patients with or without induced sustained monomorphic VT were correctly classified. When ejection fraction and syncope/presyncope were removed from the analysis, leaving late potentials as the only discriminant variable,

Table III

Sensitivity, Specificity and Predictive Accuracy of the Signal-Averaged ECG Parameters for the Induction of Sustained Monomorphic VT

	QRS-D	LAS40	RMS40	LAS40 and RMS40	QRS-D and RMS40	QRS-D and/or RMS40
Sensitivity (%)	16/22 (73)	14/22 (64)	14/22 (64)	14/22 (64)	14/22 (64)	16/22 (73)
Specificity (%)	61/83 (73)	74/83 (89)	72/83 (87)	74/83 (89)	74/83 (89)	59/83 (71)
Positive predictive accuracy (%)	16/38 (42)	14/23 (61)	14/25 (56)	14/23 (61)	14/23 (61)	16/40 (40)
Negative predictive accuracy (%)	61/67 (91)	74/82 (90)	72/80 (90)	74/82 (90)	74/82 (90)	59/65 (91)
Total predictive accuracy (%)	77/105 (73)	88/105 (84)	86/105 (82)	88/105 (84)	88/105 (84)	75/105 (71)

LAS40 = duration of low amplitude signals of <40 µV; QRS-D = filtered QRS duration; RMS40 = root mean square voltage in the last 40 msec of the QRS.

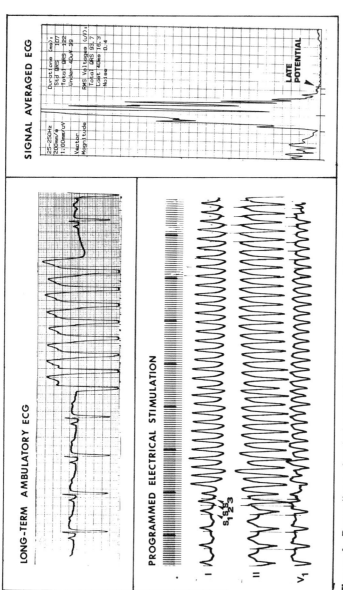

Figure 1. Recordings of ambulatory ECG, programmed electrical stimulation, and signal-averaged ECG from a 46-year-old man with coronary artery disease. The patient had a history of syncope/presyncope. The ejection fraction by radionuclide ventriculography was 35%. A 24-hour ambulatory ECG showed frequent ventricular premature complexes (average: 57/hour) and 11 runs of nonsustained monomorphic VT. The longest one is shown in the figure. It comprised 8 beats and had an averaged cycle length of 398 msec. The signal-averaged ECG was abnormal, due to the presence of prolonged QRS duration and late potentials. Programmed stimulation with two extrastimuli induced sustained monomorphic VT.

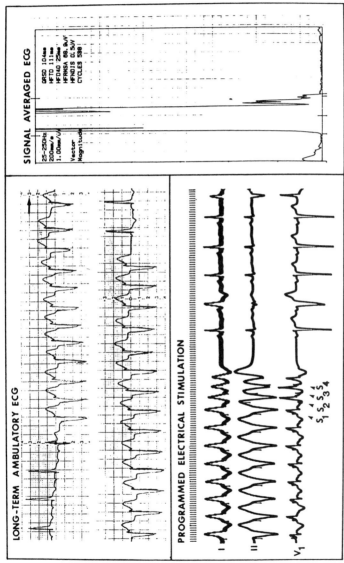

Figure 2. Recordings of ambulatory ECG, programmed electrical stimulation, and signal-averaged ECG from a 41-year-old man with nonischemic dilated cardiomyopathy. The patient had no history of syncope/presyncope. The ejection fraction by radionuclide ventriculography was 16%. A 24-hour ambulatory ECG showed frequent ventricular premature complexes (average: 240/hour) and six runs of nonsustained monomorphic VT. The longest one is shown in the figure. It comprised 26 beats and had an averaged cycle length of 452 msec. The signal-averaged ECG was normal. Programmed stimulation with up to three extrastimuli did not induce any ventricular tachyarrhythmias. (Reproduced with permission from Turitto et al, Am J Cardiol 61:1272, 1988.)

the proportion of patients correctly classified remained at 84%. When late potentials were removed from the equation, the significant variables were ejection fraction, history of syncope/presyncope, and segmental a/dyskinesia. The combination of these variables provided a predictive accuracy of 71%. Late potentials could still enter the model with a probability of improving it <0.05. Thus, the signal-averaged ECG offered predictive information above that found in clinical variables and other tests. On the other hand, no single variable or combination of variables predicted the induction of ventricular fibrillation.

In this study, the induction of sustained monomorphic VT was significantly correlated with the presence of late potentials on the signal-averaged ECG. The induction of sustained monomorphic VT has been accepted as an indication of the presence of an arrhythmia substrate based on reentry.[21] On the other hand, late potentials represent diseased myocardial zones with delayed activation potentials capable of providing the substrate for reentrant rhythms.[22] In contrast, patients with induced nonsustained VT or induced ventricular fibrillation could not be distinguished from patients with no induced ventricular tachyarrhythmias by any of the clinical variables, Holter data, left ventricular function indices, and signal-averaged ECG parameters. This suggests that the induction of ventricular fibrillation in patients with spontaneous nonsustained VT may represent a nonclinical response to programmed stimulation.

In our series of 105 patients with spontaneous nonsustained VT, concordance between the results of programmed stimulation and those of the signal-averaged ECG was observed in 84% of cases. The largest subgroup consisted of patients who had no late potentials and no induced sustained monomorphic VT (70%). In these patients, the spontaneous arrhythmia may be due to mechanisms other than reentry. The group with both late potentials and induced sustained monomorphic VT accounted for 14% of cases. The results of the two tests were discordant in the remaining 16% of cases; nine patients had late potentials but failed to develop sustained VT at programmed stimulation. This may be explained by electrophysiologic limitations of both programmed stimulation[23] and signal averaging techniques.[22] The relationship between myocardial zones with delayed conduction during sinus rhythm and the occurrence of reentrant arrhythmias is complex. Zones showing conduction delay (i.e., late potentials) during basic rhythm may completely block during premature stimulation and not participate in a reentrant pathway.

In eight patients, a sustained VT was induced in the absence of late potentials. Again, limitations of the signal-averaged ECG, for example, the inability to detect delayed activation potentials with a dynamic Wenckebach sequence, as well as the possibility that some induced VTs represent a nonspecific response to programmed stimulation can be invoked. In this regard, in four of the eight patients in this group the cycle length of induced sustained VT was 190–195 msec. In spite of these limitations, the signal-averaged ECG proved to be the single most accurate predictor for the induction of sustained monomorphic VT in patients with spontaneous nonsustained VT. Its value was independent of that of other variables, as well as of the etiology of underlying heart disease, and the site of myocardial infarction. On the other hand, induction of ventricular fibrillation could not be predicted by the signal-averaged ECG or any other variables. This suggests that induction of ventricular fibrillation may lack clinical significance in patients with spontaneous nonsustained VT. The study concluded that the signal-averaged ECG could be used for screening patients with spontaneous nonsustained VT for electrophysiologic studies. Because of the high specificity (89%) and negative predictive accuracy (90%) of the test, those patients with no late potentials may not require invasive evaluation.

Late Potentials and Prognosis

The occurrence of spontaneous nonsustained VT in patients with organic heart disease is considered a poor prognostic index.[24] However, the likelihood of sudden cardiac death may not be the same for all patients with organic heart disease and nonsustained VT. Different method have been proposed for risk stratification in this group. The use of programmed stimulation for prognostic purposes has produced contradictory results.[25–30] Although some studies have reported that patients with spontaneous nonsustained VT and no inducible ventricular tachyarrhythmias are at low risk of sudden death and may not warrant antiarrhythmic therapy,[26,27,29] others have failed to do so.[28,30] The signal-averaged ECG has been shown to predict serious arrhythmic events in survivors of myocardial infarction (see Chapters 19 and 20). On the other hand, data on long-term follow-up of patients with complex ventricular arrhythmias who underwent signal-averaged ECG are limited.[9,11,15] We prospectively studied 90 patients with organic heart disease and spontaneous nonsustained VT who had programmed stimulation, signal-averaged ECG, and left ventricular function studies to determine the role of these techniques in risk stratification and management of this group of patients.[31] The inclusion criteria, the protocol for programmed stimulation, and the technique for signal averaging are described in the previous paragraph. In this study group, 63 patients had coronary artery disease (43 with prior myocardial infarction), while 27 had nonischemic dilated cardiomyopathy (left ventricular ejection fraction <50% in the absence of stenosis >50% of any of the major coronary arteries during coronary angiography). During programmed stimulation, sustained monomorphic VT was induced in 22 cases (24%), ventricular fibrillation in 10 (11%), and no sustained ventricular tachyarrhythmias in 58 (64%). The signal-averaged ECG showed late potentials in 23 of 90 patients (26%). In the group with late potentials, 15 cases (65%) had induced sustained VT; the incidence of induced sustained VT was 68% in patients with ejection fraction <40%, and 50% in patients with ejection fraction >40% (Figure 3). On the other hand, out of 67

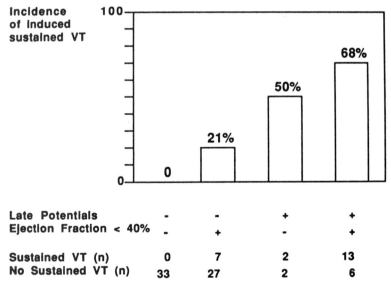

Figure 3. Correlation between the results of the signal-averaged ECG and left ventricular ejection fraction studies and the outcome of programmed stimulation in 90 patients with organic heart disease and spontaneous nonsustained VT. (Reproduced with permission from Turitto et al, Am J Med 88:1–35N, 1990.)

patients without late potentials, only 7 (10%) had induced sustained VT. All 7 cases, however, occurred in patients with ejection fraction <40% (7 of 34 patients, or 21%), while there was no induced sustained monomorphic VT among the 33 patients with ejection fraction >40% and no late potentials on the signal-averaged ECG (Figure 3).

During follow-up, all 22 patients with induced sustained monomorphic VT received therapy guided by programmed stimulation. An oral type I antiarrhythmic drug regimen capable of preventing the induction of sustained VT at repeat programmed stimulation could be identified in 10 patients. The remaining 12 cases received amiodarone therapy after they failed more than one trial with type I drugs. Amiodarone was effective by programmed stimulation and ambulatory ECG criteria (abolition of nonsustained VT and >85% reduction of ventricular ectopy) in nine patients and by ambulatory ECG criteria alone in the remaining three cases. Eight patients with induced ventricular fibrillation and all 58 patients with no induced sustained ventricular tachyarrhythmias were discharged off antiarrhythmic drugs. However, two subjects with induced ventricular fibrillation and late potentials received antiarrhythmic therapy effective by ambulatory ECG criteria, upon request of the referring physician.

All the patients were followed in our institution for a period of 30 ±10 months (range: 7 to 40). Cardiac deaths occurring during follow-up were classified as sudden, if they occurred within 1 hour of the onset of symptoms or unexpectedly during sleep, or nonsudden, if they were secondary to documented myocardial infarction or worsening congestive heart failure. During follow-up, there were 13 cardiac deaths: 6 sudden and 7 nonsudden (Table IV). Among patients with induced sustained monomorphic VT, there were four deaths: two were sudden, in patients with late potentials, and two were nonsudden, in patients without late potentials. No cardiac deaths were recorded in the group with induced ventricular fibrillation. Among patients with no induced sustained ventricular tachyarrhythmias, there were nine deaths: four were sudden (one occurred in a patient with late potentials) and five were nonsudden.

Figure 4 shows the 3-year survival analysis based on the results of programmed stimulation. The 3-year sudden death rate was 19% in the group with induced sustained VT, 0 in the group with induced ventricular fibrillation, and 9% in the group with no induced sustained VT/ventricular fibrillation. The combined 3-year sudden

Table IV

Clinical and Laboratory Data in Patients with Spontaneous Nonsustained VT Who Had Cardiac Death

Patient	Age	Heart Disease	Symptoms	Ejection Fraction (%)	Programmed Stimulation	Late Potentials	Mode of Death
1	72	CAD	Syncope	20	Sustained VT	Yes	Documented VF; in-hospital
2	72	CAD	Presyncope	30	Sustained VT	Yes	Witnessed sudden; out-of-hospital
3	65	CAD	Presyncope	20	Sustained VT	No	Worsening CHF; in-hospital
4	68	CAD	Syncope	31	Sustained VT	No	Worsening CHF; in-hospital
5	40	CMP	None	12	Monomorphic nonsustained VT	No	Worsening CHF; in-hospital
6	71	CAD	None	35	Polymorphic nonsustained VT	No	AMI with cardiogenic shock; in-hospital
7	69	CAD	None	40	Polymorphic nonsustained VT	No	Witnessed sudden; out-of-hospital
8	56	CMP	None	28	<6 repetitive ventricular responses	Yes	Witnessed sudden; out-of-hospital
9	68	CMP	Presyncope	21	<6 repetitive ventricular responses	No	Documented VF; in-hospital
10	67	CMP	None	45	<6 repetitive ventricular responses	No	Witnessed sudden; out-of-hospital
11	65	CAD	Presyncope	20	Sustained VT	No	Worsening CHF; in-hospital
12	75	CMP	Syncope	38	<6 repetitive ventricular responses	No	Worsening CHF; in-hospital
13	71	CAD	None	38	<6 repetitive ventricular responses	No	Worsening CHF; in-hospital

AMI = acute myocardial infarction; CAD = coronary artery disease; CHF = congestive heart failure; CMP = cardiomyopathy; VF = ventricular fibrillation.

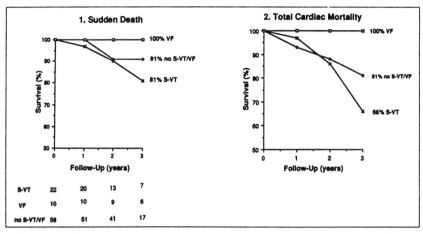

Figure 4. Three-year actuarial survival curves for sudden death and total cardiac mortality in patients with organic heart disease and spontaneous nonsustained VT classified by the outcome of programmed stimulation. The number of patients being followed at each time interval is indicated on the bottom. S-VT = sustained ventricular tachycardia; VF = ventricular fibrillation. (Reproduced with permission from Turitto et al, Am J Med 88:1–35N, 1990.)

death rate for patients without induced sustained monomorphic VT (cases with induced ventricular fibrillation or without induced sustained ventricular tachyarrhythmias) was 8% (not shown in the figure). The 3-year total cardiac mortality (including both sudden and nonsudden deaths) was, respectively, 34% in patients with induced sustained VT, 0 in those with induced ventricular fibrillation, and 19% in those with no induced sustained ventricular tachyarrhythmias.

Figure 5 shows the 3-year survival analysis of patients with no induced sustained VT based on ejection fraction. The 3-year sudden death rate was the same (7%) in those with ejection fraction <40% or ≥40%. On the other hand, the 3-year total cardiac mortality was significantly higher (27%) in those patients with ejection fraction <40% than in those with ejection fraction ≤40% (7%) (p <0.05). Risk stratification for patients with induced sustained VT based on ejection fraction was not performed because 20 of the 22 patients in this group had an ejection fraction <40%. For the whole group, the 3-year total cardiac mortality rate was significantly higher in patients with ejection fraction <40% than in those with ejection fraction ≥40% (31% vs 6%, p <0.05). The 3-year sudden death rate was,

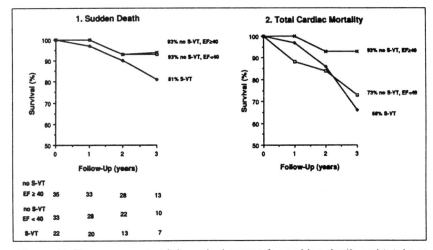

Figure 5. Three-year actuarial survival curves for sudden death and total cardiac mortality in patients with organic heart disease and spontaneous nonsustained VT who had no induced sustained VT classified by left ventricular ejection fraction. The survival curves for all patients with induced sustained VT are also shown for comparison. The number of patients, being followed at each time interval is indicated on the bottom. S-VT = sustained ventricular tachycardia; EF = ejection fraction. (Reproduced with permission from Turitto et al, Am J Med 88:1–35N, 1990.)

respectively, 13% and 6% (difference not significant). Both the 3-year total cardiac mortality and the sudden death rate were higher in patients with nonischemic dilated cardiomyopathy (25% and 14%, respectively) as compared to patients with coronary artery disease (19% and 8%, respectively), but these differences were not statistically significant.

In summary, we prospectively followed a large cohort of patients with organic heart disease and spontaneous nonsustained VT in whom no sustained monomorphic VT was induced and no antiarrhythmic treatment was administered, with a low risk of sudden cardiac death (8% at 3 years). It should be emphasized that the risk of sudden death was equally low in patients with no induced sustained ventricular tachyarrhythmias and in those with induced ventricular fibrillation, thereby confirming the lack of clinical significance of this response to programmed stimulation, in patients with spontaneous nonsustained VT. A major strength of this study was the evaluation of the role of the signal-averaged ECG in the management of patients with organic heart disease and nonsustained VT. The signal-averaged ECG provided a high negative predictive accuracy (90%) for the induction of sustained VT by programmed stimulation. The value of the signal-averaged ECG was enhanced with the combined use of left ventricular function studies. There was no case of inducible sustained monomorphic VT in 33 patients with no late potentials and ejection fraction ≥ 40%. Our data suggest that these two noninvasive tests may be used for risk stratification and management of patients with organic heart disease and spontaneous nonsustained VT according to the following guidelines (Figure 6). Patients with no late potentials on the signal-averaged ECG and ejection fraction ≥ 40% may not require programmed stimulation or antiarrhythmic therapy since the incidence of induced sustained monomorphic VT and the risk of sudden death are low in this group

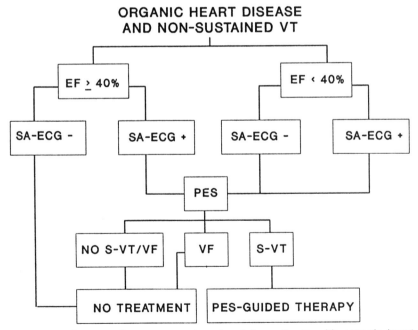

Figure 6. Suggested management protocol for patients with organic heart disease and spontaneous nonsustained VT. See text for details. EF = ejection fraction; PES = programmed electrical stimulation; SA-ECG = signal-averaged electrocardiogram; S-VT = sustained ventricular tachycardia; VF = ventricular fibrillation.

of patients. On the other hand, patients with late potentials as well as patients with no late potentials but with ejection fraction <40% may be recommended for electrophysiologic evaluation. Patients with no inducible ventricular tachyarrhythmias as well as those with inducible nonsustained VT or ventricular fibrillation could be followed while not receiving antiarrhythmic therapy, with a low risk for sudden cardiac death. If sustained monomorphic VT is induced, antiarrhythmic therapy guided by programmed stimulation may be recommended. However, this recommendation should be tempered by the fact that the value of antiarrhythmic treatment for induced sustained VT in patients with organic heart disease and spontaneous nonsustained VT has not been definitely established. This could be achieved only through randomization of therapy in a large multicenter study.

References

1. Turitto G, Fontaine JM, Ursell SN, Caref EB, Henkin R, El-Sherif N: Value of the signal-averaged electrocardiogram as a predictor of the results of programmed stimulation in nonsustained ventricular tachycardia. Am J Cardiol 61:1272, 1988.
2. Turitto G, Caref EB, Macina G, Fontaine JM, Ursell SN, El-Sherif N: Time course of ventricular arrhythmias and the signal averaged electrocardiogram in the post-infarction period: a prospective study of correlation. Br Heart J 60:17, 1988.
3. Gomes JAC, Winters SL, Stewart D, Horowitz S, Milner M, Barreca P: A new noninvasive index to predict sustained ventricular tachycardia and sudden death in the first year after myocardial infarction: based on signal-averaged electrocardiogram, radionuclide ejection fraction and Holter monitoring. J Am Coll Cardiol 10:349, 1987.
4. Buxton AE, Simson MB, Falcone RA, Marchlinski FE, Doherty JU, Josephson ME: Results of signal-averaged electrocardiography and electrophysiologic study in patients with nonsustained ventricular tachycardia after healing of acute myocardial infarction. Am J Cardiol 60:80, 1987.
5. Denes P, Santarelli P, Masson M, Uretz EF: Prevalence of late potentials in patients undergoing Holter monitoring. Am Heart J 113:33, 1987.
6. Nalos PC, Gang ES, Mandel WJ, Ladenheim ML, Lass Y, Peter T: The signal-averaged electrocardiogram as a screening test for inducibility of sustained ventricular tachycardia in high risk patients: a prospective study. J Am Coll Cardiol 9:539, 1987.
7. Poll DS, Marchlinski FE, Falcone RA, Josephson ME, Simson MB: Abnormal signal-averaged electrocardiograms in patients with nonischemic congestive cardiomyopathy: relationship to sustained ventricular tachyarrhythmias. Circulation 72:1308, 1985.

8. Coto H, Maldonado C, Palakurthy P, Flowers NC: Late potentials in normal subjects and in patients with ventricular tachycardia unrelated to myocardial infarction. Am J Cardiol 55:384, 1985.

9. Zimmermann M, Adamec R, Simonin P, Richez J: Prognostic significance of ventricular late potentials in coronary artery disease. Am Heart J 109:725, 1985.

10. Kertes PJ, Pollak SJ, Walter PF: Programmed stimulation for ventricular tachycardia: responses predicted by signal averaging in patients with and without coronary artery disease (abstr). Circulation 72(Suppl III): 111–433, 1985.

11. Denes P, Uretz E, Santarelli P: Determinants of arrhythmogenic ventricular activity detected on the body surface QRS in patients with coronary artery disease. Am J Cardiol 53:1519, 1984.

12. Denes P, Santarelli P, Hauser RG, Uretz EF: Quantitative analysis of the high-frequency component of the terminal portion of the body surface QRS in normal subjects and in patients with ventricular tachycardia. Circulation 67:1129, 1983.

13. Kanovsky MS, Falcone RA, Dresden CA, Josephson ME, Simson MB: Identification of patients with ventricular tachycardia after myocardial infarction: signal-averaged electrocardiogram, Holter monitoring, and cardiac catheterization. Circulation 70:264, 1984.

14. Pollak SJ, Kertes PJ, Bredlau CE, Walter PF: Influence of left ventricular function on signal averaged late potentials in patients with coronary artery disease with and without ventricular tachycardia. Am Heart J 110: 747, 1985.

15. Buckingham TA, Ghosh S, Homan SM, Thessen CC, Redd RM, Stevens LL, Chaitman BR, Kennedy HL: Independent value of signal-averaged electrocardiography and left ventricular function in identifying patients with sustained ventricular tachycardia with coronary artery disease. Am J Cardiol 59:568, 1987.

16. Breithardt G, Borggrefe M, Karbenn U, Abendroth R-R, Yeh H-L, Seipel L: Prevalence of late potentials in patients with and without ventricular tachycardia: correlation with angiographic findings. Am J Cardiol 49: 1932, 1982.

17. Freedman RA, Gillis AM, Keren AM, Soderholm-Difatte V, Mason JW: Signal-averaged electrocardiographic late potentials in patients with ventricular fibrillation or ventricular tachycardia: correlation with clinical arrhythmia and electrophysiologic study. Am J Cardiol 55:1350, 1985.

18. Denniss RA, Richards DA, Cody DV, Russell PA, Young AA, Ross DL, Uther JB: Correlation between signal-averaged electrocardiogram and programmed stimulation in patients with and without spontaneous ventricular tachyarrhythmias. Am J Cardiol 59:586, 1987.

19. Winters SL, Stewart D, Targonski A, Gomes JA: Role of signal averaging of the surface QRS complex in selecting patients with nonsustained ventricular tachycardia and high grade ventricular arrhythmias for programmed ventricular stimulation. J Am Coll Cardiol 12:1481, 1988.

20. Vatterott PJ, Bailey KR, Hammill SC: Improving the predictive ability

of the signal-averaged electrocardiogram with a linear logistic model incorporating clinical variables. Circulation 81:797, 1990.

21. Wellens HJJ, Brugada P, Stevenson WG: Programmed electrical stimulation of the heart in patients with life-threatening ventricular arrhythmias: what is the significance of induced arrhythmias and what is the correct protocol? Circulation 72:1, 1985.

22. El-Sherif N, Gomes JAC, Restivo M, Mehra R: Late potentials and arrhythmogenesis. PACE 8:440, 1985.

23. Mason JW, Anderson KP, Freedman RA: Techniques and criteria in electrophysiologic study of ventricular tachycardia. Circulation 75 (Suppl III):III-125, 1987.

24. Turitto G, El-Sherif N: Complex ventricular arrhythmias. Risk stratification and management. In El-Sherif N, Samet P (eds): Cardiac Pacing and Electrophysiology. Orlando: Grune & Stratton, Inc, 1990, pp. 217–232.

25. Buxton AE, Marchlinski FE, Waxman HL, Flores BT, Cassidy DM, Josephson ME: Prognostic factors in nonsustained ventricular tachycardia. Am J Cardiol 53:1275, 1984.

26. Buxton AE, Marchlinski FE, Flores BT, Miller JM, Doherty JU, Josephson ME: Nonsustained ventricular tachycardia in patients with coronary artery disease. Role of electrophysiologic study. Circulation 75:1178, 1987.

27. Gomes JAC, Hariman RI, Kang PS, El-Sherif N, Chowdry I, Lyons J: Programmed electrical stimulation in patients with high-grade ventricular ectopy. Electrophysiologic findings and prognosis for survival. Circulation 70:43, 1984.

28. Veltri EP, Platia EV, Griffith LSC, Reid PR: Programmed electrical stimulation and long-term follow-up in asymptomatic nonsustained ventricular tachycardia. Am J Cardiol 55:309, 1985.

29. Zheutlin TA, Roth H, Chua W, Steinman R, Summers C, Lesch M, Kehoe RF: Programmed electrical stimulation to determine the need for antiarrhythmic therapy in patients with complex ventricular ectopic activity. Am Heart J 111:860, 1986.

30. Sulpizi AM, Friehling TD, Kowey PR: Value of electrophysiologic testing in patients with nonsustained ventricular tachycardia. Am J Cardiol 59:841, 1987.

31. Turitto G, Fontaine JM, Ursell S, Caref EB, Bekheit S, El-Sherif N: Risk stratification and management of patients with organic heart disease and nonsustained ventricular tachycardia: role of programmed stimulation, left ventricular ejection fraction, and the signal-averaged electrocardiogram. Am J Med 88:1-35N, 1990.

23

Late Potentials in Patients with Sustained Ventricular Tachycardia/Ventricular Fibrillation

Joseph Borbola, Pablo Denes

Introduction

The routine surface electrocardiogram (ECG) during sinus rhythm has few specific warning signs to indicate the presence of electrical instability leading to ventricular tachycardia (VT) and/or ventricular fibrillation (VF). In the early 1960s, electrocardiographic studies have demonstrated distinct alterations (notching) of the high-frequency components of the ECG in patients with coronary artery disease and myocardial disease.[1,2] In the last decade, the introduction of high-gain amplification and advanced signal processing techniques of the ECG allowed recording of low amplitude, high-fre-

From El-Sherif N, Turitto G (eds): *High-Resolution Electrocardiography*. Mount Kisco, NY, Futura Publishing Co., Inc., ©, 1992.

quency signals, in the terminal portion of the surface QRS and early ST segment during sinus rhythm in patients with ventricular tachyarrhythmias, especially in those with coronary disease.[3-11] These abnormal signals have been labeled as arrhythmogenic ventricular activity, delayed depolarization waves or potentials, and most recently as ventricular late potentials (Figure 1). In recent years, there has been an explosion in the number of studies dealing with time-domain [12-45,51-78] and/or frequency-domain [46-50] analysis of signal-averaged ECG in patients with spontaneous, sustained VT/VF. The recording of a signal-averaged ECG has emerged as a clinically useful, noninvasive, inexpensive test to detect late potentials. This interest in signal averaging is related to the finding that late potentials are specific noninvasive markers for spontaneous and/or inducible VT in patients with coronary artery disease especially after myocardial infarction.[7,9,11,15,18,19,29,34,51-58] The detection of late potentials can identify those patients considered to have an anatomic substrate for the reentry circuit of sustained VT.[29,49,59-66]

Previous studies on signal-averaged ECG reported the prevalence of late potentials in normals,[9,12,15,23,24,26,27,31,36-38,49,68] in patients with coronary disease and with [9-11,15,18,19,23,25,29-31,43,44] or without sustained VT/VF[9,11,18,19,23,25,30,51,52,54-58] and those with other organic heart disease with [4,12,23,26,27,33,78] and without sustained VT.[12,26,27,33] Other reports described the utility of the signal-averaged ECG in different clinical settings such as syncope [43,46,67-69] bundle branch block,[39,40,49,70] complex ventricular arrhythmias, nonsustained [26,43,46,47,66,71,72] or sustained VT,[3-66] and sudden cardiac death.[16,24,36,41,43,44]

This chapter review summarizes the current understanding and the presently available information on late potentials in patients with documented, spontaneous sustained VT and/or VF in the setting of coronary disease and other organic heart diseases. In the context of this review, only time-domain signal averaging techniques will be discussed. The value and utility of the signal averaged ECG in the assessment of patients with sustained VT/VF has been the subject of several recent excellent reviews.[29,47,59-66] At the time of this report at least 35 major series (>10 patients) had been published including some more than 1200 patients with VT/VF.[9-12,14,15,18,19,23,25,27-46,48-50]

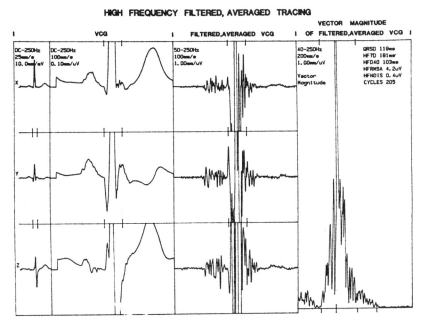

Figure 1. Recording of a ventricular late potential (LP) in a patient with documented sustained VT. The figure demonstrates an example of signal-averaged vectorcardiography (VCG). Bipolar orthogonal leads X, Y, and Z are displayed in the first three panels. The panel on the far left shows VCG leads X, Y, and Z at standard gain without signal processing. The second panel shows the signal-averaged (for 205 beats), unfiltered, and amplified (10 times the normal gain) signals. Note the presence of LP at the end of the QRS in leads X and Y. The third panel shows the further amplified (100 times the normal gain), filtered and signal-averaged VCG leads. The atrial and ventricular electrograms are seen. The panel on the far right presents a vector magnitude tracing which sums the high-frequency content of the three VCG leads. A bidirectional filter (40 to 250 Hz) is used for this presentation. The unfiltered QRS duration is 119 msec (QRS), the filtered QRS duration (HFTD) is 181 msec. The duration of the terminal signals with an amplitude of 40 μV (HFD40) is 103 msec and the amplitude of the terminal 40-msec signal (HFRMSA) is 4.2 μV. The noise level is 0.4 μV. A long low amplitude LP is present at the end of the QRS complex and extends more than 100 msec into the ST segment.

Methods, Recording Techniques, Measurements, Definitions, and Reproducibility of the Signal-Averaged ECG

Although the methods of body surface recording, the interpretations of results and definitions of late potentials differ, there is agreement that detection of a late potential can reliably identify coronary disease patients prone to sustained VT, especially after myocardial infarction.[7,9,11,15,18,19,29,34,51-66]

The problem in identifying the late potential on the surface QRS during sinus rhythm by conventional electrocardiography is that the cardiac signal of late potential is smaller than the electrical noise. Late potential are typically low amplitude (in the range of 1 to 25 µV), high-frequency (in the range of 20 to 80 Hz) signals which appear in the terminal portion of the filtered QRS complexes and extend into the ST segment of the signal-averaged ECG during sinus rhythm in patients with VT/VF.[4-66] Signal averaging is a computer based process which by aligning multiple consecutive sinus beats and then summing and averaging the waveforms, enhances the true repetitive signals and random noise tends to cancel and is removed. The diastolic noise level is under 1 µV after averaging 200 to 500 QRS complexes in most studies. The importance of the diastolic noise level is that the definition of the late potential and the reproducibility of the test depends on the actual background noise level.

Several methodological problems with the time-domain analysis of signal-averaged ECG still exist, including: differences in electrode positions; heterogeneity of signal processing methodologies and recording systems; the selection of the optimal high-pass filter settings; diverging definitions of late potentials; and limited data on short- and long-term reproducibility and stability of late potentials. For the detailed methodological aspects (filter ringing, "trigger jitter," template recognition program, optimal distance between pairs of surface electrodes, etc.) of the noninvasive recording of late potentials, we refer to the appropriate chapters of this book. A filter corner frequency ranging from 10 to 100 Hz has been utilized. In Simson's original article,[11] the high-pass filter frequency was set at 25 Hz. He demonstrated that signal processing of the surface QRS by computer can separate patients with VT from patients with VT. The sensitivity and specificity of the test were 92% and 93%, respectively. In 1983, Denes et al[15] reported that the use of a 40-Hz filter, as contrasted with a 25-Hz filter, improved the separation between normal subjects and patients with spontaneous and inducible sustained VT. Most recently, Gomes et al[38] investigated the optimal bandpass filters (10 to 100 Hz) for time-domain analysis of the signal-averaged ECG in a heterogenous patient population. The method and equipment used by Simson,[11] Denes et al,[15] and Gomes et al[38] were similar. The results of Gomes et al indicated that the sensitivity, specificity, and predictive value of quantitative signal-averaged indices assessed alone or in combination, were high-pass filter dependent. The filter frequencies tested to detect late potentials were 25, 40, and 80 Hz. Each offered advantages in regards to sensitivity as well as specificity over the other. Among the three filters, the 80-Hz high-pass filtering provided the best sensitivity.[38,50] They suggested that signal-averaged ECG should not be limited to a single high-pass filter setting, but to multiple filters for different purposes. However, as they noted, the true negative and positive results can be identified only by prospective long-term follow-up studies.

Initially, late potentials were identified qualitatively;[4,10] later Simson[11] introduced the computer-based quantitative, more objective approach based on a software program. This technique includes computer assisted measurement of a number of variables on a vector magnitude that incorporates the characteristics of three orthogonal bipolar leads. A late potential was defined by Simson et al[29] as a low amplitude signal (< 25 μV) in the last 40 msec of the filtered QRS complex. An abnormal signal-averaged ECG was defined as filtered QRS complex longer than 110 msec and/or the presence of a late potential. Later Denes et al[15] reported on the quantitative analysis of the high-frequency components of the terminal portion of the body surface QRS. They suggested the use of a new approach for delineation of late potentials: the duration of the low amplitude signals at the end of the filtered QRS (from the QRS endpoint backward to the first point where the signals reach an amplitude of 40 μV). In previous studies, abnormalities of each of the above mentioned variables were found to identify patients with VT.[11,14–18,29,64]

The following computer calculated, quantitative signal-averaged ECG variables or indices have been used for delineation of the presence of a late potential or an abnormal recording in patients with VT/VF: (1) the duration (msec) of the signal-averaged, high-frequency filtered QRS vector complex (QRSD).[11,15,39,75,76] Other abbreviations which have been used in the literature: QRSd[69]; QRSf[34,43]; and HFTD[35]; (2) the duration (msec) of the low amplitude signals at the end of the filtered QRS (LPD). This is from the QRS endpoint backward to the first point where the signals reached an amplitude of 40 µV. Other abbreviations which have been used for the description of this index in the literature: LAS[38,50,69]; LAS-40[48]; D-40[34,35,43]; and HFD40[37,39]; (3) the root mean square voltage or amplitude (microvolt) of the terminal 40 msec of the filtered QRS complex which has been used as an index of late potential, termed V-40 (Figure 2).[11,15,24,25,34,43,55,56] Other abbreviations: RMS[26,34,43,69]; RMS-40[38,48,75,76]; RMSA[35]; T40-QRS[36]; and HFRMSA.[37,39]

An abnormal signal-averaged ECG is defined if one or more of those above mentioned variables are abnormal.[58] Others require the presence of two or more abnormal variables. Ventricular activation time (millisecond) is used by Denniss et al,[28,31,33,41,54,57] and defined as the total time from earliest QRS onset in any lead to latest QRS offset in any lead. QRS offset is measured to the end of any low amplitude, high-frequency components extending into the ST segment, provided they had an amplitude more than twice that of the simultaneously displayed noise level (> 1 µV). These low amplitude signals are called delayed potentials if they extend more than 140 msec after the QRS onset. At the present time, there is no agreement on the exact definition of late potentials. The problem of standardization of late potentials is of importance. A recent multicenter study has shown that major differences in the incidence of late potentials can result from divergent definitions.[62,63] The comparison of diagnostic criteria for a late potential used by major studies in patients with VT/VF is presented in Table I. The comparison of diagnostic criteria for an abnormal signal-averaged ECG used by major studies in patients with VT/VF is shown in Table II.

Reproducibility is essential for the signal-averaged ECG especially if the effects of interventions on late potentials are to be assessed. Data on reproducibility and stability of late potentials and quantitative signal-averaged ECG variables are available mostly in normal subjects.[7,15,62] In 1981, Breithardt et al[9,62] studied the day-to-day reproducibility of late potentials (high-pass filter: 100 Hz) in 17 patients with organic heart disease. The reproducibility of the test was high, with $>90\%$ of patients still having late potentials at a second recording, provided that no change in the clinical status had taken place. In 1985, Pollak et al[25] reported on the reproducibility of the signal-averaged ECG (high-pass filter: 25 Hz) in a group of 15 patients with heterogeneous heart disease. Reproducibility of the measurements was found to be high for both QRSD and V-40. In 1986, Kuchar[61] reported on the day-to-day reproducibility of V-40 and QRSD in patients with VT (high-pass fil-

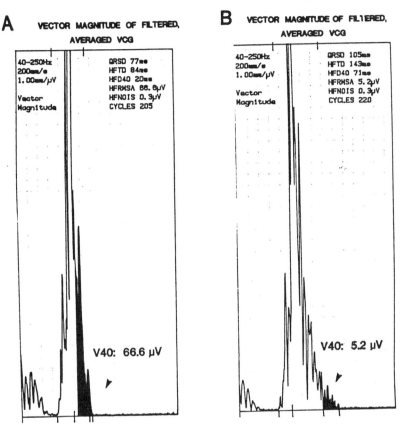

A VECTOR MAGNITUDE OF FILTERED, AVERAGED VCG

40-250Hz	QRSD 77ms
200mm/s	HFTD 84ms
1.00mm/µV	HFD40 20ms
	HFRMSA 66.6µV
Vector	HFNOIS 0.3µV
Magnitude	CYCLES 205

V40: 66.6 µV

B VECTOR MAGNITUDE OF FILTERED, AVERAGED VCG

40-250Hz	QRSD 105ms
200mm/s	HFTD 143ms
1.00mm/µV	HFD40 71ms
	HFRMSA 5.2µV
Vector	HFNOIS 0.3µV
Magnitude	CYCLES 220

V40: 5.2 µV

Figure 2. Signal-averaged electrocardiograms. (A) Normal tracing from a patient without spontaneous or inducible sustained VT. (B) Abnormal tracing from a patient with spontaneous and inducible sustained monomorphic VT. The abnormal signal-averaged electrocardiogram has a long filtered QRS complex (143 msec), a low value of V-40 (5.2 µV), and a long duration of ventricular late potential (LP). A long low amplitude signal (LP) is present at the end of the QRS complex. The baseline noise level is 0.3 µV in both recordings. V-40: the root mean square voltage of the terminal 40 msec of the filtered QRS complex.

ter: 40 Hz). They found the coefficient of variability was 6.6% for V-40 and 1.0% for QRSD (95% confidence limits of ±3.8 µV for V-40 and ±2.3 msec for QRSD). In 1987, Vatterott et al[75] reported on the hour-to-hour and day-to-day variability of the signal-averaged ECG (high-pass filter: 25 Hz) in 24 cardiac patients. They found that the signal-averaged ECG can vary considerably. In another study, the effect of residual noise on the predictive accuracy of the signal-averaged ECG was evaluated.[76] The level of residual

Table I

The Comparison of Diagnostic Criteria for Ventricular Late Potentials in Studies of Patients With VT/VF

	High-Pass Filter Used	Definition of LP
Simson et al[29]	25 Hz	A low amplitude signal (<25 μV) in the last 40 msec of the filtered QRS complex.
Breithardt et al[9]	100 Hz	Visual identification of low amplitude (>2 noise level) spikes in the high-gain averaged recordings.
Denes et al[15,18,72]	40 Hz	When two or more signal-averaged ECG indices are abnormal.
Kuchar et al[55,56]	40 Hz	A low-voltage signal (<20 μV) in the last 40 msec of the filtered QRS complex.
Denniss et al[31–33,41,54,57]		Low amplitude signals if they extend more than 140 msec after the QRS onset and have an amplitude more than twice that of the noise level.
Nalos et al[34]	67, 100 Hz	Discrete, low amplitude (<20 μV) high-frequency deflections in the terminal portion of the filtered QRS complex having an amplitude greater than twice the level of noise at both corner frequencies.
Buckingham et al[30]	25 Hz	The presence of three abnormal indices.
Hombach et al[73]		Signals within at least three or more of six possible signal-averaged leads with equal or more than twice the baseline noise and the occurrence more than 10 msec after the end of the QRS.
Kelen et al[48]	25 Hz	RMS-40 <25 μV + LAS-40 ≥40 msec
Vatterott et al[75,76]	25 Hz	QRSD 110 msec + RMS-40 <25 μV

LAS-40: the duration of the low amplitude signals at the end of the QRS where the signals reached an amplitude of 40 μV; RMS-40: the root mean square voltage of the terminal 40 msec of the filtered QRS complex; LP: late potential; VT/VF: ventricular tachycardia/fibrillation; QRSD: high-frequency, filtered QRS duration.

Table II

The Comparison of Diagnostic Criteria for an Abnormal
Signal-Averaged ECG in Studies of Patients With VT/VF

	High-Pass Filter Used	QRSD (msec)	LPD (msec)	V-40 (μV)
Simson[11]	25 Hz	>110	—	<25
Kanovsky et al[19]	25 Hz	>120	—	<25
Denes et al[15,18,72]	40 Hz	>120	>39	<20
Kuchar et al[55,56]	40 Hz	>120	—	<20
Buckingham et al[30]	25 Hz	>120	>40	<25
Vatterott et al[75,76]	25 Hz	>110	—	<25
Gomes et al[38]	25 Hz	>114	>32	<25
	40 Hz	>114	>38	<20
	80 Hz	>107	>42	<17
Pollak et al[25]	25 Hz	>120	—	<25

LPD: late potential duration at 40 μV; V-40: the root mean square voltage in the last 40 msec of the filtered QRS complex; QRSD: high-frequency, filtered QRS duration.

noise affected the signal-averaged ECG's ability to predict results of electrophysiologic study. It was suggested that averaging to a fixed low-noise level may improve the sensitivity of the signal-averaged ECG for detecting patients with sustained monomorphic VT and better characterize those without VT. Denniss et al,[57] using the ventricular activation time for the characterization of late potentials, have found that their day-to-day reproducibility exceeded 90%. The determination of ventricular activation time was free from significant interobserver variability. In the study of Nalos et al,[34] the mean intra- and interobserver variability of the filtered QRS duration was ±5 msec and for the amplitude of late potential it was ±1μV. Most recently, Borbola and Denes[77] reported on the short- (within a period of an hour) and long-term (within a period of 3.2 ±2.3 days) reproducibility of the quantitative indices of the signal-averaged ECG (high-pass filter: 40 Hz) in 60 patients with coronary artery disease (82% of patients had an old myocardial infarction). Their results suggested, that in coronary patients: (1) short- and long-term reproducibility of quantitative indices of signal-averaged ECG is excellent, when a criteria for noise level of <0.8 μV for all recordings is used; (2) the reproducibility is not affected by the presence of the late potentials; and (3) the residual noise level has significant effect on reproducibility.

Reproducibility of late potentials is affected by several factors which include electrode position, residual noise level, cardiac status, amiodarone treatment, and change in the intraventricular conduction, also dynamic changes in the terminal QRS voltage are observed during the first year after myocardial infarction.[55,62] Further studies are warranted to define factors governing reproducibility of the signal-averaged ECG.

Correlation Between Cardiac Mapping and the Signal-Averaged ECG in Patients with VT/VF

The usual mechanism of VT in the coronary and post-infarction patients is believed to be reentry associated with a fixed anatomic substrate. Berbari et al[3] and later Simson et al[17,64] have shown using epicardial mapping and endocardial recording that delayed and fractionated, low amplitude signals at the end of the surface QRS can be consistently recorded during sinus rhythm from ischemic zones adjacent to an old myocardial scar tissue. The amplitude of the delayed electrocardiogram is typically under 1 mV, when recorded directly.[6] These abnormal electrical signals bridging the diastolic interval prior to the onset of VT provide evidence for reentry. In theory, such signals should be detectable noninvasively on the body surface. Signal averaging, high-gain amplification and high-pass filtering allow the detection of these signals from the body surface. Late potentials are thought to represent delayed and inhomogeneous conduction in and around a scar tissue which is the presumed arrhythmogenic substrate of reentry.[3,17,62-64] The prerequisites of reentry are unidirectional block, slow conduction, and recovery of tissue ahead of wave front of excitation.[9,12,29] The slow conduction through the area of delay during sinus rhythm may be recorded as late potentials if the delayed activation outlasts normal ventricular activation.[17,29,57] When the fragmented electrograms are of brief duration, late potentials cannot be detected by signal averaging because it is masked by the activation of normal myocardium.[17,29] Results of clinical studies using signal-averaged ECG have demonstrated a correlation between late potentials detected from body surface and delayed ventricular activation detected during epicardial mapping or endocavitary electrode catheter recordings. Map-directed surgical excision of a ventricular scar tissue, for treatment of recurrent VT, is able to abolish or modify not only the inducible VT, but also late potential.[5,13,20,29,32,65] In 1981, Breithardt et al[9] reported a good correlation between signal averaging and epicardial mapping in coronary disease patients with left ventricular aneurysm before and after surgery. Most recently, Gomes et al[42] reported on a comparative analysis of signal averaging of the surface the QRS complex and signal averaging of the endocardial and epicardial electrograms in patients with VT. Signal averaging of right ventricular endocardial and left ventricular epicardial unipolar recordings correlated well with with signal-averaged surface QRS. There was no significant difference in the quantitative signal-averaged parameters among the three recording sites. This observation further validates the fact that the signal-averaged ECG detects delayed ventricular activation.

Ventricular Late Potentials in Patients with VT/VF

In the last few years, many centers have demonstrated that low amplitude, high-frequency signals in the terminal QRS and early ST segment identified by time-domain technique are almost never detected in normal subjects.[9,12,15,23,24,26,27,31,33,36–38,49,61] The prevalence of late potentials in the normal population is about 1% (Table III). They can be detected in about 30% of patients with chronic coronary disease in whom sustained VT and/or VF have not been previously documented.[9,11,12,18,19,23,25,30,51,52,54–58,71,77] The incidence of late potentials in this subset of patients has been reported to be in the range of 7% to 51%, depending on the presence or absence of myocardial infarction, time interval after the infarction, and the presence or absence of complex ventricular arrhythmias. In contrast, patients with chronic coronary disease and spontaneous VT and/or VF have a high incidence of late potentials (mean: 79% range: 60% to 100%) (Table IV), or abnormal signal-averaged ECG.[10–12,15,18,19,23,25,29–31,35,37,43,44,60] Among patients with coronary disease, the prevalence of late potentials is 42%–48% in the presence of a left ventricular aneurysm and 66%–100% in the presence of a history of previous sustained VT/VF[12,18,23] Late potentials have also been described in the setting of organic heart disease other than coronary disease with or without spontaneous VT/VF.[4,12,23,26,27,33,34,60,66,78]

Table III

Prevalence of Ventricular Late Potentials in Normal Subjects

	Number of Healthy Subjects	Age (Years)	Incidence of LPs (%)
Breithardt et al[9]	11	37 ±14	0
Breithardt et al[12]	27	—	0
Denes et al[15]	42	18–67	0
Coto et al[26]	50	18–36	6
Poll et al[27]	55	36 ±11	2
El-Sherif et al[60]	18	—	7
Freedman et al[24]	19	30 ±4	0
Lindsay et al[49]	28	34 ±10	0
Zimmermann et al[23]	25	24–37	0
Gang et al[68]	15	—	0
Kuchar[61]	8	—	0
Denniss et al[31]	32	22–64	0
Denniss et al[33]	16	22–55	0
Gomes et al[38]	25	34 ±10	5
Kacet et al[37]	131	29 ±11	1
Greene et al[36]	11	—	0
	513		1.4

LPs: late potentials.

Using different high-pass filter settings (25 to 100 Hz) many centers have detected abnormal signal-averaged ECG variables from patients with VT/VF. The most commonly reported distinguishing features are a significant increase in the QRSD and LPD, and a decrease in the magnitude of V-40. Previous studies[4,10–12,15,18,19,23,25,29–31,35,37,43,44,60–64] have provided convincing evidence that the presence of a late potential or an abnormal signal-averaged ECG can reliably identify patients with coronary disease and sustained VT. In the reported studies[11,30,50,60,61] the sensitivity of late potentials for detecting patients with VT varied from 64% to 92%, the specificity from 78% to 93%, and predictive accuracy from 75% to 90%, which are comparable to invasive programmed stimulation.[30] Long QRSD proved to be less sensitive (55%) but more specific for VT.[61]

Controversy, however, remains as to why late potentials cannot be detected in all patients despite previously documented sustained

Table IV

Prevalence of Ventricular Late Potentials in Patients with
Coronary Artery Disease and Documented Sustained VT/VF

	Number of Patients	Incidence of LPs (%)
Rozansky et al[10]	8	100
Breithardt et al[12]	47	79
Simson[11]	39	92
Denes et al[15]	12	83
Denes et al[18]	30	66
Kanovsky et al[19]	98	81
Zimmermann et al[23]	17	82
Pollak et al[25]	16	63
Buckingham et al[30]	14	64
Simson et al[29]	49	86
Denniss et al[31]	65	89
Nalos et al[43]	21	88
El-Sherif et al[60]	21	71
Volosin et al[35]	11	64
Kacet et al[37]	21	90
Borbola et al[44]	50	60
Total	519	79

LPs = Late potentials; VT/VF: ventricular tachycardia/fibrillation.

VT/VF and/or inducible VT. Several explanations may account for the lack of late potentials in these patients.[11,12,31,61-66] The VT which is associated with other than reentrant mechanism (long QT syndrome) would not be expected to have abnormal signal-averaged ECG. Breithardt et al[12,62,63] suggested several other possible mechanisms related to technical limitations of signal-averaged recordings by which late potentials can remain undetected in patients with documented VT/VF. Nalos et al[43] reported on the finding that in patients presenting with VT/VF while taking antiarrhythmic drugs, the signal-averaged ECG in the drug-free state can distinguish patients with possible proarrhythmic events from those who have the substrate for inducible sustained VT. Borbola et al[45] suggested that hidden or small reentry circuits, undetectable by signal averaging, may become manifest during amiodarone treatment by prolonging the late potential duration more than the QRSD.

Several studies demonstrated that the prevalence of late potentials varies according to the clinical presentation. Patients presenting with spontaneous VF have a lower incidence of late potentials (21% to 57%)[16,24,36,44] than patients with sustained VT (52% to 92%).[11,12,15,16,19,24,34,36,44,47,62,64] This difference in the prevalence of late potentials parallels the difference in inducibility of sustained VT in these conditions.[24,34,44] Denniss et al[79] recorded late potentials more frequently in patients with sustained VT (in 58% of those with rates > 270/min and in 95% of those with rate of 270/min or less) than in patients with spontaneous VF (32%). Greene et al[36] reported on the finding that late potentials were much less common in resuscitated survivors of VF (27%) than in patients with recurrent sustained VT (79%). No difference was found in the incidence of late potentials between patients with chronic recurrent VT (74%) and with a single documented episode of VT (80%).[62] Denniss et al[41] studied the differences between patients with spontaneous VT and VF assessed by signal-averaged ECG, cardiac mapping, and radionuclide ventriculography. Post-infarction patients with spontaneous VT had a longer ventricular activation time than did patients with spontaneous VF on both signal-averaged recordings (181 ±33 msec vs 152 ±23 msec; p < 0.05) and epicardial mapping (210 ±17 msec vs 192 ±17 msec; p < 0.05).

Less information is available on the relationship between the clinical presentation and the specific signal-averaged ECG indices.[24,58] Freedman et al[24] found that the mean amplitude of V-40 in patients with VT was significantly lower than in patients with VF. The value of V-40 in patients with VF was not significantly different from that in normal subjects. The mean duration of late potentials is longer in patients with VT than in those with VF.[62] Gomes et al[58] reported that in patients with acute myocardial infarction the mean values of all signal-averaged ECG indices are significantly different between patients with arrhythmic events (VT, VT/VF, sudden cardiac death) during the follow-up period compared with patients without arrhythmic events. In our study,[44] late potentials were found in 75% of patients who initially had an episode of syncope due to VT and in 46% of patients with aborted sudden cardiac death. We also demonstrated that they had a more prolonged duration in patients with syncope due to VT (50 ±16 msec) compared with those with cardiac arrest (41 ±16 msec; p < 0.05).

Regional conduction delay during sinus rhythm seems to be greatest in patients with spontaneous and inducible sustained VT and the least in patients with spontaneous and inducible VF.[41] These results suggest that in patients with aborted sudden cardiac death either a stable reentry circuit is less frequently present or cannot be detected by the signal-averaged ECG or that sudden cardiac death may result from a de novo, unstable electrophysiologic milieu.[24,44,64] Considering the fact that late potentials are less prevalent in patients with spontaneous VF compared to those with spontaneous sustained VT, they are thought to be less suitable to detect patients at risk of sudden cardiac death than of sustained VT.[62]

Data by Breithardt and coworker[62] showed that late potentials did not correlate with the frequency and complexity of spontaneous ventricular arrhythmias. Denes et al[72] demonstrated that patients with complex ventricular arrhythmias on Holter monitoring but without history of sustained VT had a low prevalence of late potentials (18%). They concluded that their presence indicates an electrical property of the heart, which is distinct from complex ventricular arrhythmias detected on Holter monitoring. Buxton et al[80] found that in patients with nonsustained VT those who had inducible sustained VT had a significantly higher incidence of late potentials (67%) than patients without inducible sustained VT (25%).

Correlation Between Late Potentials and Underlying Heart Disease in Patients with VT/VF

Data by Poll et al[27] suggest that patients with cardiomyopathy and VT frequently have an abnormal signal-averaged ECG. They studied 41 patients with nonischemic congestive cardiomyopathy with or without a history of sustained ventricular arrhythmias. An abnormal signal-averaged ECG was more frequently detected (83%) in the patients with sustained ventricular arrhythmias than in those without them (14%). The QRSD was longer and the magnitude of V-40 was lower in the cardiomyopathy patients with VT. It was concluded that the signal-averaged ECG can identify patients with nonischemic cardiomyopathy and sustained VT/VF. These findings are in agreement with other reports.[12,33,78] In contrast, Coto et al[26] reported that in nonischemic heart disease patients with VT late potentials appeared only when cardiomegaly was present. In the most recent study,[33] it was found that in patients with VT/VF not associated with ischemic heart disease late potentials are much less common than in patients with coronary artery disease and VT/VF. Endocardial late potentials recorded during sinus rhythm were detected in 96% of patients with coronary disease compared to 76% of patients with dilated cardiomyopathy. Bethe et al[81] showed that the fractionated electrograms were seen more often in patients with coronary disease (52%) than in patients with cardiomyopathy. Cassidy et al[82] showed that the cardiomyopathy group had a higher percent of normal endocardial electrograms than the coronary disease group, regardless of the type of their arrhythmias.

Rozanski et al[10] observed the presence of late potentials in eight patients with left ventricular aneurysm and VT. The administration of antiarrhythmic drugs never abolished the delayed waveform whereas ventricular resection did. They concluded that late potentials were related to the presence of an aneurysm. Breithardt et al[12] in a heterogenous group of patients demonstrated a close correlation between the presence of late potentials and left ventricular function in patients with and without previously documented VT or VF. Late potentials were not related to the extent of coronary disease, but were associated with angiographically documented regional or diffuse ventricular contraction abnormalities. In contrast, Buckingham et al[30] supported the view that late potentials are independent of left ventricular function in identifying patients with coronary disease and sustained VT. Nalos et al[34] showed that the signal-averaged ECG correlates with inducibility of VT irrespective of left ventricular function.

Correlation Between Ventricular Late Potentials and Electrophysiologic Study Findings in Patients with VT/VF

In 1983, Breithardt et al[52] reported that the incidence of inducible ventricular arrhythmias during electrophysiologic study directly correlated with increasing duration of late potentials. The incidence of nonstimulated, repetitive ventricular response (4 or more consecutive ventricular echo beats) increased from 42% in those with late potentials of <20 msec to 56% in those with late potentials of 20- to 39-msec duration and to 92% in those with late potentials of 40 msec or more. Borggrefe et al[83] found that the median value of late potentials in patients in whom VT can be induced by single or double extrastimuli during sinus rhythm was longer (60 msec) than in patients in whom it can only be induced by single or double extrastimuli at basic driven rates of 120 or more (45 and 40 msec, respectively). Freedman et al[24] found a correlation between low values of V-40 and ventricular arrhythmia inducibility. There was no significant difference in the magnitude of V-40 between noninducible patients and patients with nonsustained VT. In another study,[84] a higher prevalence of late potentials was described in patients in whom ventricular arrhythmias could be induced with one or two extrastimuli (77%) than in patients in whom three extrastimuli were required for induction (40%). The signal-averaged ECG is considered to be more useful in predicting the induction of sustained monomorphic VT than in predicting the induction of nonsustained VT or VF.[34] In another study of patients with spontaneous nonsustained VT the signal-averaged ECG predicted the inducibility of sustained VT.[66] This study suggested that it may be a useful screening test in patients with complex ventricular arrhythmias.

Our group obtained signal-averaged ECG recordings in all patients undergoing electrophysiologic study. In patients who did not have late potentials or an abnormal recording, sustained VT was rarely inducible even with three extrastimuli from the right ventricular outflow tract. On the contrary, in patients who had late potentials or an abnormal recording especially with long late potentials, sustained monomorphic VT usually was frequently inducible with one or two ventricular extrastimuli (Figure 3). Recently, our group reported on the correlation between the signal-averaged ECG and electrophysiologic findings in 50 patients with chronic coronary disease (7 women and 43 men; mean age: 59 ±9 years) and spontaneous sustained VT or VF.[44] Correlations between mode of sustained VT/VF induction (single, double, triple extrastimuli) and signal-averaged ECG indices were as follows: significant differences in these indices were found between patients who were induced with single and double extrastimuli when compared with those inducible only with triple ventricular extrastimuli. The QRSD was longer (128.5 ±11.3 vs 117.8 ±13.6 msec; p <0.01), the V-40 was lower (16.2 ±11.6 vs 23.8 ±16.3 μV; p <0.05), and the late potential was more prolonged (53.3 ±18.1 vs 41.7 ±14.1 msec; p <0.25) in patients who were inducible with single or double ventricular extrastimuli. Correlation between the induced ventricular tachyarrhythmia (sustained monomorphic VT, pleomorphic VT or VF, nonsustained VT, noninducibility) and the signal-averaged ECG indices was as follows: late potentials were present in 71% of the inducible sustained

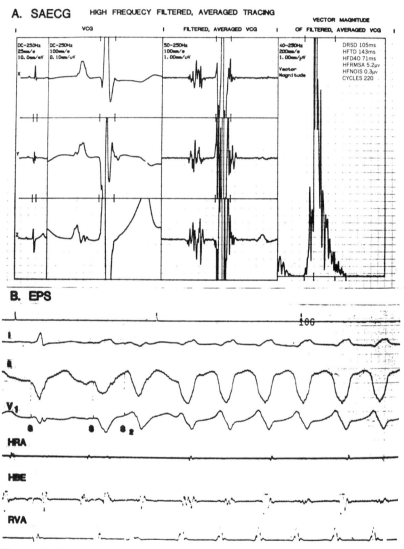

Figure 3. Representative recordings of signal-averaged electrocardiogram (SAECG) and electrophysiologic study (EPS) finding from a patient with coronary artery disease and a history of unexplained syncope. (A) The SAECG revealed the presence of a long ventricular late potential (abbreviations: see Figure 1). (B) Programmed ventricular stimulation using one extrastimulus from the right ventricular apex induced a sustained monomorphic VT (cycle length: 280 msec). HRA: high right atrium; HBE: His bundle electrogram; RVA: right ventricular apex.

monomorphic VT group; in 40% of the pleomorphic VT or VF group; in 57% of the nonsustained VT group; and in none of the noninducible group. Their prevalence was significantly higher in the sustained monomorphic VT group when compared with the remaining groups (p < 0.05). There was no significant difference between the pleomorphic VT/VF and noninducible groups. Our results support the current view that the signal-averaged ECG appears to be more useful in predicting the inducibility of sustained monomorphic VT, than in predicting other inducible ventricular tachyarrhythmias. Kuchar[61] found that the degree of prolongation of late potentials by antiarrhythmic drugs served as a useful guide to the degree of slowing of VT rate if the VT recurred. The fact that the VT cycle length correlated only with the total duration of the filtered QRS (QRSD) and not the other signal-averaged ECG indices, suggested that the localized conduction delay may not be the only determinant of the rate of VT.

Conclusions

In spite of the differences in methology among investigators for recording the signal-averaged ECG, the application of this technique to patients with sustained VT has resulted in clinically useful information. The test has a high sensitivity and specificity for detecting patients with inducible sustained monomorphic VT and it may become a useful tool for detection of high-risk patients for development of this lethal arrhythmia. The many published clinical research studies have also established a close relationship between the presence of fractionated electrograms, recorded directly from the heart (endocardial and/or epicardial) and the presence of late potentials on the signal-averaged ECG. In some cases a causal relationship has been established between late potentials and the VT by surgical ablation of the area of fractionated electrograms (site of reentry) and the disappearance of late potentials. There is also suggestive evidence that the size of the reentry area may relate to late potentials duration and determine the severity index of the induction protocol and the cycle length of induced VT. It is also clear that in patients with VT/VF who have reentrant arrhythmias, but in whom the conduction delay during sinus rhythm either does not outlast the activation time of the ventricular muscle and/or is comprised of insufficient muscle mass, it will not be detected by the signal-averaged ECG. Transient changes related to acute ischemia, drugs, or electrolytes in the reentry area are also not detectable by the current methodology. Further advances in the techniques of signal averaging, such as beat-to-beat analysis, will provide answers to some of the currently unresolved problems.

Acknowledgment: We wish to thank Ms. Lillian Linares for her invaluable secretarial help.

References

1. Langner PH, Geselowitz DB, Mausure FT: High frequency in the electrocardiograms of normal subjects and patients with coronary heart disease. Am Heart J 62:746, 1961.
2. Reynolds EW, Muller BF, Captain MC et al: High frequency components in the electrocardiogram. A comparative study of normals and patients with myocardial disease. Circulation 35:195, 1967.
3. Berbari EJ, Scherlag BJ, Hope RR, Lazzara R: Recording from the body surface of arrhythmogenic ventricular activity during the ST segment. Am J Cardiol 41:697, 1978.
4. Fontaine G, Frank R, Gallais Hamonne F, Allali I, Phan-Thuc H, Grosgogeat Y: Electrocardiography des potentials tardifs du syndrome de post-excitation. Arch Mal Coeur 71:854, 1978.
5. Uther JB, Dennett CJ, Tan A: The detection of delayed activation signals of low amplitude in the vectorcardiogram of patients with recurrent ventricular tachycardia by signal averaging. In Sandoe E, Julian DG, Bell JW (eds): Management of Ventricular Tachycardia—Role of Mexiletine. Amsterdam: Excerpta Medica, 1978, pp 80–82.
6. Breithardt G, Becker R, Seipel L: Non-invasive recording of late ventricular activation in man (abstr). Circulation 62(Suppl III):320, 1980.
7. Simson M, Horowitz L, Josephson M, et al: A marker for ventricular tachycardia after myocardial infarction (abstr). Circulation 62(Suppl III):262, 1980.
8. Hombach V, Hopp HW, Braun V, Behrenbeck DW, Tauchert M, Hilger HH: Die Bedeutung von Nachpotentialen innerhalb des ST-Segments im Oberflachen-EKG bei Patienten mit koronarer Herzkrankheit. Dtsch med Wschr 105:1457, 1980.
9. Breithardt G, Becker R, Seipel L, Abendroth RR, Ostermeyer J: Non-invasive detection of late potentials in man—a new marker for ventricular tachycardia. Eur Heart J 2:1, 1981.
10. Rozanski JJ, Mortara D, Myerburg RJ, Castellanos A: Body surface detection of delayed depolarizations in patients with recurrent ventricular tachycardia and left ventricular aneurysm. Circulation 63:1172, 1981.
11. Simson MB: Use of signals in the terminal QRS complex to identify patients with ventricular tachycardia after myocardial infarction. Circulation 64:235, 1981.
12. Breithardt G, Borggrefe M, Karbenn U, Abendroth R-R, Yeh H-L, Seipel L: Prevalence of late potentials in patients with and without ventricular

tachycardia: correlation with angiographic findings. Am J Cardiol 49:-1932, 1982.

13. Breithardt G, Seipel L, Ostermayer J, Karbenn U, Abendroth R-R, Borggrefe M, Yeh HL, Birks W: Effects of antiarrhythmic surgery on late ventricular potentials recorded by precordial signal averaging in patients with ventricular tachycardia. Am Heart J 104:996, 1982.

14. Simson MB, Spielman SR, Horowitz LN et al: Effects of antiarrhythmic drugs on body surface late potentials in patients with ventricular tachycardia. Am J Cardiol 49:1032, 1982.

15. Denes P, Santarelli P, Hauser RG, Uretz EF: Quantitative analysis of the high-frequency components of the terminal portion of the body surface QRS in normal subjects and in patients with ventricular tachycardia. Circulation 67:1129, 1983.

16. Simson MB, Falcone R, Dresden C, Buxton A, Marchlinski F, Waxman H, Josephson M: The signal-averaged ECG and electrophysiologic studies in patients with ventricular tachycardia and fibrillation (abstr). Circulation 68(Suppl III):173, 1983.

17. Simson MB, Untereker WJ, Spielman SR, Horowitz LN, Marcus NH, Falcone RA, Harken AH, Josephson ME: Relation between late potentials on the body surface and directly recorded fragmented electrograms in patients with ventricular tachycardia. Am J Cardiol 51:105, 1983.

18. Denes P, Uretz E, Santarelli P: Determinants of arrhythmogenic ventricular activity detected on the body surface QRS in patients with coronary artery disease. Am J Cardiol 53:1519, 1984.

19. Kanovsky MS, Falcone RA, Dresden CA, Josephson ME, Simson MB: Identification of patients with ventricular tachycardia after myocardial infarction: signal-averaged electrocardiogram, Holter-monitoring, and cardiac catheterization. Circulation 70:264, 1984.

20. Marcus NH, Falcone RA, Harken AH, Josephson ME, Simson MB: Body surface late potentials: effects of endocardial resection in patients with ventricular tachycardia. Circulation 70: 632, 1984.

21. Berbari EJ, Friday KJ, Jackman WM: Effects of atrial pacing on surface recorded late potentials in patients with ventricular tachycardia (abstr). Circulation 70(Suppl II):373, 1984.

22. Simson MB, Falcone R, Kindwall E: The signal-averaged electrocardiogram does not predict antiarrhythmic drug success (abstr). Circulation 72(Suppl III):7, 1985.

23. Zimmermann M, Adamec R, Simonin P, Richez J: Prognostic significance of ventricular late potentials in coronary artery disease. Am Heart J 109:725, 1985.

24. Freedman RA, Gillis AM, Keren A, Soderholm-Difatte V, Mason JW: Signal-averaged electrocardiographic late potentials in patients with ventricular fibrillation or ventricular tachycardia: correlation with clinical arrhythmia and electrophysiologic study. Am J Cardiol 55:1350, 1985.

25. Pollak SJ, Kertes PJ, Bredlau CE, Walter PF: Influence of left ventricular function on signal-averaged late potentials in patients with coronary artery disease with and without ventricular tachycardia. Am Heart J 110:747, 1985.

26. Coto H, Maldonado C, Palakurthy P, Flowers NC: Late potentials in normal subjects and in patients with ventricular tachycardia unrelated to myocardial infarction. Am J Cardiol 55:384, 1985.
27. Poll DS, Marchlinski FE, Falcone RA, Josephson ME, Simson MB: Abnormal signal-averaged electrocardiograms in patients with nonischemic congestive cardiomyopathy: relationship to sustained ventricular tachyarrhythmias. Circulation 72:1308, 1985.
28. Denniss AR, Ross DL, Richards DA, Cody DV, Russell PA, Young AA, Uther JB: Effect of antiarrhythmic drug therapy on delayed potentials detected by the signal-averaged electrocardiogram in patients with ventricular tachycardia after acute myocardial infarction. Am J Cardiol 58:261, 1986.
29. Simson MB, Kindwall E, Buxton AE, Josephson ME: Signal averaging of the ECG in the management of patients with ventricular tachycardia: prediction of antiarrhythmic drug efficacy. In Brugada P, Wellens HJJ (eds): Cardiac Arrhythmias: Where To Go From Here? Mount Kisco, NY: Futura Publishing Company, 1987, pp 299–310.
30. Buckingham TA, Ghosh S, Homan SM, Thessen CC, Redd RR, Stevens LL, Chaitman BR, Kennedy HL: Independent value of signal-averaged electrocardiography and left ventricular function in identifying patients with sustained ventricular tachycardia with coronary artery disease. Am J Cardiol 59:568, 1987.
31. Denniss AR, Richards DA, Cody DV, Russell PA, Young AA, Ross DL, Uther JB: Correlation between signal-averaged electrocardiogram and programmed stimulation in patients with and without spontaneous ventricular tachyarrhythmias. Am J Cardiol 59:585, 1987.
32. Denniss AR, Johnson DC, Richards DA, Ross DL, Uther JB: Effect of excision of ventricular myocardium on delayed potentials detected by the signal-averaged electrocardiogram in patients with ventricular tachycardia. Am J Cardiol 59:591, 1987.
33. Denniss AR, Ross DL, Johnson DC et al: Abnormalities on signal-averaged electrocardiogram and electrophysiologic study in patients with ventricular tachyarrhythmias not associated with ischemic heart disease. J Appl Cardiol 2:251, 1987.
34. Nalos PC, Gang ES, Mandel WJ, Ladenheim ML, Lass Y, Peter T: The signal-averaged electrocardiogram as a screening test for inducibility of sustained ventricular tachycardia in high risk patients: a prospective study. J Am Coll Cardiol 9:539, 1987.
35. Volosin KJ, Greenspan AJ: The effects of direct current countershock on ventricular late potentials. PACE 10:305, 1987.
36. Greene HL, Callahan DB, Dolack GL, Bardy GH: Signal-averaged electrocardiographic late potentials in resuscitated survivors of ventricular fibrillation. PACE 10(Part II):683, 1987.
37. Kacet S, Dagane J, Lacroix D et al: Quantitative analysis of signal averaged electrocardiogram in normal subjects compared to patients with sustained ventricular tachycardia. PACE 10(Part II):981, 1987.
38. Gomes JA, Winters SL, Stewart D, Targonski A, Barreca P: Optimal bandpass filters for time-domain analysis of the signal-averaged electrocardiogram. Am J Cardiol 60:1290, 1987.

39. Kacet S, Dagano J, Lacroix D et al: Results of signal averaged electrocardiogram in patients with complete right bundle branch block with and without ventricular tachycardia. PACE 10(Part II):605, 1987.
40. Edwardsson N, Lindblad A, Hirsch I: Late potentials with left bundle branch block with and without ventricular tachycardia/fibrillation. Pace 10(Part II):1005, 1987.
41. Denniss AR, Ross DL, Richards DA, Holley LK, Cooper MJ, Johnson DC, Uther JB: Differences between patients with ventricular tachycardia and ventricular fibrillation as assessed by signal-averaged electrocardiogram, radionuclide ventriculogrphy and cardiac mapping. J Am Coll Cardiol 11:276, 1988.
42. Gomes JA, Mehra R, Barreca P, Winters SL, Ergin A, Estioko M, Minditch BP: A comparative analysis of signal averaging of the surface QRS complex and signal-averaging of intracardiac and epicardial recordings in patients with ventricular tachycardia. PACE 11:271, 1988.
43. Nalos PC, Gang ES, Mandel WJ, Myers MR, Oseran DS, Lass Y, Peter T: Utility of the signal-averaged electrocardiogram in patients presenting with sustained ventricular tachycardia or fibrillation while on antiarrhythmic drug. Am Heart J 115:108, 1988.
44. Borbola J, Ezri MD, Denes P: Correlation between the signal-averaged electrocardiogram and electrophysiologic study findings in patients with coronary artery disease and sustained ventricular tachycardia. Am Heart J 115:816, 1988.
45. Borbola J, Denes P: Oral amiodarone loading therapy: I. The effect on serial signal averaged electrocardiographic recordings and the QTc in patients with ventricular tachyarrhythmias. Am Heart J 115:1202, 1988.
46. Lindsay BD, Ambos HD, Schechtman KB, Cain ME: Improved selection of patients for programmed ventricular stimulation by frequency analysis of signal-averaged electrocardiogram. Circulation 73:675, 1986.
47. Cain ME, Ambos HD, Lindsay BD: Fast Fourier transform analysis of the signal averaged electrocardiogram in the management of patients with or prone to ventricular tachycardia or fibrillation. In Brugada P, Wellens HJJ (eds): Cardiac Arrhythmias: Where To Go From Here? Mount Kisco, NY: Futura Publishing Company, 1987, pp 311–328.
48. Kelen GJ, Henkin R, Fontaine JM, El-Sherif N: Effects of analysed signal duration and phase on the results of fast Fourier transform analysis of the surface electrocardiogram in subjects with and without late potentials. Am J Cardiol 60:1282, 1987.
49. Lindsay BD, Markham J, Schechtman KB, Ambos HD, Cain ME: Identification of patients with sustained ventricular tachycardia by frequency analysis of signal averaged electrocardiograms despite the presence of bundle branch block. Circulation 77:122, 1988.
50. Machac J, Weiss A, Winters SL, Barecca P, Gomes JA: A comparative study of frequency domain and the time domain analysis of signal-averaged electrocardiograms in patients with ventricular tachycardia. J Am Coll Cardiol 11:284, 1988.
51. Breithardt G, Schwarzmaier J, Borggrefe M, Haerten K, Seipel L: Prognostic significance of late ventricular potentials after myocardial infarction. Eur Heart J 4:487, 1983.

52. Breithardt G, Borggrefe M, Quantius B, Karbenn U, Seipel L: Ventricular vulnerability assessed by programmed ventricular stimulation in patients with and without late potentials. Circulation 68:275, 1983.
53. Breithardt G, Borggrefe M, Haerten K: Ventricular late potentials and inducible ventricular tachyarrhythmias as a marker for ventricular tachycardia after myocardial infarction. Eur Heart J7 (Suppl A):127, 1986.
54. Denniss AR, Richards DA, Cody DV, Russell PA, Young AA, Cooper MJ, Ross DL, Uther JB: Prognostic significance of ventricular tachycardia and fibrillation induced at programmed stimulation and delayed potentials detected on the signal-averaged electrocardiograms of survivors of acute myocardial infarction. Circulation 74:731, 1986.
55. Kuchar DL, Thornburn CW, Sammel NL: Late potentials detected after myocardial infarction: natural history and prognostic significance. Circulation 74:1280, 1986.
56. Kuchar DL, Thornburn CW, Sammel NL: Prediction of serious arrhythmic events after myocardial infarction: signal-averaged electrocardiogram, Holter monitoring and radionuclide ventriculography. J Am Coll Cardiol 9:531, 1987.
57. Denniss AR, Ross DL, Richards DA, Uther JB: Changes in ventricular activation time on the signal-averaged electrocardiogram in the first year after acute myocardial infarction. Am J Cardiol 60:580, 1987.
58. Gomes JA, Winters SL, Stewart D, Horowitz S, Milner M, Barreca P: A new noninvasive index to predict sustained ventricular tachycardia and sudden death in the first year after myocardial infarction: based on signal-averaged electrocardiogram, radionuclide ejection fraction and Holter-monitoring. J Am Coll Cardiol 10:349, 1987.
59. El-Sherif N, Mehra R, Gomes JAC, Kelen G: Appraisal of a low noise electrocardiogram. J Am Coll Cardiol 1:456, 1983.
60. El-Sherif N, Gomes JAC, Restivo M: Late potentials and arrhythmogenesis. PACE 8:440, 1985.
61. Kuchar DL: Use of signal-averaged electrocardiography in the diagnosis of ventricular tachycardia. Practical Cardiol 12:61, 1986.
62. Breithardt G, Borggrefe M: Pathophysiological mechanism and clinical significance of ventricular late potentials. Eur Heart J 7:364, 1986.
63. Breithardt G, Borggrefe M: Recent advances in the identification of patients at risk of ventricular tachyarrhythmias: role of ventricular late potentials. Circulation 75:1091, 1987.
64. Simson MB: Signal averaging. Circulation 75(Suppl III):69, 1987.
65. Breithardt G, Borggrefe M, Karbenn U, Schwarzmaier J: Effects of pharmacological and non-pharmacological interventions on ventricular late potentials. Eur Heart J 8(Suppl A):97, 1987.
66. Fontaine JM, Turitto G, El-Sherif N: Prognostic significance of ambulatory electrocardiographic recording, programmed electrical stimulation and signal-averaged electrocardiogram in patients with complex ventricular arrhythmias. J Electrophysiol 1:204, 1987.

67. Kuchar DL, Thornburn CW, Sammel NL: Signal-averaged electrocardiogram for evaluation of recurrent syncope. Am J Cardiol 58:949, 1986.
68. Gang ES, Peter T, Rosenthal ME, Mandel WJ, Lass Y: Detection of late potentials on the surface electrocardiogram in unexplained syncope. Am J Cardiol 58:1014, 1986.
69. Winters SL, Stewart D, Gomes JA: Signal averaging of the surface QRS complex predicts inducibility of ventricular tachycardia in patients with syncope of unknown origin: a prospective study. J Am Coll Cardiol 10:775, 1987.
70. Fontaine JM, Henkin R, Howard M et al: New signal averaging criteria for determine the presence of late potentials in patients with left bundle branch block (abstr). PACE 10:451, 1987.
71. Turitto G, Macina G, Caref E et al: Lack of correlation between Holter recording and signal-averaged electrocardiogram in the post-infarction period (abstr). Circulation 74(Suppl II):402, 1986.
72. Denes P, Santarelli P, Masson M, Uretz EF: Prevalence of late potentials in patients undergoing Holter monitoring. Am Heart J 113:33, 1987.
73. Hombach V, Hopp HW, Kebbel U et al: Recovery of ventricular late potentials from body surface using the signal-averaging and high resolution ECG techniques. Clin Cardiol 9:361, 1986.
74. Faugere G, Savard P, Nadeau RA, Derome D, Shenasa M, Page PL, Guardo R: Characterization of the spatial distribution of ventricular late potentials by body surface mapping in patients with ventricular tachycardia. Circulation 74:1323, 1986.
75. Vatterott P, Hammill S, Berbari E et al: The reproducibility of the signal averaged electrocardiogram (abstr) PACE 10:450, 1987.
76. Vatterott P, Hammill S, Berbari E et al: The effect of residual noise on the predictive accuracy of the signal averaged electrocardiogram (abstr). PACE 10:450, 1987.
77. Borbola J, Denes P: Short and long-term reproducibility of the signal-averaged electrocardiogram in patients with coronary artery disease. Am J Cardiol 61:1123, 1988.
78. Iannucci G Baciariello G, Villani M et al: Late ventricular potentials in nonischemic congestive cardiomyopathy. PACE 10(Part II):690, 1987.
79. Denniss AR, Holley LK, Cody DV et al: Ventricular tachycardia and fibrillation: differences in ventricular activation times and ventricular function. J Am Coll Cardiol 1:606, 1983.
80. Buxton AE, Simson MB, Falcone R, et al: Signal-averaged ECG in patients with nonsustained ventricular tachycardia: identification of patients with potential for sustained ventricular arrhythmias. J Am Coll Cardiol 3:495, 1984.
81. Bethe KP, Genska BD, Kreuzer H et al: Endocardial late potentials recorded during sinus rhythm in man: incidence in different cardiac disease states. Clin Cardiol 11:164, 1988.
82. Cassidy DM, Vassallo JA, Miller JM, Poll DS, Buxton AE, Marchlinski FE, Josephson ME: Endocatheter mapping in patients in sinus rhythm:

relationship to underlying heart disease and ventricular arrhythmias. Circulation 73:645, 1986.

83. Borggrefe M, Karbenn U, Breithardt G: Spatpotentiale und elektrophysiologische befunde bei ventrikularen tachykardien. Z Kardiol 71:627, 1982.

84. Freedman RA, Gillis AM, Keren A et al: Signal averaged ECG late potentials correlate with clinical arrhythmia and electrophysiologic study in patients with ventricular tachycardia or fibrillation. Circulation 70(Suppl II):252, 1984.

24

Late Potentials and Syncope

Alfred E. Buxton

Introduction

Syncope is a frightening but nonspecific symptom that may be due to a variety of underlying conditions, many benign, but some potentially life-threatening. As such, it causes alarm for the patient and concern on the part of the physician. Both noncardiac and cardiac diseases may be responsible for syncope. Even among nonarrhythmic and arrhythmic cardiac mechanisms, historical descriptions of the event often fail to identify the specific cause. Thus, the patient with syncope frequently presents a difficult diagnostic and therapeutic problem for the physician. The physician must frequently reach out beyond the history and physical exam, utilizing technology to arrive at a diagnosis. The first step usually employed is the ambulatory electrocardiogram (ECG). However, episodes of syncope occur unpredictably and sporadically in most patients. Thus, the yield of one or more 24-hour ambulatory ECGs is low.[1]

In the search for greater sensitivity and specificity in determining the mechanism causing syncope, a number of centers have reported results of electrophysiologic testing in patients presenting with syncope.[2-9] While electrophysiologic studies frequently reveal abnormalities in patients with syncope, these studies are expensive, time consuming, require specially trained personnel with high de-

From El-Sherif N, Turitto G (eds): *High-Resolution Electrocardiography*. Mount Kisco, NY, Futura Publishing Co., Inc., ©, 1992.

grees of expertise, and carry some risk. Thus, it would be helpful to be able to screen patients prior to performing electrophysiologic studies by a noninvasive means in order to select those patients likely to have the highest yield from electrophysiologic studies. Programmed stimulation has frequently revealed previously unsuspected inducible ventricular tachycardia (VT) as a potential cause of syncope. Based on this, several studies have evaluated the signal-averaged ECG as a means to screen patients with syncope who should undergo electrophysiologic testing.[10–12] The purpose of this chapter is to present our own experience regarding the role of signal-averaged electrocardiography in patients referred for electrophysiologic evaluation of syncope, and to review the experience of others in this area.

Patient Population

Forty-three patients referred for evaluation of syncope of unexplained origin underwent signal-averaged ECG and complete electrophysiologic evaluation. Eight additional patients were excluded from analysis because they had bundle branch block, since criteria for abnormality of the signal-averaged ECG in patients with bundle branch block have not been established. Any patients who had documented tachyarrhythmias or bradyarrhythmias in association with episodes of syncope were excluded. Thus, we only included patients in whom at the time of electrophysiologic evaluation, the cause of syncope was completely unclear. A majority of patients had underlying structural heart disease: 25 patients had coronary artery disease; 2 patients had dilated cardiomyopathy; 2 had hypertensive cardiovascular disease; 2 had valvular heart disease; and 12 had no recognizable structural heart disease. Twenty of the 25 patients with coronary disease had a previous myocardial infarction (anterior in 9, inferior in 9, and anterior and inferior in 2). The mean left ventricular ejection fraction of the patients with coronary artery disease was 45.3%. Ten of the patients with coronary artery disease had left ventricular aneurysms. The mean age of the patients with coronary artery disease was 62.5 years while the mean age of patients without coronary artery disease was 53.2 years. Patients with coronary disease had experienced a mean of 1.9 episodes of syncope prior to study, while the patients without coronary artery disease had suffered a mean of three episodes of syncope prior to study (P = NS).

ECG monitoring had revealed nonsustained VT in 12 patients with coronary disease and in 10 patients without coronary artery disease. In no patient were symptoms reported at the time of the nonsustained VT.

Electrophysiologic Study Protocol

At least three 6 Fr quadripolar electrode catheters were inserted percutaneously for each study, and positioned in the high right atrium, His bundle area, and right ventricular apex and outflow tract. Sinus node recovery time, corrected sinus node recovery time, and sinoatrial conduction time were calculated by standard methods.[13] Atrial premature depolarizations were delivered during sinus rhythm and at two paced cycle lengths (usually 600 and 450 msec) in order to determine inducibility of supraventricular arrhythmias and atrial refractoriness. Atrial pacing was performed to the point of atrio-ventricular block in order to evaluate nodal and His-Purkinje function. Programmed ventricular stimulation utilized one to three extrastimuli during at least two drive cycle lengths (usually 600 and 400 msec). At least two right ventricular sites were stimulated utilizing previously reported methods.[14] All electrophysiologic studies were performed in the absence of antiarrhythmic medication.

Interpretation of Electrophysiologic Studies

The electrophysiologic study was considered "positive" if: uniform sustained or nonsustained VT was inducible. Nonsustained VT was considered a positive result as this may cause syncope. However, induced nonsustained VT had to last at least 15 seconds and cause hypotension in order to be considered a likely cause for syncope. Induced supraventricular tachycardias were considered a positive result if they were associated with a systolic blood pressure fall to < 80 mmHg (supine). Other positive results included a markedly prolonged sinus node recovery time (i.e., ≥ 3 seconds), prolonged response to carotid sinus massage with asystole (≥ 3 seconds), infranodal block during atrial pacing at increasing rates, or a markedly prolonged resting HV interval (≥ 100 msec). The electrophysiologic study was considered negative if no electrophysiologic abnormality likely related to syncope was demonstrated. Included in this classification was an entirely normal study, supraventricular tachycardia not associated with hypotension, and only polymorphic VT or ventricular fibrillation induced by programmed ventricular stimulation, or a resting HV interval < 100 msec.

Signal-Averaged ECG Protocol

All signal-averaged ECGs were performed in the absence of antiarrhythmic medication within 48 hours of the electrophysiologic study. Approximately 150 beats were recorded during sinus rhythm for each bipolar X, Y, and Z lead using the technique of Simson.[15] Each lead was filtered with a bidirectional, high-pass filter (band-pass 25–250 Hz), specially designed to eliminate ringing. The filtered X, Y, and Z leads were combined into a vector magnitude ($\sqrt{X^2 + Y^2 + Z^2}$) which measures the sum of the high-frequency information from all three leads and is termed the filtered QRS complex. A computer algorithm determined the onset and offset of the filtered QRS complex (the points at which the mean filtered voltage over a 5-msec interval exceeded the mean + 3 standard deviations of the noise level). A 20- to 80-msec window noise sample was located in the PR segment for the onset of the filtered QRS complex, and in the ST segment for the end of the filtered QRS complex. The noise level in each case was < 1 μV. The results of the signal-averaged ECG were expressed as two values: the filtered QRS complex duration ("normal" 110 msec or less); and RMS voltage in the last 40 msec of the filtered QRS complex ("normal" > 25 μV). A "late potential" was defined as a waveform with < 25 μV in the last 40 msec of the filtered QRS complex.

Statistical Methods

Results are expressed as mean ± standard deviation. The results of values for the signal-averaged ECG were compared using the two-tailed nonpaired $\overline{T}$-test.

Results

Results of Electrophysiologic Studies

Ventricular tachycardia having a uniform morphology was induced in 13 patients. In four patients self terminating, nonsustained VT was induced while in nine patients sustained VT requiring overdrive pacing or cardioversion was induced by programmed stimulation. Other abnormalities were noted in seven patients: infranodal block in two patients; rapid atrio-ventricular nodal reentrant tachycardia associated with hypotension in two patients; and marked sinus pauses with 3 seconds of asystole in response to carotid sinus massage in one patient. In two additional patients, nonelectrophysiologic abnormalities were precipitated by pacing: angina with electrocardiographic evidence of ischemia and hypotension in one patient; and coronary artery spasm in one patient. Overall, 19 patients demonstrated abnormalities thought to be likely etiologies of syncope during electrophysiologic testing. All 19 patients had coronary artery disease. All 13 patients with inducible VT had experienced a previous myocardial infarction. No patient without coronary artery disease had a positive electrophysiologic study. The mean left ventricular ejection fraction of patients with inducible VT was 46.0 $\pm 21.0\%$ while the ejection fraction of patients with coronary disease but no inducible VT was 45.6 $\pm 21.2\%$.

Results of Signal-Averaged ECG

The mean filtered QRS duration of all 25 patients with coronary artery disease was 118.1 ± 26.4 msec (Table I). Thirteen of 25 patients with coronary artery disease had abnormal filtered QRS durations (> 110 msec). In contrast, the mean filtered QRS duration of patients without coronary artery disease was 95.7 ± 8.3 msec (p = 0.001 vs patients with coronary artery disease). One of the 18 patients without coronary artery disease had an abnormal filtered QRS duration.

The amplitude of the last 40 msec of the filtered QRS duration

Table I
Signal-Averaged ECG Results

Patient Group	Filtered QRS Duration (msec)	Amplitude Last 40 msec (μV)
Non-CAD	95.7 ± 8.3	56.5 ± 37.1
CAD	118.1 ± 26.4	39.4 ± 27.4
CAD with inducible VT (n = 13)	130.4 ± 30.3	27.6 ± 19.6
CAD without inducible VT (n = 12)	104.8 ± 12.6	52.1 ± 29.7

p = 0.001   p = 0.01   p = 0.09   p = 0.02

CAD = coronary artery disease.

was 39.4 ± 27.4 µV in the patients with coronary disease and 56.5 ± 37.1 µV in the patients without coronary artery disease (p = 0.09). Ten of 25 patients with coronary artery disease had late potentials and 2 of 18 patients without coronary artery disease had late potentials. A total of 15 patients with coronary disease had either an abnormally prolonged filtered QRS duration or a late potential while 3 patients without coronary artery disease had either abnormality on the signal-averaged ECG.

In order to determine the ability of the signal-averaged ECG to predict patients with coronary artery disease who would have inducible VT, we then analyzed the results only for patients with coronary artery disease. The mean filtered QRS duration was significantly longer in patients with coronary disease and inducible VT than in patients without inducible VT (Table I). Nine of 13 patients with inducible VT had abnormally prolonged filtered QRS complex durations versus 3 of 12 patients without inducible VT (p = 0.03). Patients with inducible VT had significantly lower voltage in the last 40 msec of the filtered QRS complex than the patients with coronary disease without inducible VT (Table I). Eight of 13 patients with inducible VT had late potentials versus 2 of 12 without inducible VT (p = 0.03). Eleven patients with inducible VT had either signal-averaged ECG parameter abnormal while four without inducible VT had an abnormality of either signal-averaged ECG parameter (p = 0.01).

Based on the above results we then calculated the sensitivity, specificity, and predictive values of the signal-averaged ECG parameters for identifying patients with coronary disease who would have inducible VT (Table II). Considering each signal-averaged ECG parameter alone or in combination results in moderate sensitivity, specificity, and predictive values when patients with coronary disease are evaluated.

In order to determine whether the signal-averaged ECG offered a significant advantage over historical data in predicting inducibility of VT, we evaluated the sensitivity, specificity, and predictive values of knowing that a patient with syncope has coronary artery disease with a prior myocardial infarction. As can be seen (Table II) in this patient population, these historical facts are quite sensitive and carry a high negative predictive value for identifying patients with inducible VT. The positive predictive value of having a history of coronary disease with prior myocardial infarction approximates that of the signal-averaged ECG parameters.

Table II

Utility of the Signal-Averaged ECG to Identify Patients With
Ventricular Tachycardia Among Those With Coronary Artery Disease

Parameter	Sensitivity	Specificity	Positive Predictive Value	Negative Predictive Value
Filtered QRS Duration > 110 msec	69%(9/13)	75%(9/12)	77%(10/13)	75%(9/12)
+Late Potential	62%(8/13)	83%(10/12)	80%(8/10)	67%(10/15)
Either abnormal	85%(11/13)	50%(6/12)	73%(11/15)	80%(8/10)
History of CAD and MI	100%(13/13)	42%(5/12)	65%(13/20)	100%(5/5)

CAD = coronary artery disease; MI = myocardial infarction.

Comparison With Previous Studies

Three prior studies have examined the utility of the signal-averaged ECG in the evaluation of patients with syncope. Kuchar et al[10] evaluated 150 unselected patients with syncope. Only 47 of these patients underwent programmed stimulation. They used a variety of criteria to diagnose VT, including three or more consecutive ventricular complexes on ambulatory ECG monitoring, and five or more complexes of nonsustained VT induced by programmed stimulation. By their criteria VT was diagnosed in 22 patients. Only eight of these patients had VT induced by programmed stimulation and in only two patients was uniform morphology sustained VT induced. These workers did not report data on the filtered QRS duration of the signal-averaged ECG, but only the presence or absence of late potentials (defined as < 20 μV RMS in the last 40 msec). Late potentials were found in 29 patients, and 16 of these were diagnosed as having VT, resulting in a positive predictive value in this study of 54%. Of 22 patients given a diagnosis of VT, 16 had late potentials resulting in a sensitivity of 73%. In this study, 43 patients had coronary artery disease and 58 had no structural heart disease with the remainder having a variety of other types of heart disease. Of note, no patient who had a late potential without structural heart disease was given a diagnosis of VT.

Gang et al[11] using a different type of signal averaging technology than we have used, reported results in 24 consecutive patients with unexplained syncope referred for electrophysiologic studies. Eighteen of these patients had cardiovascular disease including coronary disease in eight. Eight of nine patients with inducible sustained VT had late potentials, resulting in a sensitivity of 89%. These authors did not detect late potentials in any patient without inducible VT.

Winters et al[12] studied 34 patients with syncope of unknown origin without bundle branch block using programmed stimulation and the signal-averaged ECG. Twelve patients had inducible VT. Seven of these 12 had coronary artery disease, three had cardiomyopathy, and two had no structural heart disease. Using a similar signal averaging technique as we have used, they found that 11 of their 12 patients with inducible VT had at least one abnormal signal-averaged ECG parameter, while 7 of 22 patients without VT had one or more abnormal parameters on the signal-averaged ECG.

All three of these reports concluded that the signal-averaged ECG was a useful test to screen which patients with syncope of unknown origin should undergo electrophysiologic studies.[10-12] However, all three reported values for sensitivity and specificity were based on their entire patient population, without regard for historical factors such as previous myocardial infarction and coronary artery disease.

Discussion

The present small series of patients with unexplained syncope confirms and extends previous observations by our laboratory and others. We have demonstrated that potential causes of syncope can be demonstrated during electrophysiologic studies in a majority of patients who have coronary artery disease, but rarely in patients with syncope without coronary artery disease. We have also shown that patients who have inducible VT with a uniform morphology are significantly more likely to have abnormalities of the signal-averaged ECG than the patients without inducible uniform morphology VT. As is well known, a majority of patients who have abnormalities of the signal-averaged ECG have coronary artery disease and prior myocardial infarction. Thus, it is not surprising that historical factors such as coronary artery disease with previous myocardial infarction should also predict the likelihood of inducible VT in a population of patients presenting with syncope.[9,16]

One must use caution when interpreting the results of electrophysiologic studies and the signal-averaged ECG in patients with syncope. Although we and others have used programmed stimulation as a "gold standard" by which to interpret the results of the signal-averaged ECG, both of these laboratory tests are likely to have a certain, as yet undefined incidence of false-positive and false-negative results. A primary difficulty is that syncope is a nonspecific symptom with a multitude of potential causes. Since most patients do not have their ECG monitored at the time of syncope, the significance of any abnormal finding from these laboratory tests must be examined critically. The patient with syncope of unknown etiology presents a far more difficult diagnostic problem than the patient referred for electrophysiologic studies to evaluate a documented arrhythmia.

Electrophysiologic studies encompass a range of tests capable of diagnosing a variety of disorders in addition to ventricular tachyarrhythmias. As demonstrated in this study, patients with syncope may have supraventricular tachyarrhythmias induced by programmed stimulation and disorders of the atrial ventricular conduction system revealed by an electrophysiologic study. Patients with syncope due to arrhythmias other than VT would not be expected to have abnormalities of the signal-averaged ECG. Thus, the signal-averaged ECG at best can be expected to play a complimentary role to the electrophysiologic study in the evaluation of patients with syncope. It may contribute to our understanding of mechanisms underlying VT, but should not be expected to serve as a broad screening test in patients with syncope.

The interpretation of the results of any laboratory test must take into account the patient population studied. For example, a study of patients with syncope which includes a number of patients without structural heart disease, and especially without coronary artery disease would be expected to demonstrate many patients with normal signal-averaged ECGs and many patients without inducible VT. If one then compares the results of the signal-averaged ECG in patients without heart disease and without inducible VT to patients with heart disease having inducible VT, the test is likely to look good. If, however, one compares the results of the signal-averaged ECG in a population of patients with coronary disease who present with syncope, the signal-averaged ECG is put to a more stringent test. When considering a population of patients with syncope, all of whom have coronary artery disease, the specificity of the signal-averaged ECG is likely to be lower than if patients without coronary disease are included. Our analysis and that of others[9,16] suggests that knowing that a patient with syncope has coronary disease and a prior myocardial infarction is as good a predictor of an abnormal electrophysiologic study, and more specifically inducible VT, as is the results of the signal-averaged ECG. A limitation of this study is that few patients with noncoronary cardiac disease were studied. The studies referred to above suggest that there is a significant yield of abnormal results when electrophysiologic studies are performed in patients with syncope and any structural cardiac disease.

Based on the results of this and the previous studies, we would not recommend the signal-averaged ECG be used as a screening test to determine whether or not patients with syncope should undergo electrophysiologic study. Rather, the signal-averaged ECG should be used as an adjunct to aid in interpreting the clinical significance and relevance of the electrophysiologic study. As has been noted before, electrophysiologic studies are likely to have a low yield in patients presenting with syncope who do not have structural heart disease and coronary artery disease with previous myocardial infarction.

Acknowledgment: The author acknowledges the work of Michael Simson, MD in developing the signal-averaged ECG, Rita Falcone, Roxellen Auletto, RN, and Nancy Britton, RN for performing the signal-averaged ECG, and to the technicians and nurses of the Electrophysiology Laboratory of the University of Pennsylvania for their aid in performing the studies reported. The author is indebted to Elizabeth Lomis for her secretarial and editorial assistance.

References

1. Gibson TC, Heitzman MR: Diagnostic efficacy of 24-hour electrocardiographic monitoring for syncope. Am J Cardiol 53:1013, 1984.
2. DiMarco JP, Garan H, Harthorne JW, Ruskin JN: Intracardiac electrophysiologic techniques in recurrent syncope of unknown cause. Ann Intern Med 95:542, 1981.
3. Hess DS, Morady F, Scheinman MM: Electrophysiologic testing in the evaluation of patients with syncope of undetermined origin. Am J Cardiol 50:1309, 1982.
4. Ezri M, Lerman BB, Marchlinski FE, Buxton AE, Josephson ME: Electrophysiologic evaluation of syncope in patients with bifascicular block. Am Heart J 106:693, 1983.
5. Morady F, Higgins J, Peters RW, Schwartz AB, Shen EN, Bhandari A,

Scheinman MM, Sauve MJ: Electrophysiologic testing in bundle branch block and unexplained syncope. Am J Cardiol 54:587, 1984.

6. Hammill SC, Holmes DR, Wood DL, Osborn MJ, McLaran C, Sugrue DD, Gersh BJ: Electrophysiologic testing in the upright position: improved evaluation of patients with rhythm disturbances using a tilt table. J Am Coll Cardiol 4:65, 1984.

7. Olshansky B, Mazuz M, Martins JB: Significance of inducible tachycardia in patients with syncope of unknown origin: a long-term follow-up. J Am Coll Cardiol 5:216, 1985.

8. Teichman SL, Felder SD, Matos JA, Kim SG, Waspe LE, Fisher JD: The value of electrophysiologic studies in syncope of undetermined origin: Report of 150 cases. Am Heart J 110:469, 1985.

9. Doherty JU, Pembrook-Rogers D, Grogan W, Falcone RA, Buxton AE, Marchlinski FE, Cassidy DM, Kienzle MG, Almendral JM, Josephson ME: Electrophysiologic evaluation and follow-up characteristics of patients with recurrent unexplained syncope and presyncope. Am J Cardiol 55:703, 1985.

10. Kuchar DL, Thorburn CW, Sammel NL: Signal-averaged electrocardiogram for evaluation of recurrent syncope. Am J Cardiol 58:949, 1986.

11. Gang ES, Peter T, Rosenthal ME, Mandel WJ, Lass Y: Detection of late potentials on the surface electrocardiogram in unexplained syncope. Am J Cardiol 58:1014, 1986.

12. Winters SL, Stewart D, Gomes JA: Signal averaging of the surface QRS complex predicts inducibility of ventricular tachycardia in patients with syncope of unknown origin: a prospective study. J Am Coll Cardiol 10:775, 1987.

13. Josephson ME, Seides SF: Clinical Cardiac Electrophysiology. Philadelphia: Lea & Febiger, 1979.

14. Buxton AE, Waxman HL, Marchlinski FE, Untereker WJ, Waspe LE, Josephson ME: Role of triple extrastimuli during electrophysiologic study of patients with documented sustained ventricular tachyarrhythmias. Circulation 69:532, 1984.

15. Simson MB: Use of signals in the terminal QRS complex to identify patients with ventricular tachycardia after myocardial infarction. Circulation 64:235, 1981.

16. Krol RB, Morady F, Flaker GC, DiCarlo LA, Baerman JM, Hewett J, DeBuitleir M: Electrophysiologic testing in patients with unexplained syncope: clinical and noninvasive predictors of outcome. J Am Coll Cardiol 10:358, 1987.

25

Bundle Branch Block and the Signal-Averaged Electrocardiogram

John M. Fontaine, Nabil El-Sherif

Introduction

Signal-averaged electrocardiography is a noninvasive technique that is utilized to identify low amplitude signals which are present in the terminal portion of the QRS or ST segment but not evident on the conventional surface electrocardiogram (ECG). These signals, termed late potentials, are thought to represent electrical activity in slowly conducting areas of abnormal myocardium and have been shown to be present in patients with ischemic heart disease and sustained ventricular tachycardia (VT).[1-8] More recently, the signal-averaged electrocardiogram (SAECG) has been found to be a useful marker of those patients who demonstrate spontaneous and/ or inducible sustained monomorphic ventricular tachycardia (SMVT) during programmed electrical stimulation.[9-17] The electrophysiologic basis for late potentials is derived from experimental canine models of myocardial infarction in which delayed activation potentials have been found in regions of ischemic myocardium and correlated with the occurrence of circus movement VT.[18-24]

The presence of a bundle branch block (BBB) however, has served as an exclusionary criterion when the SAECG is utilized for the identification of patients at a high risk of sustained VT.[1-11,13-16]

From El-Sherif N, Turitto G (eds): *High-Resolution Electrocardiography*. Mount Kisco, NY, Futura Publishing Co., Inc., ©, 1992.

Altered ventricular activation associated with BBB may mask or simulate late potentials. Abnormal myocardial zones generating low amplitude signals may be totally obscured by the delayed activation of normal myocardial regions during BBB. Alternatively, time-domain analysis of the SAECG may show late potentials in an otherwise normal heart as a result of applying a high-pass filter to a terminal QRS region of lower than normal amplitude and/or slope due to BBB. Although a few studies have proposed preliminary SAECG criteria which may be helpful in delineating patients with left (L) BBB and inducible SMVT from those who are noninducible, a quantitative and qualitative analysis of SAECG parameters in these patients is still lacking.[25–29]

In this chapter we will review the clinical studies of time-domain SAECG in patients with BBB. We will discuss in detail our recent study to define new time-domain SAECG criteria based on data obtained during pacing-induced LBBB that could provide the best predictive accuracy for inducible SMVT when applied to patients with intrinsic LBBB. In addition, we will report preliminary data on time-domain SAECG in patients with right (R) BBB and discuss the difference in SAECG parameters between patients with LBBB and RBBB.

The SAECG in Patients With LBBB

Methods

Study Population

The study population was comprised of a total of 87 patients. There were 78 men and 9 women. The mean age was 63 ±9.7 years (range 34–87). Forty-eight patients had ECG evidence of LBBB. The ECG criteria for the diagnosis of LBBB were: (1) QRS duration > 120 msec; (2) delayed intrinsicoid deflection of 0.06 seconds or more in leads V_5 and V_6 with or without associated notching of the R wave in these leads; and (3) the absence of "septal" Q waves in leads I, V_5, and V_6. All patients were studied because they had either nonsustained VT (≥ 3 consecutive ventricular complexes occurring at a rate of ≥ 100 beats/min and < 30 seconds in duration) or sustained

VT (VT ≥ 30 seconds in duration or associated with immediate hemo-dynamic collapse) documented on a 24-hour ambulatory ECG record-ing or 12-lead ECG with rhythm strip and associated with clinical symptoms of palpitations, lightheadedness, syncope, or near syn-cope. No patient had primary ventricular fibrillation as a clinical event. All studies were performed prior to undertaking any pharma-cologic intervention. Clinical characteristics and SAECG data for all patients are shown in Tables I–IV. Left ventricular ejection frac-tion was determined by two-dimensional echocardiography, multi-gated radionuclide scan, or left ventriculography performed at the time of coronary angiography.

Pacing-Induced LBBB

Pacing from the right ventricular apex was performed in 39 patients with a standard surface QRS duration < 120 msec. Right ventricular pacing produced the LBBB pattern that was subse-quently used for signal averaging. To avoid the presence of the P wave in the terminal portion of the QRS or ST segment, as is ex-pected in the presence of retrograde conduction or during atrio-ventricular dissociation, we performed atrio-ventricular sequential pacing at a rate slightly above the sinus mechanism. Atrio-ventricu-lar intervals of 0 to 50 msec were chosen to preclude anterograde conduction of the paced atrial complex while assuring the P wave's position relative to the QRS and ST segment.

Electrophysiologic Study

All patients underwent electrophysiologic evaluation using standard techniques and in the post-absorptive, nonsedated state.[12] Informed consent was obtained in all patients. The stimulation pro-tocol consisted of the administration of an 8-beat S_1 drive at paced cycle lengths of 600, 500, and 400 msec followed by the introduction of single, double, and triple extrastimuli at two right ventricular sites. Electrophysiologic study guided pharmacologic therapy was reserved for patients with inducible SMVT. Termination of VT was achieved via overdrive pacing or direct current cardioversion. In-ducible SMVT was defined as VT induced during programmed ven-tricular stimulation that was of uniform QRS morphology with a

Table I

Clinical Characteristics and SAECG Data for Patients With Inducible Sustained Monomorphic VT

		Clinical Characteristics			Pacing-Induced LBBB Patients SAECG				Surface QRS <120 msec SAECG			
Patient #	Age	Cardiac DX	Arrhythmia	EF	QRS (msec)	LAS 40 (msec)	RMS 40 (µV)	LP	QRS (msec)	LAS40 (msec)	RMS 40 (µV)	LP
1	72	ASHD	VT-NS	20%	272	84	7.7	+	183	47	8	+
2	76	ASHD	VT-NS	59%	135	49.5	17	+	108	38	10.4	+
3	72	ASHD	VT-NS	23%	242	72	9	+	195	72	3	+
4	75	ASHD	VT-NS	29%	195	78	5	+	136.5	49.5	5.7	+
5	73	ASHD	VT-NS	45%	192	87	15	+	132	51	6	+
6	48	ASHD	VT-NS	30%	287	47	14	+	168	73	9	+
7	57	ASHD	VT-NS	18%	229	87	12	+	153	69	12	+
8	64	ASHD	VT-NS	45%	255	20	71	−	135	46.5	18.9	+
9	68	ASHD	VT-NS	40%	160.5	10.5	73.6	−	117	39	16	+
10	71	CM	VT-NS	45%	190.5	31.5	28.6	−	111	42	14	+
11	69	ASHD	VT-NS	30%	219	59	11	+	130.5	60	10	+
12	68	ASHD	VT-NS	31%	186	57	12.6	−	112.5	18	34	−
13	68	ASHD	VT-NS	43%	145.5	33	27	−	97.5	30	87	−
14	78	ASHD	VT-NS	33%	201	32	30	−	120	3	108	−

Table I *(Continued)*

Pacing-Induced LBBB Patients

					SAECG				Surface QRS <120 msec SAECG			
		Clinical Characteristics										
Patient #	Age	Cardiac DX	Arrhythmia	EF	QRS (msec)	LAS 40 (msec)	RMS 40 (µV)	LP	QRS (msec)	LAS40 (msec)	RMS 40 (µV)	LP
15	56	ASHD	VT-NS	32%	168	19.5	44.6	–	114	9	113	–
16	70	CM	VT-NS	38%	215	40.5	11.7	+	102	27	26.6	–
17	52	ASHD	VT-S	34%	300	78	7	+	151.5	48	12.9	+
18	40	ASHD	VT-S	25%	197	18	23	+	151.5	56	8	+
19	50	ASHD	VT-S	28%	284	69	5	+	184	99	2	+
20	63	ASHD	VT-S	40%	310.5	93	3.1	+	178.5	73	12	+
21	53	ASHD	VT-S	38%	245	112	7	+	136	52	11.9	+
22	47	ASHD	VT-S	45%	193.5	79.5	8.3	+	100.5	22.5	40	–
23	55	ASHD	VT-S	32%	214	63	7.7	+	139	64	7.9	+
mean ±SD				34.9 ±9%	218.9 ±48	57 ±28	19.6 ±19		137 ±29	47 ±22	25 ±32	

Clinical characteristics of patients undergoing right ventricular pacing induced LBBB are shown on the left; whereas the prepaced SAECG parameters in those patients with a normal surface QRS duration are shown on the right. Late potentials (LP) are defined as RMS40 ≤25 µV or LAS40 ≥38 msec during LBBB aberration. + = Present; – = absent; ASHD = atherosclerotic heart disease; CM = idiopathic cardiomyopathy; DX = diagnosis; EF = ejection fraction; NS = nonsustained; S = sustained; SAECG = signal-averaged electrocardiogram; SD = standard deviation; VT = ventricular tachycardia.

Table II

Clinical Characteristics and Signal-Averaged Electrocardiogram (SAECG) Data for Patients With No Inducible Sustained VT

Pacing-Induced LBBB Patients

Patient #	Age	Cardiac DX	Arrhythmia	EF	SAECG QRS (msec)	LAS 40 (msec)	RMS 40 (µV)	LP	Surface QRS <120 msec SAECG QRS (msec)	LAS 40 (msec)	RMS 40 (µV)	LP
1	57	NL	VT-NS	54%	155	68	18	+	93	32	57	−
2	65	LVH	VT-NS	55%	171	9	49	−	111	39	18	+
3	59	NL	VT-NS	60%	143	50	14	+	96	24	32	−
4	73	ASHD	VT-NS	55%	170	56	21	+	93	20	70	−
5	75	ASHD	VT-NS	45%	162	21	39	−	81	17	154	−
6	75	ASHD	VT-NS	72%	164	35	23	+	99	30	35	−
7	68	ASHD	VT-NS	17%	138	27	28	−	111	24	27	−
8*	51	AI	VT-NS	50%	186	5	55	−	95	17	209	−
9	59	ASHD	VT-NS	73%	165	33	37	−	98	20	138	−
10	66	AI	VT-NS	75%	219	86	9	+	107	18	77	−
11	66	ASHD	VT-NS	44%	151	60	12	+	107	33	44	−
12	34	CM	VT-NS	50%	175	62	12	+	111	30	40	−
13	66	ASHD	VT-NS	23%	249	62	14	+	137	23	76	−
14	67	ASHD	VT-NS	60%	162	37	16	+	105	26	64	−
15	63	CM	VT-NS	42%	182	77	19	+	98	33	41	−
16	48	CM	VT-NS	22%	203	37	28	−	121	39	22	+
mean ±SD				49.8 ±17%	174 ±28	45 ±23	24 ±13		103 ±13	26.5 ±7	69 ±53	

Clinical characteristics of patients undergoing right ventricular pacing-induced LBBB are shown on the left; the prepaced SAECG parameters with a normal surface QRS duration are shown on the right. AI = aortic insufficiency. All other abbreviations are the same as in Table I. Late potentials are defined as RMS 40 ≤25 µV or LAS40 ≥38 msec during LBBB aberration.

Table III

Clinical Characteristics and Signal-Averaged Electrocardiogram (SAECG) Data for Patients With Intrinsic Left Bundle Branch Block and Inducible Sustained Monomorphic Ventricular Tachycardia

| | Clinical Characteristics | | | | SAECG | | | |
Patient #	Age	Cardiac DX	Arrhythmia	EF	QRS (msec)	LAS40 (msec)	RMS40 (µV)	LP
1*	61	ASHD	VT-S	25%	159	44	19.5	+
2	55	ASHD	VT-S	30%	159	54	10.8	+
3	65	ASHD	VT-NS	40%	138	52	17.3	+
4	59	ASHD	VT-S	13%	166.5	45	13.6	+
5	60	CM	VT-S	18%	217.5	67.5	15.2	+
6	54	ASHD	VT-NS	15%	134	46	16.4	+
7	68	ASHD	VT-S	36%	215	71	6.2	+
8	63	ASHD	VT-NS	22%	192	56	11.8	+
9	66	ASHD	VT-NS	20%	172	59	9.7	+
10	41	ASHD	VT-S	24%	125	23	32.7	–
11	55	ASHD	VT-S	37%	202	72	7.1	+
12	72	ASHD	VT-NS	34%	174	42	20.4	+
13	42	ASHD	VT-S	26%	145	38	20.4	+
14*	62	ASHD	VT-NS	37%	148	7	47.1	–
15	48	ASHD	VT-S	20%	181	111	9.7	+
16	65	ASHD	VT-S	15%	192	88	5.3	+
mean ±SD				25.7 ±9%	170 ±28	54.7 ±25	16.5 ±11	

All abbreviations are the same as in the prior tables. Late potentials are defined as RMS40 ≤25 µV or LAS40 ≥38 msec. * denotes a female patient.

Table IV

Clinical Characteristics and Signal-Averaged Electrocardiogram (SAECG) Data For Patients With Intrinsic Left Bundle Branch Block and No Inducible VT

Patient #	Clinical Characteristics				SAECG			
	Age	Cardiac DX	Arrhythmia	EF	QRS (msec)	LAS40 (msec)	RMS40 (µV)	LP
1*	58	NL	VT-NS	57%	150	51	18	+
2	76	CM	VT-NS	40%	151	6	43.6	−
3*	50	CM	VT-NS	27%	153	38	25	+
4*	63	CM	VT-NS	12%	171	32	41	−
5	65	ASHD	VT-NS	22%	120	26.5	24.7	+
6	60	ASHD	VT-NS	65%	177	45	22.1	+
7	74	CM	VT-NS	20%	168	76.5	12.9	+
8	63	ASHD	VT-NS	21%	148.5	46.5	14.9	+
9	66	CM	VT-NS	18%	147	43.5	19.5	+
10	62	CM	VT-NS	21%	151.5	61.5	15.2	+
11	62	ASHD	VT-NS	15%	162	9	54	−
12	74	ASHD	VT-NS	40%	186	37	28.8	−
13	76	ASHD	VT-NS	35%	128	32.8	20	+
14	67	ASHD	VT-NS	15%	165	23	31.9	−
15	68	ASHD	VT-NS	36%	121	49	21.6	+
16	87	ASHD	VT-NS	52%	156	36	19.8	+
17	51	ASHD	VT-NS	62%	151	18	27.4	−
18	68	ASHD	VT-NS	36%	129	37	19.7	+

Table IV (Continued)

| Patient # | Clinical Characteristics | | | | SAECG | | | LP |
	Age	Cardiac DX	Arrhythmia	EF	QRS (msec)	LAS40 (msec)	RMS40 (µV)	
19	61	LVH	VT-NS	65%	170	9	29.8	−
20	54	ASHD	VT-NS	14%	133	43	16.6	+
21	48	ASHD	VT-NS	55%	153	21	27.1	−
22	60	ASHD	VT-NS	20%	160	49	4.4	+
23*	66	ASHD	VT-NS	25%	163	28	23.3	+
24*	54	ASHD	VT-NS	30%	174	28	25.6	−
25	64	ASHD	VT-NS	40%	133	20	26.3	−
26	71	ASHD	VT-NS	20%	146	6	45.5	+
27	66	ASHD	VT-NS	44%	128	40	15.2	+
28	59	ASHD	VT-NS	38%	145	46	19.2	+
29*	73	CM	VT-NS	40%	159	43	21.5	+
30	71	LVH	VT-NS	65%	181	34	18.3	−
31	54	CM	VT-NS	25%	142	10.2	41	−
32	70	ASHD	VT-NS	35%	184	9	40.1	−
mean ± SD				34.7 ±16%	153 ±18	32.9 ±16	25 ±10	

LVH = left ventricular hypertrophy; NL = normal. All other abbreviations are the same as in Table I. Late potentials are defined as RMS 40 ≤25 µV or LAS 40 ≥38 msec. * denotes a female patient.

cycle length > 200 msec and lasting ≥ 30 seconds in duration or associated with immediate hemodynamic collapse.

Signal-Averaged Electrocardiography

The SAECG was performed utilizing a commercially available system (Arrhythmia Research Technology, ART, model 101 PCD) or a custom designed unit. Although the custom designed unit was used infrequently, it was occasionally necessary since the ART system did not always identify the ventricular pacing spike in patients undergoing atrio-ventricular sequential pacing. Data derived from the custom designed system has been previously published.[30] In a study from our laboratory, no significant difference in SAECG parameters were noted when the two systems were compared provided that the same filter settings were utilized.[31]

The SAECG was recorded with standard bipolar X, Y, and Z orthogonal leads. Signals were amplified, averaged, and filtered with a four-pole Butterworth, bidirectional bandpass filter with cut-off frequencies of 25 to 250 Hz. The filtered signals were combined into a vector magnitude $\sqrt{X^2 + Y^2 + Z^2}$ and the QRS duration, the duration of low amplitude signals < 40 µV (LAS40) and the root mean square voltage of the signals in the last 40 msec of the filtered QRS (RMS40) calculated. Recordings with a noise level > 1 µV were rejected. The SAECG was considered to be abnormal if QRS duration was ≥ 120 msec, RMS40 ≤ 25 µV, and LAS40 ≥ 38 msec.

Statistics

Continuous variables are presented as the mean ± 1 standard deviation. Multiple comparisons of SAECG parameters were performed via analysis of variance. Tests for differences among the group means for SAECG parameters for nonparametric data were performed utilizing the Kruskal-Wallis test. Comparison of SAECG parameters between groups were made employing the Student's t-test for paired and unpaired data. Nonparametric data between groups were compared using the Mann-Whitney U test (rank sum test). The Chi square test with Yates correction factor (where appropriate) was used for the comparisons of two proportions (late potentials and inducible VT). The Fisher's exact test was substituted where appropriate. The sensitivity, specificity, negative and positive predictive values, and the total predictive accuracy of the various SAECG parameters for inducible VT were defined as follows:

$$\text{Sensitivity} = \frac{\text{patients with late potentials + inducible VT}}{\text{total patients with inducible VT}}$$

$$\text{Specificity} = \frac{\text{patients without late potentials + no inducible VT}}{\text{total patients without inducible VT}}$$

$$\text{Positive Predictive Value} = \frac{\text{patients with late potentials + inducible VT}}{\text{total patients with a positive SAECG for late potentials}}$$

$$\text{Negative Predictive Value} = \frac{\text{patients without late potentials or inducible VT}}{\text{total patients with a negative SAECG for late potentials}}$$

$$\text{Total Predictive Accuracy} = \frac{\text{true positives + true negative patients}}{\text{total patients evaluated}}$$

A p value of <0.05 was considered statistically significant.

Results

Electrophysiologic Study

Sustained monomorphic VT was induced in 16 of 48 (33%) patients with intrinsic LBBB and 23 of 39 (59%) patients without BBB (standard QRS duration <120 msec). Programmed ventricular stimulation induced VT in all 17 patients with clinical sustained VT. The difference in the mean VT cycle length between patients with intrinsic LBBB (300 ±40, range 250–380 msec) and those with standard QRS duration <120 msec (290 ±54, range 210–410 msec) was not statistically significant. In patients with intrinsic LBBB, the mean ejection fraction was significantly lower in those patients with inducible SMVT (26 $\pm8\%$) than in those who were noninducible (35 $\pm16\%$; p <0.01). The difference in the mean ejection fraction between inducible and noninducible patients without LBBB was also significant (35 $\pm9\%$ vs 50 $\pm17\%$, respectively; p <0.005).

Comparison of the SAECG in Patients Without BBB During Normal Conduction and Pacing-Induced LBBB

In patients without BBB and during normal conduction, the mean filtered total QRS duration, RMS40 and LAS40 values for inducible and noninducible patients were 137 ± 29 msec, 25 ± 32 μV, 47 ± 22 msec, and 104 ± 13 msec, 69 ± 53 μV and 27 ± 7 msec, respectively. The difference in all three SAECG parameters for the two groups was statistically significant (see Figure 1).

Late potentials were present in 17 of 23 (74%) patients with inducible SMVT and 2 of 16 (13%) patients who were noninducible (see Figure 2).

The sensitivity, specificity, and total predictive accuracy for

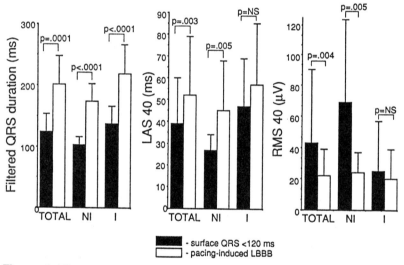

Figure 1. The mean total filtered QRS duration, RMS40 and LAS40 for all patients with a normal surface QRS duration and during pacing-induced LBBB are shown. NI = noninducible; I = inducible; total = the mean values for the sum of inducible and noninducible patients with a surface QRS < 120 msec or during pacing-induced LBBB. A statistically significant difference in the mean total filtered QRS duration, RMS40 and LAS40 values was noted between the total number of patients with a surface QRS < 120 msec and those with pacing-induced LBBB irrespective of inducibility status. In inducible patients, differences between mean RMS40 and LAS40 values were not significant whereas in noninducible patients differences between these values were. See text for details.

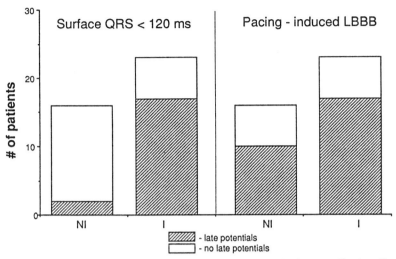

Figure 2. Illustrated is the incidence of late potentials in those patients with a surface QRS < 120 msec and during pacing-induced LBBB when SAECG criteria of RMS40 ≤25 µV or LAS40 ≥38 msec were utilized. Late potentials were present in 17 of 23 patients with a surface QRS duration < 120 msec who had inducible sustained VT and 2 of the remaining 16 patients without inducible VT. Pacing-induced LBBB was not associated with a change in the incidence of late potentials in the inducible patients whereas 10 of 16 patients who were noninducible developed late potentials. RMS40 and LAS40 criteria were associated with a low specificity and positive predictive value for inducible VT during pacing-induced LBBB (see Table V).

inducible VT when using all three SAECG parameters in those patients with a normal surface QRS duration were 74%, 88%, and 79%, respectively (Table V).

In the same group of patients the SAECG was analyzed during pacing-induced LBBB. The mean total filtered QRS duration, RMS40 and LAS40 values in the inducible and noninducible VT patients were 219 ±48 msec, 20 ±19 µV, 57 ±28 msec, and 175 ±28 msec, 25 ±13.7 µV, 45 ±23 msec, respectively (see Figure 1). Employing the "standard" RMS40 and LAS40 criteria to the SAECG during pacing-induced LBBB, late potentials were present in 17 of 23 (74%) patients with inducible SMVT and in 10 of 16 (63%) without inducible VT (see Figure 2).

The sensitivity, specificity, positive and negative predictive values, and predictive accuracy for inducible SMVT of the SAECG

Table V

Statistical Accuracy of SAECG Parameters in Predicting Inducible Sustained Monomorphic VT in Patients With a Normal Surface QRS Duration and that of RMS40 and LAS40 in Pacing-Induced LBBB Patients

Surface QRS <120 msec		Pacing-Induced LBBB	
		RMS40 (≤25 µV)	LAS40 (≥38 msec)
Sensitivity	74%	74%	70%
Specificity	88%	38%	50%
Positive Predictive value	89%	63%	67%
Negative Predictive value	70%	50%	53%
Total Predictive Accuracy	79%	59%	62%

during pacing-induced LBBB are shown in Table V. Pacing-induced LBBB resulted in lower specificity and negative predictive value for inducible SMVT when "standard" RMS40 and LAS40 criteria were applied. Pacing-induced LBBB was generally associated with a lower RMS40 and longer LAS40 than that noted during normal conduction. Pacing-induced LBBB resulted in no significant change in the mean RMS40 (from 25 to 20 µV, a decrease of 21%) or in LAS40 (from 47 to 57 msec, an increase of 25%) in patients with inducible SMVT. In contrast, there was a significant decrease in the mean RMS40 (from 69 to 25 µV or 60%) along with a significant increase in the mean LAS40 (from 27 to 45 msec or 71%) in patients with no inducible VT (Figure 1). These data highlight the similarities of RMS40 and LAS40 in those patients with inducible SMVT as well as illustrate the significant differences in the same SAECG parameters for those individuals with pacing-induced LBBB who do not have inducible VT.

Examples of the SAECG during pacing-induced LBBB in one patient with late potentials and in another patient without late potentials during control (standard QRS duration <120 msec) are shown in Figures 3 and 4.

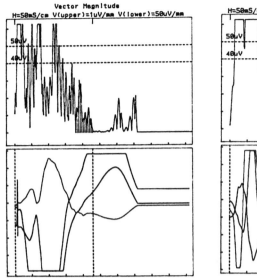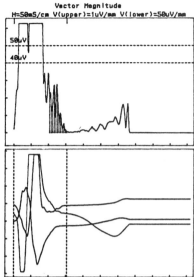

Figure 3. SAECGs from a patient who underwent pacing-induced LBBB (patient #7 of Table I) are shown. This patient had inducible sustained monomorphic VT and late potentials during the baseline period (QRS <120 msec) and during pacing-induced LBBB. The total filtered QRS duration, RMS40 and LAS40 values during the baseline and pacing-induced LBBB were 153.0 msec, 11.8 μV, 69.0 msec, and 229 msec, 12.0 μV, 87.0 msec, respectively. LBBB aberration did not result in the loss of late potentials. Considerable fragmentation of the filtered QRS complex was characteristic of LBBB aberration. The stimulus artifact precedes the QRS complex and is evident in the lower left quadrant in the figure.

The SAECG in Spontaneous LBBB

Substantiation of the pacing data was provided by two patients who developed spontaneous LBBB, in the absence of any clinical event, and who underwent the same directional change in RMS40 and LAS40 produced during pacing-induced LBBB. The SAECG and 12-lead ECG of one of these patients (patient #29, Table IV), obtained during normal intraventricular conduction and during spontaneous LBBB, are shown in Figure 5. In the absence of LBBB, the SAECG does not reveal late potentials nor is there fragmentation of the signals in the terminal portion of the filtered QRS complex.

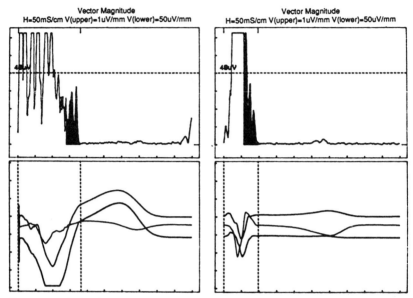

Figure 4. SAECGs from a patient without inducible VT or late potentials recorded during a surface QRS duration < 120 msec or pacing-induced LBBB are shown. The total filtered QRS duration, RMS40 and LAS40 values for the normal surface QRS duration recording and pacing-induced LBBB recording were 97.5 msec, 40.7 µV, 33 msec, and 181.5 msec, 19.0 µV, 76.5 msec, respectively. Although this patient did not have inducible VT, late potentials would be present if RMS40 ≤25 or 20 µV were considered abnormal. LBBB aberration revealed the characteristic fragmentation or increase in the number of terminal deflection seen in the latter part of the filtered QRS. The stimulus artifact precedes the QRS complex and is evident in the lower left quadrant in the figure.

During LBBB, a marked decrease in the RMS40 and prolongation of the LAS40 occurred. There was also obvious fragmentation of the signals in the terminal portion of the filtered QRS. When standard SAECG criteria for late potentials in patients without BBB were applied, late potentials were present. The RMS40 and LAS40 parameters changed from 110 to 21.5 µV and 12 to 43 msec, respectively, as a consequence of LBBB aberration. Figure 6 illustrates the SAECG of another patient who had late potentials during normal intraventricular conduction and continued to exhibit late potentials (using standard criteria) when spontaneous LBBB developed.

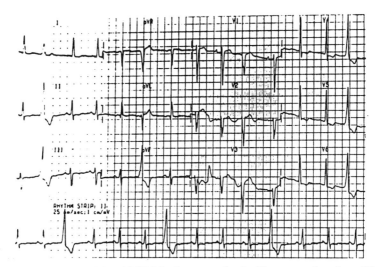

Figures 5A–D. The 12-lead SAECGs from a patient with a normal surface QRS duration and after the spontaneous development of LBBB are shown. Panel A reveals an ECG with a normal QRS duration.

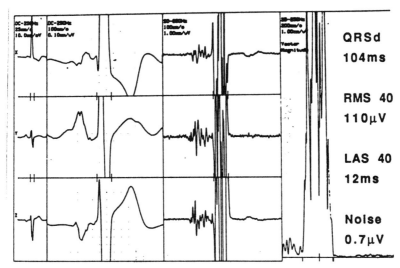

Figure 5B. The corresponding SAECG recording is shown in panel B. In panel B the total filtered QRS duration, RMS40, and LAS40 during normal conduction are 104 msec, 110 μV, and 12 msec.

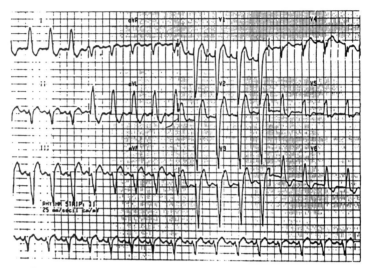

Figure 5C. Panel C reveals an ECG from the same patient during intrinsic LBBB.

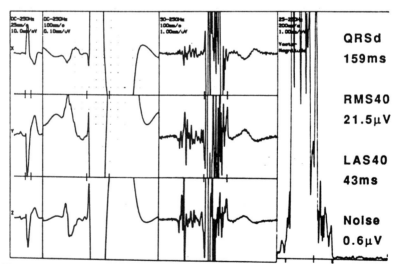

QRSd
159ms

RMS40
21.5μV

LAS40
43ms

Noise
0.6μV

Figure 5D. The corresponding SAECG recording is shown in panel D. During LBBB the total filtered QRS duration, RMS40, and LAS40 were 159 msec, 21.5 μV, and 43 msec. Although this patient did not have inducible sustained VT or late potentials during normal intraventricular conduction, late potentials were present during LBBB when standard RMS40 < 25μV or LAS 40 ≥ 38 msec criteria were used. The characteristic decrement in RMS40 and increment in LAS40 values were noted. These changes were similar to those seen during pacing-induced LBBB. Fragmentation of the filtered QRS complex associated with LBBB was also noted. QRSd = total filtered QRS duration.

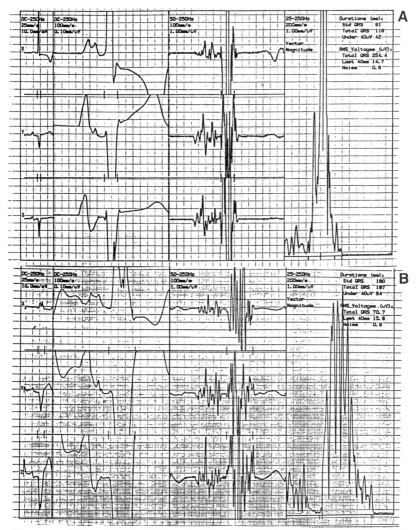

Figure 6. Signal-averaged electrocardiograms during a normal surface QRS duration (panel A) and spontaneous LBBB (panel B) in a patient with clinical nonsustained VT after a myocardial infarction are illustrated. Late potentials were present during normal conduction and intrinsic LBBB. The total filtered QRS duration, RMS40, and LAS40 values during normal conduction and spontaneous LBBB were 116 msec, 14.7 μV, 42 msec, and 187 msec, 15.8 μV, and 64 msec, respectively. The characteristic fragmentation of the signals in the terminal portions of the filtered QRS during LBBB is evident. Late potentials recorded during normal surface QRS duration were not affected by the development of LBBB aberration, as was noted in the pacing model of LBBB (Fig. 3). This patient, however, was not included in this study, since programmed ventricular stimulation was not performed. Both SAECG recordings were obtained within a few hours of each other.

SAECG Parameters in Patients with Intrinsic LBBB

The mean filtered QRS duration, RMS40 and LAS40 values for inducible and noninducible patients with intrinsic LBBB were 170 ± 28 msec, 16 ± 10 μV, 55 ± 24 msec, and 153 ± 18 msec, 25 ± 10 μV and 33 ± 16.9 msec, respectively. These differences achieved statistical significance (p < 0.04, < 0.009, and < 0.007, respectively; see Figure 7). Application of "standard" RMS40 (≤ 25 μV) and LAS40 (≥ 38 msec) criteria for late potentials revealed the presence of late potentials in 14 of 16 (88%) patients with inducible SMVT and in 19 of 32 (59%) patients without inducible SMVT (see Figure 8). The sensitivity, specificity, and positive and negative predictive values for inducible VT using these criteria were 88%, 41%, 42%, and 87% (for RMS40); and 88%, 59%, 52%, and 90% (for LAS40). The specificity of RMS40 and LAS40 in patients with intrinsic LBBB was reduced when compared with patients without BBB.

No significant difference was noted in the mean RMS40 and LAS40 values between inducible VT patients with intrinsic LBBB and those with a standard QRS duration. These data revealed marked similarities in RMS40 and LAS40 parameters in the inducible VT patients regardless of the presence of LBBB. In contrast, in patients who were noninducible, the difference in the mean RMS40 and LAS40 values between those with intrinsic LBBB and those with a standard QRS duration < 120 msec was statistically significant. This difference was similar to that observed in patients with a standard QRS duration < 120 msec and no inducible VT when the SAECGs during normal intraventricular conduction and pacing-induced LBBB were compared.

New SAECG Criteria For Patients With Intrinsic LBBB

In this study the objective was to derive SAECG parameters which would best discriminate patients with intrinsic LBBB with and without inducible SMVT. Pacing-induced LBBB provided information regarding directional and quantitative changes in SAECG parameters useful in separating patients with inducible from those without inducible SMVT when applied to those patients with intrinsic LBBB. The parameters sought were those that would at least provide similar sensitivity, specificity, and predictive accuracy as those noted in the study group devoid of LBBB.

The results of Chi square analysis of selected values for all three SAECG parameters, used singly and in combinations, which yielded a total predictive accuracy of 60% or better in patients with intrinsic LBBB are shown in Table VI. An RMS40 ≤ 17 μV provided the

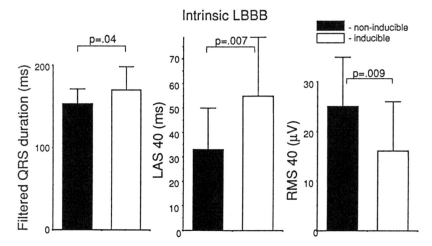

Figure 7. The mean total filtered QRS duration, RMS40 and LAS40 for all patients with intrinsic LBBB are shown. A statistically significant difference was noted for all three SAECG parameters between inducible and noninducible patients.

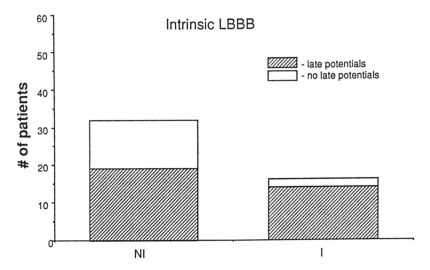

Figure 8. The incidence of late potentials in inducible and noninducible patients with intrinsic LBBB are shown. NI = noninducible; I = inducible. Of those patients who were inducible, 14 of 16 had late potentials whereas 19 of 32 patients without inducible VT had late potentials when standard criteria (RMS40 ≤ 25 µV or LAS40 ≥ 38 msec) were used. These criteria demonstrated low specificity and positive predictive value for inducible VT.

Table VI

Predictive Statistics of Selected SAECG Criteria for Late Potentials Applied to Patients with Intrinsic LBBB

SAECG Criteria	Sensitivity (%)	Specificity (%)	(+) Predictive Value (%)	(−) Predictive Value (%)	Total Predictive Value (%)	Chi Square P Value (Two Tailed)	Odds Ratio
RMS40 ≤20	87.5	59.3	51.8	90.4	69	0.005	10.2:1
RMS40 ≤17	68.7	81.2	64.7	83.8	77	0.001	9.5:1
RMS40 ≤15	56.2	84.3	64.2	79.4	75	0.005	6.9:1
RMS40 ≤12	43.7	96.8	87.5	77.5	79	0.001	24.0:1
LAS40 ≥38	87.5	59.3	51.8	90.4	69	0.005	10.2:1
LAS40 ≥40	81.2	62.5	52	86.9	69	0.01	7.2:1
LAS40 ≥45	68.7	75.0	57.8	82.7	73	0.009	6.6:1
LAS40 ≥50	56.2	90.6	75	80.5	79	0.0008	12.4:1
LAS40 ≥55	43.7	93.7	77.7	76.9	77	0.003	11.6:1
QRS ≥160	56.2	62.5	42.8	74.0	—	NS	—
QRS ≥170	50.0	78	53.3	75.7	—	NS	—
QRS ≥180	37.5	90.6	66.6	74.3	73	0.04	5.8:1

Table VI (Continued)

SAECG Criteria	Sensitivity (%)	Specificity (%)	(+) Predictive Value (%)	(−) Predictive Value (%)	Total Predictive Value (%)	Chi Square P Value (Two Tailed)	Odds Ratio
RMS40 ≤20 + LAS40 ≥38	87.5	46.8	45.1	88.2	60	0.04	6.1:1
RMS40 ≤20 + LAS40 ≥40	87.5	50	46.6	88.8	63	0.02	7.0:1
RMS40 ≤20 + LAS40 ≥45	87.5	53.1	48.2	89.4	65	0.01	7.9:1
RMS40 ≤20 + LAS40 ≥50 or 55	87.5	59.3	51.8	90.4	69	0.005	10.2:1
RMS40 ≤17 or ≤15 + LAS40 ≥38	87.5	59.3	51.8	90.4	69	0.005	10.2:1
RMS40 ≤17 or ≤15 + LAS40 ≥40	81.2	62.5	52	86.9	69	0.01	7.2:1
RMS40 ≤17 + LAS40 ≥45	68.7	68.7	52.3	81.4	69	0.03	4.8:1
RMS40 ≤17 + LAS40 ≥50	68.7	78.1	61.1	83.3	75	0.004	7.8:1
RMS40 ≤17 + LAS40 ≥55	68.7	81.2	64.7	83.8	77	0.001	9.5:1
RMS40 ≤15 + LAS40 ≥45	68.7	71.8	55	82.1	71	0.01	5.6:2
RMS40 ≤15 + LAS40 ≥50	62.5	81.2	62.5	81.2	75	0.006	7.2:1
RMS40 ≤15 + LAS40 ≥55	56.2	84.3	64.2	79.4	75	0.006	6.9:1

RMS40 ≤17 μV when used singly yielded the best overall statistical results. The combination of RMS40 ≤17 μV and LAS40 ≥55 msec yielded the best overall sensitivity and specificity and the highest total predictive accuracy among the various combinations. The total filtered QRS duration was not more useful alone or when combined with the other parameters. + = positive; − = negative. The units of QRS duration, RMS40, and LAS40 values are msec, μV, and msec, respectively. See text for details.

best overall sensitivity (69%) and specificity (81%) for this parameter and a total predictive accuracy of 77%. Although an RMS40 <12 μV provided a slightly higher total predictive value of 79%, it had a much lower sensitivity of 44%. In addition, an LAS40 ≥50 msec offered the highest total predictive accuracy (79%), but had a moderate sensitivity (56%). When the total filtered QRS duration between ≥120 msec and ≥180 msec was evaluated, only a filtered QRS duration ≥180 msec allowed separation of inducible from noninducible VT patients at a statistically significant level. This parameter had a high specificity (91%) but a low sensitivity (38%).

When combined RMS40 and LAS40 parameters were assessed an RMS40 ≤17 μV plus LAS40 ≥55 msec yielded the highest total predictive accuracy (77%) with the best overall sensitivity (69%) and specificity (81%). Thus the SAECG parameters that would appear to be clinically most useful are RMS40 ≤17 μV alone or in combination with LAS40 ≥55msec. The addition of filtered QRS duration >180 msec to those parameters did not improve the total predictive accuracy.

Study Conclusions

In this study, simulation of LBBB pattern with right ventricular apical pacing provided useful data regarding the qualitative and quantitative directional changes in SAECG parameters associated with this activation pattern. The justification for the implementation of this pacing model was based on data derived from studies of left ventricular activation in normal conduction and in the presence of LBBB.[32] Endocardial and epicardial mapping studies of patients with intrinsic LBBB have revealed that LBBB aberration is generally associated with early activation of the right ventricle preceded by right to left septal activation and followed by left ventricular activation.[33,34] The inferoposterior and posterobasal regions of the left ventricle are generally the latest sites activated. Vassallo et al performed endocardial catheter mapping during right ventricular pacing in 40 patients in order to study left ventricular activation and the influence of the site of infarction on the activation sequence.[32] They concluded that right ventricular pacing yielded activation patterns similar to those observed during intrinsic LBBB and that the left ventricular activation patterns and conduction times were influenced by the site of previous infarction.

Pacing-induced LBBB showed that the conduction abnormality is usually associated with a decrease of RMS40 and an increase of LAS40 of the SAECG. These changes explain the high incidence of false-positive late potentials when the standard criteria utilized in the absence of a BBB (i.e., RMS40 $\leq 25 \mu V$ and LAS40 ≥ 38 msec) are employed. Interestingly enough applying the standard criteria did not result in a significant change in the incidence of false-negative results. The directional changes in the SAECG illustrated during pacing-induced LBBB were corroborated by the observations in patients who developed spontaneous LBBB (Figures 5 and 6).

Among the 39 patients in the present study with a standard QRS duration < 120 msec, late potentials were present in 17 of 23 patients with inducible SMVT. The sensitivity, specificity, and total predictive accuracy of the combined SAECG parameters for inducible sustained VT were 74%, 88%, and 79%, respectively. When the standard criteria were applied to the SAECG during pacing-induced LBBB, they produced the same incidence of late potentials among inducible patients (74%) but resulted in a decrease to 63% of the positive predictive value among noninducible patients. When these same SAECG parameters were applied to 48 patients with intrinsic LBBB, a 59% false-positive incidence of late potentials was noted. Thus, although RMS40 ($\leq 25 \mu V$) and LAS40 (≥ 38 msec) parameters yielded acceptable sensitivity, specificity, and total predictive accuracy in patients with a standard QRS duration < 120 msec; these values were less than optimal when applied to patients with pacing-induced or intrinsic LBBB.

Comparison With Previous Studies

Previous studies have proffered opposing views regarding the utility of the SAECG in the presence of LBBB. Gomes et al performed SAECG and programmed ventricular stimulation in patients with either RBBB or LBBB and found no significant difference in SAECG parameters between those with and without VT regardless of the pattern of BBB or filter setting.[29] They concluded that patients with BBB should probably be excluded from studies assessing the role of the SAECG in predicting arrhythmic events. However, the study was a preliminary report and the small sample size of the study population was a significant limitation.

In another study, Nalos et al prospectively evaluated 12 patients with LBBB, 7 of whom had inducible VT.[11] Although the authors did not specifically differentiate patients with RBBB or LBBB, they reported that the number of terminal deflections and the QRS duration ≤ 20 μV could be used to differentiate those with VT from those without (p <0.001). However, it is not clear whether patients with RBBB or LBBB could be grouped together in view of the obvious difference in conduction patterns and its potential influence on the SAECG.

Kindwall et al studied 37 patients with LBBB patterns of which 24 had inducible VT and 13 did not.[27] Applying an RMS40 value of <30 μV as abnormal, they were able to distinguish the two groups with a sensitivity, specificity, and positive predictive value of 79%, 61%, and 79%, respectively. The authors, however, made no specific recommendation for SAECG criteria in patients with LBBB.

In a larger study, Buckingham et al evaluated the effects of conduction defects on the SAECG and the ability of the SAECG to identify patients at risk for VT.[28] Among the total number of patients evaluated were 79 patients with BBB. Seven of 47 patients with BBB and 14 of 32 patients with LBBB had VT. Their recording technique and analysis appeared comparable to that used in the present study with the exception of their usage of a 40-Hz high-pass filter setting as compared to 25 Hz. The authors found that the SAECG in the presence of a BBB is characterized by longer duration of the filtered QRS and LAS40 as well as a lower RMS40. The presence of LBBB in patients without VT was associated with an increase in the duration of the filtered QRS and a decrease in RMS40, which was similar to changes seen in patients with VT and normal conduction. Their findings are concordant with the data presented in this study. They also described an increase in fragmentation of signals and in the number of terminal deflections in patients with LBBB, similar to the findings in the present study. However, the authors did not specify SAECG values that define late potentials in patients with BBB. Although they recognized that differences between RBBB and LBBB in the SAECG may exist, they chose to analyze the two conduction disorders jointly and suggested that uniform criteria may be applicable to both. A difference between their results and ours is expected, since they utilized different high-pass filter settings. This may be due to an attenuation or loss of voltage in the total filtered QRS and RMS40 associated with the use of high-pass filter settings above 25 Hz.[35,36]

The SAECG in Patients with RBBB

Although only a few studies have analyzed the role of the SAECG in predicting the risk of spontaneous and inducible SMVT in patients with BBB, these studies have not separated patients with RBBB from those with LBBB in their analysis.[11,28,29] The sequence of ventricular activation is markedly different in these two conduction defects and hence the results of the SAECG may be markedly different. In this chapter we present data from our preliminary investigation of the SAECG in patients with RBBB and compare these data with those from patients with LBBB. The objectives of this study were to determine: (1) whether a difference in SAECG parameters exists between patients with RBBB or LBBB; and (2) whether the SAECG in patients with RBBB would be predictive of inducible sustained VT.

Study Patients

Eighteen patients who met standard electrocardiographic criteria for RBBB and had either nonsustained or sustained VT underwent time-domain SAECG and programmed ventricular stimulation according to the previously described protocol. The mean age of the patients with RBBB was 71 ±7 years. Coronary heart disease was present in 15 of 18 patients and hypertensive heart disease in the remaining 3 patients. Nonsustained VT was present in 14 patients, and sustained VT was present in 4. No patient had clinical ventricular fibrillation. Data are expressed as a mean ± the standard deviation. Comparison of SAECG parameters between patients with RBBB who were inducible and those who were noninducible was performed using the Student's t-test.

Results

The clinical characteristics of the study group are shown in Table VII. Seven of the 18 patients with RBBB had inducible SMVT. All patients with spontaneous SMVT had inducible SMVT requiring pharmacologic therapy. The mean total filtered QRS duration,

Table VII
Clinical Characteristics of Patients With RBBB and VT

Pt	Age	Dx	Arrhythmia	PVS	EF (%)	QRS (msec)	LAS40 (msec)	RMS40 (µV)
1	69	ASHD	VT-S	IN	25	173	18	151.4
2	71	ASHD	VT-S	IN	30	176	15	41.9
3	67	ASHD	VT-NS	IN	37	157.5	43.5	14.4
4	79	ASHD	VT-S	IN	20	162	22	100.4
5	81	ASHD	VT-NS	IN	25	184	46	20
6	61	ASHD	VT-NS	IN	20	183	29	28
7	66	ASHD	VT-S	IN	15	160	25	107
8	76	ASHD	VT-NS	Non-IN	45	153	26	28
9	71	ASHD	VT-NS	Non-IN	45	174	20	41.4
10	69	ASHD	VT-NS	Non-IN	30	135	27	31.7
11	60	ASHD	VT-NS	Non-IN	60	124	22	69.4
12	82	HTN	VT-NS	Non-IN	40	125	12	123.2
13	73	ASHD	VT-NS	Non-IN	15	150	15	72.9
14	69	ASHD	VT-NS	Non-IN	32	134	21	51
15	77	HTN	VT-NS	Non-IN	50	134	21	93
16	77	HTN	VT-NS	Non-IN	57	137	36	30
17	63	ASHD	VT-NS	Non-IN	50	159	21	73
18	69	ASHD	VT-NS	Non-IN	42	132	21	80

SAECG parameters and results of programmed ventricular stimulation (PVS) are shown. ASHD = atherosclerotic heart disease; Dx = diagnosis; EF = ejection fraction; HTN = hypertension; IN = inducible; NS = nonsustained; S = sustained.

RMS40 and LAS40 values in RBBB patients with and without inducible SMVT were 171 $\pm$ 11 msec, 65 $\pm$ 53 µV, 28 $\pm$ 12 msec, and 142 $\pm$ 16 msec, 63 $\pm$ 30 µV, 22 $\pm$ 6 msec, respectively. SAECG parameters for RBBB patients with inducible and noninducible SMVT are shown in the bar graphs in the right panels in Figures 9–11. The difference between RMS40 or LAS40 in inducible and noninducible patients was not statistically significant. In patients with RBBB, only the difference between the total QRS duration appeared useful in separating those with inducible VT from those without. Figure 12 illustrates a patient with spontaneous and inducible SMVT who showed late potentials in the SAECG during normal intraventricular conduction. The late potentials disappeared when the patient developed RBBB in the absence of a new clinical event. This demonstrates the

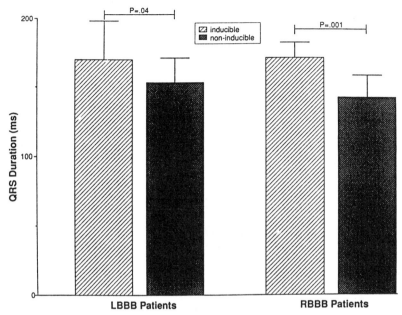

Figure 9. Comparison of the total filtered QRS duration in patients with LBBB (left panel) or RBBB (right panel) with or without inducible sustained monomorphic VT. See text for details.

propensity for masking late potentials with a high amplitude signal, which corresponds with late right ventricular activation in the presence of RBBB.

In LBBB patients the mean total filtered QRS duration, RMS40 or LAS40 values in inducible and noninducible patients were 170 ± 28 msec, 16 ± 10 µV, 54 ± 24 msec, and 153 ± 18 msec, 25 ± 10 µV, 32 ± 16 msec, respectively. (The left panels in Figures 9–11.) In contrast to patients with RBBB, the difference between each of the three SAECG parameters in inducible and noninducible patients with LBBB was statistically significant. Quantitatively, the SAECG in patients with LBBB reveals a lower mean RMS40 and longer mean LAS40 when compared with the inducible and noninducible counterpart with RBBB. Conversely, patients with RBBB tend to have larger terminal deflections and thus a higher RMS40 value as well as a lower RMS (QRS) to RMS40 ratio than those with LBBB. Consequently, LAS40 tends to be shorter in patients with RBBB than in those with LBBB.

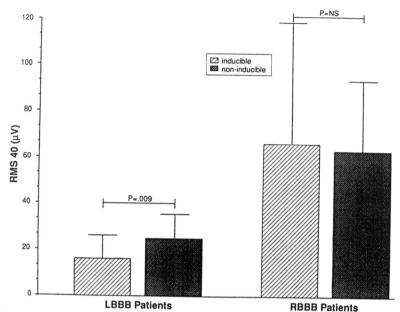

Figure 10. Comparison of the root mean square voltage of the last 40 msec of the filtered QRS (RMS40) in patients with LBBB (left panel) and RBBB (right panel) with or without inducible sustained monomorphic VT. See text for details.

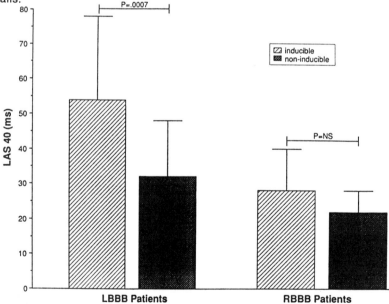

Figure 11. Comparison of the duration of low amplitude signals <40 µv (LAS40) in patients with LBBB (left panel) and RBBB (right panel) with or without inducible sustained monomorphic VT. See text for details.

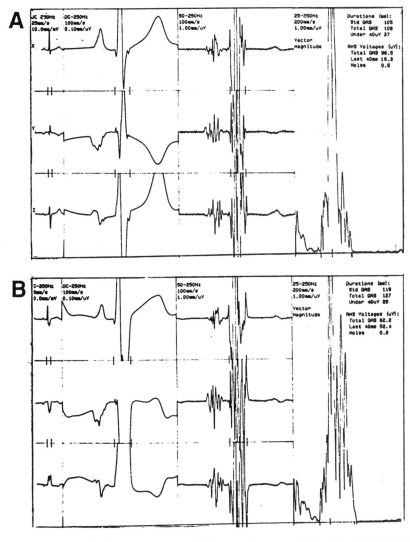

Figure 12. SAECGs during normal QRS duration (panel A) and spontaneous RBBB (panel B) in a patient with spontaneous and induced sustained monomorphic VT are shown. The total filtered QRS duration, RMS40, and LAS40 values during normal conduction and spontaneous RBBB were 108 msec, 16.3 µV, 37 msec, and 127 msec, 52.4 µV, 29 msec, respectively. Note that late potentials were present during normal conduction and disappeared during RBBB.

Summary and Conclusions

Few studies, including our own, have suggested that time-domain analysis can be reliable in patients with LBBB provided that the appropriate adjustment in criteria for abnormality is undertaken. On the other hand, the presence of a RBBB on the surface ECG appears to present a significant limitation to this method of SAECG analysis. It is apparent from the data presented in this chapter that the delayed left ventricular activation associated with LBBB does not preclude accurate delineation of inducible SMVT patients from those who are noninducible based upon SAECG parameter. However, in patients with RBBB, RMS40 or LAS40 could not be utilized to distinguish those patients with inducible SMVT from those who are not inducible. Spectral analysis of the SAECG has been been utilized to improve the predictive accuracy of the technique in patients with BBB. [37-40] Currently, there is no standardized methodology or acceptable criteria for abnormality. These techniques, however, may prove to be more useful than time-domain analysis of the SAECG in patients with BBB.

Acknowledgments: We would like to thank Matthew Avitable, Ph.D. of the Biostatistics Department and Mrs. Theresa Luppowitz, Medical Secretary, for their assistance in the preparation of this manuscript. This study was supported in part by the National Institutes of Health Grant HL 31341 and Veterans Administration Medical Research Funds.

References

1. Simson MB: Use of signals in the terminal QRS complex to identify patients with ventricular tachycardia after myocardial infarction. Circulation 64:235, 1981.
2. Denes P, Santarelli P, Hauser RG, Uretz EF: Quantitative analysis of the high frequency components of the terminal portion of the body surface QRS in normal subjects and in patients with ventricular tachycardia. Circulation 67:1129, 1983.
3. Breithardt G, Borggrefe M, Karbenn U, Abendroth RR, Yeh HL, Seipel L: Prevalence of late potentials in patients with and without ventricular tachycardia: correlation with angiographic findings. Am J Cardiol 49: 1932, 1982.
4. Uther JB, Dennett CJ, Tan A: The detection of delayed activation signals of low amplitude in the vectorcardiogram of patients with recurrent ventricular tachycardia by signal averaging. In Sandoe E, Julian DG,

Bell JW (eds): Management of Ventricular Tachycardia–Role of Mexiletine. Amsterdam: Excerpta Medica, 1978, p80.

5. Rozanski JJ, Mortara D, Myerburg RJ, Castellanos A: Body surface detection of delayed depolarizations in patients with recurrent ventricular tachycardia and left ventricular aneurysm. Circulation 63:1172, 1981.

6. Kanovsky MS, Falcone R, Dresden CA, Josephson ME, Simpson MB: Identification of patients with ventricular tachycardia after myocardial infarction: signal-averaged electrocardiogram, Holter monitoring, and cardiac catheterization. Circulation 70:264, 1984.

7. Gomes JAC, Mehra R, Barreca P, El-Sherif N, Hariman R, Holtzman R: Quantitative analysis of the high frequency components of the signal averaged QRS complex in patients with acute myocardial infarction: a prospective study. Circulation 72:105, 1985.

8. Hombach V, Braun V, Hopp HW, et al: The applicability of the signal averaging technique in clinical cardiology. Clin Cardiol 5:107, 1982.

9. Breithardt G, Borggrefe M, Karbenn QU, Seipel L: Ventricular vulnerability assessed by programmed ventricular stimulation in patients with and without late potentials. Circulation 68:275, 1983.

10. Buxton AE, Simson MS, Falcone RA, Marchlinski FE, Doherty JU, Josephson ME: Results of signal-averaged electrocardiography and electrophysiologic study in patients with nonsustained ventricular tachycardia after healing of acute myocardial infarction. Am J Cardiol 60:80, 1987.

11. Nalos PC, Gang ES, Mandel WJ, Ladenheim ML, Lass Y, Peter T: The signal-averaged electrocardiogram as a screening test for inducibility of sustained ventricular tachycardia in high risk patients: a prospective study. J Am Coll Cardiol 9:539, 1987.

12. Turitto G, Fontaine J, Ursell S, Caref EB, Henkin R, El-Sherif N: Value of the signal averaged electrocardiogram as a predictor of programmed stimulation in nonsustained ventricular tachycardia. Am J Cardiol 61:-1272, 1988.

13. Fontaine JM, Turitto G, El-Sherif N: Prognostic significance of ambulatory electrocardiographic monitoring, programmed electrical stimulation and signal averaging in patients with complex ventricular arrhythmias. J Electrophysiol 1:204, 1987.

14. Denniss AR, Richards DA, Cody DV, Russell PA, Young AA, Cooper MJ, Ross DL, Uther JB: Prognostic significance of ventricular tachycardia and fibrillation induced at programmed stimulation and delayed potentials detected on the signal averaged electrocardiograms of survivors of acute myocardial infarction. Circulation 74:731, 1986.

15. Winters S, Stewart D, Targonski A, Gomes JA: Role of signal averaging of the surface QRS complex in selecting patients with nonsustained ventricular tachycardia and high grade ventricular arrhythmias for programmed ventricular stimulation. J Am Coll Cardiol 12:1481, 1988.

16. Gomes JA, Winters SL, Martinson M, Machac J, Stewart D, Targonski A: The prognostic significance of quantitative signal-averaged variables relative to clinical variables, site of myocardial infarction, ejection fraction and ventricular premature beats: a prospective study. J Am Coll Cardiol 13:377, 1989.

17. Turitto G, Fontaine JM, Ursell S, Caref EB, Bekheit S, El-Sherif N: Risk stratification and management of patients with organic heart disease and nonsustained ventricular tachycardia: role of programmed stimulation, left ventricular ejection fraction, and the signal-averaged electrocardiogram. Am J Med 88:1–35N, 1990.
18. El-Sherif N, Scherlag BJ, Lazzara R: Electrode catheter recordings during malignant ventricular arrhythmias following experimental acute myocardial ischemia. Circulation 51:1003, 1975.
19. El-Sherif N, Hope RR, Scherlag BJ, Lazzara R: Reentrant ventricular arrhythmias in the late myocardial infarction period. II. Patterns of initiation and termination of reentry. Circulation 55:702, 1977.
20. Waldo AL, Kaiser GA: A study of ventricular arrhythmias associated with myocardial infarction in the canine heart. Circulation 47:1222, 1973.
21. Boineau JP, Cox JL: Slow ventricular activation in acute myocardial infarction. A source of reentrant premature ventricular contractions. Circulation 48:702, 1973.
22. Mehra R, Zeiler RH, Gough WB, El-Sherif N: Reentrant ventricular arrhythmias in the late myocardial infarction period. 9. Electrophysiologic anatomical correlation of reentrant circuits. Circulation 67:11, 1983.
23. Simson MB, Untereker WJ, Spielman SR, Horowitz LN, Marcus NH, Falcone RA, Harken AH, Josephson ME: Relation between late potentials on the body surface and directly recorded fragmented electrograms in patients with ventricular tachycardia. Am J Cardiol 51:105, 1983.
24. El-Sherif N, Gomes, JAC, Restivo M, Mehra R: Late potentials and arrhythmogenesis. PACE 8:440, 1985.
25. Fontaine J, Henkin R, Howard M, El-Sherif N: Establishing criteria for the presence of late potentials in patients with left bundle branch block (abstr). PACE 10:75, 1987.
26. Fontaine JM, Henkin R, Howard M, Turitto G, Ursell S, El-Sherif N: New signal averaging criteria for determining the presence of late potentials in patients with left bundle branch block (abstr). PACE 10:451, 1987.
27. Kindwall KE, Auletto R, Falcone R, et al: Abnormalities in the signal averaged electrocardiogram in patients with ventricular tachycardia and left bundle branch block (abstr). J Am Coll Cardiol 7:103, 1986.
28. Buckingham TA, Thessen CC, Stevens LL, Redd RM, Kennedy HL: Effect of conduction defects on the signal averaged electrocardiographic determination of late potentials. Am J Cardiol 61:1265, 1988.
29. Gomes JAC, Stewart D, Winters SL, Barreca P: The signal averaged electrocardiogram in patients with ventricular tachycardia and bundle branch block (abstr). J Am Coll Cardiol 9:208A, 1987.
30. Kelen G, Henkin R, Fontaine JM, El-Sherif N: Effects of analyzed signal duration and phase on the results of Fast Fourier Transform analysis of the surface electrocardiogram in subjects with and without late potentials. Am J Cardiol 60:1282, 1987.
31. Henkin R, Caref EB, Kelen G, El-Sherif N: The signal-averaged elec-

trocardiogram and late potentials. A comparative analysis of commercial devices. J Electrocardiol 22(Suppl):19, 1990.

32. Vassallo JA, Cassidy DM, Miller JM, Buxton AE, Marchlinski FE, Josephson ME: Left ventricular endocardial activation during right ventricular pacing: effect of underlying heart disease. J Am Coll Cardiol 7:1228, 1986.

33. Vassallo JA, Cassidy DM, Marchlinski FE, Buxton AE, Waxman HL, Doherty JU, Josephson ME: Endocardial activation of left bundle branch block. Circulation 69:914, 1984.

34. Wyndham CRC, Smith T, Meeran MK, Mammana R, Levitsky S, Rosen KM: Epicardial activation in patients with left bundle branch block. Circulation 61:696, 1980.

35. Gomes JA, Winters JL, Stewart D, Targonski A, Barreca P: Optimal bandpass filters for time domain analysis of the signal-averaged electrocardiogram. Am J Cardiol 60:1290, 1987.

36. Caref EB, Turitto G, Ibrahim BB, Henkin R, El-Sherif N: Role of bandpass filters in optimizing the value of the signal-averaged electrocardiogram as a predictor of the results of programmed stimulation. Am J Cardiol 64:16, 1989.

37. Cain ME, Ambos D, Witkowski FX, Sobel BE: Fast-Fourier transform analysis of signal averaged electrocardiograms for identification of patients prone to sustained ventricular tachycardia. Circulation 69:711, 1984.

38. Cain ME, Ambos HD, Markham J, Fischer AE, Sobel BE: Quantification of differences in frequency content of signal-averaged electrocardiograms in patients with compared to those without sustained ventricular tachycardia. Am J Cardiol 55:1500, 1985.

39. Lindsay BD, Ambos HD, Schectman KB, Cain ME: Improved selection of patients for programmed ventricular stimulation by frequency analysis of signal-averaged electrocardiograms. Circulation 73:675, 1986.

40. Haberl R, Jilge G, Steinbeck G: Multisegment frequency analysis of the electrocardiogram with Fourier transform for identification of patients with sustained ventricular tachycardia (abstr). Circulation 78:II-302, 1988.

26

Antiarrhythmic Drug Therapy and the Signal-Averaged Electrocardiogram

Jonathan S. Steinberg,
Roger A. Freedman,
J. Thomas Bigger, Jr, and the ESVEM
Investigators*

Introduction

The signal-averaged electrocardiogram (ECG) is more sensitive than the standard ECG for detecting low amplitude potentials[1] and may be a more accurate measure of the duration of ventricular activation. When recorded with the signal-averaged ECG, the QRS will include the terminal low amplitude signals that are presumed to arise from delayed depolarization of damaged segments of the ventricular myocardium. Prolonged low amplitude signals in the terminal portion of the QRS on the signal-averaged ECG have been termed "late potentials." The presence of ventricular late potentials

*Please see Appendix p. 587.
From El-Sherif N, Turitto G (eds): *High-Resolution Electrocardiography*. Mount Kisco, NY, Futura Publishing Co., Inc., ©, 1992.

has been associated with increased risk of ventricular tachyarrhythmias in post-myocardial infarction populations[2,3] and greater likelihood for induced ventricular tachycardia (VT) in patients with unexplained syncope[4] or unsustained VT.[5]

Antiarrhythmic agents with Class I action decrease the rate of rise of the action potential and retard conduction velocity, which may be their mechanism of action particularly for reentrant arrhythmias.[6] Many antiarrhythmic drugs increase or prolong tissue refractoriness and thus modify the electrophysiologic properties necessary for reentrant arrhythmias.[7] The signal-averaged ECG may be especially well suited to assess changes in the ventricular activation process mediated by pharmacologic intervention, especially if conduction is slowed, because of its sensitivity for detecting low amplitude potentials and the ability to measure activation of damaged ventricular myocardium.

We evaluated antiarrhythmic drug effects on the signal-averaged ECG in a group of patients who were undergoing serial drug testing for sustained ventricular tachyarrhythmias. We had the following aims: (1) to determine whether antiarrhythmic drugs prolong or shorten depolarization as measured by the signal-averaged ECG in the time domain and if so, whether these changes are antiarrhythmic class specific; and (2) to examine whether the baseline signal-averaged ECG or changes during drug therapy predict the outcome of drug testing.

Methods

Study Population

Patients who had experienced sustained ventricular tachyarrhythmias and were undergoing serial antiarrhythmic drug testing as part of the Electrophysiologic Study versus Electrocardiographic Monitoring study (ESVEM) at three participating institutions (Columbia-Presbyterian Medical Center, University of Oklahoma Health Sciences Center, University of Utah Medical Center) were eligible for this study. ESVEM is sponsored by the National Institutes of Health and is currently in progress. It is designed to compare the predictive accuracy, efficiency, and cost of electrophysiologic study with continuous ECG monitoring and stress testing for predicting arrhythmic event-free survival in three groups of patients: (1) patients with documented sustained VT; (2) survivors of cardiac arrest; and (3) patients with unexplained syncope who have sustained VT induced at electrophysiologic study. The clinical characteristics of the 31 patients who participated in this signal-averaged ECG substudy are shown in Table I.

Table I
Clinical Characteristics of Study Subjects

Gender	
Male	23(74%)
Female	8(26%)
Age (years)	61 ±8
Structural Heart Disease	
Coronary heart disease	24(77%)
Idiopathic dilated cardiomyopathy	3(10%)
Hypertensive cardiomyopathy	2(6%)
None	2(6%)
*Left Ventricular Ejection Fraction**	0.31 ±0.08
Presenting Arrhythmic Event	
Sustained VT	21(68%)
VF	5(16%)
Syncope	3(10%)
Aborted sudden death	2(6%)
Baseline Electrophysiologic Study	
Inducible sustained VT	28(90%)
Inducible VF	3(10%)
Cycle length of arrhythmia (msec)	268 ±68
Number of extrastimuli	2.1 ±0.6
Baseline 48-Hour ECG	
Ventricular premature depolarizations/hour	279 ±408
Ventricular couplets/hour	14 ±40
VT runs/hour	4.6 ±19.3

ECG = electrocardiogram; VT = ventricular tachycardia; VF = ventricular fibrillation; *in 28 subjects only.

Study Design

Details of the ESVEM protocol have been previously published.[8] Briefly, patients with sustained VT, after cardiac arrest or with syncope, who had sustained VT induced at a drug-free electrophysiologic study and who had an average of > 10 ventricular premature complexes (VPCs)/hour during 48-hour continuous ECG recording were eligible for participation in the trial. Patients were randomized to one of two evaluation arms; one arm utilized serial electrophysiologic studies and the other arm utilized serial continuous ECG recordings. Antiarrhythmic drug treatment consisted of a random sequence of up to six drugs. Dose titration was continued until target doses or trough plasma concentrations of individual drugs were achieved. Therapeutic efficacy by electrophysiologic study was defined as noninducibility of sustained VT, and by ECG monitoring, as 70% reduction of VPCs, 80% reduction of ventricular couplets, 90% reduction of VT runs on ambulatory ECG, and abolition of VT runs > 15 beats on both ambulatory ECG and treadmill testing. If the evaluation predicted the drug would be ineffective, the patient was randomized to the next drug. The process was repeated until an effective drug was found. If an effective drug was identified, and tolerated, the patient was discharged. The antiarrhythmic agents used in this study represented four classes of action: IA (imipramine, procainamide, quinidine); IB (mexiletine); IC (propafenone); and III (sotalol). For the purposes of this substudy, the antiarrhythmic drugs will be so classified, although they could instead be grouped according to their 12-lead ECG effects, e.g., QRS prolongation, QTc prolongation, etc.

Patients in the electrophysiologic study limb also had 24-hour continuous ECG recording while receiving their first and last drugs. The results of these recordings were not available to ESVEM investigators, nor were they used for determination of drug efficacy. The results of these recordings were made available for this substudy to increase the endpoints available for analysis.

Within 24 hours of therapeutic assessment by the assigned method, during drug steady state, a signal-averaged ECG was performed for 83 drug trials. We also analyzed a standard 12-lead ECG, which was recorded during drug steady state in 56 drug trials.

Signal-Averaged Electrocardiography

The signal-averaged ECGs were recorded with the Corazonix Predictor system (Oklahoma City, OK) or the Arrhythmia Research Technology Model 1200 EPX (Austin, TX). The subject's skin was cleansed with alcohol pads and abraded with gauze. An orthogonal lead arrangement was used. Three electrode pairs were placed in the following locations: (1) X, at the fourth intercostal space in both midaxillary lines; (2) Y, in the midclavicular line, just inferior to the clavicle and to the left of the umbilicus; and (3) Z, in the fourth intercostal space, to the left of the sternum and to the left of the vertebral column. Positive electrodes were left, inferior, and anterior. The electrodes used throughout the study were silver-silver chloride. The QRS signal was amplified with a gain of 1000, 2000, or 5000 without saturating the analog/digital converter. The signal was digitized at a frequency of 2000 samples/sec with 16-bit accuracy. This system utilizes a cross correlation program to select QRSs for averaging; a template was selected by the operator and QRS complexes that did not match the template with a 99% correlation coefficient were rejected automatically. With this feature, QRS complexes were accurately aligned (± 2.5 msec jitter). From 200 to 600 complexes were acquired to ensure a low-noise recording, preferably ≤ 0.3 μV.[9]

A bidirectional filter with a bandpass cut-off of 40–300 Hz was applied to the three bipolar leads. The filtered QRS complexes of the three bipolar leads were combined into a vector magnitude[10] by the formula $\sqrt{(X^2 + Y^2 + Z^2)}$. The result was amplified to improve visualization of the low amplitude components. The QRS onset and offset were calculated automatically by a computer algorithm when the voltage exceeded the mean of the baseline by 3 standard deviations. The end of the QRS was detected as an increment in voltage relative to baseline, scanning backward from the end of the sampling window toward the QRS. The beginning of the QRS was similarly detected by scanning in a forward direction.

Three signal-averaged ECG variables were calculated for each study: (1) the total duration of the filtered QRS vector magnitude, fQRS; (2) the root mean square voltage of the terminal 40 msec of the vector complex, V40; and (3) the low amplitude signal duration <40 μV in the terminal portion of the vector complex, LAS. The fQRS was considered prolonged if it was >120 msec. Late potentials were considered present if the V40 was <20 μV or the LAS was ≥39 msec.

The percent change of signal-averaged ECG variables on drug as compared to baseline was expressed as ΔfQRS, ΔV40, and ΔLAS, and defined as ([baseline value-drug value]/baseline value) × 100.

The QRS duration on the 12-lead standard ECG was defined as the longest manually measured value from beats of supraventricular origin in the limb leads. ΔQRS was defined in an identical fashion to the signal-averaged ECG values.

Statistical Analysis

Data are expressed as mean ±1 SD. Analysis was performed using the Student t-test for paired and unpaired data. A p value <0.05 was deemed statistically significant.

Results

Results of the Drug–Free Signal-Averaged ECG Study

There were 31 study subjects and 28 (90%) met the criteria for the presence of late potentials. The fQRS measured 133 ±22 msec, the V40 11 ±12 μV, and the LAS 56 ±21 msec in the 31 subjects. The fQRS was abnormal in 21/31 patients (68%); the V40 was abnormal in 19/31 patients (61%); the LAS was abnormal in 25/31 patients (81%). Only 2/31 patients (6%) had normal values for all three measurements.

Results of the Signal-Averaged ECG During Antiarrhythmic Drug Therapy

The number of trials, the method of assessment, the mean dose for each drug, and the mean plasma concentration of each drug are shown in Table II. Some drugs were evaluated by electrophysiologic

Table II
Antiarrhythmic Drug Therapy

	Number of Patients	Daily Dose (mg)	Plasma Drug Concentration (µg/mL)	Number of Drug Trials	
				EPS	24-hour ECG
Imipramine	13	261 ±125	0.21 ±0.07*	10	10
Procainamide	9	5444 ±1424	8.1 ±1.9	8	3
Quinidine	7	2368 ±928	3.3 ±1.1	5	2
Mexiletine	10	960 ±190	1.3 ±0.4	8	4
Propafenone	10	982 ±311	0.94 ±0.70	7	3
Sotalol	17	456 ±119	2.0 ±0.7	12	11

EPS = Electrophysiologic study; *sum of imipramine and desipramine levels.

study and continuous ECG methods, and these results will be treated as separate drug trials. There were a total of 66 drug trials, and each patient had 1–6 drug trials (mean = 2.1).

Table III contains the signal-averaged ECG results for each antiarrhythmic drug. The fQRS was significantly prolonged by antiarrhythmic drug therapy with quinidine, procainamide, imipramine, and propafenone. Drug therapy with mexiletine and sotalol did not result in fQRS prolongation. The most marked QRS change from baseline was seen during propafenone treatment, a 20% increase. Moderate prolongation was observed for each drug with IA action (12% for quinidine, 10% for procainamide, 8% for imipramine).

No drug caused a statistically significant change in V40, but propafenone resulted in a fall in V40 of borderline statistical significance (p = 0.06). The LAS lengthened modestly after procainamide and imipramine (15% and 13%, respectively), but markedly after propafenone (60%). Only propafenone caused a statistically significant (p <0.005) increase in LAS.

The prolongation of the fQRS that was observed in the imipramine, procainamide, propafenone, and quinidine trials was often predominantly accounted for by the change in LAS, however there was significant variability of this relationship. By specific drug, the most consistent relationship of ΔLAS and ΔfQRS was observed in the propafenone trials. The average contribution of ΔLAS to ΔfQRS

Table III
Signal-Averaged ECG Results During Steady State Antiarrhythmic Drug Therapy

	fQRS (msec)		V40 (µV)		LAS (msec)		ΔfQRS (%)	ΔV40 (%)	ΔLAS (%)
	B	D	B	D	B	D			
Imipramine (n = 13)	132 ± 18	142 ± 20*	10 ± 6	10 ± 7	52 ± 19	59 ± 21	8 ± 9	18 ± 99	15 ± 27
Procainamide (n = 9)	132 ± 27	145 ± 31*	15 ± 18	10 ± 7	58 ± 24	65 ± 28	10 ± 9	−3 ± 39	13 ± 15
Quinidine (n = 7)	130 ± 25	146 ± 26†	15 ± 21	14 ± 20	56 ± 22	64 ± 29	12 ± 5	−4 ± 39	13 ± 25
Mexiletine (n = 10)	130 ± 16	134 ± 19	8 ± 5	8 ± 5	56 ± 13	60 ± 14	3 ± 7	7 ± 50	8 ± 16
Propafenone (10)	126 ± 19	150 ± 20§	13 ± 12	8 ± 7	52 ± 24	71 ± 22†	20 ± 11	−31 ± 31	60 ± 83
Sotalol (n = 17)	136 ± 17	136 ± 16	9 ± 6	10 ± 7	59 ± 23	60 ± 16	−0.6 ± 8	29 ± 75	10 ± 41

B = drug-free baseline; D = during drug therapy; fQRS = total duration of the filtered QRS vector magnitude; LAS = low amplitude signal duration (<40 µV) in the terminal portion of the vector complex; V40 = root mean square voltage of the terminal 40 msec of the vector complex; *p <0.01; †p <0.005; §p <0.0005 versus control studies.

(expressed as the ratio of ΔLAS/ΔfQRS) was 0.9 $\pm$ 0.7 for the propafenone trials.

The conventional ECG also was analyzed for QRS changes during drug therapy in 56 drug trials. Procainamide and propafenone elicited significant QRS prolongation, 9% and 15%, respectively. Quinidine, imipramine, mexiletine, and sotalol did not. The change in QRS on the standard ECG was moderately correlated with the change in the fQRS on the signal-averaged ECG ($r = 0.61$, $p < 0.001$).

Prediction of Efficacy by Baseline Signal-Averaged ECG

There were 50 drug trials assessed by the electrophysiologic study approach. Of these 50 trials, 7 (14%) were effective and 43 (86%) were ineffective by the study definitions. There were 45 drug trials in patients who had late potentials in their baseline recording of which 7 (16%) were effective and 38 (84%) were ineffective. In the 5 drug trials in patients without baseline late potentials, none proved effective.

There were 33 drug trials assessed by the 24-hour ECG recordings. Of these 33 trials, 20 (61%) were effective and 13 (39%) were ineffective by the study definitions. There were 31 drug trials in the patients with baseline late potentials of which 18 (58%) were effective and 13 (42%) were ineffective. There were 2 drug trials in patients without baseline late potentials; 2 (100%) were effective.

A drug was effective by at least one approach or the other in 22 of 60 trials (37%) and ineffective by the designated approach in 38 of 60 trials (63%) in patients with baseline late potentials. In those without them, 2 of 6 trials (33%) were deemed effective and 4 of 6 trials (67%) were not.

Six patients (32%) of the 19 tested by electrophysiologic study went on to have at least 1 effective drug trial, and 13 (68%) did not. The fQRS, V40, and LAS measured at baseline were similar between patients with and without drug efficacy found at electrophysiologic study (Figure 1). Nineteen patients (73%) of the 26 tested by 24-hour continuous ECG recordings had an effective drug trial, and 7 (27%) did not. There was a trend for a longer fQRS ($p = 0.13$) and LAS ($p = 0.10$) to be present at baseline in the patients who ultimately had at least 1 effective drug trial as judged by the continuous ECG (Figure 2).

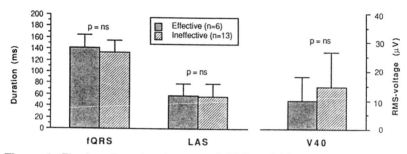

Figure 1. The baseline signal-averaged ECG variables are contrasted between patients who had ≥1 successful drug trial (effective group) guided by electrophysiologic study, and patients who had no successful drug trials (ineffective group).

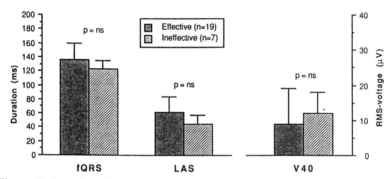

Figure 2. The baseline signal-averaged ECG variables are contrasted between patients who had ≥1 successful drug trial (effective group) guided by continuous ECG, and patients who had no successful drug trials (ineffective group).

Prediction of Drug Efficacy by Signal-Averaged ECG Recorded During Treatment

The signal-averaged ECG was recorded during antiarrhythmic therapy prior to drug testing. There were 50 trials assessed by electrophysiologic study; 7 (14%) were deemed effective and 43 (86%) were deemed ineffective. The absolute values of fQRS, V40, and LAS on treatment were similar regardless of test results as assessed by electrophysiologic study in 50 trials (Figure 3A). Although there was no statistically significant change from baseline to treatment value of the signal-averaged ECG variables (Figure 3B), the ΔfQRS tended

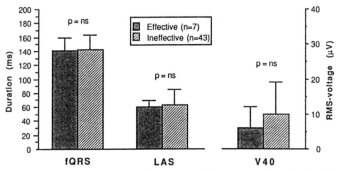

Figure 3A. The signal-averaged ECG recorded during antiarrhythmic therapy is contrasted for the effective and ineffective drug trials guided by electrophysiologic study.

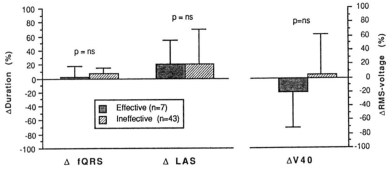

Figure 3B. The change from baseline of signal-averaged ECG variables is contrasted.

to be smaller for effective trials than for ineffective trials (p = 0.14). When the results of individual drugs were examined, sotalol therapy appeared to account for this finding.

A post-hoc comparison of sotalol results was made separately. In trials that were judged effective due to sotalol therapy (n = 4), there was a significant absolute decrease (p <0.05) in fQRS compared to the ineffective trials (n = 6). A cutpoint of 5% change from baseline fQRS appeared to divide the sotalol group into effective and ineffective outcomes. If the fQRS was diminished by 5% or more, three of four of the sotalol-effective and all six of the sotalol-ineffective patients were correctly predicted. The dose and plasma level of sotalol did not differ between these groups. The ΔV40 and ΔLAS did not exhibit significant differences between effective and ineffective groups. Other drugs were associated with too few successes to warrant subgroup analysis.

There were 33 drug trials that were assessed by 24-hour ECG recordings. Of these 33, 20 (61%) met efficacy criteria and 13 (39%) did not. Similar to the trials guided by electrophysiologic studies, there was no significant difference between signal-averaged ECGs (absolute values) recorded during effective versus ineffective therapy (Figure 4A). Of note, however, was the ΔLAS which showed divergent changes when examining treatment outcomes (Figure

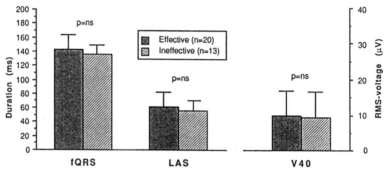

Figure 4A. The signal-averaged ECG recorded during antiarrhythmic therapy is contrasted for the effective and ineffective drug trials guided by continuous ECG.

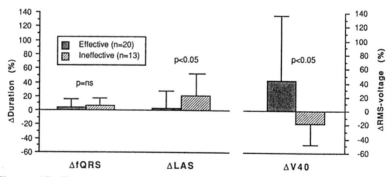

Figure 4B. The change from baseline of signal-averaged ECG variables is contrasted.

4B). The effective trials were associated with no change in the LAS, whereas the ineffective trials were associated with an increase in LAS (p <0.05). The V40 also showed a similar pattern; the V40 increased during effective trials and decreased during ineffective trials (p <0.05) (Figure 4B). Although for all drugs there was too much overlap of ΔLAS and ΔV40 to find a value that separated effective and ineffective outcomes, a negative ΔLAS (with one exception) was seen only with effective trials. Two individual drugs, sotalol and imipramine, had statistically significant differences in the ΔLAS values when comparing effective and ineffective outcomes, and accounted for the vast majority of evaluated trials. Sotalol therapy, when effective, was associated with a decrease in the LAS, but not fQRS, as compared to ineffective studies. All seven patients with sotalol-effective trials had no greater than a 9% increase in LAS, whereas all six patients with sotalol-ineffective trials had a prolongation of LAS by >17%. Similarly in 3 of 4 imipramine-effective trials the LAS did not change or shortened, and in all 6 ineffective trials the LAS lengthened by at least 18%. The doses and plasma levels of sotalol and imipramine were slightly greater in the ineffective groups, but the differences were not statistically significant.

No drug trial evaluated by 24-hour continuous ECG recordings met arbitrary arrhythmia aggravation criterion (three-fold increase in VPCs), and therefore no analysis could be performed regarding the relationship between the signal-averaged ECG and the development of proarrhythmia.

It was rare for the late potentials in the baseline recording to be abolished by drug therapy. In no instance did the fQRS shorten to <120 msec, in 1 trial the LAS shortened to < 39 msec, and the V40 increased to more than 20 μV on two occasions. When the signal-averaged ECG variable was normal at baseline, it was common for an abnormality to develop during treatment with antiarrhythmic drugs. The fQRS became abnormal in 11 of 18 trials, the LAS in 9 of 14 trials, and the V40 in 4 of 8 trials.

An example of a baseline signal-averaged ECG and the signal-averaged ECG recorded during drug therapy is shown in Figure 5. Note the effects on all three variables during treatment with propafenone at 1012 mg/day. The fQRS lengthened by 70 msec and the LAS by 75 msec. The V40 decreased by 2.1 μV.

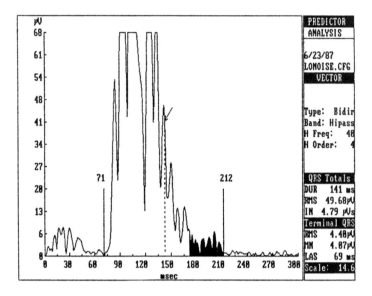

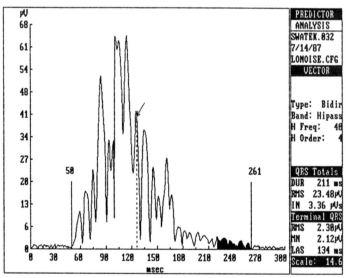

Figure 5. An example of a patient's baseline signal-averaged ECG and one recorded during steady state propafenone therapy. Note the prolongation of fQRS and LAS.

Discussion

In a population of patients with life threatening ventricular arrhythmias, the following observations were made: (1) the signal-averaged ECG demonstrates a late potential in 90% of these patients and is abnormal (either late potential or prolonged fQRS) in almost all (94%) patients; (2) Class IA and IC drugs are generally associated with prolongation of fQRS and LAS, indexes of ventricular conduction; and (3) the signal-averaged ECG during drug therapy was usually not useful in predicting treatment outcome, with the possible exception of recordings made during sotalol and imipramine therapy. The observations described in this substudy are preliminary, and data will continue to be collected until ESVEM is completed. This report is limited to analysis of the signal-averaged ECG in the time domain.

Previous Studies

Simson et al[11] examined 38 patients with recurrent sustained VT who were undergoing serial drug testing with Class IA or IB drugs, or amiodarone. The late potentials observed in most of these patients in the drug-free study were present during antiarrhythmic drug therapy. The QRS on the signal-averaged ECG was prolonged by procainamide, quinidine, and amiodarone. The authors were unable to identify a change in the signal-averaged during antiarrhythmic therapy that indicated drug success. Small changes in late potential duration were recorded by Jauernig et al[12] in 13 of 16 patients who were exposed to antiarrhythmic drugs with Class I action or amiodarone. When heart rate was kept constant with atrial pacing, consistent, but small, late potential changes were seen. However, the authors concluded that the signal-averaged ECG did not appear to be of value for predicting drug efficacy. In a group of 39 patients with a history of VT studied by Denniss et al,[13] treatment with either quinidine, mexiletine, or metoprolol did not significantly alter the signal-averaged QRS duration or the frequency of abnormal low amplitude signals. The signal-averaged ECG did not yield useful information for predicting noninducible VT or clinical efficacy. The technique of Denniss et al[13] differs from ours and from that of Simon et al[11] in that the signal-averaged QRS was analyzed visually and was not subjected to filtering. The absence of filtering, which effectively eliminates the ST segment and T wave, might limit the possibility of detecting QRS prolongation by drugs, particularly if it is due to prolongation of low amplitude signals that are occurring during the ST segment.

These prior reports were limited to determinations of drug efficacy by electrophysiologic study and not by noninvasive methods.

Present Study

The observations described in this report confirm and extend those made in prior studies.[11-13] As others have noted, ventricular conduction throughout the myocardium (i.e., as measured by the fQRS) or limited to the late segments (i.e., as measured by the LAS) is slowed or delayed further by antiarrhythmic drugs that are known to most potently interfere with sodium conductance and action potential upstroke. Drugs with Class IA action, imipramine, procainamide, and quinidine, and the IC drug, propafenone, all prolonged the fQRS. Propafenone elicited marked increases in LAS, while imipramine and procainamide elicited smaller changes. In addition, the change from a normal signal-averaged ECG measurement during drug treatment to an abnormal one, occurred frequently. Previous studies have not reported the frequency with which signal-averaged ECG abnormalities are precipitated by antiarrhythmic drugs. This observation suggests that interpretation of the signal-averaged ECG may be problematic if it is recorded only during antiarrhythmic drug therapy.

The prolongation of conduction observed on the signal-averaged ECG, however, did not correlate with drug success. There are several possible explanations for the general lack of correlation between findings on the signal-averaged ECG recorded during drug therapy and drug treatment success: (1) the recording is obtained with the patient in sinus rhythm, and it may be that "stress" (e.g., increased rate or following premature beats[11]) on conduction is required to bring out changes that are characteristic or predictive of drug response; (2) changes on the signal-averaged ECG may take the form of loss of late potential or greater prolongation. When the late potential persists (which was observed in almost all trials), this might reflect localized conduction with exit block, so that segments critical to reentry are capable of being activated in sinus rhythm, but incapable of activating neighboring segments;[14] (3) the late potential is possibly only a marker of conduction characteristics or diseased myocardium.[15] Only a fraction of the diseased tissue generating the late potential is involved in reentry, so changes in the late potential may be an insensitive marker for changes in tissue involved in reentry; (4) successful antiarrhythmic treatment is mediated by effects on normal tissue, rather than damaged tissue that is responsible for the registration of the late potential[11]; (5) pharmacologic effects might be most pronounced on the interface between normal and damaged tissue, and mediated by impedance mismatch; (6) effects of drugs might be directed at passive properties of conduction, i.e., cell coupling,[16] which may not be present or difficult to record with the signal-averaged ECG in sinus rhythm. These explanations all assume that reentry is the mechanism for chronic VT in the population under study, and that pharmacologic control is achieved by modification of conduction characteristics of the reentrant circuit; and (7) changes in refractoriness, not measured by the signal-averaged ECG, are responsible for drug efficacy.

Treatment with sotalol, a drug that has Class II and Class III, but not Class I actions,[17] was associated with a different set of signal-averaged ECG results. Prior studies have not described the results seen with drugs whose major effect is Class III activity such as sotalol. When treatment was effective, conduction was abbreviated compared to the trials when treatment was ineffective. Effective sotalol therapy was associated with a decrease in fQRS in the electrophysiologic study guided trials, and a decrease in LAS in the 24-hour continuous ECG guided trials. The mechanism responsible for these results is unclear; the change in refractoriness may foster a beneficial change in the activation sequence with entrance block to areas of slow conduction. It is also possible that when sotalol therapy is associated with a small decrease in conduction velocity,[18] which is seen on the signal-averaged ECG as an increase in fQRS, it allows tissue recovery to occur and offset the beneficial effects of increased tissue refractoriness. These observations were few in number, and additional study seems warranted with sotalol and other Class III agents.

Given the history of a sustained ventricular arrhythmia, the presence of late potentials on the baseline signal-averaged ECG suggested a greater chance of finding an effective treatment when guided by electrophysiologic study. Conversely, the absence of late potentials suggested greater difficulty in treatment. However, the number of patients who did not have a late potential is small, and further experience is needed before these findings could be considered conclusive. Extrapolations to mechanistic implications are again difficult; the absence of significant activation delay in sinus rhythm may thus require conduction stress for reentry to occur, and in turn may be relatively immune to the effects of antiarrhythmic drugs. Alternatively, the signal-averaged ECG may be insensitive to conduction in certain myocardial regions, by virtue of their location in the chest relative to lead placement, by virtue of their intermittent activation,[19] or by virtue of their total amplitude transmitted to the body surface. Why these regions would be relatively resistant to the effects of antiarrhythmic drugs is not clear.

Recent work by de Langen et al[16] provides experimental observations regarding the effects of pharmacologic agents on epicardial and body surface electrical recordings. In their canine experimental model of myocardial infarction, procainamide proved more effective than lidocaine and acetylstrophanthidin in preventing VT. Procainamide prolonged the epicardial electrograms that occurred during the main body of the QRS on the signal-averaged ECG, as well as those that occurred during the terminal tail of the QRS, compared to the other two drugs. Similar to our findings with propafenone, the terminal portion of the QRS on the signal-averaged recordings prolonged to a greater degree than the rest of the QRS. Although this differential effect is a possible explanation for the greater procainamide efficacy noted in this study, data were not presented demonstrating that dogs who had their arrhythmia suppressed differed in their electrographic or electrocardiographic manifestations from dogs who did not have their arrhythmias suppressed.

Although the signal-averaged ECG may reflect antiarrhythmic drug effects on the heart, it has as yet no defined role for assessing drug efficacy. Several hypothetical uses can be generated from the currently available data and suggest the directions future research may take. The signal-averaged ECG may be useful as a noninvasive approach to arrhythmia or antiarrhythmic mechanism, or as a guide to drug concentrations. The baseline recording may help predict the likelihood of successful drug treatment, and thus aid decisions regarding drug or alternate forms of therapy, but it has not yet been shown that information obtained from the signal-averaged ECG is independent of variables previously shown to predict successful drug treatment when guided by the electrophysiologic study such as left ventricular function.[20] The findings presented in this chapter paper are preliminary, and a larger database will need to be examined in the future to fully understand the relationship of the signal-averaged ECG and the effects of antiarrhythmic drug therapy.

Acknowledgment: This work was supported in part by grant HL-34071 from the National Heart, Lung and Blood Institute, by grant RR-00645 from the Research Resources Administration, Bethesda, Maryland, and by a grant from the American Heart Association, Montana Affiliate, and by a gift from David and Lydia Wolf, New York, New York.

Appendix
The ESVEM Investigators

Principal Investigator: Jay W. Mason—University of Utah

Collaborating Investigators (listed by institution in order of number of subjects enrolled)
University of Utah: Jay W. Mason, M.D., Jeffrey L. Anderson, M.D., Kelley P. Anderson, M.D., Roger A. Freedman, M.D., David A. Rawling, M.D.
Columbia University: J. Thomas Bigger, M.D., James Coromilas, M.D., Frank D. Livelli, Jr, M.D., James Reiffel, M.D., Jonathan S. Steinberg, M.D.
University of Arizona: Frank I. Marcus, M.D., Lionel Faitelson, M.D.
University of Oklahoma: Ralph Lazzara, M.D., Karen J. Friday, M.D., Warren M. Jackman, M.D.
University of New Mexico: Richard C. Klein, M.D.
Baylor College of Medicine: Craig Pratt, M.D., Antonio Pacifico, M.D., Christopher R.C. Wyndham, M.D.
University of Colorado: Michael J. Reiter, M.D., David Mann, M.D.
University of California, San Francisco: Jerry C. Griffin, M.D., John M. Herre, M.D., Melvin Scheinman, M.D.
University of Oregon: John H. McAnulty, Jr, M.D., Jack Kron, M.D.
Presbyterian-University of Pennsylvania Medical Center: Leonard Horowitz, M.D.
Newark Beth Israel Medical Center: Sanjeev Saksena, M.D., Ryszard B. Krol, M.D., Nicholas G. Tullo, M.D.
University of Massachusetts: Shoei K. Stephen Huang, M.D., Charles I. Haffajee, M.D.
University of British Columbia: Charles R. Kerr, M.D., John A. Yeung, M.D.

Northwestern University: Richard Kehoe, M.D., Thomas Mattioni, M.D., Terry Ann Zheutlin, M.D.

Nurse Coordinators: University of Utah: Marian Bartholomew, Lori Bedont, Melinda Hutson, Diane Mannis
Columbia University: Annmarie Squatrito, Karen Nieminski
University of Arizona: Zee Garcia, Kathy Gear, MaryKay Pierce
University of Oklahoma: Chris Carter, Tammy Deaton, Shelly Harris, Adrienne Oden
University of New Mexico: Patti Doherty, Nancy Rushforth
Baylor College of Medicine: Peggy Keus, Madeline Madden
University of Colorado: Elissa Barpal, Susan Breckinridge, Kathy Freeman, Cathleen Kenny
University of California, San Francisco: Hugh Sharkey, Christ Titus
University of Oregon: Kris Sinner
Presbyterian-University of Pennsylvania Medical Center: Christine Vrabel
Newark Beth Israel Medical Center: Ann Marie Mauro
University of Massachusetts: Gina M. Gasdia
University of British Columbia: Shirley Vorderbrugge
Northwestern University: Cathy Dunnington

Data Coordinating Center: University of Arizona: Thomas Moon, Ph.D. (Principal Investigator), Elizabeth Hahn, Vern Hartz, Ann Rico, Richele Schaffer

Safety Monitoring Committee: Rubin Bressler, M.D., Eugene Morkin, M.D., Michael Lebowitz, Ph.D., Leon Greene, M.D.

References

1. Simson MB, Euler D, Michelson EL, Falcone RA, Spear JF, Moore EN: Detection of delayed ventricular activation on the body surface in dogs. Am J Physiol 241:H363, 1981.
2. Gomes JA, Winters SL, Stewart D, Horowitz S, Milner M, Barreca P: A new noninvasive index to predict sustained ventricular tachycardia and sudden death in the first year after myocardial infarction: based on signal-averaged electrocardiogram, radionuclide ejection fraction and Holter monitoring. J Am Coll Cardiol 10:349, 1987.
3. Kuchar DL, Thornburn CW, Sammel NL: Prediction of serious arrhythmic events after myocardial infarction: signal-averaged electrocardiogram, Holter monitoring and radionuclide ventriculography. J Am Coll Cardiol 9:531, 1987.

4. Winters SL, Stewart D, Gomes JA: Signal averaging of the surface QRS complex predicts inducibility of ventricular tachycardia in patients with syncope of unknown origin: a prospective study. J Am Coll Cardiol 10:775, 1987.
5. Turitto G, Fontaine JM, Ursell SN, Caref EB, Henkin R, El-Sherif N: Value of the signal-averaged electrocardiogram as a predictor of the results of programmed stimulation in nonsustained ventricular tachycardia. Am J Cardiol 61:1272, 1988.
6. Hoffman BF, Rosen MR, Wit AL: Electrophysiology and pharmacology of cardiac arrhythmias. III. The causes and treatment of cardiac arrhythmias. Part A. Am Heart J 89:115, 1975.
7. Rensma PL, Allessie MA, Lammers WJEP, Schalij MJ: Length of the excitation wave and susceptibility to reentrant atrial arrhythmias in normal conscious dogs. Circ Res 62:395, 1988.
8. The ESVEM Investigators: The ESVEM Trial: electrophysiologic study versus electrocardiographic monitoring for selection of antiarrhythmic therapy of ventricular tachyarrhythmias. Circulation (in press).
9. Steinberg JS, Bigger JT Jr: Importance of the endpoint of noise reduction in analysis of the signal averaged electrocardiogram. Am J Cardiol 63:556, 1989.
10. Simson MB: Use of signals in the terminal QRS complex to identify patients with ventricular tachycardia after myocardial infarction. Circulation 64:235, 1981.
11. Simson MB, Waxman HL, Falcone R, Marcus NH, Josephson ME: Effects of antiarrhythmic drugs on noninvasively recorded late potentials. In Breithardt G, Loogen F (eds): New Aspects in the Medical Treatment of Tachyarrhythmias. Role of Amiodarone. Munich: Urban and Schwarzenberg, 1983, pp 80–87.
12. Jauernig RA, Senges J, Lengpelder W, Kizos I, Hoffman E, Brachmann J, Kubler W: Effect of antiarrhythmic drugs on ventricular late potentials at sinus rhythm and at constant atrial rate. In Steinbach K, Glogar D, Laczkovics A, Scheibelhofer W, Weber H (eds): Cardiac Pacing. Darmstadt: Steinkopff, 1983, pp 767–772.
13. Denniss AR, Ross DL, Richards DA, Cody DV, Russell PA, Young AA, Uther JB: Effect of antiarrhythmic therapy on delayed potentials detected by the signal-averaged electrocardiogram in patients with ventricular tachycardia after acute myocardial infarction. Am J Cardiol 58:261, 1986.
14. Breithardt G, Borggrefe M: Pathophysiological mechanisms and clinical significance of ventricular late potentials. Eur Heart J 7:364, 1986.
15. Poll DS, Marchlinski FE, Falcone RA, Josephson ME, Simson MB: Abnormal signal-averaged electrocardiograms in patients with nonischemic congestive cardiomyopathy: relationship to sustained ventricular tachyarrhythmias. Circulation 72:1308, 1985.
16. de Langen CDJ, Hanich RF, Michelson EL, Kadish AH, Levine JH, Blake CW, Spear JF, Moore EM: Differential effects of procainamide, lidocaine and acetylstrophanthidin on body surface potentials and epicardial conduction in dogs with chronic myocardial infarction. J Am Coll Cardiol 11:403, 1988.

17. Echt DS, Berte LE, Clusin WT, Samuelsson RG, Harrison DC, Mason JW: Prolongation of the human cardiac monophasic action potential by sotalol. Am J Cardiol 50:1082, 1982.
18. Carmeliet E: Electrophysiologic and voltage clamp analysis of sotalol on isolated cardiac muscle and Purkinje fibers. J Pharmacol Exp Ther 232:817, 1985.
19. El-Sherif N, Scherlag BJ, Lazzara R: Electrode catheter recordings during malignant ventricular arrhythmia following experimental acute myocardial ischemia. Circulation 51:1003, 1975.
20. Kuchar DL, Rottman J, Berger E, Freeman CS, Garan H, Ruskin JN: Prediction of successful suppression of sustained ventricular tachyarrhythmias by serial drug testing from data derived at the initial electrophysiologic study. J Am Coll Cardiol 12:982, 1988.

Section VI.

Frequency-Domain Analysis of the Signal-Averaged Electrocardiogram

27

Value of Frequency-Domain Analysis in Identifying Patients with Ventricular Tachyarrhythmias

Michael E. Cain, Bruce D. Lindsay,
H. Dieter Ambos

Introduction

Sudden cardiac death from sustained ventricular arrhythmias remains a major health issue throughout the world. Reduction of the incidence of sudden cardiac death will require accurate identification of those at risk and accurate, prospective determination of the effectiveness of specific antiarrhythmic interventions in individual patients. Noninvasive detection of the patient at risk for developing sustained ventricular tachycardia (VT) or ventricular fibrillation (VF) has been attempted with clinical and electrocardiographic criteria including frequent and complex ventricular ectopy detected in the course of ambulatory electrocardiographic monitoring.[1–12] Although certain patterns of ventricular ectopy predict higher cardiac mortality in large groups, none specifically predicts risk for development of sustained VT or VF when applied to individuals.

From El-Sherif N, Turitto G (eds): *High-Resolution Electrocardiography*. Mount Kisco, NY, Futura Publishing Co., Inc., ©, 1992.

Thus, institution of prophylactic antiarrhythmic therapy based solely on the detection of ventricular ectopy exposes many patients to potent drugs unnecessarily. Moreover, antiarrhythmic treatment directed toward suppressing nonspecific arrhythmias has not proved successful in preventing sustained VT or VF.[13-20]

Results of laboratory[21-29] and clinical[30-37] studies implicate reentrant mechanisms, at least in part, in the genesis of sustained VT complicating ischemic heart disease. Derangements of ventricular activation during sinus rhythm have been observed consistently in regions bordering the infarct and overlying epicardial regions and appear temporally related to the development of VT or VF. Recently, several groups[38-45] have applied advanced signal processing techniques in the time domain to extract this occult yet clinically relevant information present during sinus rhythm from the surface electrocardiogram (ECG). The reported incidences of abnormal signals detected during sinus rhythm from patients with a history of sustained VT have ranged from 60% to 90% depending on the methods of signal processing and data analysis, the definition of abnormal results, and the patient group studied.

We have developed, tested, and implemented a signal processing system using fast Fourier transform (FFT) analysis in order to determine whether frequency analysis of signal-averaged ECGs facilitates objective, noninvasive identification of an electrophysiologic substrate conducive to the development of reentrant ventricular arrhythmias, and to determine whether results of frequency analysis can be used to prospectively stratify patients with structural heart disease at high and low risk for developing life-threatening ventricular arrhythmias.[46-54] This chapter describes the evolution of this approach and summarizes the results of clinical studies.

Methods

Basis for Using Frequency Analysis

FFT analysis is a powerful analytic method for signal processing in the frequency domain that allows some of the inherent limitations of high-gain amplification and signal filtering required for analysis in the time domain to be avoided.[55,56] Moreover, frequency analysis facilitates identification and characterization of frequencies independent of signal amplitude and provides flexibility for analyzing different ECG segments. ECG waveforms, like other periodic physical and biologic signals, may be represented by the mathematical summation of a series of sine and cosine components of differing amplitudes and periods. FFT analysis is a computer-based mathematical algorithm whereby the amplitudes of the various frequency components that comprise a complex periodic waveform are determined. The Fourier transform is unique since for each time-domain representation there is one and only one frequency-domain presentation.

The computer-based model shown in Figure 1 illustrates one example of how frequency analysis facilitates identification of low amplitude potentials in the ECG.[46] To mathematically simulate a small oscillatory waveform superimposed on the trailing edge of a QRS complex, two complete cycles of a 40-Hz sine wave of variable voltage and onset have been superimposed on a ramp function with a negative voltage versus time slope starting at a fixed voltage of 1 mV and reaching 0 mV at 50 msec. In this computer generated mathematical model, the ramp function and 40-Hz sine wave have been premultiplied by a first-order Hanning window function to avoid edge discontinuities. Classic Fourier series analysis was performed

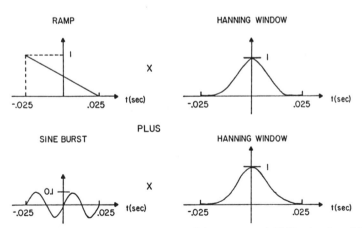

Figure 1. Time-domain representation of the ramp and 40-Hz sine burst functions used to simulate a small oscillatory waveform superimposed on the trailing edge of the QRS complex. To exclude edge discontinuities both functions are multiplied by a first-order Hanning window function before frequency analysis. (Reproduced with permission of the American Heart Association, from Cain et al, Circulation 69:711, 1984.)

on both functions, the spectra generated being verified by time-domain reconstruction of the original waveform (Figure 2). As shown in Figure 2C, the amplitude (0 to peak) of the sine burst is 0.1 mV and the peak amplitude of the ramp function is 1 mV. The time-domain perturbation that reflects the 40-Hz sine burst contribution is minimal but clearly detectable in the frequency domain. Moreover, the sine burst component is easily detectable at levels as low as 10 µV in the frequency domain as a bump in the spectra near 40 Hz. However, it is not evident at these low levels in the time domain without prefiltering regardless of gain.

The effects of gain and prefiltering in the time domain are illustrated in Figure 3. In each panel, the original time-domain waveform and idealized filtered waveform are shown. In the top panel, the display gain has been doubled when compared to Figure 2C. When

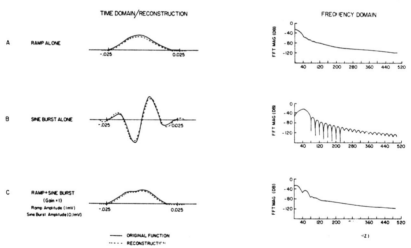

Figure 2. Comparison of results of time- and frequency-domain analyses. Right: the spectral analysis (after Hanning window multiplication) of the ramp function (A), 40-Hz sine burst function (B), and the sum of the ramp and sine burst functions (C) are shown. Left: the original time-domain waveforms (solid lines) of these functions are shown along with the time-domain reconstruction (broken lines) from the Fourier series. (C) The amplitude (0 to peak) of the sine burst is 0.1 mV, and the peak amplitude of the ramp function is 1 mV. The time-domain perturbation that reflects the sine burst contribution is minimal without prefiltering. However, the contribution from the 40-Hz sine wave is easily detectable in the frequency domain. (Reproduced with permission of the American Heart Association, from Cain et al, Circulation 69:711, 1984.)

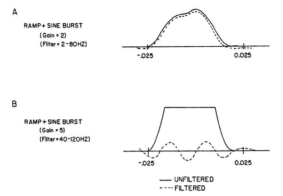

Figure 3. Effect of gain and prefiltering in the time domain. In (A) and (B), the original time-domain waveform (solid line) and the idealized filtered waveform (broken line) are shown. (A) The display gain is twice that in Figure 2C. When the filter used in the reconstruction is 2 to 80 Hz, the filtered waveform and original waveform correlate closely. However, the sine burst contribution is still only minimally apparent. (B) The display gain is five times that in Figure 2C. The filter used in the reconstruction is 40 to 120 Hz. With high-gain amplification and prefiltering the sine burst can be adequately visualized in the time domain. However, selection of the high- and low-pass filters requires *a priori* knowledge of the frequency content of the signal of interest. (Reproduced with permission of the American Heart Association, from Cain et al, Circulation 69:711, 1984.)

the filter used in the reconstruction is 2 to 80 Hz, the filtered waveform and original waveform correlate closely. However, the sine burst contribution is still only minimally apparent. In the bottom panel, the display is five times that in Figure 2C and the filter used in the reconstruction was 40 to 120 Hz. Thus, only after high-gain amplification and specific filtering was the 40-Hz sine burst adequately visualized in the time domain. A limitation of filtering is that the selection of the high- and low-pass filter requires *a priori* knowledge of the frequency content of the signal of interest. Filtering may exclude potentially significant signals. Furthermore, filtering may modify the amplitude and phase of signals of interest.[56]

Derangements of ventricular conduction during sinus rhythm have been observed consistently in regions bordering the infarct and overlying epicardial regions and appear temporally related to the development of VT. Figure 4 illustrates the variety of electrogram patterns recorded from the epicardium of the left ventricle during the course of computerized intraoperative mapping during sinus

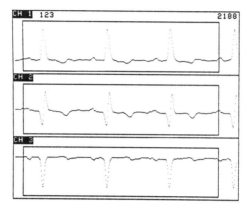

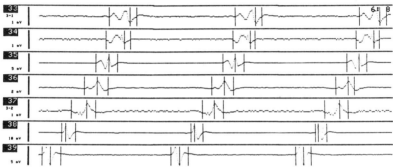

Figure 4. Representative electrograms recorded simultaneously during 3 consecutive sinus beats with a 96-button sock electrode from the left ventricular epicardial surface overlying a remote myocardial infarction from a patient with recurrent sustained VT. Cursors identify electrogram onset, peak activation, and offset, respectively.

rhythm from a patient with sustained VT. Figure 5 demonstrates abnormalities of transmural ventricular activation detected with plunge needles during sinus rhythm from a patient with recurrent sustained VT. Results of clinical studies using catheter mapping techniques during sinus rhythm have demonstrated that delayed ventricular activation is more profound and detectable at more cardiac sites from patients with, compared with those without, sustained VT.[57-59]

Because the surface ECG reflects total activation of the heart, we hypothesized that the frequency content of signal-averaged ECGs obtained during sinus rhythm from patients with a history of

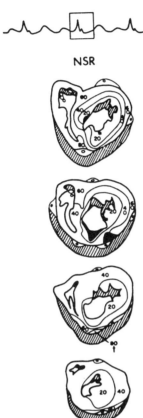

NSR

Figure 5. Three-dimensional isochronous activation map (20-msec isochronal lines) during normal sinus rhythm obtained intraoperatively from a patient with a remote anterior myocardial infarction. Levels I to III indicate 2- to 3-cm thick, short-axis slices of the ventricles from base to apex, respectively. The anterior surface and left anterior descending coronary artery are at the lower margin of each slice. The right ventricle is at the left of each slice. During sinus rhythm, early activation (*) spreads throughout the endocardial layer and proceeds toward the epicardium; (+) denotes latest activation. Solid areas and bold lines indicate the locations of conduction block.

sustained VT would differ quantitatively from that from patients without sustained VT.

Signal Processing

Standard Frank X, Y, and Z ECG leads are recorded simultaneously using a Hewlett-Packard 1507A vectorcardiogram modified to give a specific frequency response of 0.05 to 470 Hz with a rolloff of 18 dB per octave.[46,47] ECG signals are amplified 1000-fold to optimize the maximum ±2.5 V input range of the A/D converter. Normalized signals are digitized at 1 kHz using a 12-bit A/D converter providing a 72-dB range. The digitized data are processed with a

DEC VT103 LSI 11/23 microcomputer system with 64 kbytes of memory, two serial communication ports, a dual floppy disk system, and a Selanar Raster graphics board with joystick control that operates with an RT-11 operating system.

Signal Averaging

The X, Y, and Z ECG signals are averaged after passage through a template recognition program generated from a 3-second display of normal sinus rhythm.[46,47] The lead having the largest R wave amplitude in relation to the P and T waves is selected, the RR interval and fiducial point (peak of the R wave) set with an adjustable cursor, and the QRS amplitudes calculated for all three leads. During averaging, 3 seconds of X, Y, and Z lead data are stored in a circular memory buffer consisting of three individual 1-K buffers per lead. Usually the data contained in the central buffer are compared with the template beat generated initially. The RR interval is checked forward and backward with the beat in the first and last buffers, respectively. If the RR interval is not within 20% of the template value, the beat is rejected. Otherwise, the peak-to-peak QRS amplitudes of the X, Y, and Z leads are compared with the stored template values. The amplitudes must be within 5% of the template values for the beat to be considered further for averaging. If the RR interval and amplitudes are acceptable, a 40-point cross correlation of the R wave is performed about the fiducial point. If the correlation coefficient is <98%, the beat is rejected. Reference jitter cannot exceed 1 msec. The beat immediately after a rejected beat is rejected also. Signal averaging is performed in real time and uses double precision arithmetic. Routinely, the data from 100 beats are averaged and stored on a floppy disk for further processing. A 100-beat average reduces inherent noise to <1.5 μV, approximately equal to the 1.2 μV quantization error of the A/D converter. The X, Y, and Z leads are monitored continuously in real time during averaging to allow detection of changes in heart rate, QRS morphology, or amplitude. After averaging is complete, the double precision values are changed to single precision values and stored on floppy disk.

Fast Fourier Transform Analysis

Technical Considerations and Performance Limitations

Several major sources of artifactual frequency shifts must be excluded before reliable differences in spectral content of ECG signals from patients with and without a history of sustained VT can be accepted. The first and most obvious is the contribution of random background noise, which with our current system configuration is reduced to 1.5 μV by signal averaging.

The bandwidth of our analog amplifiers extends from 0.05 to 470 Hz. However, some inherent limitations of frequency analysis and signal averaging can alter the ability to definitely detect discrete signals over this broad range of frequencies. First, frequency resolution is inversely proportional to sample size (QRS complex, terminal 40 msec of the QRS complex, ST segment, terminal QRS and ST segment, and T wave). Frequency resolution is theoretically 6.6 Hz for a 150-msec data sample comprised of the terminal QRS and ST segment. High-frequency signals may be attenuated further during signal averaging due to reference jitter, a limitation encountered with time- and frequency-domain analysis. Jitter is ±1msec in our system and comparable to the 0.5- to 2.0-msec jitter reported by other investigators.[60] Jitter in this range can operate as a low-pass filter and mask high-frequency signals.[60] In our system, with the worse case of reference jitter being ±1 msec, the −3 dB point is 134 Hz.

Another source of possible artifact relates to introducing step discontinuities between regions of interest (terminal QRS, ST segment, and T wave). Fourier analysis assumes that the signal contained in a sample window interval is a periodic function. However, if the initial and final sampling points are not at zero potential, a sharp discontinuity may be introduced between the end of one cycle and the beginning of the next that may artificially add both high- and low-frequency harmonics to the original signal. To obviate this source of error, mathematical window functions are used that smooth the windowed data to zero at the boundaries. Since multiplication by the window function in the time domain leads to convolution in the frequency domain, care must be taken to choose a window function that allows detection of nearby components of significantly different amplitudes without compromising resolution, dynamic range, or ease of implementation. Spectral leakage is most marked for the detection of low amplitude signals in the presence of nearby large amplitude signals. The ability of a window function to diminish spectral leakage is directly related to its sidelobe level. The four-term Blackman-Harris window (Figure 6) has a 92-dB sidelobe level and sidelobe falloff of 6 dB per octave.[61] The contribution of artifactual frequencies due to spectral leakage is apparent only at decibel drops > 92 dB which is below the 72-dB dynamic range of the 12-bit A/D converter.

This smoothing function, however, can attenuate resolution of frequency peaks. Figure 7 compares the amplitude spectra of the

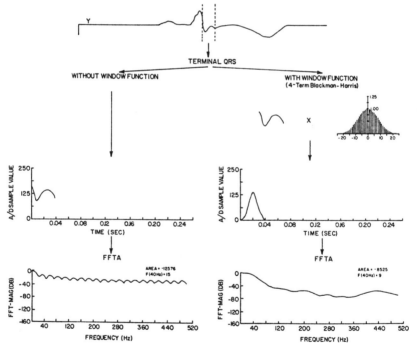

Figure 6. Parallel data processing of the terminal 40 msec of the QRS with (right) and without (left) the four-term Blackman-Harris window function. Left: the edge discontinuity between the initial and final sample point of the terminal QRS is readily apparent and adds artifactual frequency information to the signal of interest. As shown in the middle panel, right, multiplication by the four-term Blackman-Harris window eliminates these edge discontinuities and the initial sample points are now isopotential. (Reproduced with permission of the American Heart Association, from Cain et al, Circulation 69:711, 1984.)

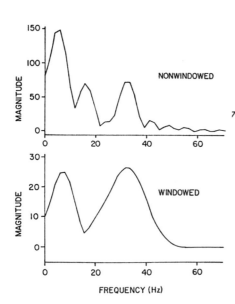

Figure 7. Fast Fourier transforms computed from a nonwindowed (upper panel) and windowed (lower panel) 150-msec composite signal generated by summing sine waves of unit amplitude with frequencies 5, 7, 10, 15, and 32 Hz. Frequency resolution of the 150-msec nonwindowed signal is 6.6 Hz precluding the ability to distinguish individual frequency peaks at 5, 7, and 10 Hz. The four-term Blackman-Harris window markedly reduces the contribution of artifactual high-frequency components due to edge discontinuities but further decreases resolution making it difficult to resolve individual frequency peaks. Importantly, the areas under each spectral curve are comparable. Composite signals that have durations of 100, 200, and 300 msec were also tested. As expected, resolution improves as the duration of the data segment increases.

FFT computed from a windowed and nonwindowed 150-msec composite signal generated by summing sine waves of unit amplitude with frequencies 5, 7, 10, 15, and 32 Hz. The Blackman-Harris window markedly reduces the contribution of artifactual high-frequency components due to edge discontinuities but decreases resolution making it difficult to resolve individual frequency peaks with data segment durations < 150 msec. Importantly, the areas under the spectral curves of the windowed and nonwindowed data are comparable. Accordingly, differentiation of patient groups has been based on a range of frequency components rather than individual frequencies.

The Fourier transform assumes that signals of interest are composed of continuous sine waves. However, biologic signals contributing to altered frequency components may be present in only a portion of the terminal QRS/ST segment or other ECG intervals undergoing analysis. To determine the extent to which signals of short duration can be detected reliably by analysis of larger data segments, we generated 200- and 500-msec test signals comprised of 7-, 10-, and 15-Hz sine waves each having an amplitude of unity. The FFTs of these composite signals were computed and compared to

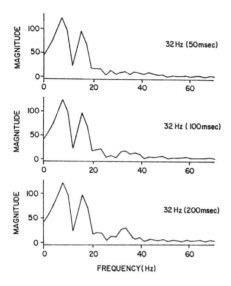

Figure 8. Fast Fourier transforms of 200-msec composite signals comprised of 7-, 10-, and 15-Hz sine waves each having an amplitude of 1- and 32-Hz sine bursts with variable amplitudes and durations. The 32-Hz sine bursts in this example have amplitudes of 0.25 and durations of 50 msec (top panel), 100 msec (middle panel), and 200 msec (bottom panel). The 32-Hz sine burst is easily detectable when present for 100 and 200 msec but is not readily apparent when the duration is <50 msec. Thus, detection of a low amplitude signal that is a component of a complex, large amplitude signal is a function of the duration of the low amplitude component.

that obtained when 32-Hz sine wave bursts of varying amplitude and duration were added to the test signals. As shown by the example in Figure 8, as the amplitude of the 32-Hz sine wave decreases, detection using the FFT becomes a function of signal duration.

Log Transformation

Spectral estimates of the entire QRS complex, the terminal 40 msec of the QRS complex, the ST segment, and the T wave of each signal-averaged X, Y, and Z lead were computed initially from the log transformation to determine the optimal ECG interval for detecting altered frequency components that distinguish patients with from those without sustained VT.[46,47] For each region of interest, a 512-point FFT was calculated after multiplication by a four-term Blackman-Harris window to reduce spectral leakage. After multiplication by the window function, the selected sample values were placed at the beginning of the 512-point array and the remaining values set to zero. This step permitted maintenance of the same frequency scale in the output data but allowed a varying number of input values to be analyzed with the same system software. Since data were obtained at 1-msec intervals, samples up to 512 msec in length could be analyzed.

Power Spectral Density

To quantify and characterize further the differences in frequency content between patients with and without sustained VT, the power spectral density was computed by squaring the magnitudes of the FFT data.[48] This computation was used to expose frequencies with high amplitude components and differentiate their contribution to the signal-averaged raw data from the contributions of frequencies with low amplitude components. To enhance frequency resolution, analysis was performed on the terminal 40 msec of the QRS complex and ST segment as a single unit.

FFT Magnitude

Initial studies were performed on ECG signals obtained from patients during sinus rhythm in the absence of bundle branch block or marked abnormalities of intraventricular conduction.[46-48] The ECGs from many patients with a history of sustained VT, however, exhibit marked abnormalities of intraventricular conduction during sinus rhythm. Moreover, the ECGs from such patients demonstrate a wide range of QRS durations and ST segment lengths when compared with ECGs from patients without intraventricular conduction abnormalities. As mentioned previously, frequency resolution is proportional to the duration of the signal analyzed. Before the clinical application of this noninvasive approach can be expanded, methods of data analysis must be relatively insensitive to physiologic and pathologic variations in ST segment length. To determine the effect of the ST segment length on the FFT in order to develop a method of analysis that would enable the reliable comparison of FFT results in patients over a broad range of physiologic and pathologic ST segment lengths, changes in the energy distribution between 0 to 50 Hz were computed at 10-Hz intervals from the energy spectrum and FFT magnitude during progressive shortening of the ST segment.[52] The area under the curve for each 10-Hz interval was calculated and normalized by dividing the area of each interval by the value of the maximum magnitude. The relative contribution of peak magnitudes in this range to the frequency content of the entire interval of interest was computed by dividing the peak magnitudes by the maximum magnitude.

A comparison of the energy distribution between 0 to 50 Hz for a 160-point and 148-point data segment from a signal-averaged X lead computed using the energy spectrum is shown in Table I. As demonstrated, shortening the ST segment by 12 msec increased substantially the proportion of frequency components in the 10- to 20-Hz and 20- to 30-Hz ranges while the proportion of components in the 0- to 10-Hz range decreased. The values for the areas under the curve between 30 to 50 Hz changed only modestly. In each subject, the largest relative change occurred between 20 to 30 Hz where area values increased by 200% to 1400%. Since the ST segment is composed predominantly of low-frequency components, shortening the ST segment resulted in a change in the proportion of low and high frequencies. Previously, we calculated an area ratio, 20–50 Hz/0–20 Hz, from the energy spectrum as a measure of the relative contribution of high-frequency components to the terminal QRS and ST segment. This ratio has been shown to reliably distinguish patients with and without sustained VT in whom ST segment lengths during sinus rhythm are comparable. However, the changes in frequency distribution when the length of the ST segment is shortened were accentuated because the FFT magnitudes were squared. As shown in Table I, the area ratio increased by 122% from 9 to a value of 20.

Results of detailed analysis of ECGs from normal subjects of the changes in energy distribution during alterations of signal duration have indicated that indices computed from the FFT magnitude are less sensitive to ST segment length and thus may be more appropriate for comparing the frequency content of signal-averaged ECGs having a broad range of physiologic or pathologic ST segment durations. Table II demonstrates the effect of shortening the ST segment on the frequency distribution when the same data are expressed as a FFT magnitude and not as the energy spectrum. When the ST segment was shortened by 12 msec, the area from 10 to 20 Hz and 20 to 30 Hz increased, but less substantially when compared with the changes observed in the energy spectrum. Only modest changes were observed in the 30- to 50-Hz intervals. Thus, the shift in frequency distribution of the FFT magnitude due to shortening the ST segment was much less than observed in the energy spectrum.

Results of studies in several subjects demonstrated that as the ST segment was progressively shortened, the energy distribution from 0 to 10 Hz changed disproportionately to that observed from 10 to 30 Hz; and as a result, the 20–50 Hz/0–20 Hz ratio would change dramatically with changes in the ST segment length. [52,53] To avoid this inherent variable, the approach was modified and a new ratio

Table I

Influence of Signal Duration on Energy Distributions Between 0 to 50 Hz Computed from the Energy Spectrum

160 Points
Maximum Magnitude (MAX MAG) = 3034.9 at 0.00 Hz

Frequency (Hz)	Area	Area/Max Mag
0–10	18005.98	0.593E + 01
10–20	796.78	0.263E + 00
20–30	1.17	0.386E − 03
30–40	0.47	0.154E − 03
40–50	0.06	0.181E − 04

$$\text{Area Ratio} = \frac{\text{area 20–50 Hz}}{\text{area 0–20 Hz}} \times 10000 = 9$$

148 Points
Maximum Magnitude = 2706.9 at 0.00 Hz

Frequency (Hz)	Area	Area/Max Mag
0–10	16812.96	0.621E + 01
10–20	993.16	0.367E + 00
20–30	3.14	0.116E − 02
30–40	0.37	0.138E − 03
40–50	0.05	0.190E − 04

$$\text{Area Ratio} = \frac{\text{area 20–50 Hz}}{\text{area 0–20 Hz}} \times 10000 = 20$$

Table II

Influence of Signal Duration on Energy Distributions between 0 to 50 Hz Computed from the FFT Magnitude

160 Points

Maximum Magnitude (MAX MAG) = 55.09 at 0.00 Hz			Maximum Magnitude = 52.03 at 0.00 Hz		
Frequency (Hz)	Area	Area/Max Mag	Frequency (Hz)	Area	Area/Max Mag
0–10	408.35	0.741E+01	0–10	397.48	0.764E+01
10–20	68.54	0.124E+01	10–20	79.53	0.153E+01
20–30	2.86	0.519E−01	20–30	4.38	0.842E−01
30–40	2.13	0.386E−01	30–40	1.90	0.366E−01
40–50	0.71	0.129E−01	40–50	0.66	0.128E−01

$$\text{Area Ratio} = \frac{\text{area 20–50 Hz}}{\text{area 10–50 Hz}} \times 1000 = 77$$

$$\text{Area Ratio} = \frac{\text{area 20–50 Hz}}{\text{area 10–50 Hz}} \times 1000 = 80$$

was calculated whereby the area between 20 to 50 Hz was divided by the area from 10 to 50 Hz. Thus, the numerator and denominator contain data pertinent to the frequency distribution between 20 to 30 Hz, the range of frequencies most affected by changes in the length of the ST segment. As demonstrated, values for the new ratio changed by only 4% from 77 to 80 when the ST segment was shortened by 12 msec. Values for these areas were calculated using the trapezoidal scale with linear interpolation used to compute FFT magnitudes at points between actual FFT data.

Data Analysis

Presently, FFT analysis is performed on the terminal 40 msec of the QRS complex and ST segment of each signal-averaged X, Y, and Z lead.[53] The region of interest is identified with the use of the computer graphics cursor and standard electrocardiographic criteria. To enhance frequency resolution, FFT analysis is performed on the terminal QRS and ST segment as a single unit. This region of interest is multiplied by a four-term Blackman-Harris window to reduce spectral leakage. The averaged signal is scaled before computation of the FFT to reduce variations in the magnitude of the transformed data by scaling the maximum magnitude to unity. A 512-point FFT is calculated. Transformed data are expressed as a FFT magnitude and plotted on a scale defined by the maximum value of the data. To detect smaller peaks that might be obscured by the dominant amplitudes of low-frequency components, a second plot is generated by dividing the initial scale by 10. Values exceeding those on the reduced scale are analyzed but not plotted. For each magnitude versus frequency plot, three parameters are defined by the computer system. First, the data are analyzed for amplitude peaks between 20 and 50 Hz. Peaks are defined by an increase in magnitude for at least two points followed by a decreased in magnitude for at least one point. A frequency range of 20 to 50 Hz was chosen based on results of previous studies. Second, each peak amplitude is divided by the maximum magnitude of the entire signal (peak magnitude ratio). This ratio is computed to determine the relative proportion of frequencies between 20 and 50 Hz that comprise the terminal 40 msec of the QRS complex and ST segment, an approach shown previously to reduce the influence of signal duration on results in normal subjects. For patient-to-patient comparisons, the individual X, Y, and Z values for the peak magnitude and area ratios are averaged arithmetically. The mean peak frequency magnitude is multiplied by 1×10^4 and the mean area ratio is multiplied by 1×10^3 to facilitate graphic display.

The reproducibility of the results of frequency analysis of signal-averaged ECGs from normal subjects and patients with sustained VT are shown in Figure 9. Two separate recordings were made within an interval of 30 minutes and the results compared. Results demonstrate only modest changes in values for the 20–50/10–50 Hz ratio. Pearson's correlation coefficient is 0.94 for area ratio values and 0.81 for peak magnitude ratio values. Importantly, by the established criteria to distinguish normal (area ratio ≤ 107, peak frequency magnitude ≤ 150) from abnormal frequency content, none of the FFT values obtained from this group of patients resulted in a change of classification. The reproducibility in this sample size yields 95% certainty that the actual population reproducibility of the normal-abnormal classification exceeds 87% for recordings that are not subject to changes in lead position or temporal variation.

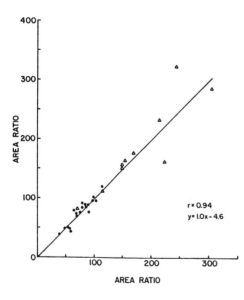

Figure 9. Comparison of the values for the area ratio obtained during two separate recordings made within an interval of 30 minutes from 19 normal subjects, shown by the closed circles, and from 10 patients with sustained VT, shown by the open triangles (r = 0.94). Importantly, by the established criteria to distinguish normal from abnormal frequency content, none of the FFT values obtained resulted in a change of patient classification. Δ = VT; • Normal subjects.

Clinical Studies

Qualitative Differences in Frequency Content

Prior to performing studies in patients, the signal processing system was validated by analyzing test signals of known amplitudes and frequency.[46,47] During initial studies in patients, FFT analysis was performed on the entire QRS complex, the terminal 40 msec of the QRS complex, the ST segment, and the T wave of each signal-averaged X, Y, and Z ECG lead. Results demonstrated a significant (p < 0.0001) increase in high-frequency components in the terminal 40 msec of the QRS complex and of the ST segment of sinus beats from patients with histories of prior myocardial infarction, and subsequent sustained VT when compared with results from patients with prior infarction without sustained VT and with those from normal subjects. Representative plots of results of FFT analysis of the terminal QRS complex and of the ST segment from a signal-averaged Y lead from a patient with and from one without sustained VT are shown in Figure 10. The major differences in the terminal QRS and the ST segment were observed at frequencies < 120 Hz.

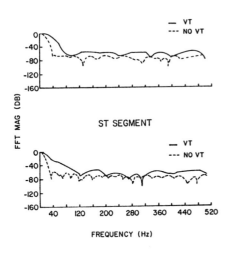

Figure 10. Representative spectral plots of the terminal QRS complexes (top panel) and the ST segments (bottom panel) from a patient with prior myocardial infarction and sustained VT (solid curves) and from a patient with prior infraction without VT (broken curve). Shown in each panel are power versus frequency plots of signal-averaged ECGs recorded from a bipolar Y lead. Distinguishing qualitative features in the frequency content of the terminal QRS and ST segment between the two patients are apparent.

With this approach, there were no significant differences in the high-frequency content of the entire QRS complex or T wave among the three patient groups.

Quantitative Analysis of Frequency Content

The results of more quantitative analysis of the terminal QRS and ST segments from patients with sustained VT demonstrated a greater proportion of components in the 20- to 50-Hz range compared with the proportion in corresponding ECG segments from patients without VT.[48]

Figure 11 illustrates the power spectral density computed with the energy spectrum of the terminal QRS and ST segment from a patient with and from a patient without sustained VT. In these studies, the data are expressed as a ratio of the area under the spectral plot between 20 to 50 Hz divided by the area under the spectral plot between 0 to 20 Hz and as a magnitude ratio that

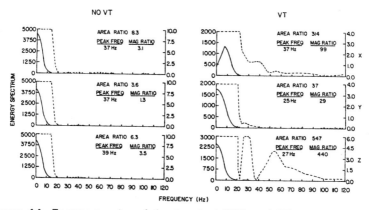

Figure 11. Energy spectra of the terminal QRS and ST segments from a patient with prior myocardial infarction and sustained VT (right) and from a patient with prior infarction without sustained VT (left). Shown in each panel are the initial (left scale) and magnified (right scale) energy versus frequency plots of the terminal QRS and ST segment of signal-averaged X, Y, and Z ECG leads, values for the area ratio, peak frequencies, and values for the magnitude ratios. In each lead, the combined terminal QRS and ST segment from the patient with VT contains a 10- to 100-fold greater proportion of components in the 20- to 50-Hz range compared with corresponding values from the patients without VT.

quantifies the relative magnitudes of frequency peaks identified between 20 to 50 Hz. In each lead, the terminal QRS and ST segment from the patient with VT contains a 10- to 100-fold greater proportion of frequencies in the 20- to 50-Hz range compared with corresponding values from the patient without VT. Importantly, these distinguishing features are independent of QRS duration, left ventricular ejection fraction, or complexity of spontaneous ventricular ectopy.

Figure 12 illustrates the mean peak frequencies detected between 20 to 50 Hz and the corresponding magnitude ratios in the terminal QRS and ST segment from patients with and without VT

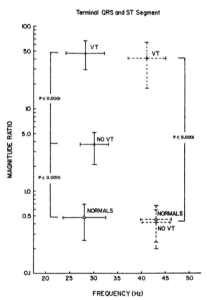

Figure 12. Peak frequencies between 20 and 50 Hz and values for the magnitude ratios for patients with prior infarction who had sustained VT (dots), patients with prior infarction without sustained VT (circles), and normal subjects (triangles). Two frequency peaks (solid and broken lines) were detected regularly in each group. There were no significant differences in the distribution of components defined by peak frequencies between patients with and without sustained VT. However, the relative contribution of the amplitudes of components to the overall magnitude of the spectral plot of the terminal QRS and ST segments of patients with sustained VT was ten- to one hundred-fold greater for components in the 20- to 50-Hz range in patients with sustained VT. (Reproduced with permission from Cain et al, Am J Cardiol 55:1500, 1985.)

and from normal subjects. There were no significant differences in the peak frequencies among patients in the three groups. However, the relative contribution of the magnitudes of these peak frequencies to the overall magnitude of the spectrum of the terminal QRS and ST segments differed significantly (p < 0.0001). No frequencies above 50 Hz contributed substantially to the ECG segments in any group. Thus, differences in the power spectral density of the terminal QRS/ST segment from patients with and without sustained VT do not result primarily from differences in the frequencies of components, but instead are attributable primarily to differences in the amplitudes of components within a relatively narrow range of frequencies.

Detection of Vulnerability to Sustained VT

To test the hypothesis that FFT results would improve selection of patients for programmed ventricular stimulation, FFTs of signal-averaged ECGs were obtained prospectively from patients with spontaneous sustained VT, patients with nonsustained VT, and patients with syncope, and results were compared with those of programmed stimulation.[50] Representative FFT magnitudes of the terminal QRS and ST segments from two patients who had nonsustained VT clinically are shown in Figure 13. In each lead, the terminal QRS and ST segment from the patient in whom sustained monomorphic VT was induced during programmed ventricular stimulation contains relatively more high-frequency components than the complex from the patient in whom sustained VT was not induced. Overall, the results of FFT analysis correctly predicted the response to programmed stimulation in 88% of patients studied and in 82% of patients with nonsustained VT or syncope. The sensitivity of the prediction of inducibility was 100%, and specificity was 77%. Results of multivariate analysis demonstrated that results of FFT analysis were independent of other determinants of inducibility, including left ventricular ejection fraction and prior myocardial infarction. Thus, this approach offers promise for improving the identification of patients in whom sustained VT will be induced during programmed ventricular stimulation.

Bundle Branch Block During Sinus Rhythm

Studies were performed in 28 normal subjects (group I) and 141 patients grouped according to clinical characteristics.[53] Group II

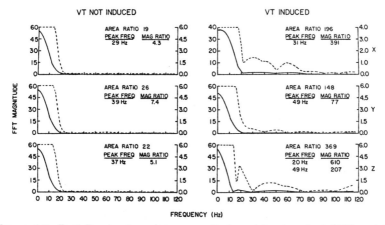

Figure 13. Fast Fourier transform magnitudes of the terminal QRS and ST segments from a patient having nonsustained VT clinically in whom sustained VT was induced during programmed ventricular stimulation (right), and from a patient having nonsustained VT clinically in whom sustained VT was not induced (left). Shown in each panel are the initial (left scale, solid curve) and magnified (right scale, broken curve) magnitude versus frequency plots of the terminal 40 msec of the QRS complex and ST segment of signal-averaged X, Y, and Z ECG leads, values for the area ratio (20–50 Hz/10–50 Hz), frequency peaks if detected, and peak magnitude ratio. To facilitate graphic display, values for the area ratio and peak magnitude ratio have been multiplied by constants.

comprised 40 patients with prior myocardial infarction without sustained VT, in whom the QRS duration during sinus rhythm was <120 msec. Group III included 21 patients with organic heart disease without a history of sustained VT whose ECG during sinus rhythm demonstrated a QRS duration of 120 msec or greater. Left bundle branch block was present in the ECGs from 6 patients, right bundle branch block in 11, and a nonspecific intraventricular conduction delay in 4. Group IV included 43 consecutive patients referred to the arrhythmia service at Barnes Hospital with a history of spontaneous sustained VT in whom the QRS duration during sinus rhythm was <120 msec. Group V comprised 37 consecutive patients with a history of spontaneous sustained VT having ECGs with QRS durations during sinus rhythm of 120 msec or greater. Left bundle branch block was present in the ECGs from 13 patients, right bundle branch block in 11, and nonspecific intraventricular conduction delays in 13.

Studies were performed first in normal subjects to define the normal range of area ratio and peak magnitude values. Values for the individual mean XYZ area and peak magnitude ratios in these 28 normal subjects are illustrated in Figures 14 and 15, along with those from the other four study groups. As demonstrated, values of the mean area ratio from normal subjects have a normal distribution (mean 73 ± 20). An abnormal area ratio value was defined based on a one-sided upper confidence limit for which only high values are abnormal, as that exceeding the mean plus 1.65 times the standard deviation (abnormal value > 107). Values for the peak magnitude ratio of normal subjects demonstrated a nonnormal distribution (mean 51 ± 38). These values were ordered, and by the theory of ordered statistics, the maximum value was found to be the best estimate of the 95th percentile. Accordingly, peak magnitude ratios exceeding a value of 150 were defined as abnormal. Results derived from normal subjects were then applied to patients in the other four study groups. Overall, results of FFT analysis were defined as abnormal if either the mean area ratio or mean peak magnitude ratio was abnormal.

Representative magnitude versus frequency plots from patients in groups II and III, and from patients in groups IV and V are shown in Figures 16 and 17, respectively. Overall, as summarized in Figure 18, the FFT magnitude was abnormal in 4% of normal subjects, 20% of those without sustained VT or QRS prolongation, and 19% of those without VT whose QRS duration during sinus rhythm was 120 msec or greater. There were no significant differences in the percentage of normal subjects with an abnormal frequency content compared with those in group II or III. Among patients with sustained VT, the FFT magnitude was abnormal in 91% of those with a QRS duration <120 msec and 95% of those with a QRS duration of 120 msec or greater. The percentage of patients with an abnormal frequency content in groups IV and V was significantly different from that observed in either group II or III (p <0.001). Within groups III and V, the type of conduction abnormality (left bundle branch block, right bundle branch block, nonspecific intraventricular conduction delay) did not affect results. Moreover, results were independent of QRS duration (Figure 19) and independent of the duration of the signal analyzed (Figure 20). Thus, differentiation of patients with and without sustained VT by means of indices derived from the FFT magnitude can be performed accurately over a wide range of physiologic and pathologic QRS durations and ST segment lengths.

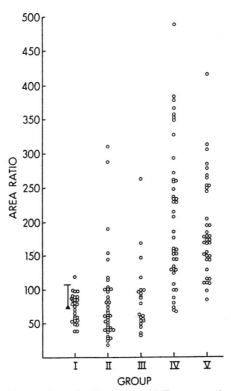

Figure 14. Individual values for the mean XYZ area ratio from 28 normal subjects (group I), and 40 patients with prior myocardial infarction without sustained VT in whom the QRS duration during sinus rhythm was < 120 msec (group II), 21 patients with organic heart disease without a history of sustained VT whose ECG during sinus rhythm demonstrated a QRS duration of 120 msec or greater (group III), 43 patients with sustained VT in whom the QRS duration during sinus rhythm was < 120 msec (group IV), and 37 patients with sustained VT having ECGs with QRS durations during sinus rhythm of 120 msec or greater (group V). In group I, values for the area ratio had a normal distribution. The closed triangle represents the mean XYZ area ratio for this group. An abnormal area ratio was defined as a value exceeding 1.65 times the standard deviation and is demarcated by the vertical line (abnormal area ratio > 107). (Reproduced with permission of the American Heart Association, from Lindsay et al, Circulation 77:122, 1988.)

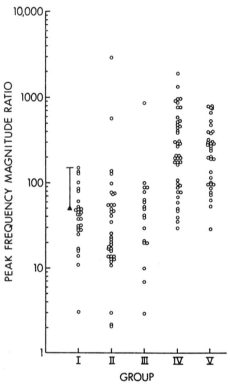

Figure 15. Individual values for the peak frequency magnitude ratio from 28 normal subjects (group I) and from 141 patients. Groups II to V are the same as those defined in Figure 14. In group I, the values for the mean peak magnitude, shown on a logarithmic scale, had a nonnormal distribution. The values in group I were ordered and the maximum value was found to be the best estimate of the 95th percentile. Peak magnitudes above this value (vertical line) were defined as abnormal (abnormal peak magnitude > 150). (Reproduced with permission of the American Heart Association, from Lindsay et al, *Circulation* 77:122, 1988.)

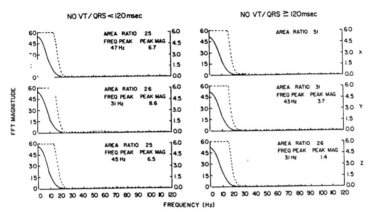

Figure 16. Fast Fourier transform magnitudes of the terminal QRS and ST segments from a patient without sustained VT having a right bundle branch block during sinus rhythm (right), and from a patient without sustained VT or QRS prolongation (left). Data are displayed in a format similar to that used in Figure 13. In each lead, values for the area ratio and peak magnitude ratio are normal irrespective of the presence or absence of bundle branch block. (Reproduced with permission of the American Heart Association, from Lindsay et al, Circulation 77:122, 1988.)

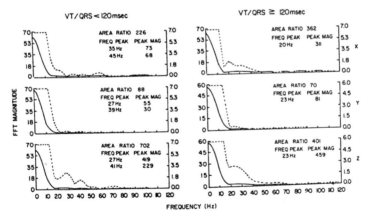

Figure 17. Fast Fourier transform magnitudes of the terminal QRS and ST segments during sinus rhythm from a patient with sustained VT having right bundle branch block (right), and from a patient with sustained VT without QRS prolongation (left). Data are displayed in a format similar to that used in Figure 13. Increased contributions of frequencies between 20 and 50 Hz are evident in the plots from both patients, particularly in the X and Z leads. (Reproduced with permission of the American Heart Association, from Lindsay et al, Circulation 77:122, 1988.)

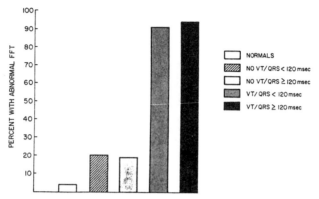

Figure 18. Comparison of the percentage of patients in each of the five groups with abnormal FFT results. Results are shown from left to right in normal subjects (group I), patients without VT having a QRS duration during sinus rhythm <120 msec (group II) or ≥120 msec (group III), and patients with sustained VT having QRS durations during sinus rhythm <120 msec (group IV) or ≥120 msec (group V). (Reproduced with permission of the American Heart Association, from Lindsay et al, Circulation 77:122, 1988.)

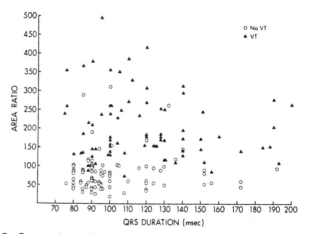

Figure 19. Comparison of values for the area ratio and QRS duration. Patients with a history of sustained VT are depicted by closed triangles, and patients without VT are depicted by open circles. As shown, values for the area ratio are independent of QRS duration. (Reproduced with permission of the American Heart Association, from Lindsay et al, Circulation 77:122, 1988.)

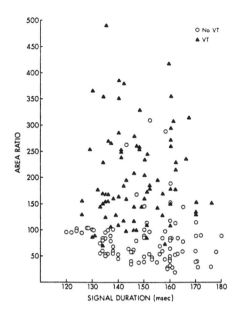

Figure 20. Comparison of values for the area ratio and duration of the signal analyzed. Patients with a history of sustained VT are depicted by closed triangles, and patients without VT are depicted by open circles. As shown, values for the area ratio are independent of the duration of the data signal analyzed. (Reproduced with permission of the American Heart Association, from Lindsay et al, Circulation 77:122, 1988.)

Frequency Domain Versus Time Domain

Results of studies in the time domain using signal processing techniques developed by several investigators have demonstrated characteristic features that differentiate patients with from those without sustained VT.[38-45] Signal processing systems have now become commercially available. We prospectively compared, in the same group of patients, the results of frequency analysis of signal-averaged ECGs with those obtained in the time domain from a commercially available device.[62]

Twenty-six patients having sustained VT or VF were studied. Most had a history of remote myocardial infarction. The locus of the infarct was anterior in 13 patients and inferior in 7. Six had a nonischemic cardiomyopathy. The mean left ventricular ejection fraction was 35%. Seventeen normal subjects were also evaluated. In each, signal-averaged ECGs were analyzed in the frequency and time domains and results compared.

For frequency analysis, Frank X, Y, and Z leads were recorded and averaged. The transformed data were expressed as a FFT magnitude.[53] For time-domain analysis, bipolar X, Y, and Z ECG leads were recorded, averaged, and combined into a vector magnitude using the Arrhythmia Research Technology Model 101PCD signal processing system. The vector magnitude was analyzed for filter QRS duration, the duration of signals < 40 µV in amplitude, and the root mean square voltage in the terminal 40 msec of the QRS complex. Analysis was performed using both a 25-Hz and a 40-Hz high-pass filter. QRS complexes were averaged until diastolic noise was below 1 µV.

The results obtained from normal subjects and from patients with sustained VT with both methods are summarized in Table III. Overall, 6% of normal subjects had either an abnormal area ratio or peak magnitude value. For time-domain studies, a filtered QRS duration > 110 msec, a duration of low amplitude signal duration > 40 msec, and a root mean square voltage of < 25 µV were defined as abnormal. When a 25-Hz high-pass filter was used, 24% of normal subjects demonstrated at least one abnormal index. No subject, however, had both an abnormal filtered QRS duration and a root mean square voltage. When analyzed with a 40-Hz high-pass filter, 0% to 18% of normal subjects had an abnormal index.

Comparisons of the results of frequency- and time-domain analysis from two patients with a history of sustained VT are shown in Figures 21 and 22. Overall, 89% of patients with VT had abnormal FFT magnitudes (Table III). In contrast, when data were analyzed with a 25-Hz high-pass filter, 69% of patients demonstrated at least one abnormal index. Only 31% had both an abnormal filtered QRS duration and root mean square voltage. With analysis after use of a 40-Hz high-pass filter, 40% to 82% of patients appeared to be abnormal.

Patients in whom results of analysis in the frequency- and time-domains were discordant (Figure 22), often exhibited abnormal frequency components in one or two of the ECG leads suggesting that analysis of multiple ECG leads individually is superior to analysis of derived signals including the vector magnitude. This concept has been reinforced by the results of a recent study performed to determine the extent to which FFT analysis of individual X, Y, and Z ECG leads and of the vector magnitude contributes to the differentiation of patients with from those without sustained VT.[54] Spectra of the X lead, the Y lead, and the Z lead, the vector magnitude, and the mean XYZ results were significantly different in patients with VT compared to results from normal subjects and patients without VT (p < 0.001). Results were abnormal in multiple leads from 71% of patients with VT and from only 5% of normal subjects (p < 0.0001). In many patients with VT, abnormalities were identified in two of the three leads indicating a selective spatial distribution of altered ECG

Table III
Comparison of Results in the Time
and Frequency Domains

Results in Normal Subjects

Frequency Domain

Index	% Abnormal
20–50/10–50 Hz	6%
Peak Magnitude	0%
Either	6%

Time Domain

Index	% Abnormal (25–250 Hz)	% Abnormal (40–250 Hz)
QRSD >110 msec	12%	0%
HFD >40 msec	6%	12%
HFRMSA <25 µV	12%	18%
QRSD or HFD or HFRMSA	24%	12%
QRSD and HFRMSA	0%	0%

Results in Patients with VT/VF

Frequency Domain

Index	% Abnormal
20–50/10–50 Hz	85%
Peak Magnitude	62%
Either	89%

Time Domain

Index	% Abnormal (25–250 Hz)	% Abnormal (40–250 Hz)
QRSD >110 msec	58%	68%
HFD >40 msec	27%	41%
HFRMSA <25 µV	27%	68%
QRSD or HFD or HFRMSA	69%	82%
QRSD and HFRMSA	31%	55%

HFD = duration of the high-frequency components in terminal 40 msec of filtered QRS; HFRMSA = root mean square voltage in terminal 40 msec of filtered QRS; QRSD = QRS duration.

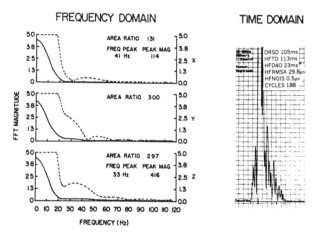

Figure 21. Comparison of the results of frequency- and time-domain analysis from a patient with sustained VT. Results are concordant. Analysis of the FFT magnitudes demonstrated an abnormal contribution of 20- to 50-Hz frequencies in each lead. Abnormal time-domain indices included a filtered QRS duration of 138 msec, a low amplitude signal duration of 52 msec, and a root mean square voltage of 10.4 μV.

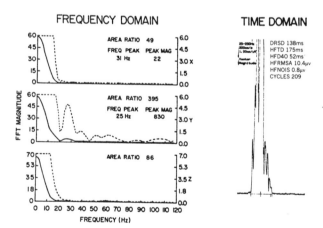

Figure 22. Comparison of the results of frequency- and time-domain analysis from another patient with sustained VT. Results are discordant. The mean FFT magnitude is abnormal, primarily because of profound abnormalities in the signal-averaged Y lead. Results of analysis in the time-domain, however, are normal for all indices.

signals that elicit abnormal frequency components. The specific lead or number of leads abnormal was independent of the locus of infarction. Differentiation of patient groups was best achieved by combining results obtained from individual X, Y, and Z ECGs when compared to results based on analysis of each lead alone or of the vector magnitude. These results support our approach of analyzing multiple ECG leads and making patient-to-patient comparisons based on mean XYZ results.

These results demonstrate that frequency analysis with the approach under development provides better differentiation of patients with and without sustained VT compared with time-domain analysis with a commercially available processing system. Overall, 91% of individuals in this study were classified correctly with the use of frequency analysis. In contrast, only 58% and 74% of individuals were classified correctly with the use of time domain when a 25-Hz or 40-Hz high-pass filter was used. Differences between the two techniques were most apparent for patients with VT and prior anterior myocardial infarction.

On the other hand, such comparisons using commercially available systems typify the limitations encountered in studies purported to establish the superiority of one approach over that of another.[63,64] The Arrhythmia Research Technology Model 101PCD is patterned after but not identical to that developed initially by Simson.[42] Our results in the time domain are comparable to those reported by others using the 101PCD device[63,64] but not as good as those reported in studies in which the original device developed by Simson was employed.[42,43] Thus, comparisons using currently available commercial systems cannot determine whether discrepancies of results are due to problems with data processing or conceptual deficiencies of the overall method. Furthermore, time-domain analysis is performed on the vector magnitude computed from bipolar, orthogonal ECG leads. In contrast, in our laboratory, frequency analysis is performed on Frank X, Y, and Z ECG leads individually.

Similar issues are pertinent to interpreting studies in which frequency analysis has been performed using commercially available systems designed for analysis in the time domain.[63,64] The frequency content of ECG signals is spatially variable and thus lead dependent.[65] Results of spectral analysis of Frank XYZ ECG signals may not be comparable to results of spectral analysis of bipolar XYZ ECG signals. Moreover, the frequency content of ECG signals recorded with commercial units equipped with nonlinear (four-pole Butterworth) and notch filters known to distort phase and magnitude information[56] is not comparable to that of ECG signals recorded in the absence of these perturbations. The Fourier transform is unique since for each time-domain representation there is one and only one frequency-domain presentation. In instances of a discrepancy between the results of frequency- and time-domain analysis of the same ECG signals, suboptimal data recording or an inadequate analytic method must be assumed because no information is lost in changing from one domain to another.

Summary

Frequency analysis of signal-averaged Frank X, Y, and Z ECGs is an accurate, noninvasive method for distinguishing patients with prior myocardial infarction with from those without sustained ventricular arrhythmias.[46,48,53,54] Altered frequency components have been detected in ECGs from 93% of patients with prior infarction and subsequent sustained VT, 20% of those with prior infarction without documented sustained VT, and 4% of normal subjects. Moreover, results are not affected by the presence of bundle branch block during sinus rhythm.[53] The power of frequency analysis in distinguishing patients with and without sustained VT has been reported by others.[66] In addition, this approach is a sensitive method for identifying patients who have sustained VT induced during programmed stimulation.[50] Importantly, FFT results are independent of more conventional determinants of prognosis and inducibility.[46,48] Results of pilot studies have demonstrated that frequency analysis of signal-averaged ECGs offers promise as a noninvasive method to stratify risk for developing sustained VT in patients convalescing from acute myocardial infarction,[67] distinguish patients with noninvasive cardiomyopathy having sustained VT,[68] and to assess the efficacy of antiarrhythmic drugs.[69]

Methods of frequency analysis of signal-averaged ECGs have evolved from qualitative to more quantitative techniques having broad clinical applicability. In the studies cited, spectral estimates computed from the FFT of the terminal QRS complex and ST segment have been the major focus to permit us to compare our results with those of others using time-domain procedures. The area and peak magnitude ratios are indices derived from the FFT magnitude that, to date, best distinguish patients with from those without sustained VT.

These findings indicate that abnormal FFT results reflect an anatomic/electrophysiologic substrate conducive to the development of sustained VT or VF. Results of studies using signal processing systems in the time domain have demonstrated a correlation between abnormal late potentials detected in the signal-averaged ECG and delayed ventricular activation detected during the course of epicardial mapping.[38,39,57] Delineation of the pathophysiologic determinants of the altered frequency components in ECG signals from patients with sustained VT is paramount to determining its optimal clinical application. Studies are in progress in our laboratory utilizing a computer mapping system[70,71] and morphometric analytic techniques[29] to define the anatomic/electrophysiologic substrate responsible for the genesis of the altered frequencies detected by FFT analysis of the terminal QRS and ST segments of signal-averaged ECGs. Although delayed ventricular activation is likely to be responsible in part for the differences in frequency content between patients with and without sustained VT, our finding that results are independent of QRS width suggests that derangements in ventricular conduction in addition to the total duration of ventricular activation contribute to the generation of abnormal frequency components.[53] Heterogeneity in the pattern and phase of ventricular activation caused by the concomitant excitation of normal myocardium and myocardium that has undergone infarction will generate QRS complexes resulting from more heterogeneous activation even though the total duration of ventricular activation may be comparable to that of ventricles from patients without VT or VF. Accordingly, late potentials may not be the only hallmark of an anatomic/electrophysiologic substrate conducive to the development of sustained ventricular arrhythmias; and such a substrate may be present despite the absence of late potentials. Results of our studies comparing time- and frequency-domain techniques in the same patients help support these assumptions.[62] Moreover, methods of spectral estimation in addition to the FFT should be of value in further defining the temporal aspects of the altered frequency components detected in ECG signals from patients with life-threatening ventricular arrhythmias.[72]

Each year more than 400,000 Americans die suddenly from sustained ventricular arrhythmias. Interrogation of ECG signals by signal processing techniques in the frequency domain offers promise as a noninvasive method of improved identification of patients at high risk for VT or VF and more specific selection of patients who may benefit from prophylactic antiarrhythmic therapy.

Acknowledgment: This work was supported in part by NIH Grant HL 17646, SCOR in Ischemic Heart Disease.

References

1. Tominaga S, Blackburn H: The Coronary Drug Project Research Group: prognostic importance of premature beats following myocardial infarction. J Am Med Assoc 223:116, 1973.
2. Schulze RA Jr, Strauss HW, Pitt B: Sudden death in the year following myocardial infarction: relation to ventricular premature contractions in the late hospital phase and left ventricular ejection fraction. Am J Med 62:192, 1977.
3. Vismara SA, Vera A, Foerster JM, Amsterdam IA, Mason DT: Identification of sudden death risk factors in acute and chronic coronary artery disease. Am J Cardiol 39:821, 1977.
4. Anderson KP, DeCamilla J, Moss AJ: Clinical significance of ventricular tachycardia (3 beats or longer) detected during ambulatory monitoring after myocardial infarction. Circulation 57:890, 1977.
5. Moss AJ, Davis HT, DeCamilla J, Bayer LW: Ventricular ectopic beats and their relation to sudden and nonsudden cardiac death after myocardial infarction. Circulation 60:998, 1980.
6. Kleiger RE, Miller JP, Thanavaro S, Province MA, Martin TF, Oliver GC: Relationships between clinical features of acute myocardial infarction and ventricular runs 2 weeks to 1 year after infarction. Circulation 63:64, 1981.
7. Ruberman W, Weinblatt E, Goldberg JD, Frank CW, Chaudhary BS, Shapiro S: Ventricular premature complexes and sudden death after myocardial infarction. Circulation 64:297, 1981.
8. Moss AJ, The Multicenter Postinfarction Research Group: Risk stratification and survival after myocardial infarction: the Multicenter Postinfarction Research Group. N Engl J Med 309:331, 1983.
9. Bigger JT Jr, Fleiss JL, Kleiger R, Miller JP, Rolnitzky LM: The relationships among ventricular arrhythmias, left ventricular dysfunction, and mortality in the 2 years after myocardial infarction. Circulation 69:250, 1984.
10. Mukharji J, Rude RE, Poole WK, Gustafson N, Thomas LJ, Strauss HW, Jaffe AS, Muller JE, Roberts R, Raabe DS, Croft CH, Passamani E, Braunwald E, Willerson JT, the Milis Study Group: Risk factors for sudden death after acute myocardial infarction: two-year follow-up. Am J Cardiol 54:31, 1984.
11. Maisel AS, Scott N, Gilpin E, Ahnve S, LeWinter M, Henning H, Collins D, Ross J: Complex ventricular arrhythmias in patients with Q wave versus non Q wave myocardial infarction. Circulation 72:963, 1985.
12. Kostis JB, Byington R, Friedman LM, Goldstein S, Furberg C: Prognostic significance of ventricular ectopic activity in survivors of acute myocardial infarction. J Am Coll Cardiol 10:231, 1987.
13. Collaborative Group: Phenytoin after recovery from myocardial infarction: controlled trial in 568 patients. Lancet 2:1055, 1971.

14. Peter T, Ross D, Duffield A, Luton M, Harper R, Hunt D, Sloman G: Effect on survival after myocardial infarction of long-term treatment with phenytoin. Br Heart J 40:1356, 1978.

15. Hugenholtz PG, Hagemeijer F, Lubsen J, Glazer B, Van Durme JP, Bogaert MG: One year follow-up in patients with persistent ventricular dysrhythmias after myocardial infarction treated with aprindine or placebo. In Sandoe E, Julian DG, Pell JW (eds): Management of Ventricular Tachycardia: Role of Mexiletine. Amsterdam: Excerpta Medica, 1978, pp. 572–578.

16. Bastian BC, MacFarlane PW, McLaughlan JH, Ballantyne D, Clark R, Hillis WS, Rae AP, Hutton I: A prospective randomized trial of tocainide in patients following myocardial infarction. Am Heart J 100:1017, 1980.

17. Chamberlain DA, Julian DG, Boyle D, Jewitt DE, Campbell RWF, Shanks RG: Oral mexiletine in high-risk patients after myocardial infarction. Lancet 2:1324, 1980.

18. Ryden L, Arnman K, Conradson TB, Hofvendahl S, Mortensen O, Smedgard P: Prophylaxis of ventricular tachyarrhythmias with intravenous and oral tocainide in patients with and recovering from acute myocardial infarction. Am Heart J 100:1006, 1980.

19. Impact Research Group: International mexiletine and placebo antiarrhythmic coronary trial: I. Report on arrhythmias and other findings. J Am Coll Cardiol 4:1148, 1984.

20. Gottlieb SH, Achuff SC, Mellits ED, Gerstenblith G, Baughman KL, Becker L, Chandra NC, Henley S, Humphries JO, Heck C, Kennedy MM, Weisfeldt ML, Reid PR: Prophylactic antiarrhythmic therapy of high-risk survivors of myocardial infarction: lower mortality at 1 month but not at 1 year. Circulation 75:792, 1987.

21. El-Sherif N, Scherlag BJ, Lazzara R, Hope RR: Reentrant ventricular arrhythmias in the late myocardial infarction period. I. Conduction characteristics in the infarction zone. Circulation 55:686, 1977.

22. Karaguezian HS, Fenoglio JJ, Weiss MB, Wit Al: Protracted ventricular tachycardia induced by premature stimulation of the canine heart after coronary artery occlusion and reperfusion. Circ Res 44:833, 1979.

23. Michelson EL, Spear JF, Moore EN: Electrophysiologic and anatomic correlates of sustained ventricular tachyarrhythmias in a model of chronic myocardial infarction. Am J Cardiol 45:583, 1980.

24. El-Sherif N, Smith RA, Evans K: Canine ventricular arrhythmias in the late myocardial infarction period. 8. Epicardial mapping of reentrant circuits. Circ Res 49:255, 1981.

25. Wit AL, Allessie MA, Bonke FIM, Lammers W, Smeets J, Fenoglio JJ: Electrophysiologic mapping to determine the mechanism of experimental ventricular tachycardia initiated by premature impulses. Experimental approach and initial results demonstrating reentrant excitation. Am J Cardiol 49:166, 1982.

26. Mehra R, Zeiler R, Gough WB, El-Sherif N: Reentrant ventricular arrhythmias in the late myocardial infarction period. 9. Electrophysiologic-anatomic correlation of reentrant circuits. Circulation 67:11, 1983.

27. El-Sherif N, Mehra R, Gough WB, Zeiler RH: Reentrant ventricular arrhythmias in the late myocardial infarction period. Interruption of

reentrant circuits by cryothermal techniques. Circulation 68:644, 1983.

28. Cardinal R, Savard P, Carson DL, Perry JB: Mapping of ventricular tachycardia induced by programmed stimulation in canine preparations of myocardial infarction. Circulation 70:136, 1984.

29. Kramer JB, Saffitz JE, Witkowski FX, Corr PB: Intramural reentry as a mechanism of ventricular tachycardia during evolving canine myocardial infarction. Circ Res 56:736, 1985.

30. Wellens HJJ, Duren DR, Lie KI: Observations on the mechanisms of ventricular tachycardia in man. Circulation 54:237, 1976.

31. Josephson ME, Horowitz LN, Farshidi A, Kastor JA: Recurrent sustained ventricular tachycardia. 1. Mechanisms. Circulation 57:431, 1978.

32. Josephson ME, Horowitz LN, Farshidi A: Continuous local electrical activity: a mechanism of recurrent ventricular tachycardia. Circulation 57:659, 1978.

33. Josephson ME, Horowitz LN, Farshidi A, Spielman SR, Michelson EL, Greenspan AM: Sustained ventricular tachycardia: evidence for protected localized reentry. Am J Cardiol 42:416, 1978.

34. Josephson ME, Spielman SR, Greenspan AM, Horowitz LN: Mechanism of ventricular fibrillation in man. Observations based on electrode catheter recordings. Am J Cardiol 44:623, 1979.

35. Almendral JM, Gottlieb CD, Rosenthal ME, Stamato NJ, Buxton AE, Marchlinski FE, Miller JM, Josephson ME: Entrainment of ventricular tachycardia: explanation for surface electrocardiographic phenomena by analysis of electrograms recorded within the tachycardia circuit. Circulation 77:569, 1988.

36. DeBakker JMT, VanCapelle FJL, Janse MJ, Wilde AAM, Coronel R, Becker AE, Dingeman KP, VanHemel NM, Hauer RNW: Reentry as a cause of ventricular tachycardia in patients with chronic ischemic heart disease: electrophysiologic and anatomic correlation. Circulation 77: 589, 1988.

37. Hoyt RH, Pogwizd SM, Corr PB, Cain ME, Cox JL, Saffitz JE: Electrophysiologic and morhologic determinants of intramural reentry in human ventricular tachycardia (abstr). J Am Coll Cardiol 11:113A, 1988.

38. Berbari EJ, Scherlag BJ, Hope RR, Lazzara R: Recording from the body surface of arrhythmogenic ventricular activity during the S-T segment. Am J Cardiol 41:697, 1978.

39. Simson MB, Euler D, Michelson EL, Falcone RA, Spear JF, Moore EN: Detection of delayed ventricular activation on the body surface in dogs. Am J Physiol 241:H363, 1981.

40. Breithardt G, Becker R, Seipel L, Abendroth RR, Ostermeyer J: Noninvasive detection of late potentials in man: a new marker for ventricular tachycardia. Eur Heart J 2:1, 1981.

41. Rozanski JJ, Mortara D, Myerburg RF, Castellanos A: Body surface detection of delayed depolarizations in patients with recurrent ventricular tachycardia and left ventricular aneurysm. Circulation 63:1172, 1981.

42. Simson MB: Use of signals in the terminal QRS complex to identify patients with ventricular tachycardia after myocardial infarction. Circulation 64:235, 1981.

43. Denes P, Santarelli P, Hauser RG, Uretz EF: Quantitative analysis of the high-frequency components of the terminal portion of the body surface QRS in normal subjects and in patients with ventricular tachycardia. Circulation 67:1129, 1983.
44. Kanovsky MS, Falcone RA, Dresden CA, Josephson ME, Simson MB: Identification of patients with ventricular tachycardia after myocardial infarction: signal-averaged electrocardiogram, Holter monitoring, and cardiac catheterization. Circulation 70:264, 1984.
45. Freedman RA, Gillis AM, Keren A, Soderholm-Difatte V, Mason JW: Signal-averaged electrocardiographic late potentials in patients with ventricular fibrillation or ventricular tachycardia: correlation with clinical arrhythmia and electrophysiologic study. Am J Cardiol 55:1350, 1985.
46. Cain ME, Ambos HD, Witkowski FX, Sobel BE: Fast Fourier transform analysis of signal-averaged electrocardiograms for identification of patients prone to sustained ventricular tachycardia. Circulation 69:711, 1984.
47. Ambos HD, Markham J, Cain ME: Use of fast Fourier transform analysis to detect patients prone to sustained ventricular arrhythmias. In: Computers in Cardiology. Los Angeles: IEEE Computer Society Press, 1984, pp. 181–184.
48. Cain ME, Ambos HD, Markham J, Fischer AE, Sobel BE: Quantification of differences in frequency content of signal-averaged electrocardiograms between patients with and without sustained ventricular tachycardia. Am J Cardiol 55:1500, 1985.
49. Cain ME, Ambos HD. Detection of patients with malignant ventricular arrhythmia by frequency analysis of signal-averaged electrocardiograms. In: Computerized Interpretation of the Electrocardiogram—Proceedings of the 1984 Engineering Foundation Conference. New York: Engineering Foundation, 1985, pp. 51–63.
50. Lindsay BD, Ambos HD, Schechtman KB, Cain ME: Improved selection of patients for programmed ventricular stimulation by frequency analysis of signal-averaged electrocardiograms. Circulation 73:675, 1986.
51. Cain ME, Ambos HD, Lindsay BD: Fast-Fourier transform analysis of the signal-averaged electrocardiogram in the management of patients with or prone to ventricular tachycardia or fibrillation. In Brugada P, Wellens HJJ (eds): Cardiac Arrhythmias: Where to Go from Here? Mount Kisco, NY: Futura Publishing, 1987, pp. 311–328.
52. Ambos HD, Markham J, Lindsay BD, Cain ME: Spectral analysis of signal-averaged electrocardiograms from patients with and without sustained ventricular tachycardia. In: Computers in Cardiology, 1986. Los Angeles: IEEE Computer Society Press, 1987, pp. 529–532.
53. Lindsay BD, Markham J, Schechtman KB, Ambos HD, Cain ME: Identification of patients with sustained ventricular tachycardia by frequency analysis of signal-averaged electrocardiograms despite the presence of bundle branch block. Circulation 77:122, 1988.
54. Lindsay BD, Ambos HD, Schechtman KB, Cain ME: Improved differentiation of patients with and without ventricular tachycardia by fre-

quency analysis of multiple electrocardiographic leads. Am J Cardiol 62:556, 1988.

55. Oppenheim A, Schafer R: Digital Signal Processing. Englewood Cliffs, NJ: Prentice Hall, 1975.

56. Cadzow JA: Foundations of Digital Signal Processing and Data Analysis. New York: Macmillan Publishing Co., 1987.

57. Simson MB, Untereker WJ, Spielman SR, Horowitz LN, Marcus NH, Falcone RA, Harken AH, Josephson ME: Relation between late potentials on the body surface and directly recorded fragmented electrograms in patients with ventricular tachycardia. Am J Cardiol 51:105, 1983.

58. Wiener I, Mindich B, Pitchon R: Determinants of ventricular tachycardia in patients with ventricular aneurysms: results of intraoperative epicardial and endocardial mapping. Circulation 65:856, 1982.

59. Klein H, Karp RB, Kouchoukos NT, Zorn GL, James TN, Waldo AL: Intraoperative electrophysiologic mapping of the ventricles during sinus rhythm in patients with a previous myocardial infarction. Identification of the electrophysiologic substrate of ventricular arrhythmias. Circulation 66:847, 1982.

60. Ros HH, Koeleman ASM, Akker TJ: The technique of signal averaging and its practical application in the separation of atrial and His-Purkinje activity. In Hombach V, Hilger HH (eds): Signal Averaging Technique in Clinical Cardiology. New York: Schattauer Verlag, 1981, pp 3–14.

61. Harris FJ: On the use of windows for harmonic analysis with the discrete Fourier transform. Proc IEEE 66:51, 1978.

62. Cain ME, Lindsay BD, Fischer AE, Ambos HD, Sobel BE: Prospective comparison of frequency- and time-domain analysis of signal-averaged ECGs from patients with ventricular tachycardia (abstr). Circulation 74:II–471, 1986.

63. Machac J, Weiss A, Winters SL, Barreca P, Gomes JA: A comparative study of frequency domain and time domain of signal-averaged electrocardiograms in patients with ventricular tachycardia. J Am Coll Cardiol 11:284, 1988.

64. Worley SJ, Mark DB, Smith WM, Wolf P, Califf RM, Strauss HC, Manwaring MG, Ideker RE: Comparison of time domain and frequency domain variables from the signal-averaged electrocardiogram: a multivariable analysis. J Am Coll Cardiol 11:1041, 1988.

65. Nichols TL, Mirvis DM: Frequency content of the electrocardiogram. Spatial features and effects of myocardial infarction. J Electrocardiol 18:185, 1985.

66. Haberl R, Jilge G, Pulter R, Steinbeck G: Comparison of frequency and time domain analysis of the signal-averaged electrocardiogram in patients with ventricular tachycardia and coronary artery disease: methodologic validation and clinical relevance. J Am Coll Cardiol 12:150, 1988.

67. Lindsay BD, Ambos HD, Fischer AE, Cain ME: Predictive values of frequency analysis of signal-averaged ECGs at specific intervals after myocardial infarction (abstr). Circulation 72:III-164, 1985.

68. Lindsay BD, Fischer AE, Ambos HD, Markham J, Cain ME: Detection of patients with nonischemic cardiomyopathy prone to sustained ven-

tricular arrhythmias by frequency analysis of signal-averaged electrocardiograms (abstr). Circulation 76:IV-345, 1987.

69. Cain ME, Ambos HD, Fischer AE, Markham J, Schechtman KB: Noninvasive prediction of antiarrhythmic drug efficacy in patients with sustained ventricular tachycardia from frequency analysis of signal-averaged ECGs (abstr). Circulation 70:II-253, 1984.

70. Witkowski FX, Corr PB: An automated transmural cardiac mapping system. Am J Physiol 247:H661, 1984.

71. Kramer JB, Corr PB, Cox JL, Witkowski FX, Cain ME: Simultaneous computer mapping to facilitate intraoperative localization of accessory pathways in patients with Wolff-Parkinson-White syndrome. Am J Cardiol 56:571, 1985.

72. Kay SM, Marple SL Jr: Spectrum analysis—a modern perspective. Proc IEEE 69:1380, 1981.

28

Spectro-Temporal Mapping of the Surface Electrocardiogram

Ralph Haberl, Gerhard Jilge, Peter Steinbigler, Gerhard Steinbeck

Time Domain Versus Frequency Domain

The time domain is the traditional way to look at a signal: the amplitude of a signal is plotted versus time as in the conventional electrocardiogram (Figure 1). The frequency domain is another perspective to look at a signal: the amplitude of the components is plotted versus frequency in Hertz. Both perspectives are interchangeable and bear the same information. However, sometimes a difficult problem might be solved quite easily, if the perspective is switched from one domain to the other.[1,2]

Delayed ventricular activation in the early ST segment of the electrocardiogram can be recorded from the body surface with a small amplitude (1–10µV). The detection of these small signals is still at the limits of technical performance and separation from noise interference is a difficult problem. The current methods in the time

From El-Sherif N, Turitto G (eds): *High-Resolution Electrocardiography*. Mount Kisco, NY, Futura Publishing Co., Inc., ©, 1992.

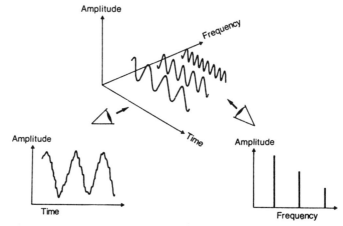

Figure 1. Time and frequency domain. Both domains are different perspectives to a signal: in the time domain the sine waves add up to a complex signal, the amplitude is plotted versus time (view from the left). The frequency domain is characterized by spectral lines, the amplitude is plotted versus frequency in Hertz (view from below).

domain after signal averaging and high amplification have severe limitations: the signals have to be high-pass filtered and the results are influenced by the type of the filter and the cut-off frequencies.[3-5] In most systems the definition of abnormal uses the start and end point of the filtered QRS complex which are calculated relative to the noise level.[6] Different noise levels may thereby directly influence the classification of patients. Subjects with complete bundle branch block in general have to be excluded from time-domain analysis. Finally, the signal-to-noise ratio is not adequate for single beat analysis of delayed ventricular activation.

These problems inherent to time-domain analysis are the major reason for discrepancies between working groups and results even differed strikingly, when several commercially available systems were applied to the same patients.[7] To overcome some of these limitations, a change of the perspective to the frequency domain has been proposed.[8,9] This approach is based on the idea that delayed ventricular activation should be characterized by a higher frequency content than the otherwise low frequent ST segment. The Fourier transform is the mathematical algorithm mostly used to calculate the power spectrum of a periodic time series.[1,10-12]

Fourier Transform of the Electrocardiogram

In 1920, Baron Jean Baptiste Josef Fourier showed that every real signal is composed of sine waves with different amplitude, phase, and frequency. Correspondingly, each periodic signal can be split up into those sine waves.[1] The Fourier transform gives excellent results, if a signal is periodic and infinitely long. The ECG does not meet these criteria: the segments of interest (i.e., QRS, ST segment, etc.) are of finite sample size. There is a reciprocal relationship between the segment size and the frequency resolution in Hertz. In principle, delayed ventricular activation can be detected by frequency analysis, if the frequency resolution of the algorithm is good enough to distinguish high-frequency components within the ST segment and if the dynamic range allows evaluation of small deflections (a few microvolts) in the segment. Nonperiodic signals like the electrocardiogram may also be analyzed with Fourier transform, however, some methodological prerequisites have strictly to be considered:

1. Fourier transform of which time segment? The length of the time segment is one major determinant of frequency resolution. Long segments result in good frequency resolution, but might be inappropriate for detection of short signal components such as late potentials: the relative spectral contribution of these signals is the smaller the longer the segment. Another problem arises when parts of the QRS complex are located within the segment as a transient. In our experience, artificial frequencies appear as soon as > 20msec of the terminal QRS complex are included in a segment.[13]
2. Which window to analyze the ST segment? Window functions are cosinoidal curves which are superimposed to the segment of interest: the signal is multiplied point by point with the window function. This is necessary to make a nonperiodic signal "pseudoperiodic" and thereby eliminating artificial frequencies due to edge discontinuities of the segment. Figure 2 shows the effect of different window functions on the analysis of the ST segment of the ECG. A Blackman-Harris window proved to give best results due to a big dynamic range, although frequency resolution is deteriorated.[14]

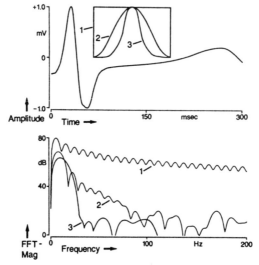

Figure 2. Influence of the window function on the frequency analysis of the ST segment. One hundred twenty milliseconds of the ST segment are multiplied point by point with a rectangular window (1), a Hanning window (2), or a Blackman-Harris window (3) (top panel). The fast Fourier transform of the windowed segments is shown in the lower panel. The rectangular window has the best frequency resolution (narrow peak at 9 Hz), but prominent spectral leakage which makes analysis of high-frequency components impossible. The Hanning window reduces spectral leakage, however, low amplitude components might also be overshadowed by the side lobes. The Blackman-Harris window causes broad peaks (poor frequency resolution), but low spectral leakage.

3. Influence of a direct current (DC) offset. A DC offset is present, if the mean of all signal values of a segment is unequal to zero. The DC component leads to a peak at zero frequency which might become so broad and big that high-frequency components might be overshadowed. Elimination of the DC offset before Fourier transform is mandatory, but has been disregarded in most previous studies (Figure 3).

4. Normalization or nonnormalization of spectra? In most previous studies [16–19] the frequency spectra have been normalized by setting the fundamental frequency equal to 0 dB. The spectral peak at the fundamental frequency (= lowest predominant frequency), however, depends on the segment length, the steepness of the ST segment, and the relative direction of the termi-

INFLUENCE OF DC - OFFSET

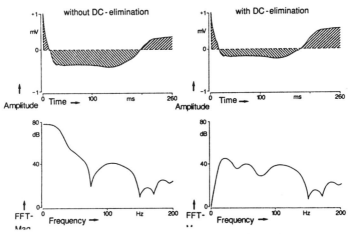

Figure 3. Effect of DC components in the time domain on the power spectrum of the terminal QRS and ST segment. Left panel: the mean of all data samples is non-zero (different areas below and above zero potential). The corresponding spectrum starts at a high value at 0 Hz (lower left), which makes it impossible to analyze components in the range up to 70 Hz. Right panel: after removing the DC component (area below and above zero potential is equal), the value at 0 Hz is zero, and the frequency components between 0 Hz and 60 Hz are displayed correctly.

nal QRS complex and T wave (concordant or discordant S and T wave). Thus, many factors that are not related to delayed ventricular activation may influence the results when spectra are normalized. For the same reason, area ratios which include the fundamental peak are not recommended.

Spectral Mapping of the Electrocardiogram

In Figure 4 the single spectrum analysis of two patients is shown: on the left side, the high-gain recording of the ST segment clearly reveals late potentials at the end of the QRS complex. The corresponding power spectrum shows a peak at the fundamental frequency (15 Hz) and prominent high-frequency components in the range above 50 Hz. After elimination of the late potentials with the computer cursor (stippled line), the high-frequency components dis-

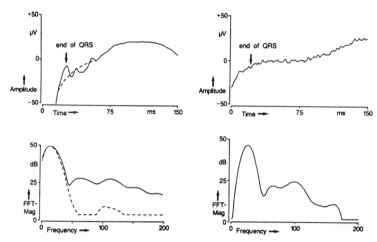

Figure 4. Single spectrum analysis of the ST segment. Left panel: a patient after myocardial infarction with late potentials at the end of the QRS complex (upper left); the corresponding spectrum shows a fundamental peak at 10 Hz and high-frequency components above 50 Hz. After elimination of late potentials with the computer cursor (stippled line) the high-frequency components disappear. Right panel: a noisy signal without late potentials. The frequency spectrum also reveals high-frequency components which cannot be differentiated from late potentials.

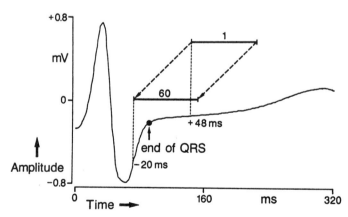

Figure 5. Spectro-temporal mapping with Fourier transform: 60 segments are defined within the ST wave (segment size 80 msec). The first segment starts 48 msec after the end of QRS (segment 1), the last segment starts 20 msec within the QRS complex.

appear. On the right side, a somewhat noisy signal of a healthy volunteer without late potentials was analyzed. The power spectrum also reveals high-frequency components. Thus, a single spectrum analysis does not allow differentiation between late potentials and noise. We therefore developed the analysis with spectro-temporal mapping (Figure 5): 60 segments slightly shifted in time were analyzed with Fourier transform. The first segment started 48 msec after the end of QRS (segment size 80 msec), the subsequent segments started progressively earlier in the ST segment, and the 60th segment started 20 msec inside the QRS complex. The frequency components of each subsegment were calculated with Fourier transform after multiplication with a Blackman-Harris window and elimination of DC offset. The 60-frequency spectra were combined into a three-dimensional plot (Figure 6). The frequency spectrum of segment 1 (which started far outside the QRS) was defined as a reference spectrum; the spectra of segments 2–60 were compared with this reference spectrum by cross correlation in the frequency range 40–150 Hz. The similarity of spectra was expressed by the correlation

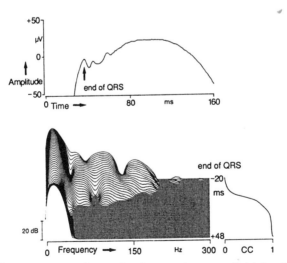

Figure 6. Spectro-temporal mapping in a post-myocardial infarction patient with sustained ventricular tachycardia. In segments far outside the QRS complex, there are no high-frequency components, however, analysis of segments at the end of the QRS complex reveals progressively higher spectral peaks in the range 40–220 Hz. Right panel: the correlation coefficient (CC) drops to zero in these segments. The factor of normality is 2%.

coefficient (Figure 6, right panel). It was 0, if two spectra showed no similarity, it was 1, if two spectra were identical. A "factor of normality" (NF) was calculated: the mean of the correlation coefficient of segments 40–45 was divided by the mean of the correlation coefficients of spectra 1–15, multiplied by 100. High-frequency content at the end of QRS (spectra 20–55) which was absent far outside the QRS (spectra 1–15) caused NF to be low. NF ranges between 0% and 100% (0% = strong evidence of late potentials, 100% = no evidence of late potentials). NF below 30% was considered abnormal.

Analysis of Representative Patients

Patient 1 (Figure 6) experienced a myocardial infarction 2 years ago and presented now with sustained ventricular tachycardia. In a high-gain recording (channel Y) late potentials with an amplitude of 10 µV can be seen at the end of the QRS complex (definition of late potentials: deflection > 1 µV after the end of the QRS complex in all three leads). Spectro-temporal mapping with FFT reveals that in segments far outside the QRS complex (segments 1–34) only the fundamental peak is present and high-frequency components are missing. In segments at the end of QRS (35–60) high-frequency components appear as soon as late potentials become part of the subsegments. The better the late potentials pass the window function, the higher the frequency peaks in the range 40–220 Hz. The correlation coefficient (right panel) drops towards 0 in spectra at the end of the QRS complex. The factor of normality is 2%. This is a characteristic pattern of late potentials which cause high-frequency components only in segments at the end of the QRS complex and which are absent in segments far outside the QRS complex. The definition of abnormal does not depend upon the absolute localization of the end the QRS complex which in many cases is difficult to determine.

Patient 2 (Figure 7) had also suffered from previous myocardial infarction, but he was free of arrhythmias. The high-gain recording of the ST waves does not reveal late potentials. Spectro-temporal mapping does not show any high-frequency components in the range above 50 Hz. The correlation coefficient is 1 for all spectra (all spectra are identical), the factor of normality is 100%. There is no indication of late potentials.

Patient 3 (Figure 8) was a patient after myocardial infarction without arrhythmias; the figure demonstrates the advantages of

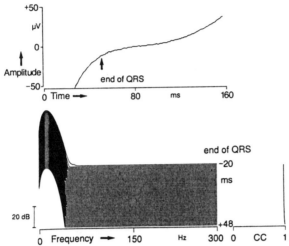

Figure 7. Spectro-temporal mapping in a patient after myocardial infarction without ventricular tachycardia. None of the spectra shows high-frequency components above 50 Hz. The correlation coefficient is one for all spectra, the factor of normality is 100%.

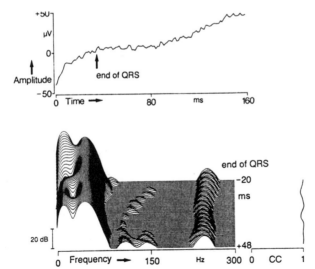

Figure 8. Spectro-temporal mapping of a noisy signal. High-frequency components at 50 and 170 Hz uniformly spread through all spectra. They are caused by noise interference. The correlation coefficient does not fall below 0.9, and the factor of normality is 90%. There is no indication of delayed ventricular activation.

spectro-temporal mapping. Even after signal averaging noise interference is present, because the recording conditions were bad. The patient was obese, the skin was dry (electrode impedance 15kOhm), and the recording was done in the coronary care unit. In the time domain it is impossible to decide whether late potentials are present or not. Spectro-temporal mapping with fast Fourier transform reveals high-frequency components (peaks at 50 Hz and 240 Hz), however, these peaks are not only present in segments at the end of the QRS complex, but were uniformly present in all spectra. Therefore, these components did not represent localized delayed ventricular activation, but noise interference (i.e., line disturbance and muscle noise). The correlation coefficient between the spectra (right panel) did not fall below 0.9 in this patient, the factor of normality was 90%. Thus, there was no indication of late potentials in this patient.

A difficult, but realistic example is shown in Figure 9. In this post-myocardial infarction patient, the quality of recording again is

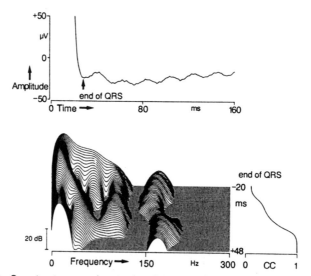

Figure 9. Spectro-temporal mapping in a post-myocardial infarction patient with ventricular tachycardia. In the time domain, late potentials cannot be identified because of noise interference. Spectro-temporal mapping shows high-frequency components at 70 and 170 Hz which are present in all spectra; they are due to noise interference. Additionally, frequency components at 40–65 Hz are present in segments only at the end of the the QRS complex; they are due to late potentials. The correlation coefficient drops towards zero in these segments. The factor of normality is 10%.

poor. In the time domain, late potentials cannot be identified at the end of the QRS complex. The Simson method was normal (filtered QRS duration 105 msec, RMS 33 μV). Spectro-temporal mapping revealed two different types of peaks: at 50 Hz and 170 Hz high-frequency components exist which spread throughout all segments. Additionally, frequency components between 40 and 100 Hz are present only in segments at the end of the QRS complex. The correlation coefficient indicates a change of the spectra at the end of the QRS complex, and the factor of normality was 15%. Thus, in this patient late potentials could be identified despite the presence of noise interference. The Simon method failed because the high-noise level caused an incorrect determination of the QRS limits.

Results of Patient Groups

Three groups of patients were studied (Figure 10):

1. Group 1 consisted of 38 patients in the chronic phase of myocardial infarction (3- to 200-months old, median 24 months) with documented, sustained ventricular tachycardia. The clinical

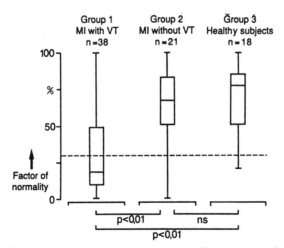

Figure 10. Results in patients from groups 1–3. The median of the factor of normality is plotted for each group. The box represents 50% of all data values, the bars indicate the whole range. In group 1 patients the factor of normality is significantly lower than in group 2 and 3 patients.

data are given in Table I. Each patient was recorded in the absence of antiarrhythmic drugs and beta blockers. Cardiac catheterization and an electrophysiologic study were performed in all patients. Single and double extrastimuli were applied at the right ventricular apex and pulmonary outflow tract (basic drive 100, 120, 150, and 180 beats/min, rectangular pulses, twice diastolic threshold, duration 2 msec). In 30 patients a sustained monomorphic ventricular tachycardia (duration >30 seconds or termination necessary because of hemodynamic deterioration) could be induced, in 4 patients primary ventricular fibrillation, and in 4 patients only a nonsustained ventricular tachycardia (7–12 beats) could be induced.

2. Group 2 consisted of 21 patients after myocardial infarction (2- to 100-months old, medium 20 months). None had arrhythmias, syncope, or palpitation. A 24-hour ambulatory electrocardiogram revealed <10 ventricular ectopic beats per hour and no ventricular pairs.

3. Group 3 comprised 18 healthy volunteers.

Patients with bundle branch block (QRS duration >0.12 seconds) were not excluded. Statistical evaluation was done with the Wilcoxon rank sign test for unpaired data.

	Group 1 MI With VT	Group 2 MI Without VT	Group 3 Healthy Persons
Table I Patient Data			
n	38	21	18
Sex (m/f)	29/9	18/3	11/7
Age (years)	60 ± 13	55 ± 11	29 ± 11
Site of infarction			
anterior	28	15	—
posterior	15	10	—
Ejection fraction (%)	44 ± 20	49 ± 14	—
Bundle branch block	11	7	1

MI = myocardial infarction; VT = ventricular tachycardia

Results in Patients Without Heart Disease (Group 3)

In 2 out of 18 patients, spectro-temporal mapping was abnormal. Both patients had an incomplete right bundle branch block with an rSr'-complex. The r' caused the high-frequency components. In patients after myocardial infarction this is a rare finding. The Simson method was abnormal in three patients.

Results in Patients After Myocardial Infarction Without Arrhythmias (Group 2)

Spectro-temporal mapping revealed high-frequency components in 3 out of 21 patients (Table II). Two of them also showed late potentials in the time domain. Seven patients with bundle branch block had normal spectra. The Simson method was abnormal in 3 out of 14 patients (7 patients with bundle branch block excluded). In 2 out of 3 of these patients, frequency analysis showed a typically noisy pattern (as in Figure 8).

Results in Patients After Myocardial Infarction With Ventricular Tachycardia (Group 1)

Frequency analysis was abnormal in 26 out of 38 patients (67%). Channels with abnormal frequency analysis also showed late potentials in the time domain in most cases (22 records could not be evaluated in the time domain because of a steep ST wave). The Simson method was abnormal in 16 out of 27 patients (11 patients with bundle branch block excluded), and in 9 out of 27 cases there was a discrepancy between the Simson method and frequency analysis. In all cases the reason of discrepancy could be identified, the most common reason was incorrect determination of the QRS limits due to noise interference (thereby five patients were incorrectly classified as normal).

The presence of late potential, its amplitude and frequency content did not correlate with the ejection fraction, the localization of myocardial infarction, and the presence of an aneurysm.

Table II
Results in Patients After Myocardial Infarction Without Ventricular
Tachycardia (Group 2)

Patient No.	Age(yr) Sex	Infarction Site	EF (%)	LP + in Lead	Simson Method	X	Y	Z
				Time Domain		FFT NF (%)		
1	58 m	A	60	? ? ?	-	53	87	70
2	53 m	P+	35	- - -	p	85	96	79
3	74 m	P	-	- - -	n	100	100	40
4	57 m	AP	64	- ? ?	n	82	32	100
5	58 m	A+	31	+ + -	p	17	5	36
6	49 m	A	49	- - -	n	80	40	66
7	45 m	AP	42	- ? -	n	78	60	95
8	68 m	P	61	- - ?	-	75	76	100
9	55 f	A	44	? - -	n	100	92	100
10	50 f	AP	45	- - ?	n	100	64	38
11	56 m	A	52	? - ?	p	100	82	75
12	60 m	P	52	- - ?	-	100	100	100
13	61 m	P	29	? - ?	n	47	71	35
14	70 m	A+	-	- - -	n	76	57	51
15	62 m	A	44	- - -	-	100	100	100
16	71 m	P	54	? - -	n	100	32	38
17	70 m	A	35	- ? ?	p	100	100	26
18	52 f	A	46	- + +	-	78	53	22
19	60 m	AP	66	- - -	-	100	65	73
20	61 m	A	55	- - -	n	45	100	33
21	67 m	A+	43	- - ?	-	100	100	78

LP+ =Late potentials present; NF=Factor of Normality; A=anterior infarction; EF=Ejection fraction; P=posterior infarction; Simson Method: p=abnormal, n=normal - not to be evaluated; + =Aneurysm present

Clinical Relevance

Frequency analysis proved to be a powerful analytic method for detection of late potentials in the surface electrocardiogram. Frequency analysis of multiple segments (spectro-temporal mapping) considerably enhances the evaluation of delayed ventricular activation in patients after myocardial infarction.[20,21]

Table III

Results in Patients After Myocardial Infarction With Ventricular
Tachycardia (Group 1)

Patient No.	Age (yr) Sex	Ejection Fraction (%)	Infarction Site	LP + in Lead	Simson Method	FFT NF (%)		
						X	Y	Z
1	60 m	83	A+	x - ?	n	3	72	17
2	55 f	64	P	- y -	p	100	100	100
3	68 m	48	A	- - -	p	100	62	61
4	58 f	84	P	- y -	p	100	23	100
5	65 m	40	A	- y ?	-	100	9	35
6	74 m	30	A	x y z	-	1	6	25
7	54 m	35	A+	- y -	n	75	23	70
8	55 f	25	A	- - -	p	83	100	71
9	62 m	34	A+	- - -	n	100	100	58
10	70 m	32	AP+	x - ?	p	15	85	100
11	66 m	68	P	- - -	n	100	92	100
12	54 m	15	A+	- y -	p	99	13	100
13	51 m	72	A	- - -	p	100	100	53
14	68 f	20	A+	- - -	n	55	82	75
15	75 m	44	A	- y -	p	99	29	97
16	62 m	20	AP+	- y -	n	100	100	100
17	53 f	24	A+	x y ?	p	30	15	37
18	59 m	41	P	x y z	p	23	18	30
19	73 m	43	A+	- - z	-	100	32	2
20	39 m	70	P	? - z	-	100	100	15
21	58 m	52	A	- - -	n	100	47	97
22	59 m	40	P	x y ?	n	79	2	65
23	66 m	48	AP	- y z	p	100	15	1
24	59 f	60	A	? ? ?	-	69	7	5
25	61 m	62	A	- - -	p	81	100	100
26	79 m	27	AP	x y z	-	0	2	4
27	69 m	63	P	? y -	-	94	30	100
28	54 m	-	A	- - ?	n	100	100	84
29	36 m	65	A	- - ?	n	79	39	70
30	49 m	28	P	? ? ?	-	18	100	69
31	65 f	39	P	? y -	p	12	18	100
32	75 f	45	P+	x y ?	p	24	16	14
33	52 m	21	A+	- - z	n	57	100	29

Table III *(Continued)*

Patient No.	Age (yr) Sex	Ejection Fraction (%)	Infarction Site	LP + in Lead	Simson Method	FFT NF (%)		
						X	Y	Z
34	79 f	31	A +	- ? z	-	100	97	30
35	66 m	15	A	x y z	-	6	25	1
36	52 m	27	A	? ? ?	p	83	10	100
37	71 m	26	AP	x ? -	p	15	89	98
38	64 m	85	A	- y -	-	35	2	34

LP + = Late potentials present; NF = Factor of Normality; A = anterior infarction; EF = Ejection fraction; P = posterior infarction; Simson Method: p = abnormal, n = normal - not to be evaluated; + = Aneurysm present

The method has distinct advantages:

1. Spectro-temporal mapping allowed a good discrimination between late potentials and noise, which both have a typical spectral representation.[20–23] Thereby sensitivity and specificity of the method is increased compared to conventional time-domain analysis. Even single-beat analysis is possible.[24,25] In contrast, the definitions of the Simson method depend directly upon the noise level, a possible source of error (example in Figure 9).

2. Our results suggest that patients with bundle branch block need not to be excluded.[26,27] Bundle branch block is a common finding in patients with organic heart disease and impaired left ventricular function (up to 30% of patients). Since time-domain analysis is limited to patients without intraventricular conduction abnormalities, frequency analysis considerably increases clinical applicability. Our data are also supported by Lindsay et al,[28] who also found that patients with bundle branch block need not be excluded.

3. Spectro-temporal mapping of the ST segment does not require exact definition of the onset and end of the QRS complex, which often is difficult to determine. The calculation of a "factor of normality" gives a simple and reliable parameter for distinction between normal and abnormal. This factor is independent on the noise level and the fundamental peak.

4. Complex high-pass filtering is not necessary, and discussion about filter artifacts, signal distortion, and the choice of adequate cut-off frequencies can be avoided.[4]

Comparison With Previous Studies

Our data differ in part from the results obtained by Cain et al.[8,29-31] They found an increased band in the range of 20 to 50 Hz and a higher area ratio (20 to 50 Hz)/(0 to 20 Hz) of the power spectrum in patients with ventricular tachycardia and coronary artery disease. However, their method differs from our technique: they used a long segment, included the terminal portion of the QRS complex in the segment, utilized a variable segment length, and normalized the spectra apparently without compensation of direct current components (spectra started with the highest point at 0 Hz). We found that long segments and area ratios in the frequency domain including the fundamental peak, did not correlate with delayed ventricular activation in the time domain. Furthermore, they use single spectrum analysis which does not allow precise differentiation between noise and late potentials in our opinion.

Conclusions

Spectro-temporal mapping significantly improves recent approaches with single spectrum evaluation of the electrocardiogram. Some limitations of conventional time-domain analysis might be overcome. Single-beat analysis is possible which offers a diagnostic approach in cases when signal averaging is not possible: analysis of extrasystoles and during electrophysiologic study. This method should now be tested prospectively in larger groups of patients using the criteria worked out in this study. It might enhance identification of patients prone to sustained ventricular tachycardia after myocardial infarction.

References

1. Brigham EO: The Fast Fourier Transform. Englewood Cliffs, New Jersey: Prentice Hall, 1974.
2. Martini H: Methoden der Signalverarbeitung. München: Franzis Verlag, 1987.
3. El-Sherif N, Mehra R, Gomes JA, Kelen G: Appraisal of a low noise electrocardiogram. J Am Coll Cardiol 1:456, 1983.
4. Gomes JA, Winters SL, Stewart D, Targonski A, Barreca P: Optimal bandpass filters for time-domain analysis of the signal-averaged electrocardiogram. Am J Cardiol 60:1290, 1987.
5. Gomes JA, Mehra R, Barreca P, Winters SL, Ergin A, Estioko M, Min-

ditch BP: A comparative analysis of signal averaging of the surface QRS complex and signal averaging of intracardiac and epicardial recordings in patients with ventricular tachycardia. PACE 11:271, 1988.

6. Simson MB: Use of signals in the terminal QRS complex to identify patients with ventricular myocardial infarction. Circulation 64:235, 1981.

7. Oeff M, von Leitner ER, Sthapit R, Breithardt G, Borggrefe M, Karbenn U, Meinertz T, Zotz R, Clas W, Hombach V, Hopp H.-W: Methods for non-invasive detection of ventricular late potentials: a comparative multicenter study. Eur Heart J 7:25, 1986.

8. Cain ME, Ambos HD, Witkowski FX, Sobel BE: Fast-Fourier transform analysis of signal-averaged electrocardiograms for identification of patients prone to sustained ventricular tachycardia. Circulation 69:711, 1984.

9. Haberl R, Hengstenberg E, Steinbeck G: Single beat analysis of frequency content in the surface ECG for identification of patients with ventricular tachycardia. Circulation 72(Suppl III):433, 1985.

10. Cooley JW, Tukey JW: An algorithm for the machine computation of complex Fourier series. Math Comput 19:297, 1965.

11. Hewlett Packard: The fundamentals of signal analysis. Application Note 243, 1985.

12. Kay SM, Marple SL: Spectrum analysis. A modern perspective. IEEE Proc 69:1380, 1981.

13. Haberl R, Pulter R, Hengstenberg E, Steinbeck G: Frequency analysis of single beat electrocardiograms for identification of patients with sustained ventricular tachycardia. New Trends in Arrhythmias I:475, 1985.

14. Harris FJ: On the use of windows for harmonic analysis with the discrete Fourier transformation. IEEE Proc 66:51, 1978.

15. Ramirez RW: The FFT. Fundamentals and Concepts. Englewood Cliffs, New Jersey: Prentice Hall Inc, 1985.

16. DeCaro M, Volosin KJ, Friedman O, Greenspon AJ: Frequency analysis of the signal averaged QRS-ST complex in patients with ventricular tachycardia (abstr). Circulation 74(Supp II):209, 1986.

17. Kelen GJ, Henkin R, Fontaine JM, El-Sherif N: Effects of analyzed signal duration and phase on the results of fast Fourier transform analysis of the surface electrocardiogram in subjects with and without late potentials. Am J Cardiol 60:1282, 1987.

18. Machac J, Weiss A, Winters SL, Barreca P, Gomes JA: A comparative study of frequency domain and time domain analysis of signal-averaged electrocardiograms in patients with ventricular tachycardia. J Am Coll Cardiol 11:284, 1988.

19. Worley SJ, Mark DB, Smith WM, Wolf P, Califf RM, Strauss HC, Manwaring MG, Ideker RE: Comparison of time domain and frequency domain variables from the signal-averaged electrocardiogram: a multivariable analysis. J Am Coll Cardiol 11:1041, 1988.

20. Haberl R, Jilge G, Steinbeck G: Multisegment frequency analysis of the electrocardiogram with Fourier transform for identification of patients with sustained ventricular tachycardia. Circulation 78 (Suppl II):302, 1988.

21. Haberl, R, Jilge G, Pulter R, Steinbeck G: Spectral mapping of the electrocardiogram with Fourier transform for identification of patients with sustained ventricular tachycardia and coronary artery disease. Eur Heart J 10:316, 1989.

22. Haberl R, Jilge G, Pulter R, Steinbeck G: Direct comparison between frequency and time domain analysis of the surface ECG in patients with ventricular tachycardia. New Trends in Arrhythmias 4:423, 1988.

23. Haberl R, Jilge G, Steinbeck G: Spectral mapping of electrocardiogram with Fourier transform for identification of patients with sustained ventricular tachycardia. Eur Heart J 9(Suppl 1):109, 1988.

24. Haberl R, Hengstenberg E, Steinbeck G: Frequenzanalyse des Einzelschlag-EKG zur Erkennung von Patienten mit ventrikulären Tachykardien bei dilativer Kardiomyopathie. Z Kardiol 76:15, 1987.

25. Haberl R, Jilge G, Pulter R, Steinbeck G: Frequency analysis of the surface ECG versus late potentials in the time domain: direct comparison in patients with ventricular tachycardia. Eur Heart J 8(Suppl 2):21, 1987.

26. Haberl R, Hoffmann E, Steinbeck G: Low-frequency components in patients with delayed ventricular activation. Circulation 72(Suppl III):6, 1985.

27. Hoffmann E, Haberl R, Steinbeck G: Frequenzanalyse des Oberflächen-EKG von Patienten mit intraventrikulärer Leitungsstörung. Z Kardiol 75(Suppl 1):122, 1986.

28. Lindsay BD, Markham J, Schechtman KB, Ambos HD, Cain ME: Identification of patients with sustained ventricular tachycardia by frequency analysis of signal-averaged electrocardiograms despite the presence of bundle branch block. Circulation 77:122, 1988.

29. Cain ME, Ambos HD, Boerner JA, Martin TC, Fischer AE, Sobel BE: Prospective identification of patients with inducible sustained ventricular tachycardia with fast Fourier transform analysis of signal averaged electrocardiograms. J Am Coll Caardiol 3:495, 1984.

30. Cain ME, Ambos HD, Markham J, Fischer AE, Sobel BE: Quantification of differences in frequency content of signal-averaged electrocardiograms in patients with compared to those without sustained ventricular tachycardia. Am J Cardiol 55:1500, 1985.

31. Lindsay BD, Ambos HD, Schechtman KB, Cain ME: Improved selection of patients for programmed ventricular stimulation by frequency analysis of signal-averaged electrocardiograms. Circulation 73:675, 1986.

29

Improved Noninvasive Identification of the Substrate for Inducible Sustained Monomorphic Ventricular Tachycardia by Spectral Turbulence Analysis

George Kelen, Raphael Henkin,
Anne-Marie Starr, Edward B. Caref,
Dennis Bloomfield, Nabil El-Sherif

Introduction

Demonstration of late potentials in the terminal QRS region of the signal-averaged surface electrocardiogram (SAECG) has been shown in numerous studies to be a clinically useful predictor of vulnerability to ventricular tachyarrhythmias.[1-10] Current techniques for time-domain late potential analysis are not however without shortcomings. There is a lack of agreement in the literature as to optimal filter characteristics, as well as to the best numerical

From El-Sherif N, Turitto G (eds): *High-Resolution Electrocardiography*. Mount Kisco, NY, Futura Publishing Co., Inc., ©, 1992.

criteria of abnormality.[11] The numeric measurements are sensitive to the specific algorithm used for determining QRS termination.[12] In the presence of intraventricular conduction defect and/or bundle branch block, which many patients at potential risk have, interpretation of late potentials may be difficult[13]—most published studies have specifically excluded such patients. In a recent review of the literature,[14] the predictive value of time-domain SAECG analysis ranged between 28%–95% with an average of 64%.

Several authors have reported promising results employing frequency analysis techniques for ventricular tachycardia (VT) risk assessment.[15-20] The group of Cain et al, in multiple publications, claimed improved noninvasive definition of risk for development of sustained VT[15-20] and even ventricular fibrillation[21] using frequency analysis. Their technique consisted of performing a Fast Fourier transform, after Blackman Harris windowing, upon a variable length of signal-averaged ECG from each orthogonal lead X, Y, and Z comprising the terminal 40 msec of the QRS complex in addition to the whole of the ST segment. Abnormality was indicated by the presence of increased signal components in the 20- to 50-Hz range as measured by a variety of indices, whose numerical definitions have been somewhat modified over the course of their various publications. The indices proposed included an increased proportion of power between 20–50 Hz compared with 0–20 Hz or 10–50 Hz ("Area Ratio"), and the presence of frequency peaks between 20–50 Hz with increased power compared with the magnitude of the entire signal over this range ("Magnitude Ratio"). The region of signal analyzed ("region of interest") was selected by the operator using a computer graphics cursor and "standard electrocardiographic criteria."

In 1987 Kelen et al[22] reported inability to use Cain's technique in any usefully reproducible fashion owing to the effect of variable analyzed signal segment length swamping out the contribution of any abnormal high-frequency components that the signal might or might not contain. In our hands, area and magnitude ratios were exquisitely sensitive to the length of signal analyzed which depended upon the exact operator designated position of QRS termination and T wave onset. We confirmed this technical pitfall using mathematically synthesized signals as well as real recordings from subjects with and without known time-domain late potentials.

Worley et al[23] reported in 1988 that using a fixed analyzed signal

normality is represented by "abnormally high" or "abnormally low" frequencies, anywhere throughout the whole QRS complex. None of the abnormality criteria invoke any arbitrary value for signal amplitude, duration, or frequency. The hallmark of arrhythmogenic abnormality is postulated to be frequent and abrupt changes in the frequency signature of the QRS wave front velocity as it propagates throughout the ventricle around and across areas of abnormal conduction resulting in a high degree of spectral turbulence. This may provide a more accurate marker for the anatomic-electrophysiologic substrate of reentrant tachyarrhythmias.

Study Subjects

Our study was carried out retrospectively on the SAECG of 142 subjects, divided into four groups based upon presence or absence of time-domain late potentials, and inducibility of sustained monomorphic ventricular tachycardia (SMVT) at electrophysiologic study. Patients with bundle branch blocks and intraventricular conduction defect were included in the study.

Group A—"Time-Domain True Negatives"—71 Subjects

These were healthy adult volunteers (mostly hospital staff) with no known history or symptoms of heart disease, absent time-domain late potentials, and normal 12-lead ECG. Subjects with bundle branch block including incomplete right bundle branch block, intraventricular conduction defect, and/or a QRS duration > 120 msec were specifically excluded from this group.

Group B—"Time-Domain True Positives"—33 Subjects

All patients in this group had positive time-domain late potentials and inducible SMVT at electrophysiologic study. All had a history of prior myocardial infarction and documented spontaneous SMVT (> 120 beats/min for > 30 sec: 24 patients) or nonsustained VT (> 3 beats, < 30 sec, at > 120 beats/min: 9 patients). Subjects with

QRS duration >120 msec and/or bundle branch block were not included in this group.

Group C—"Time-Domain False-Positives"—28 Subjects

This group comprised subjects with positive time-domain late potentials in two clinical categories. Nine were "normal" volunteers without evidence or symptoms of heart disease, but with a complete or incomplete right bundle branch block pattern on their 12-lead ECG. The remaining 19 were patients with ventricular tachyarrhythmias referred for electrophysiologic study in whom SMVT could NOT be induced. In this group, the 12-lead ECG showed a complete right bundle branch block pattern in three, complete left bundle branch block in four, and intraventricular conduction defect with QRS duration >120 msec in six patients.

Group D—"Time-Domain False-Negatives"—10 Subjects

These were all patients with nonsustained or sustained VT in whom time-domain late potentials were ABSENT, but who had inducible SMVT at electrophysiologic study. Two patients had a left bundle branch block pattern on the 12-lead ECG, and two an intraventricular conduction defect with QRS duration >120 msec.

Thus in groups C and D combined, 26 of 38 subjects had an ECG pattern of intraventricular conduction defect or bundle branch block.

Methods

Acquisition of Signal-Averaged Electrocardiograms

Recordings of three lead orthogonal signal-averaged ECGs were made using an ART Model 1200 EPX unit (123 subjects) or a prototype Del Mar Avionics Model 183 Cardiac Early Warning System (CEWS) (19 subjects) and stored on floppy diskettes. The 183 CEWS has been compared with the ART model 1200 EPX and found to give closely similar results. X lead electrodes were placed in the 5th intercostal space in the anterior axillary line, Y lead at the top and bottom sternal border, and Z lead anteriorly and posteriorly at the level of the 4th intercostal space just to the left of the midline. Sampling frequency of the signal was 1,000 Hz for both acquisition devices.

Time-Domain Analysis

Time-domain analysis was performed using four-pole bidirectional Butterworth filters at 25–250 Hz and 40–250 Hz with calculation of the vector magnitude. The Del Mar 183 CEWS was utilized for analysis of all recordings. The number of beats averaged ranged between 215 and 600. Root mean square (RMS) noise level of the vector magnitude was < 1 µV in all recordings. Late potentials were deemed present if the RMS amplitude of the terminal 40 msec (RMS40) of the vector magnitude was < 25 µV using 25-Hz high-pass filtering and < 16 µV at 40-Hz high-pass filtering.

Electrophysiologic Study

The programmed stimulation protocol consisted of up to three extrastimuli delivered at two right ventricular sites during three ventricular pacing drives. Inducible SMVT was defined as VT with uniform QRS morphology lasting at least 30 seconds at a cycle length of > 200 msec or requiring termination because of hemodynamic compromise.

Frequency-Domain Analysis

Spectral analysis was performed on a Del Mar Avionics CEWS 183 system using custom software running on a desktop computer to generate adjacently drawn frequency plots of relatively short, consecutive, and overlapping segments of ECG signals spanning the entire QRS region and ST segment from three bipolar signal-averaged surface leads. We refer to the three-dimensional frequency plots as "spectrocardiograms," since they represent the relative contributions of differing frequencies to the ECG waveform throughout the cardiac cycle.

Spectrocardiogram derivation was achieved as follows:

Delineation of Region of Interest:

So as to include all high and low power QRS activity in subsequent frequency analysis, the region commencing 25 msec before the onset of the QRS complex (referred to as T1) and terminating 125 msec after the end of the QRS complex (referred to as T2) of the SAECG was selected by computer algorithm for spectrocardiogram generation. The precise determination of QRS onset and offset was actually performed separately for each lead, using the frequency-domain data, as described later in this section.

Spectrocardiogram Calculation for Each Lead (X, Y, and Z):

(A) *Signal Segmentation:* Commencing at point T1, overlapping signal segments of 24-msec duration (i.e., 25 data points 1 msec apart) were analyzed, in steps of 2 msec. Thus each 24-msec analyzed segment commenced 2 msec later than its predecessor. The end of the last analyzed segment coincided with point T2. If the total region span (T2 − T1) was, for example 375 msec, the number of segments processed would be $((T2-T1) - 25) / 2$ or 175 segments.

(B) *Differentiation:* Each 25-point signal segment was differentiated according to the following formula[34]:

$$y[t] = [(x[t+1] - x[t-1]) / 2] + [(x[t+2] - x[t-2]) / 8]$$

where y[t] is the new (differentiated) value of the signal at time t, while x[t] is the original amplitude of the signal (from any lead X, Y, or Z) at time [t]. This equation is one of many available approximations for calculating the first derivative of a time sampled signal. It is less sensitive to the effect of random high-frequency noise than some simpler alternatives. Thus all further calculations were performed upon the velocity (not amplitude) of the ECG wave front. This step of differentiation has critical importance for the rest of the analysis. First, it is the abrupt changes in velocity (not amplitude) of the wave front signal which we hypothesize to correlate with an arrhythmogenic substrate. Second, differentiation has the convenient characteristic of shifting the frequency content of the signal upward in a precise mathematical way, so that Fourier analysis of relatively short segments of signal may have sufficient frequency resolution to be useful. The Fourier transform of a segment length of 24 msec has a fundamental frequency of 42 Hz, which may be virtually useless for analyzing an ECG amplitude signal. However, by first differentiating the signal, its power spectrum is spread and shifted upward so that harmonic multiples of 42 Hz disclose visually and numerically significant differences between normal and abnormal subjects.

(C) *Mean Subtraction:* The arithmetical mean of the differentiated signal segment was next calculated and subtracted from each (differentiated) data point to remove the effect of DC offset.

(D) *Windowing:* After differentiation and mean subtraction, each 24-msec signal segment was multiplied by a 4-term Blackman-Harris window of equal duration. The choice of window was based upon its excellent concentration of central lobe with low side-lobe structure.[35] A detailed discussion of the need for windowing, or the relative merits of various window types has been addressed before by several authors[15-30] and is beyond the scope of this chapter.

(E) *Fast Fourier Transformation:* The windowed 25-point signal was next moved to the beginning of a 64-point data array, padded with zeroes for points 26 to 64 and a double precision 64 point Fast Fourier transform performed. The power spectral density (PSD) at each frequency harmonic was calculated in standard fashion as the sum of the squares of the corresponding real and imaginary Fourier coefficients.

(F) *Normalization:* After separate calculation of PSD for each data segment for each ECG lead (X, Y, and Z), the maximum PSD at any frequency in any lead was arbitrarily designated as representing "100%" PSD, and all other PSDs were scaled correspondingly.

(G) *Spectrocardiogram Plotting:* CEWS software automatically generates three-dimensional spectral plots of each lead. Because of the three-dimensional nature of the spectral information, multiple views assist in identifying features not apparent in any single projection. Figure 1 illustrates different projections of the spectrocardiogram from a normal subject in group A. The conventional time-domain plot is also shown for comparison. On each view, T1 to T2 indicate the time axis with T1 being nearer the P wave and T2 nearer the T wave. PSD is always plotted vertically while the remaining axis

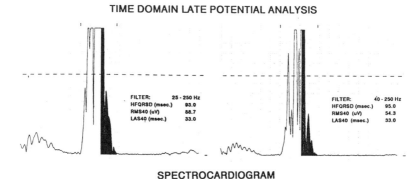

Figure 1. Time-domain plots (top) and spectral plots (bottom) of the signal-averaged electrocardiogram of a normal 28-year-old subject. Note absence of late potentials in the time-domain plots (time-domain true negative). The signal in last 40 msec is highlighted. The spectrocardiogram is displayed in different views: an oblique view in the bottom left panel, a horizontal view at both low and high gains in the bottom middle panel, and a "transparent" view in the bottom right panel. There is a low degree of spectral turbulence throughout the ventricular depolarization signal with a turbulence score of 0. See text for details. In this and subsequent figures: HFQRSD = high-frequency filtered QRS duration; RMS 40 = root mean square voltage of the signal in the last 40 msec; LAS40 = duration of the low amplitude signal <40 μV; T_1-T_2, the region commencing 25 msec before the onset of the QRS complex and terminating 125 msec after the end of the QRS complex; PSD = power spectral density. The horizontal dotted line in the time-domain late potential plots represents 40 μV.

represents frequency from 0 to 500 Hz. The left-hand lower panel is an oblique view from the T wave end of the QRS complex. The lower center panel illustrates a horizontal view with the QRS time axis running from left to right at both low and high magnifications. This view is the most convenient for estimating the duration of "late potentials." The right lower panel shows the ST segment viewed from the T wave and unlike the previous two views shows complete spectral contours within the whole QRS region, unhidden by time slices closer to the viewer. This is termed the "transparent" view. The last two views are best for gauging the overall level of spectral turbulence.

(H) *Numeric Calculations:* The normalized PSDs for each 25-point signal segment, for each lead X, Y, and Z were stored in a separate table for each lead, with rows containing the Fourier PSDs for a single 24-msec signal segment varying with frequency, while columns contained the PSDs at a particular frequency varying in time through the ECG signal.

The PSDs in each row were next summed to form an extra column containing the total PSD at all frequencies of each time slice.

Next the 40 msec (20 consecutive slices) region with lowest total PSD was assigned as the "baseline noise level" and its mean and standard deviation calculated.

The beginning and end of the QRS complex were designated as the time slices having total PSD at least five standard deviations above mean baseline noise, sustained for at least two slices.

The hypothesis tested was that the hallmark of normality was a generally smooth transition between frequency contours from one time slice to the next. Conversely the plots of abnormal subjects showed a high degree of spectral turbulence with relatively frequent and abrupt dissimilarities among the spectral contours of nearby slices. These regions of "lumpiness" appeared to be present not only in the late potentials region of abnormal subjects (in those who had late potentials) but, significantly, seemed scattered throughout much of the QRS complex proper. Calculations were based on correlations of PSD values among time slices. Four parameters of spectral turbulence were chosen to encompass different variants of abnormality observed visually on the spectrocardiogram plots. In some abnormal subjects, spectral turbulence was intense but of relatively short duration, while in others it was less marked but more prolonged. The four parameters of spectral turbulence analyzed were:

i. *"Inter-slice Correlation Mean."* This is the average degree to which ADJACENT time slices agree with respect to their frequency makeup. It is calculated as the mean Pearson correlation coefficient of each time slice with its neighbor, i.e., the average correlation between one row of the PSD table with the row immediately below it, multiplied by 100.

ii. *"Inter-slice Correlation SD."* The standard deviation of the correlation of each slice with its neighbor multiplied by 100, represents the lack of homogeneity in correlation around an average value.

iii. *"Low-slice Correlation Ratio."* The percentage of adjacent slice pairs with correlation coefficient < 0.985.

iv. "Spectral Entropy". This is the average discordance (i.e., 1 − correlation coefficient) of each slice with an imaginary "average slice," multiplied by 100. The "average slice" to which each real slice is correlated is the arithmetic mean of the PSDs at each frequency over the whole QRS region.

Averaging of Numerical Results From Each Lead:

After separate computation of each parameter for each lead (X, Y, and Z) the average of the three leads was computed for each correlation parameter.

Statistical Analysis:

Using software written expressly for the purpose, the "normals" (group A + group C) and "inducible SMVT" (group B + group D) subject groups were analyzed and the criterion of abnormality for each correlation parameter which yielded the best total predictive accuracy was established. Using these optimized normality criteria, each subject in each study group was scored for "spectral abnormality," with a score of 1 awarded for each abnormal correlation parameter. The lowest possible score was zero (most normal) and the highest 4 (most abnormal). Predictive values, sensitivity, and specificity statistics were computed for each subject group. Statistics were separately calculated for time-domain late potentials analysis, for each correlation parameter separately, and for the "Spectral Abnormality Score."

Results

Qualitative

In subjects with time-domain late potentials (Figures 2 and 3), regions of low power (<1% peak PSD) were clearly visible on the spectral plots extending beyond the end of the higher power main QRS region, their duration corresponding approximately to the low-amplitude signal <40 μV (LAS40) of time-domain analysis. When associated with inducible SMVT as in Figure 2, the spectral contours of nearby time slices varied markedly in shape (i.e., correlated poorly with each other). By contrast, when the late potentials were due to right bundle branch block as in Figure 3, the transition from one time slice to the next was smoother. Further, late potentials seemed to contain generally LOWER frequencies than the rest of the QRS complex.

In subjects with inducible SMVT (Figure 2 with late potentials and Figure 4 without late potentials) there was an increased degree of spectral turbulence over much of the QRS region as a whole. This corresponded visually to the degree of apparent disorganization in the "transparent" spectrocardiogram plots.

Quantitative

Table I summarizes the optimal sensitivity, specificity, and total predictive accuracy of individual spectral turbulence parameters based on comparison of "normals" (group A + group C) and "inducible VT" (group B + group D). Calculations were made separately for each of the X, Y, and Z leads and their average. The parameters with the highest total predictive accuracies were the inter-slice correlation mean and low slice correlation ratio for the average of the three leads, and the inter-slice correlation mean of the X lead alone. Since for each turbulence parameter, the total predictive accuracy of the three leads was superior to that of any single lead, the values for the average of the three leads were used for the rest of the statistical analysis.

Table II summarizes the results of spectral analysis by parameters and subject groups. For classification purposes, spectral abnor-

TIME DOMAIN LATE POTENTIAL ANALYSIS

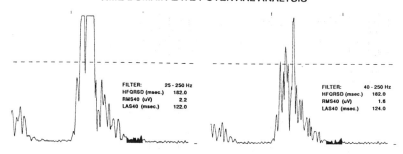

FILTER:	25 - 250 Hz
HFQRSD (msec.)	182.0
RMS40 (uV)	2.2
LAS40 (msec.)	122.0

FILTER:	40 - 250 Hz
HFQRSD (msec.)	182.0
RMS40 (uV)	1.6
LAS40 (msec.)	124.0

SPECTROCARDIOGRAM

SPECTROCARDIOGRAM GENERATION PARAMETERS

TIME SLICE DURATION	24.0 MSEC.
TIME SLICE STEP INTERVAL	2.0 MSEC
SIGNAL PRE-PROCESSING	VELOCITY
DC OFFSET SUBTRACTION	PRE-WINDOW
FFT POINTS	64
WINDOW	BLACKMAN-HARRIS

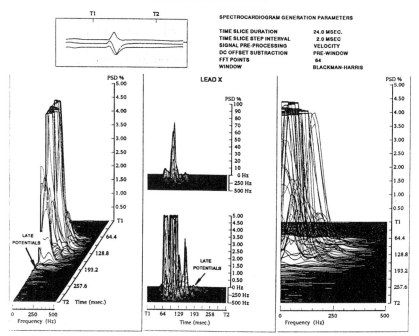

Figure 2. Time-domain plots (top) and spectral plots (bottom) of the signal-averaged electrocardiogram (ECG) from a 63-year-old male with prior myocardial infarction and recurrent sustained monomorphic ventricular tachycardia that was inducible by programmed stimulation (time-domain true positive). The time-domain plots show long, low amplitude late potentials. The spectrocardiogram shows a high degree of spectral turbulence throughout most of the ventricular depolarization signal with a turbulence score of 4. The arrows refer to segments in the spectral plots that correspond in time to the region where late potentials are evident in the time-domain signal averaged ECG. See text for details.

TIME DOMAIN LATE POTENTIAL ANALYSIS

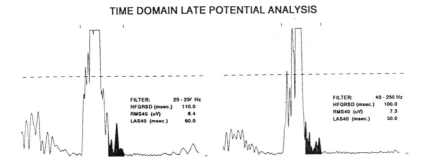

FILTER: 25 - 25ʹ Hz
HFQRSD (msec.) 110.0
RMS40 (uV) 8.4
LAS40 (msec.) 60.0

FILTER: 40 - 250 Hz
HFQRSD (msec.) 100.0
RMS40 (uV) 7.3
LAS40 (msec.) 50.0

SPECTROCARDIOGRAM

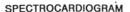

SPECTROCARDIOGRAM GENERATION PARAMETERS

TIME SLICE DURATION	24.0 MSEC.
TIME SLICE STEP INTERVAL	2.0 MSEC
SIGNAL PRE-PROCESSING	VELOCITY
DC OFFSET SUBTRACTION	PRE-WINDOW
FFT POINTS	64
WINDOW	BLACKMAN-HARRIS

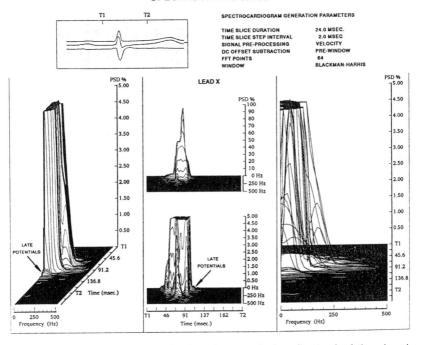

Figure 3. Time-domain plots (top) and spectral plots (bottom) of the signal-averaged electrocardiograms of a 36-year-old normal subject who had an incomplete right bundle branch block pattern in the 12-lead electrocardiogram. The time-domain plots show late potentials (time-domain false-positive). The position of late potentials in the spectrocardiogram is marked by arrows. However, there is a low degree of spectral turbulence throughout the ventricular depolarization signal with a turbulence score of 0 as in normal subjects without bundle branch block. See text for details.

TIME DOMAIN LATE POTENTIAL ANALYSIS

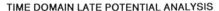

FILTER:	25 - 250 Hz
HFQRSD (msec.)	99.0
RMS40 (uV)	129.0
LAS40 (msec.)	18.0

FILTER:	40 - 250 Hz
HFQRSD (msec.)	100.0
RMS40 (uV)	67.7
LAS40 (msec.)	20.0

SPECTROCARDIOGRAM

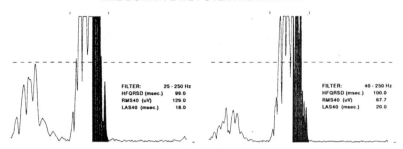

SPECTROCARDIOGRAM GENERATION PARAMETERS

TIME SLICE DURATION	24.0 MSEC.
TIME SLICE STEP INTERVAL	2.0 MSEC
SIGNAL PRE-PROCESSING	VELOCITY
DC OFFSET SUBTRACTION	PRE-WINDOW
FFT POINTS	64
WINDOW	BLACKMAN-HARRIS

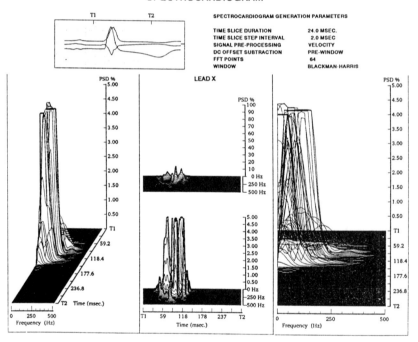

Figure 4. Time-domain plots (top) and spectral plots (bottom) of the signal-averaged electrocardiogram of a 75-year-old male with prior myocardial infarction, spontaneous nonsustained ventricular tachycardia (VT) and inducible sustained monomorphic VT. The time-domain plots do not show late potentials (time-domain false-negative). On the other hand, the spectrocardiogram reveals a high degree of spectral turbulence throughout most of the ventricular depolarization signal with a turbulence score of 4. See text for details.

Table I

Statistical Analysis of Individual Spectral Turbulence Parameters—Normals versus VT-Inducible Groups

Average of X, Y, and Z Leads

Spectral Turbulence Parameter	P-Mean	P-SD	N-Mean	N-SD	p	CRIT	TPA	SENS	SPEC
Interslice correlation mean	91	1	94	1	<.001	<92	91	91	91
Interslice correlation S.D.	121	20	85	20	<.001	>105	84	84	84
Low slice correlation ratio	77	5	67	6	<.001	>73	90	88	91
Spectral entropy	18	5	11	3	<.001	>14	87	79	90

Lead X

Spectral Turbulence Parameter	P-Mean	P-SD	N-Mean	N-SD	p	CRIT	TPA	SENS	SPEC
Interslice correlation mean	91	2	95	2	<.001	<93	90	88	91
Interslice correlation S.D.	122	33	72	33	<.001	>110	80	67	86
Low slice correlation ratio	77	6	62	9	<.001	>70	84	95	80
Spectral entropy	19	7	9	4	<.001	>14	84	72	89

Table I (Continued)

Lead Y

Spectral Turbulence Parameter	P-Mean	P-SD	N-Mean	N-SD	p	CRIT	TPA	SENS	SPEC
Interslice correlation mean	91	2	93	2	<.001	<92	77	77	78
Interslice correlation S.D.	125	32	90	34	<.001	>131	77	46	90
Low slice correlation ratio	76	7	70	8	<.001	>78	75	49	87
Spectral entropy	18	7	12	4	<.001	>20	77	35	96

Lead Z

Spectral Turbulence Parameter	P-Mean	P-SD	N-Mean	N-SD	p	CRIT	TPA	SENS	SPEC
Interslice correlation mean	91	2	93	2	<.001	<92	76	74	77
Interslice correlation S.D.	116	29	93	32	<.001	>114	71	53	79
Low slice correlation ratio	77	7	70	9	<.001	>83	75	28	96
Spectral entropy	18	7	13	4	<.001	>16	75	49	86

P-MEAN = Mean of VT-Inducible groups; N-MEAN = Mean of Normal groups; p = Significance statistic (Student's test); P-SD = Standard Deviation of VT-Inducible groups; N-SD = Standard Deviation of Normal groups; CRIT = Criterion of abnormality; TPA = Total Predictive Accuracy; SENS = Sensitivity; SPEC = Specificity.

Table II

Results of Spectral Turbulence Scoring by Subject Group

Criterion	A (%)	B (%)	Subject Group C (%)	D (%)	A+C (%)	B+D (%)
Abnormal interslice correlation mean	3(4)	32(97)	6(21)	7(70)	9(9)	39(91)
Abnormal interslice correlation S.D.	10(14)	31(94)	9(32)	7(70)	19(19)	38(88)
Abnormal low slice correlation ratio	1(1)	32(97)	8(29)	6(60)	9(9)	38(88)
Abnormal spectral entropy	3(4)	32(97)	6(21)	7(70)	9(9)	39(91)
Total spectral abnormality score = 0	58(82)	0	12(43)	3(30)	70(70)	3(7)
Total spectral abnormality score = 1	9(13)	0	7(25)	0	16(16)	0
Total spectral abnormality score = 2	4(6)	1(3)	5(18)	1(10)	9(9)	2(5)
Total spectral abnormality score = 3	0	6(18)	3(11)	1(10)	3(3)	7(16)
Total spectral abnormality score = 4	0	26(79)	1(4)	5(50)	1(1)	31(72)
Total spectral abnormality score = 3 or 4	0	32(97)	4(14)	6(60)	4(4)	38(88)
Total spectral abnormality score = <3	71(100)	1(3)	24(86)	4(40)	95(95)	5(12)
Total number of subjects	71	33	28	10	99	43

mality scores of 2 or less have been designated as "normal" while scores of 3 or 4 were considered "abnormal."

Of the 71 clinically normal volunteers without time-domain late potentials (group A), all (100%) had spectral abnormality scores of 2 or less. Of 32 patients with both time-domain late potentials and inducible SMVT at electrophysiologic study (group B), 31 had spectral abnormality scores of 3 or 4, while one had a score of 2. Of the 28 subjects with time-domain late potentials in whom there was no evidence of SMVT by either clinical history (i.e., they were normal volunteers) or at electrophysiologic study (group C, time-domain false-positives), 24 subjects (86%) had spectral abnormality scores of 2 or less (normal), while 4 subjects (14%) had abnormal scores of 3 or 4. Of ten patients with inducible SMVT at electrophysiologic study in whom time-domain analysis was negative for late potentials (group D, time-domain false-negatives), six (60%) had abnormal scores of 3 or 4 while four patients (40%) had normal scores of 2 or less. Combining the results of groups C and D, spectral analysis correctly classified 30 of the 38 patients (79%) incorrectly classified by time-domain late potentials analysis. Of the 26 subjects in groups C and D who had an ECG pattern of intraventricular conduction defect or bundle branch block, 20 (77%) were correctly classified by spectral turbulence analysis.

Table III compares the overall predictive characteristics of spectral versus time-domain analysis and shows the significantly higher predictive accuracy of spectral estimation.

Table III

Comparison of Predictive Accuracy for Ventricular Tachycardia Inducibility of Spectral Analysis and Time Domain Late Potential Analysis (All Subject Groups Combined)

Predictive Statistic	Spectral Analysis	Time Domain
Total Predictive Accuracy	94%	73%
Positive Predictive Accuracy	90%	54%
Negative Predictive Accuracy	95%	88%
Sensitivity	88%	77%
Specificity	96%	72%

Discussion

The present study tested the hypothesis that abrupt changes in wave front velocity as the ventricular activation wave front traverses regions with abnormal conduction characteristics could be quantified by spectral analysis of the body surface QRS complex and that these changes could represent a more accurate marker for the anatomic-electrophysiologic substrate of reentrant ventricular tachyarrhythmias. Our results show that the spectral analysis technique is superior to conventional time-domain analysis of late potentials.

Unlike conventional time-domain analysis of the SAECG in which the signals from three orthogonal leads are usually summed so as to include contributions of signals in all vectorial directions, the spectral abnormalities analyzed by the present technique may actually be masked by vector summation. This is consistent with the hypothesis that abnormal spectral turbulence results from changes in depolarization wave front velocity. The term "velocity" as used here is a vector with both amplitude and direction in three dimensions, whereas the "vector sum" is a scalar quantity expressing magnitude but with no directional component. Changes in direction of QRS wave front propagation without a change in speed could therefore be concealed by combining the three leads into a single directionless quantity.

Electrophysiologic Limitations of Late Potential Analysis

The results of analysis of spectral turbulence occurring throughout the entire ventricular depolarization period suggest a possible modification to some basic concepts as to the role played by late potentials in the arrhythmogenic process. Late potentials have been thought to correspond to delayed and fragmented signals which have been observed in epicardial or endocardial electrograms recorded in post-infarction animal models,[36-39] and in patients with ventricular tachyarrhythmias.[40] Some studies suggested that the fragmented electrograms may represent the electrical signals of disorganized, but sometimes electrophysiologically normal, surviving myocardial fibers in areas with extensive fibrosis.[39] It was assumed that myocardial zones generating late potentials during sinus rhythm could provide the anatomic-electrophysiologic substrate for reentrant tachyarrhythmias. However, reentrant excitation has not been shown to occur in areas of extensive fibrosis with isolated uncoupled myocardial bundles in which slow and possibly discontinuous conduction could be demonstrated. Several studies from this laboratory also tend to challenge these assumptions. In a study in the canine post-infarction heart,[41] late potentials in the time-domain SAECG were shown to correspond temporally with the region of latest epicardial activation during a relatively slow basic cardiac rhythm. However, subsequent signal averaging during a reentrant rhythm revealed that the sites of late potentials during the basic rhythm were not always responsible for late potentials detected during reentrant activation. Myocardial regions with marked conduction delay, Wenckebach, or 2:1 conduction could manifest as significant late potentials during the basic rhythm yet develop conduction block and fail to participate in the reentrant circuit induced by premature stimulation. In another study,[42] the correlation between myocardial sites critical for prevention of initiation and/or termination of reentrant tachycardia by cryothermal techniques and sites of late activation during sinus rhythm was investigated in the canine post-infarction model. These sites correlated well in only 25% of the cases studied. The lack of correlation was explained by the fact that the critical sites during reentry were intimately related to the location and extent of the arcs of functional conduction block (one of two essential prerequisites for circus movement reentry besides slow conduction) while sites of delayed activation during sinus rhythm were not. Thus, late potentials during sinus rhythm may represent only indirect markers for the potential to develop reentrant tachyarrhythmias, rather than actually taking part in the clinically important reentrant circuit.

Another limitation of late potential analysis arises from the concept that these potentials may sometimes (or even usually) represent "the visible tip of an iceberg" of myocardial regions with abnormal activation having most of the electrical activity from such regions buried partially or totally within the QRS complex proper. Partial obscuring of late potentials may occur if the abnormal myocardial region begins to be activated relatively early during the QRS complex, for example, in anterior as compared to inferior wall myocardial infarction.[43] During bundle branch block, myocardial zones with abnormal activation may be totally obscured by the delayed activation of normal myocardial regions. On the other hand, time-domain analysis of the SAECG may show "late potentials" in otherwise normal hearts as a result of applying a high-pass filter to a terminal QRS region of lower than normal amplitude and/or slope due to bundle branch block.

Advantages of Spectral Turbulence Analysis

The present study strongly suggests that a high degree of spectral turbulence of the ventricular activation wave front during sinus rhythm reflects the presence of myocardial regions with abnormal conduction characteristics that may provide the anatomic-electrophysiologic substrate for reentrant tachyarrhythmias. The activation of these myocardial regions may occur totally within the QRS complex or may extend beyond the activation of the rest of the ventricular mass. The spectral turbulence generated by the activation wave front traversing these regions is not expected to be obscured by the delayed, possibly slower, but still largely synchronous and uniform activation wave front in the presence of bundle branch block. Conversely, the delayed but smooth activation process of bundle branch block in normal hearts will not be reflected as a high degree of spectral turbulence. The technique could be thus applied to all patients irrespective of QRS duration and the presence or absence of intraventricular conduction abnormality or bundle branch block.

Limitations of the Study

The concept that myocardial regions with abnormal conduction characteristics can result in a quantifiable degree of spectral turbulence, the nature and extent of these conduction abnormalities both anatomically and electrophysiologically, and their relationship to spontaneous and/or inducible reentrant tachyarrhythmias need elucidation by future basic and clinical studies. The present technique for quantifying and scoring spectral turbulence requires prospective testing in a large series of patients. Selection of the inducibility of SMVT at electrophysiologic study as the standard against which the spectral technique was evaluated is supported on electrophysiologic grounds. [44,45] However, the relationship between a fixed anatomic-electrophysiologic reentry substrate and spontaneous tachyarrhythmias is more complex and other noninvasive techniques that can detect additional factors capable of triggering and modulating the arrhythmogenic potential need to be developed.

References

1. Simson MB: Use of signals in the terminal QRS complex to identify patients with ventricular tachycardia after myocardial infarction. Circulation 64:235, 1981.
2. Breithardt G, Becker R, Seipel L, Abendroth R-R, Ostermeyer J: Noninvasive detection of late potentials in man—a new marker for ventricular tachycardia. Euro Heart J 2:1, 1981.
3. El-Sherif N, Mehra R, Gomes JAC, Kelen G: Appraisal of a low noise electrocardiogram. J Am Coll Cardiol 1:456, 1983.
4. Denes P, Santarelli P, Hauser RG, Uretz EF: Quantitative analysis of the high frequency components of the terminal portion of the body surface QRS in normal subjects and in patients with ventricular tachycardia. Circulation 67:1129, 1983.
5. Kaovsky MS, Falcone RA, Dresden CA, Josephson ME, Simson MB: Identification of patients with ventricular tachycardia after myocardial infarction. Signal-averaged electrocardiogram, Holter monitoring, and cardiac catheterization. Circulation 70:264, 1984.
6. Kuchar DL, Thorburn CW, Sammel NL: Prediction of serious arrhythmic events after myocardial infarction: signal averaged electrocardiogram, Holter monitoring and radionuclide ventriculography. J Am Coll Cardiol 9:531, 1981.
7. Gomes J, Winters SL, Stewart D, Horowitz S, Milner M, Barreca P: A new noninvasive index to predict sustained ventricular tachycardia and sudden death in the first year after myocardial infarction. J Am Coll Cardiol 10:349, 1987.
8. Turitto G, Fontaine JM, Ursell SN, Caref EB, Henkin R, El-Sherif N: Value of the signal averaged electro-cardiogram as a predictor of the results of programmed stimulation in non-sustained ventricular tachycardia. Am J Cardiol 61:1272, 1988.
9. El-Sherif N, Ursell SN, Bekheit S, Fontaine J, Turitto G, Henkin R, Caref EB: Prognostic significance of the signal-averaged electrocardiogram depends on the time of recording in the post-infarction period. Am Heart J 118:256, 1989.
10. Turitto G, Fontaine JM, Ursell SN, Caref EB, Bekheit SB, El-Sherif N: Risk stratification and management of patients with organic heart disease and non-sustained ventricular tachycardia: role of programmed stimulation, left ventricular ejection and the signal averaged electrocardiogram. Am J Med 88:35N, 1990.
11. Caref EB, Turitto G, Ibrahim B, Henkin R, El-Sherif N: Role of bandpass filters in optimizing the value of the signal averaged electrocardiogram as a predictor of the results of programmed stimulation. Am J Cardiol 64:16, 1989.

12. Henkin R, Caref EB, Kelen GJ, El-Sherif N: The signal averaged electrocardiogram: a comparative analysis of commercial devices. J Electrocardiol 22 (Suppl 1):19, 1990.

13. Buckingham TA, Thessen CC, Stevens LL, Redd RM, Kennedy HL: Effect of conduction defects on the signal-averaged electrocardiographic determination of late potentials. Am J Cardiol 61:1265, 1988.

14. Hall PAX, Atwood JE, Myers J, Froelicher VF: The signal averaged surface electrocardiogram and the identifiation of late potentials. Prog Cardiovasc Dis 31:295, 1989.

15. Cain ME, Ambos HD, Witkowski FX, Sobel BE: Fast Fourier Transform analysis of signal averaged ECGs for identification of patients prone to sustained ventricular tachycardia. Circulation 69:711, 1984.

16. Cain ME, Ambos HD, Markham J, Fischer AE, Sobel BE: Quantitation of differences in frequency content of signal-averaged ECGs in patients with compared to those without sustained ventricular tchycardia. Am J Cardiol 55:1500, 1985.

17. Lindsay BD, Ambos HD, Schechtman KB, Cain ME: Improved selection of patients for programmed ventricular stimulation by frequency analysis of signal-averaged electrocardiograms. Circulation 73:675, 1986.

18. Lindsay BD, Markham J, Schechtman KB, Ambos HD, Cain ME: Identification of patients with sustained ventricular tachycardia by frequency analysis of signal-averaged electrocardiograms despite the presence of bundle branch block. Circulation 77:122, 1988.

19. Lindsay BD, Ambos HD, Schechtman KB, Cain ME: Improved differentiation of patients with and without ventricular tachycardia by frequency analysis of multiple ECG leads. Am J Cardiol 62:556, 1988.

20. Cain MC, Ambos HD, Lindsay BD, Markham J, Arthur RM: Spectral and temporal interrogation of signal-averaged electrocardiograms: the best is yet to come. J Am Coll Cardiol 14:1741, 1989.

21. Lindsay BD, Ambos HD, Schechtman KB, Arthur RM, Cain ME: Noninvasive detection of patients with ischemic and nonischemic heart disease prone to ventricular fibrillation. J Am Coll Cardiol 16:1656, 1990.

22. Kelen G, Henkin R, Fontaine JM, El-Sherif N: Effects of analyzed signal duration and phase on the results of Fast Fourier transform analysis of the surface electrocardiogram in subjects with and without late potentials. Am J Cardiol 60:1282, 1987.

23. Worley SJ, Mark DB, Smith WM, Wolf P, et al: Comparison of time domain and frequency variables from the signal-averaged electrocardiogram: a multivariable analysis. J Am Coll Cardiol 11:1041, 1988.

24. Machac J, Weiss A, Winters SL, Barecca P, Gomes JA: A comparative study of frequency domain and time domain analysis of signal-averaged electrocardiograms in patients with ventricular tachycardia. J Am Coll Cardiol 11:184, 1988.

25. Buckingham TA, Thessen CM, Hertweck D, Janosik DL, Kennedy HL: Signal-averaged electrocardiography in the time and frequency domains. Am J Cardiol 63:820, 1989.

26. Pierce DL, Easley AR Jr, Windle JR, Engel TR: Fast Fourier transformation of the entire low amplitude late QRS potential to predict ventricular tachycardia. J Am Coll Cardiol 14:1731, 1989.

27. Haberl R, Jilge G, Pulter R, Steinbeck G: Comparison of frequency and time domain analysis of the signal-averaged electrocardiogram in patients with ventricular tachycardia and coronary artery disease. Methodologic validation and clinical relevance. J Am Coll Cardiol 12:150, 1988.

28. Haberl R, Jilge G, Pulter R, Steinbeck G: Spectral mapping of the electrocardiogram with Fourier transform for identification of patients with sustained ventricular tachycardia and coronary artery disease. Eur Heart J 10:316, 1989.

29. Haberl R, Schels HF, Steinbigler P, Jilge G, Steinbeck G: Top-resolution frequency analysis of electrocardiogram with adaptive frequency determination: identification of late potentials in patients with coronary artery disease. Circulation 82:1183, 1990.

30. Lander P, Albert DE, Berbari EJ: Spectrotemporal analysis of ventricular late potentials. J Electrocardiol 23:95, 1990.

31. Kelen G, Henkin R, Lannon M, Bloomfield D, El-Sherif N: Correlation between the signal-averaged electrocardiogram from Holter tapes and from real-time recordings. Am J Cardiol 63:1321, 1989.

32. Kelen GJ, Henkin R, Caref E, Starr A-M, Bloomfield DA, El-Sherif N: Spectral turbulence analysis of the high resolution ECG—A new concept and technique with higher predictive accuracy for inducible sustained monomorphic ventricular tachycardia than detection of late potentials. (abstr) Circulation 82:III–740, 1990.

33. Kelen GJ, Henkin R, Starr A-M, Caref E, Bloomfield DA, El-Sherif N: Spectral turbulence analysis of the signal averaged electrocardiogram and its predictive accuracy for inducible sustained monomorphic ventricular tachycardia. Am J Cardiol 67:965, 1991.

34. Gerald CF, Wheatley PO: Applied Numerical Methods. Addison Wesley Pub. Co., Reading MA 1985, p 243.

35. Harris FJ: On the use of windows for harmonic analysis with the discrete Fourier Transform. Proceedings IEEE 66:51, 1978.

36. El-Sherif N, Scherlag BJ, Lazzara R, Hope RR: Reentrant ventricular arrhythmias in the late myocardial infarction period. Conduction characteristics in the infarction zone. Circulation 55:686, 1977.

37. Berbari EJ, Scherlag BJ, Hope RR, Lazzara R: Recording from the body surface of arrhythmogenic ventricular activity during the ST-segment. Am J Cardiol 41:697, 1978.

38. Simson MB, Euler D, Michelson EL, Falcone RA, Spear JF, Moore EN: Detection of delayed ventricular activation on the body surface in dogs. Am J Cardiol 241:H363, 1981.

39. Gardner PI, Ursell PC, Fenoglio JJ Jr, Wit AL: Electrophysiologic and anatomic basis for fractionated electrograms recorded from healed myocardial infarcts. Circulation 72:596, 1985.

40. Simson MB, Untereker WJ, Spielman SR, et al: The relationship between late potentials on the body surface and directly recorded fragmented electrograms in patients with ventricular tachycardia. Am J Cardiol 51:105, 1983.

41. El-Sherif N, Gough WB, Restivo M, Craelius W, Henkin R: Electrophysiologic basis of ventricular late potentials. In: Santini M, Pistolese M, Alliegro A (eds): Progress in Clinical Pacing. Excerpta Medica, 1988, pp 209–24.
42. Assadi M, Restivo M, Gough WB, El-Sherif N: Reentrant ventricular arrhythmias in the late myocardial infarction period. 17. Correlation of activation patterns of sinus and reentrant ventricular tachycardia. Am Heart J 119:1014, 1990.
43. Breithardt G, Borggrefe M: Pathophysiological mechanisms and clinical significance of ventricular late potentials. Eur Heart J 7:364, 1986.
44. Wellens HJJ, Brugada P, Stevenson WG: Programmed electrical stimulation of the heart in patients with life-threatening ventricular arrhythmias: what is the significance of induced arrhythmias and what is the correct protocol? Circulation 72:1, 1985.
45. El-Sherif N, Gomes JAC, Restivo M, Mehra R: Late potentials and arrhythmogenesis. PACE 8:440, 1985.

Index

685

time-domain analysis versus, 674
See also Spectro-temporal mapping of surface ECG
Spectrocardiogram, 662–666
Spectro-temporal mapping of surface ECG, 122–125, 639, 648, 651, 662–666
advantages, 650
arrhythmias and, 647
bundle branch block and, 650
myocardial infarction and, 642, 644–646
procedure, 641–642
Simson method and, 645, 647
sustained ventricular tachycardia and, 642, 647
time-varying spectra and, 122–123
See also Spectral turbulence analysis
Stress test, the signal-averaged ECG during, 453–460
Sudden cardiac death, 227–230, 419–420, 593–594
nonsustained ventricular tachycardia and, 487
post-infarction, 227–228, 412–415
recurrent, 228–230
Summation-averaging, 10–13
Super Conducting Quantum Interference Devices, 148, 150–151, 153
Super conducting sensor, 150–151
Surface His bundle electrogram, 252–253, 255–257
Sustained ventricular tachyarrhythmias, 570–572, 614 *See also* Ventricular tachycardia
Swept sine wave, 122
Syncope, 383, 521–522
coronary artery disease and, 522–525, 527–531
electrophysiologic studies and, 521, 523–525, 528–529
nonsustained ventricular tachycardia and, 478, 480
signal-averaged ECG and, 524–525, 527

TECA electrode electrolyte, 262
Thrombolytic therapy, the signal-averaged ECG after, 415–416, 460–467
Time-bandwidth product, 115
Time-domain analysis
computer calculated indices and, 499–500
coronary artery occlusion and, 303, 305, 310–311
filters and, 76–101, 499
frequency-domain analysis versus, 621–622, 625–626
limitations, 635–636
methodological problems, 498
post-infarction period and, 431–433

Time-ensemble averaging, 67–68
Time-varying spectra, 120, 122–123
swept sine wave and, 121–122
See also Spectro-temporal mapping

Ventricular activation time, 394, 397
Ventricular arrhythmias, 96–101, 356–358, 365–366
experimental myocardial infarction and, 356–358
high-grade, 476
inducible, 96–101, 475–485
inducible in the canine post-infarction model, 283–287
late potentials post-infarction and, 377
localization by magnetocardiography of, 161, 163
myocardial infarction and, 433–434
myocardial ischemia and, 448–449
noninvasive index in predicting, 380–381
See also Ventricular tachyarrhythmias
Ventricular fibrillation, 228, 230–231, 356, 361, 495–496
acute myocardial infarction and, 361
cardiac mapping and, 504–505
electrophysiologic studies and, 510–511
experimental myocardial infarction and, 356
heart disease and, 509–510
inducible in the post-infarction canine model, 284
inducible in the post-infarction period, 394, 397
inducible, prognostic significance of, 487, 489–492
late potential prediction of, 228, 477–478, 484
late potential prevalence in, 228, 505–509
post-infarction period and, 393–394
Ventricular late potentials, 8–14, 22–26, 279–280
bandpass filters and, 265
beat-to-beat recording of, 204–205, 226–228, 230–237
chronic coronary artery disease and, 227–228, 324–328
dynamic changes in, 23–25, 232, 270–271, 431
electrophysiologic limitations, 273, 433
experimental recordings, 22–25, 283–287
fractionated electrograms and, 291, 293–294
high-resolution ECG and, 260–261
lead selection and, 264–265
noise reduction and, 262, 264
periodicity analysis, 44

Ventricular late potentials (*Continued*)
post-myocardial infarction, 226–227,
283–284
signal-averaged ECG and, 232, 294–296
sinus and reentrant rhythms and, 280,
282–283, 285, 287, 289
sudden death and, 226–228, 230
ventricular tachyarrhythmias and,
283–284
See also Late potentials
Ventricular stimulation, programmed,
475–478, 480, 484–485 *See also*
Programmed ventricular stimulation
Ventricular tachyarrhythmias, 393–394,
397, 593–595
clinical implications, 419–420
inducible, in the post-infarction canine
model, 283–287
late potentials and, 406–408, 409,
412–415
malignant, 96–97, 100
post-infarction period and, 393
See also Ventricular arrhythmias
Ventricular tachycardia, 96–101, 355–356,
495–496
cardiac mapping and, 504–505
electrophysiologic study and, 510–511
FFT analysis and, 235, 611–614
frequency-domain analysis and,
621–622, 625–626
heart disease and, 509–510
inducible, in the post-infarction canine
model, 283
inducible, prediction by late
potentials, 96–101, 382–387, 394, 397,
475–485
inducible, prognostic significance, 487,
489–492
late potential body surface mapping
and, 342–343, 345–346

late potential prevalence in, 505–509
mapping, in the experimental animal,
23–25
post-infarction, 227, 393
spectro-temporal mapping and, 642,
647, 667, 674
spontaneous, prevalence of late
potentials in, 228
spontaneous sustained, predictive
value of late potentials for, 227,
412
See also Nonsustained ventricular
tachycardia
Verapamil, 219
Volume conductor electrode, 198–200

Wall motion abnormalities, 375–377
Wenckebach block, 220
Wenckebach conduction pattern,
230–231, 270, 287, 289, 295, 356
Windowing, 111, 601, 637, 663
Fourier analysis and, 111–113
spectral resolution and, 115, 117–118
Window trigger, 34, 36 *See also* QRS
alignment
Wolff-Parkinson-White syndrome, 129
ajmaline and, 139–140
electrocardiographic features of, 140
filters and, 140, 143–144
His bundle recording in, 137–140
Kent bundle localization and, 158–160
magnetocardiography and, 158–160,
164–165
signal averaging and, 130–132,
134–135

XYZ leads, 60–64, 264 *See also* Frank X,
Y, and Z leads

Zero-padding, 113

690